Tropical Lung Disease

Second Edition

LUNG BIOLOGY IN HEALTH AND DISEASE

Executive Editor

Claude Lenfant

Former Director, National Heart, Lung, and Blood Institute
National Institutes of Health
Bethesda, Maryland

The opinions expressed in these volumes do not necessarily represent the views of the National Institutes of Health.

Tropical Lung Disease

Second Edition

Edited by

Om P. Sharma
University of Southern California
Los Angeles, California, U.S.A.

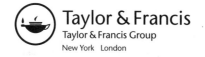

Taylor & Francis
Taylor & Francis Group
New York London

Published in 2006 by
Taylor & Francis Group
270 Madison Avenue
New York, NY 10016

International Standard Book Number-10: 0-8247-2687-1 (Hardcover)
International Standard Book Number-13: 978-0-8247-2687-4 (Hardcover)
Library of Congress Card Number 2005052897

Library of Congress Cataloging-in-Publication Data

Tropical lung disease / edited by Om Sharma.-- 2nd ed.
   p. ; cm. -- (Lung biology in health and disease ; v. 211)
   Rev. ed. of.: Lung disease in the tropics. Dekker, c1991.
  Includes bibliographical references and index.
  ISBN-13: 978-0-8247-2687-4 (alk. paper)
  ISBN-10: 0-8247-2687-1 (alk. paper)
  1. Lungs--Diseases. 2. Tropical medicine. I. Sharma, Om P. II. Lung disease in the tropics. III. Series.
  [DNLM: 1. Tropical Medicine. 2. Lung Diseases--diagnosis. 3. Lung Diseases--epidemiology. 4. Lung Diseases--therapy. WC 680 T8569 2005]

RC732.L84 2005
616.2'4--dc22   2005052897

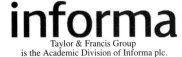

Taylor & Francis Group
is the Academic Division of Informa plc.

Visit the Taylor & Francis Web site at
http://www.taylorandfrancis.com

Introduction

In 2002, Dr. Brundtland, the Director General of the World Health Organization, wrote in her "message" introducing the 16th Program Report of Tropical Disease Research: Progress 2001–2002:

> Research is not always visible, and often does not have "immediacy." Results may take years to manifest themselves, and I commend the programme and its committed donors for continuing their work. But research remains essential if goals are to be achieved.

> *—Dr. Gro Harlem Brundtland*
> *World Health Organization.*

Tropical diseases in general, and tropical lung diseases in particular, are enormous public health problems affecting millions of people, residing in many countries, located in nearly all regions and continents of the world. Furthermore, one should not believe that if he/she lives outside these countries, he/she is protected against these diseases. As pointed out in the Preface of this volume, with the continuous migration of people and the ever-increasing interest and frequency of intercontinental travel, it is likely that many health professionals are now seeing diseases that "once occurred (only) in tropical and subtropical areas."

Considerable research on tropical diseases is being pursued world-wide and significant new outcomes are reported frequently. However, it is not always evident that these research outcomes are transported to and made available in the areas where they are likely to give better care or better health benefits. In the tropical disease area, as in many other fields of medicine, poor dissemination or translation of the knowledge where it should be used are poor and slow at best, if not actually nonexistent.

The goals of the series of monographs Lung Biology in Health and Disease are first to present ongoing research or "states of the art" and to stimulate new investigations, and second, and no less important, to bring research outcomes to practicing physicians to benefit their patients.

This new volume, edited by Dr. Om P. Sharma and titled Tropical Lung Disease, second edition, is truly a presentation of the latest research outcomes in the area of significant public health interest. The contributors chosen by Dr. Sharma are well-recognized experts, who are highly respected and commended for their work. As the Executive Editor of the series, I express my gratitude and my thanks to the editor and the contributors for the opportunity to present this volume, which has the potential to improve the care given to patients with tropical lung diseases.

Claude Lenfant, MD
Gaithersburg, Maryland, U.S.A.

Preface

Social, political, and economical upheavals of the modern era have smudged Nature's boundaries that demarcate tropical, subtropical, temperate, and the arctic land masses. With increasing intercontinental migration, rapid and unplanned industrialization, breakdown in sanitation and public health, and persistent human misery, physicians and other health workers in the developed countries encounter previously unfamiliar diseases that once occurred in tropical and subtropical areas. Several of these illnesses manifest in the lungs; whereas, others involve the respiratory organs only in conjunction with other tissue systems of the body. The modern clinician is now forced to recognize, diagnose, and treat tropical lung disease.

The authors of these 22 chapters on various aspects of *Lung Disease in the Tropics* include national and international authorities specializing in tropical pulmonary medicine. Dr. Shanu Gupta and Dr. D. G. James reinforce the importance of history and physical examination required, perhaps, more in tropical medicine than any other medical specialty. The authors provide a succinct and pragmatic account of the methods pursued in analyzing and assessing patients with tropical pulmonary disease. Dr. Om P. Sharma traces the history of zoonotic illnesses and their impact on human civilization. There are many zoonotic diseases besides HIV syndrome that have appeared or reappeared during the last few decades including Lassa fever, Marburg and Hanta virus infections, Q fever,

Brucellosis, Babesiosis, and most recently, severe acute respiratory syndrome (SARS) and chicken flu. Dr. Carlos Luna and his team from Argentina provide a refreshing insight into these unusual pneumonias.

Dr. Chaim Jacob paints a clear picture of the complex immune responses generated by the mammalian immune system in order to protect itself from exceedingly evasive and sophisticated microorganisms and parasites.

Malaria remains a threat. Annually, more than a million people die of the illness. The estimated number of infected individuals varies from 150 to 500 million. Treatment of malaria remains inadequate and inadequately available to those who need it the most. Dr. S. K. Jindal has condensed enormous information of immuno-pathogenesis of malaria into a succinct and easy to understand review. Dr. Fein and his colleagues, on the other hand, delve in the issues pertaining to respiratory failure in malaria. Eosinophilic diseases abound in tropical and subtropical countries. Dr. Vannan Kandi Vijayan from Vallabhbhai Patel Chest Institute, Delhi, gives an authoritative account of the pulmonary eosinophilic syndromes.

Endemic in 70 countries, schistosomiasis affects more than 200 million people in the world. Dr. Eli Schwartz describes two types, early and late, of pulmonary schistosomiasis. Artemether, a new Chinese antimalarial drug, has been shown to be active against the early or juvenile form of the disease; whereas, praziquantel remains the drug of choice for the late or chronic type. Dr. Bruno Gottstein describes diagnosis and pathogenesis of hydatid lung disease. Although chemotherapy is used, removal of the cyst remains the cornerstone of therapy.

Behçet's disease was first described by Hulusi Behçet, a Turkish ophthalmologist. It is also called Silk Road or Silk Route disease because of its distribution in the area of the old Silk Road between China and the Middle East. Dr. Ahmet Gül and colleagues have amassed impressive data on this disease. Their review is pragmatic and educational.

Paragonimiasis caused by lung flukes of genus *Paragonimus* has a wide distribution including most of Asia, Russia, Indonesia, Papua New Guinea, Mexico, Central and South America, and Nigeria. Because of its complex life history, its eradication has been unsuccessful so far. The disease is often confused with tuberculosis and lung cancer. Drs. Fukumi Nakamura-Uchiyama and Yukifumi Nawa discuss this complex topic. Various forms of granulomatous diseases occur and have different forms in the tropics, Drs. Mihailovic-Vucinic and Sharma provide a discussion of how to diagnose these disorders. Dr. Tshibwabwa and colleagues in an overview of imaging services in the developing countries emphasize variations in radiological features of the common conditions seen in tropical and temperate areas of the world. Dr. Avi Livneh updates the recent advances in diagnosing and treating Familial Mediterranean fever (FMF), a fascinating multisystem disease. Dr. Carla Lamb stresses the importance of bronchoscopy, bronchoalveolar lavage, and transbronchial lung biopsy in diagnosing tropical lung diseases.

Pulmonary leptospirosis used to be a relatively mild illness. Dr. Eduardo Bethlem, however, tells us that the disease has begun to show its ugly face. The disease can cause fatal respiratory failure. He provides an insight into its immuno-pathogenesis and genetic transmission. Dr. Patricio Escalante and Brenda Jones inform that approximately 1.8 million people die of tuberculosis every year with a global fatality rate of about 23%, but this figure doubles in some African countries. The main goal of global tuberculosis control is to reduce this spiraling mortality by prompt and judicious use of directly observed treatment, short course (DOTS), particularly in areas of high prevalence of tuberculosis and HIV infection. As yet, there is no vaccine universally effective against the disease. Dr. George Sarosi points out that the fungal infections of the lung are as prevalent in the tropics as they are in temperate zones. Acute pulmonary disease is a common complication of the sickling disorders, with a frequency of several hundred times than that of the general population. Dr. Cage Johnson charts the clinical course of the acute chest syndrome in children and adults and provides an algorithm to diagnose and treat the illness. Amebiasis has a worldwide distribution and the number of cases seen in some of the large metropolitan county hospitals in this country is impressive. Dr. Alejandro Sanchez and his team emphasize the importance of including pleuro-pulmonary amebiasis in the differential diagnosis of patients with unexplained pleural effusion or consolidation, particularly individuals who either live in or have come from an endemic area.

Pleural inflammation with or without effusion is a common malady in the tropics. Dr. Arunabh Talwar and his colleagues provide a logical algorithm to diagnose common and uncommon illnesses that cause pleural effusion.

This collection of highly selected topics provides a succinct and clear description of those conditions that affect significant numbers of people. I sincerely hope that this effort will assist those who face practical pulmonary and pleural problems related to tropical medicine, whatever their station may be.

Om P. Sharma, F.R.C.P.

Contributors

Gautam Ahluwalia   Department of Medicine, Dayanand Medical College and Hospital, Ludhiana, India

Zelena-Anne Aziz   Department of Radiology, King's College Hospital, London, U.K.

Eduardo P. Bethlem   Division of Pulmonary Medicine, Federal University of Rio de Janeiro State—UNI-RIO, Rio de Janeiro, Brazil

Carlos Roberto Ribeiro Carvalho   Division of Respiratory Diseases—Heart Institute (InCor), University of São Paulo Medical School, São Paulo, Brazil

Nancy F. Crum   Division of Infectious Disease Medicine, Naval Medical Center, San Diego, California, U.S.A.

Feyza Erkan   Department of Chest Diseases, Istanbul University, Istanbul, Turkey

Patricio Escalante   Division of Pulmonary and Critical Care Medicine, Keck School of Medicine, University of Southern California, Los Angeles, California, U.S.A.

Carmen Faure Division of Pulmonary Medicine, Hospital de Clinicas "Jose de San Martin," Universidad de Buenos Aires, Argentina

Alan M. Fein Division of Pulmonary and Critical Care Medicine, Department of Internal Medicine, North Shore University Hospital, Manhasset, New York, U.S.A.

Bruno Gottstein Institute of Parasitology, Vetsuisse Faculty and Faculty of Medicine, University of Bern, Bern, Switzerland

Ahmet Gül Division of Rheumatology, Department of Internal Medicine, Istanbul University, Istanbul, Turkey

Shanu Gupta University of Southampton, Southampton, U.K.

Chadi A. Hage Indiana University-School of Medicine, and Roudebush VA Medical Center, Indianapolis, Indiana, U.S.A.

Takateru Izumi Central Clinic in Kyoto, Kyoto, Japan

Chaim Oscar Jacob Department of Medicine, Keck School of Medicine, University of Southern California, Los Angeles, California, U.S.A.

D. G. James York Terrace East Regents Park, London, U.K.

Edgar Jan Department of Radiology, McMaster University Medical Centre, Hamilton, Ontario, Canada

S. K. Jindal Department of Pulmonary Medicine, Postgraduate Institute of Medical Education and Research, Chandigarh, India

Cage S. Johnson Comprehensive Sickle Cell Center, Keck School of Medicine, University of Southern California, Los Angeles, California, U.S.A.

Brenda E. Jones Division of Infectious Diseases, Keck School of Medicine, University of Southern California, Los Angeles, California, U.S.A.

Masanori Kitaichi Department of Anatomical Pathology, Kyoto University Hospital, Kyoto, Japan

Carla R. Lamb Interventional Pulmonary Medicine, Pulmonary and Critical Care Department, Lahey Clinic Tufts University, Burlington, Massachusetts, U.S.A.

Pnina Langevitz Internal Medicine "F" and the Heller Institute for Medical Research, Sheba Medical Center, Tel Hashomer, Israel

Edith R. Lederman Head of Clinical Medicine, Parasitic Disease Program, US Naval Medicine Research Unit 2, Jakarta, Indonesia

Avi Livneh Tel Aviv University, Sackler School of Medicine, Tel Aviv, Israel

Carlos M. Luna Division of Pulmonary Medicine, Hospital de Clinicas "Jose de San Martin," Universidad de Buenos Aires, Argentina

Violeta Mihailovic-Vucinic Medical School, University of Belgrade, Serbia and Institute of Pulmonary Diseases, University Clinical Center, Belgrade, Serbia

Sonoko Nagai Department of Respiratory Medicine, Kyoto University, Kyoto, Japan

Fukumi Nakamura-Uchiyama Parasitic Diseases Unit, Department of Infectious Diseases, Faculty of Medicine, Miyazaki University, Kiyotake, Miyazaki, Japan

Yukifumi Nawa Parasitic Diseases Unit, Department of Infectious Diseases, Faculty of Medicine, Miyazaki University, Kiyotake, Miyazaki, Japan

Einat Rabinovich Internal Medicine "F" and the Heller Institute for Medical Research, Sheba Medical Center, Tel Hashomer, Israel

Jürg Reichen Department of Clinical Pharmacology, University Hospital of Bern, Bern, Switzerland

Jonathan L. Richenberg Department of Radiology, The Royal Sussex County Hospital, Brighton, U.K.

Alejandro Sanchez Los Angeles County-University of Southern California Medical Center, Los Angeles, California, U.S.A.

George A. Sarosi Indiana University-School of Medicine, and Roudebush VA Medical Center, Indianapolis, Indiana, U.S.A.

Eli Schwartz Center for Geographic and Tropical Medicine, Sheba Medical Center, Tel-Hashomer, Israel and Division of Internal Medicine, Sackler Faculty of Medicine, Tel Aviv University, Tel Aviv, Israel

Om P. Sharma   Keck School of Medicine, University of Southern California, Los Angeles, California, U.S.A.

Sat Somers   Department of Radiology, McMaster University Medical Centre, Hamilton, Ontario, Canada

Arunabh Talwar   Division of Pulmonary and Critical Care Medicine, Department of Internal Medicine, North Shore University Hospital, Manhasset, New York, U.S.A.

Shraddha Tongia   Division of Pulmonary and Critical Care Medicine, Department of Internal Medicine, North Shore University Hospital, Manhasset, New York, U.S.A.

Eli Tumba Tshibwabwa   Department of Radiology, McMaster University Medical Centre, Hamilton, Ontario, Canada

Atadan Tunaci   Department of Radiology, Istanbul University, Istanbul, Turkey

Nurit Tweezer-Zaks   Internal Medicine "F" and the Heller Institute for Medical Research, Sheba Medical Center, Tel Hashomer, Israel

V. K. Vijayan   Vallabhbhai Patel Chest Institute, University of Delhi, Delhi, India

A. Wilcox   Los Angeles County-University of Southern California Medical Center, Los Angeles, California, U.S.A.

Ensar Yekeler   Department of Radiology, Istanbul University, Istanbul, Turkey

Contents

1

Pulmonary Zoonoses

OM P. SHARMA

Keck School of Medicine, University of Southern California,
Los Angeles, California, U.S.A.

I. Introduction

Zoonoses or zoonotic illnesses are infections that are transmitted between vertebrate animals and humans. This large group includes infections that man acquires from lower animals and also those that travel from man to lower animals. The zoonotic illnesses have an immense impact on the economy because the disorders not only cause significant morbidity and mortality in humans, but they have an infinite capacity to devastate the livestock industry. Most of the zoonotic illnesses are multisystem, but lung involvement is important and it may dictate the course and prognosis of most of these illnesses.

II. Historical Comment

Throughout human history, zoonotic illnesses have played a significant role. The earliest reference to a zoonotic illness occurs in a Mesopotamian code from 2000 B.C. in which the owner of a dog was fined because the dog, later found to be rabid, had bitten someone. Early Hebrew, Greek, Roman, and

1

Hindu writings provide accurate descriptions of anthrax. Plague, arguably the most devastating zoonosis, was recorded as early as 3000 years ago. The three major pandemics of plague that have occurred since the beginning of the Christian era decimated large segments of the population and stunted the development of European culture from the 14th to 17th century. It has been estimated that 25 million people—almost one-quarter of the European population—succumbed to the Black Death.

During the 18th and 19th centuries, several outbreaks of yellow fever spread via shipping routes to many major ports on the Western Hemisphere. Yellow fever, primarily a disease of monkeys, was a major obstacle during the construction of the Panama Canal. In the 20th century, HIV disease completely changed the cultural, philosophical, and medical outlook. There are many other zoonotic epidemics besides HIV disease that have been recognized during the last few decades including Lassa fever, Marburg and Hanta virus infections, Q-fever, Brucellosis, and Babesiosis. Severe acute respiratory syndrome (SARS), first diagnosed in Guangdong Province, China in November 2002, is now recognized in patients on all five continents, although a relatively new addition to the growing list of zoonotic illnesses (1). The existing knowledge originating from veterinary research tells us that the new SARS-corona virus did not emerge through mutation or recombination, but it has probably been transmitted from an as yet unidentified animal species (2). As the human population increases and man proceeds to usurp and develop those areas that have been inhabited by the lower animals, the opportunities for contact between man and animals increase. It is certain that additional zoonotic illnesses will be recognized in the future and these disorders will influence our social and cultural existence (3).

III. Epidemiology

The epidemiology of zoonotic illnesses is complex; the following factors must be understood to comprehend the cycle of infection.

1. Infection
2. Host
3. Route of transmission
4. Environment

A. Infection

There are more than 150 different zoonotic illnesses on record. The agents that cause these infections range from unicellular organisms to complex helminths.

B. Host

The natural reservoir host of a zoonotic illness is usually a wild or domestic animal or both. In general, human beings are not necessary for the transmission of zoonoses, but they may serve as a reservoir for some zoonotic diseases. Man, however, is often a dead end in the chain of infection. With diseases such as leishmaniasis, trypanosomiasis, and the viral encephalitis, person to person transmission does occur but is uncommon and of little epidemiological importance. Arthropods act as host as well as vector for certain infectious diseases. The rickettsial organism of Rocky Mountain spotted fever can be maintained for several years in the tick vector. *Babesia microti* apparently spends its winters in the tick vector and then during the following spring it moves over to the susceptible rodent host.

In many zoonotic illnesses, there exist more than one animal host. Primary reservoir hosts serve as the permanent reservoir of infection in nature; whereas, secondary reservoir hosts, a domestic or a wild animal that comes in contact with man and the wild primary host, is usually not necessary for survival of the infectious agent. Plague is a good example of this phenomenon. There are more than 200 different natural hosts for the plague bacillus. The primary hosts are wild rodents; the organism is transmitted between them by the bite of an infected flea. Sporadic human cases may arise when man enters a natural focus of the disease and is bitten by an infected flea or handles an infected wild animal as many hunters and trappers do. From these sylvatic foci, the disease may spread to urban areas where the secondary reservoir hosts (rats and mice) live in close association with man.

Most farm animals carry organisms that can cause human illness. A careful history and physical examination augmented by selected and appropriate laboratory tests can establish the diagnosis in most cases. Exposure to horses may result in *Coxiella burnetti* (Q-fever) or *Rhodococcus equi* infection. The placenta of horses, cattle, sheep, goats, and rodents may be a site for bacterial growth and contamination. Ranchers and farm workers assisting with delivery of animals are at risk. Q-fever may be acute or chronic. The acute illness may manifest as pneumonia, fever, or jaundice; whereas, chronic involvement consists of bacterial endocarditis, hepatitis, and meningitis. The presence of serum antibodies in acute and convalescent specimens establishes the diagnosis. Doxycycline is most effective in treating the illness. *R. equi*, a small bacillus, acquired from horses and cattle, rarely causes an illness in the immunocompetent individuals, but may cause cavitary pneumonia in an immunosuppressed host. Biopsy with culture of the lesion leads to the diagnosis. Pigeons, parakeets, budgerigars, and psittacine birds are associated with a variety of febrile syndromes with lung involvement. Psittacosis results from contact with sick parrots, macaws, and parakeets. As many as 10% of asymptomatic birds may harbor *Chlamydia psittaci*, the causative agent of psittacosis. About 25% of the patients diagnosed with psittacosis do not recall having exposure to birds. A characteristic pink, maculopapular, blanching rash may be seen in some patients; whereas a few patients may have erythema nodosum. The diagnosis, however, depends on acute and convalescent serological studies (4).

Cryptococcus neoformans, a fungus, is frequently found in pigeon droppings. It causes a number of clinical syndromes ranging from an asymptomatic pulmonary nodule to prolonged cough with fever and pneumonia. Fungal cultures of blood, sputum, and broncho-alveolar lavage or measurement of cryptococcal antigen from serum or cerebrospinal fluid result in accurate diagnosis. *Histoplasma capsulatum* is found in bird droppings, particularly chickens, blackbirds, and starlings and bat guana.

C. Transmission

There are four basic routes of disease transmission:

1. Contact
2. Airborne
3. Vector-borne
4. Common-vehicle

The route of transmission of an organism between the natural animal hosts may be different from the way the organism moves from the reservoir host to man. In tularemia, for example, tick transmission is the major route of spread among wild animals, but man generally acquires the infection by direct contact with infected animals. The virus of yellow fever is maintained within the jungle between monkeys, the primary reservoir hosts, and various forest species of mosquitoes that rarely bite man. Spread to urban areas may occur when infected monkeys carry the virus to areas near the perimeter of the forest and are bitten by different mosquito species that live in close association with man and preferentially feed on humans.

D. Environment

Environmental factors are important in the epidemiology of all zoonotic illnesses particularly with wild animal reservoirs. The concept of "focality" or "nodality" emphasizes that infectious diseases are not evenly distributed geographically (5). Instead, they tend to remain "focal." The pattern is defined by habitats of hosts and vectors. When man intrudes on one of these "foci," he exposes himself to the infection. The term "landscape epidemiology" has been used to emphasize the physical characteristics of a locality and may suggest the likelihood of a given disease being present or not.

Tularemia is an excellent example of disease "locality." Eight different foci of tularemia have been defined in the world, each with its typical host–vector–infectious agent relationship. In the eastern North American continent, the cycle is maintained between cottontail rabbits and hard ticks. In the western part of the continent, the jack-rabbit is the major reservoir host, and either hard ticks or deer flies may serve as vectors. In Scandinavia, mosquitoes transfer the organism between lemmings and in the area around the Black Sea, the water rat is the major reservoir.

Many zoonotic illnesses are occupational hazards for example, leptospirosis in rice field workers, anthrax in carpet weavers, Q-fever in abattoir workers, and cutaneous larva migrans in plumbers.

An environmental change may alter the epidemiologic landscape of an illness. Monsoon season in India and the heavy rains in Brazil are frequently associated with epidemics of leptospirosis because of the sewer overflow and water contamination.

Similarly, melioidosis is a disease of the rainy season in endemic areas affecting the individuals who have direct contact with wet soil. Sporadic cases of American cutaneous leishmaniasis in hunters and woodsmen are common when the forest habitat of the rodent host and sand fly is relatively undisturbed. However, small epidemics may occur in early settlers when small communities are created within the forest.

IV. Important Pulmonary Zoonoses

A. Brucellosis

Brucellosis is a zoonotic infection caused by bacteria of the genus *Brucella*. The disease has a serious medical impact worldwide (6). *Brucella* is rare in the United States with less than 100 cases reported annually. It is largely an occupational hazard of slaughterhouse workers and veterinarians (7). It is common in the Far East, the Middle East (particularly in Kuwait and the Gulf countries), South America, Mexico, and the Mediterranean region. There are four species of *Brucella* that cause human illness. Each is confined to its major animal host; *Brucella melitensis* to goats, *Brucella suis* to hogs, *Brucella abortus* to cattle, and *Brucella canis* to dogs. In the body, the bacteria is engulfed by macrophages and broken down rapidly, but a residual of 20% remains unchanged. Low solubility and poor degradability of the antigen ensures the prolonged stimulus necessary for maintaining the chronic granulomatous inflammation. Granulomas are small and poorly formed. The *Brucella* species are slow growing and can be cultured on a peptone-based medium that has been enriched with blood or serum. The optimal specimens for finding *Brucella* are blood, bone marrow, and pus from septic arthritis and osteomyelitis (8).

The illness may be acute or chronic. The organism principally causes fever, chills, aches and pains, and weakness. Respiratory symptoms may occur in as many as 31% of the patients with brucellosis. These patients have normal chest radiographs. The symptoms are usually mild and include cough with or without sputum, transient bronchitis, and vague chest discomfort.

Pulmonary brucellosis may be classified into acute and chronic depending on whether the duration of the lung involvement is less or more than 3 months. In an endemic area, acute, pulmonary brucellosis occurs as a complication of acute systemic illness; whereas, in non-endemic areas chronic pulmonary disease predominates. Patients with chronic pulmonary brucellosis are usually asymptomatic and are discovered during a routine chest X-ray or physical examination. Abnormal chest radiographs are seen in about 1% of the patients. A variety of radiographic abnormalities are observed including bronchopneumonia, lobar consolidation, miliary infiltration, hilar adenopathy, pleural effusion, hilar adenopathy, and calcification.

The diagnosis of pulmonary brucellosis is based on a combination of epidemiological information, occupational history, clinical features, culture, and serological tests. The organisms can be recovered from blood, bone marrow, body fluids, and tissue specimens. A four-fold increase in serum antibody titers or the presence of high titers is diagnostic. Monitoring the antibody titers is helpful in assessing the effect of therapy and diagnosing relapses. The application of polymerase chain reaction provides a good alternative to conventional methods used in diagnosing brucellosis. But the disadvantages include low detection limit of bacterial DNA in blood samples, increased risk of carry-over contamination, and expense (9).

Treatment of brucellosis is prolonged; the organism is intracellular and relatively inaccessible to antibiotics. Many different drugs have been used including tetracycline, doxycycline, rifampicin, trimethoprim-sulfamethoxazole, ceftriaxone, cefotaxime, streptomycin, and aminoglycosides. The prognosis of treated patients is excellent. In patients with unexplained pulmonary manifestations or undiagnosed granulomatous disease, brucellosis should be considered in the differential diagnosis, especially in the patients who either live near or have been to an endemic area.

B. Melioidosis

Burkholderia pseudomallei is a motile, aerobic, nonspore forming, soil-saprophyte, Gram-negative bacillus. Gram stain shows a typical bipolar staining resembling a safety pin. The organism grows on most agar media forming the characteristic rugose colonies resembling cornflower heads that take up crystal-violet dye from the media. The organism is oxidase positive, uses glucose by an oxidative pathway, and can be recognized by its biochemical profile.

Melioidosis is endemic in Vietnam, Thailand, Malaysia, Singapore, northern Australia, Madagascar, Guam, and Hong Kong. Human subjects acquire the illness by direct contact with the organism either through an open wound or aspiration or inhalation of the contaminated water/soil. The disease presents with a variable course ranging from a dramatic, systemic septicemia with a high mortality of about 50% to a chronic, indolent, debilitating localized infection. The lungs are the most commonly involved organs. About 80% of the patients with acute disseminated disease have bilateral, patchy infiltrates with consolidation. These pneumonic areas may cavitate if the disease advances. In the patients who recover and survive, the chest roentgenogram completely clears. In the nondisseminated localized melioidosis, the chest X-ray appearance closely resembles pulmonary tuberculosis. These patients usually have a long history of cough and expectoration. Hemoptysis and chest pain may occur. Unilateral or bilateral upper lobe infiltration may occur in about 70–90% of the cases; cavity formation is seen in more than half of these patients. Pleural effusion is found in 5–15% of the patients with localized melioidosis. Hilar adenopathy is rare occurring less than 5% of the patients.

Melioidosis should be suspected in any severely ill patient with fever and pneumonia or a septicemic illness who lives in or has traveled from an endemic area. The diagnosis can be confirmed by using one of the following criteria: (a) presence of *B. pseudomallei* from body fluids including blood, pus, sputum or urine or (b) positive serologic test for the organism (e.g., IHA titer greater than 1:80, CF titers greater than 1:4, or four-fold rising titer of either test in the convalescent serum).

Melioidosis is difficult to treat. The antibiotic of choice is ceftazidime. Other third-generation cephalosporins are less effective. Carbapenems are efficient bactericidals against *B. pseudomallei*. Meropenem is used in northern Australia. In disseminated septicemic melioidosis, parenteral amoxicillin-clavulanate is an appropriate empirical treatment in areas where melioidosis is endemic, but the treatment should be changed to ceftazidime or a carbapenem once the diagnosis is confirmed. High-dose parenteral treatment should be given for at least 10 days for systemic infections and the switch to oral agents should only be made when there is clear evidence of clinical improvement. Oral treatment is with a four-drug combination of chloremphenicol, doxycycline, trimethoprim, and sulfamethoxazole. Chloremphenicol is usually given for the first 8 weeks of oral treatment, and doxycycline and co-trimexazole are continued for a full 20 weeks of therapy. The prognosis of melioidosis is better in children. Adult patients require follow-up for the rest of their lives (10).

C. Melioidosis Acute Suppurative Parotitis

Melioidosis acute suppurative parotitis is an unusual clinical syndrome that occurs predominantly in children. It is unilateral, but in 10% of the cases it may be bilateral. Management is with antibiotic, incision and drainage. Delay in drainage may cause Bell's palsy. In Japan, Kimura's disease, an uncommon chronic inflammatory condition that causes tumor-like lesions on the head and in the neck regions, can also involve the parotid glands. The characteristic features of parotid gland biopsy in Kimura's disease are periductal sclerosis and an infiltrate rich in lymphocytes, plasma cells, and eosinophils. Pentoxyfylline has been found to be effective.

D. Tularemia (Rabbit Fever, Hare Fever, Deerfly Fever, and Lemming Fever)

Francisella tularensis causes tularemia, a serious and occasionally fatal disease of humans and animals. Its name comes from Tulare County, CA, USA, where an outbreak of a plague-like disease in rodents led to the first isolation of a small gram-negative bacterium then named *Bacterium tularensis*, now a sole member of a new genus called *Francisella* (11).

The natural hosts of *F. tularensis* include mammals, birds, amphibians, fish, and even some invertebrates. Tularemia occurs only in the Northern Hemisphere most frequently in Scandinavia, northern America, Japan, and Russia. Recently, cases have been reported from Turkey, Yugoslavia, Spain, Kosovo, and Switzerland. The organism is principally maintained in the environment by various terrestrial and aquatic animals such as ground squirrels, rabbits, hares, voles, muskrats, water rats, and other rodents. Outbreaks of the disease in humans often run parallel with outbreaks of the illness in animals. A number of arthropod vectors transmit the disease. In central Europe, the ticks *Dermacentor reticulatus* and *Ixodes ricinus* are important vectors. In the United States, biting flies are the most common vectors in Utah, Nevada, and California, but white ticks are the most common transmitters east of the Rocky Mountains. In Russia, the organism is transmitted by mosquitoes and Ixodes ticks.

E. Amebiasis

Amebiasis is the second leading cause of death from parasites worldwide. The causative protozoan, *Entamoeba histolytica* secretes proteinases that dissolve the tissue, kill host cells, and engulf red cells. *E. histolytica* trophozoites invade the intestinal mucosa, causing amebic colitis. The organisms then breach the mucosal barrier and travel through the portal, circulating to the liver causing abscesses.

Individuals can present with amebic liver abscess months to years after travel or residency in an endemic area. The lung, after the liver, is the second most common extraintestinal organ involved in amebiasis. From the intestine, amebas reach the lung in one of the following ways: progression of the liver abscess may incorporate the diaphragm and pleuropulmonary complications may then occur by direct extension. A perforation through the pleural space leads to empyema, in which a rupture into the lung may produce an abscess, a consolidation, or a hepato-bronchial fistula. Most pleuro-pulmonary complications are due to direct extension of amebic liver abscess. Hematogenous dissemination occasionally occurs and takes place either through the portal system and the hepatic veins or through the inferior hemorrhoidal veins and inferior vena cava. In rare cases, the route is via lymphatic system locally or through the thoracic and then to the superior vena cava, producing lung lesions. Pleuro-pulmonary amebiasis should be included in the differential diagnosis of the patients with unexplained right-sided pleural effusion, particularly in individuals who either live in or have come from an endemic area (12,13).

F. Echinococcosis

Echinococcosis is caused by adult or larval stages of cestodes belonging to the genus *Echinococcus*. The two major species of medical importance are *Echinococcus granulosa* and *Echinococcus multilocularis*. *E. granulosa* is found on all continents, with highest prevalence in Mediterranean countries, the Russian Federation and adjacent states, China, north and east Africa, Australia, South America, and parts of India. *E. multilocularis* seems to have a wider distribution including parts of the Near East, Russia, and the central Asian Republics, China, Northern Japan, and Alaska. The definitive hosts of *E. granulosa* are carnivores such as dogs and wolves, which are infected by ingestion of offal containing protoscoleces. In the canine intestinal mucosa, these organisms develop into adult stages. Eggs or gravid proglottids are shed in the feces. Following ingestion by a human or ungulate intermediate host, an oncosphere larva is released from the egg. The larva then penetrate the lamnia propria and is transported to distant organs including the liver, lungs, spleen, and the brain, where it develops into a hydatid cyst. The initial phase of primary infection is always asymptomatic. The infection becomes symptomatic if the cysts either rupture or exert a mass effect. The definitive diagnosis for most cases of echinococcosis in man is by radiology, ultrasonography, computed axial tomography (CT scanning), and magnetic resonance imaging. Immuno-diagnosis is useful as a primary diagnostic tool and also for follow-up of patients after surgical or medical treatment. Recently, the World Health Organization (WHO) introduced a standardized classification of the ultra-sonographic images of echinococcal cysts enabling the clinician to select appropriate treatment. For management purposes, cysts are divided into three main groups: active, transitional, and inactive. Active cysts are simple cysts or cysts containing daughter cysts. The typical active cysts have intra-cystic sedimentation echoes (hydatid sand), double-layered cyst membranes, and/or intracystic daughter cysts. Inactive cysts are semisolid and calcified. I was brought up in the tradition of never puncturing a hydatid cyst. However, percutaneous puncture, aspiration, alcohol injection, and reaspiration (PAIR) technique, developed in the 1980s, has shown to be safe as long adequate antiparasitic coverage with albendazole is provided. PAIR and other less invasive procedures are now developed for treating large cysts containing multiple daughter cysts (14–17).

G. Trypanosomiases

The trypanosomiases consist of a group of animal and human diseases caused by protozoal parasites of the genus *Trypanosoma*. There are many species of trypanosome; several of the group cause disease in animals, but only two seem to effect man.

In sub-Saharan Africa, *Trypanosoma brucei* causes sleeping sickness and in South and Central America *Trypanosoma cruzei* causes Chagas' disease. Both *T. brucei* and *T. cruzei* are transmitted by the biting insects. *T. brucei* are known as saliveria because they are transmitted in tsetse saliva, *T. cruzei* belongs to the stercoraria because the transmission is by vector feces (Table 1) (18).

Human African trypanosomiasis manifests as stage 1 or 2 depending on whether parasites have invaded the cerebrospinal fluid or not. In the first stage, after their entry into the skin, parasites proliferate at the site leading to an inflammatory nodule or ulcer. This trypanosomal chancre occurs frequently in rhodesiense infection and is rare in gambiense illness. From the site parasites spread to the draining lymph nodes and reach the blood. The patient soon develops headache, malaise, and undulating fever. Diffuse generalized lymph node enlargement is characteristic of gambiense infection. The presence of markedly enlarged lymph nodes in the posterior triangle of the neck is called Winterbottom's sign, after Thomas Masterman Winterbottom who noted that slave traders in the late 18th century used neck swelling as indicator of sleeping sickness rendering the particular slaves undesirable. In the second stage of the illness, parasites invade internal organs including the central nervous system. The exact mechanism with which parasites involve the CNS is unclear. The patient develops headaches, nighttime insomnia, daytime sleepiness, and severe personality changes. Kerandel's is a curious sign consisting of a definite delay in response to firm pressure on the tissues overlying a bone such as the tibia. Coma and death soon follow in untreated cases.

Table 1 Two Types of Trypanosomiases

Features	African trypanosomiasis	American trypanosomiasis (Chagas' disease)
Distribution	Sub-Saharan Africa	Central and South America
Organisms	*T. brucei* gambiense	*T. cruzei*
	T. brucei rhodesiense	
Vector	*Glossina fuscipes*	Triatomine bugs
	Glossina morsitans	
Habitat	Forested river banks and savannah	Roofs, huts, palm trees
Hosts	Ungulates, mammals	Mammals

American trypanosomiasis (Chagas' disease) is transmitted by an infected reduviid bug that gorges itself on blood from a sleeping host and then deposits on the skin feces containing trypnomastigotes. These organisms enter the body through the microabrasions caused by scratching by the individual. In about 6–10 days, at the site of infection a nodule or chagoma appears. Romana's sign is a swelling of the eyelids after inoculation at the site. Usually, the acute phase passes unnoticed. In about 30% of the patients, chronic manifestations of the disease appear in the form of electrocardiographic abnormalities, enlarged heart and heart failure, megaesophagus, megacolon, and bronchiectasis.

1. Leishmaniasis

Two million new cases of leishmaniasis appear annually in 88 of the world's poorest countries. In these countries 80% earn less than $2 a day. Neglected by researchers and funding agencies, the global burden of the disease has remained unchanged for some years. Human infections with Leishmania protozoan parasites, transmitted by the bite of a sand fly, cause visceral, cutaneous, and mucocutaneous leishmaniasis. The most important vertebrate hosts of *Leishmania donovani* are dogs, wild canines, jackals, rodents, and man.

The generalized infection by *L. donovani* leads to fever, usually slow or subacute, and intense sweating. The fever is irregular and intermittent at first, but later it becomes remittent. Massive enlargement of the spleen is followed by enlargement of the liver. Lymphadenopathy is not an important feature. The gold standard for diagnosing visceral leishmaniasis (kala azar) is recognizing parasites in tissue smears, but the serological tests and pentavalent antimonials are commonly used. The second-line drugs include amphotericin-B and pentamidine isetionate. It is hoped that the first leishmaniasis vaccine will become available within a decade (19).

2. Trichinellosis

Trichinellosis is a helminth zoonosis that has been re-emerging in many parts of the world because of the breakdown of hygienic conditions and veterinary services. The disease is caused by a nematode of the genus *Trichinella*. Species of trichinella are widely distributed, including the Arctic, temperate lands and the tropics. Although all mammals are susceptible to infection by one or more of the species, humans appear to be particularly prone to developing clinical disease. When, the skeletal muscle containing infective larvae is ingested by another mammal, the larvae are released by the action of gastric juices and pass into the small intestine. In the intestine, the larvae sexually mature. The newly born larvae penetrate into the submucosa and are carried by the blood to various organs, including the heart, brain, lungs, retina, and lymph nodes. The larvae that invade the skeletal muscle survive. The severity of the clinical course depends on the species causing the disease. The number of larvae ingested, and sex, age, and ethnic group of the host also influence the course of the illness. The diagnosis is easier if the disease occurs as an outbreak. Exposure to infected, raw, or incompletely cooked meat, the presence of gastroenteritis, myalgia, facial edema, and eosinophilia, and conjunctival hemorrhages should suggest trichinosis. Death, although rare, may occur due to heart failure, pneumonitis, and adrenal gland insufficiency (20–22).

V. Conclusions

Zoonotic illnesses, new and old, occur all over the world. Modern medicine has failed to control many of the old illnesses that were thought to be easy to subdue with advanced technology. Several factors are responsible for the failure. These include human demographics, rapid and unplanned industrialization, increased international travel and commerce, microbial mutation, breakdown in sanitation and public health, social and political upheavals, and persistent, pervasive poverty (23–25). Several zoonotic agents have become potential biological weapons. In order to prevent and control these zoonoses, we need to develop educational tools to recognize them, scientific tools to diagnose them early, vaccines to prevent them, and new drugs to treat them. Above all, we need to instill social and scientific awareness of the impact of these diseases on our lives.

References

1. Zhong N, Zheng B, Li Y, Poon L, Xie Z, Chan K, Li P, Tan S, Chang Q, Xie J, Liu X, Xu X, Li D, Yuen K, Peiris J, Guan Y. Epidemiology and cause of severe acute respiratory syndrome (SARS) in Guandong, People's Republic of China, in February, 2003. Lancet 2003; 362:1352–1358.
2. Tobler K, Akermann M, Griot C. SARS, possible zoonosis in the area of conflict of pathogenic coronaviruses of animals. Schweizer Arch fur Tierheilkunde 2003; 145:316–322.
3. Comer J, Paddock C, Childe J. Urban zoonoses caused by *Bartonella, Coxiella, Ehrlichia*, and *Rickettsia* species. Vector Borne Zoonotic Dis 2001; 1:91–118.
4. Gregory D, Schaffner W. Psittacosis. Semin Respir Infect 1997; 12:7–13.
5. Anan'ina Iuv. Bacterial zoonoses with natural focality: current trends in epidemic manifestations. Zhurnal Mikrobiologii, Epidemiologii, Immunobiologii 2002; 6:86–90.
6. Capasso L. Bacteria in two-millennia-old cheese, and related epizoonoses in Roman populations. J Infect 2002; 45:122–127.
7. Von Matthiessen P, Sansone R, Meier B, Gaither G, Shrader J. Zoonotic diseases and at-risk patients: a survey of veterinarians and physicians. AIDS 2003; 17:1404–1406.

8. Sauret J, Vilissova N. Human brucellosis. J Am Board Fam Pract 2002; 15:401–406.
9. Cirak M, Hizel K. The value of polymerase chain reaction methods targeting two different gene regions for the diagnosis of brucellosis. Mikrobiyologii Bulteni 2002; 36:271–276.
10. White N. Melioidosis. Lancet 2003; 361:1715–1722.
11. Feldman K. Tularemia. J Am Vet Assoc 2003; 222:275–330.
12. Pandya K, Sharma O. Pleuropulmonary amebiasis. In: Sharma OP, ed. Lung Disease in the Tropics. Lung Biology in Health and Disease. New York: Dekker, 1991; 51:225–250.
13. Shamsuzzaman S, Hashiguchi Y. Thoracic amebiasis. Clin Chest Med 2002; 23:479–492.
14. Richter J, Hatz C, Haussinger D. Ultrasound in tropical and parasitic diseases. Lancet 2003; 362:900–902.
15. WHO-IWGE (WHO Informal Working Group on Echinococcosis). International classification of ultrasound images in cystic echinococcosis for application in clinical and field epidemiological settings. Acta Trop 2003; 85:253–261.
16. Brunetti E, Filice C. Radio-frequency thermal ablation of echinococcal liver cysts. Lancet 2001; 358:1464.
17. McManus D, Zhang W, Li J, Bartley P. Echinococcosis. Lancet 2003; 362:1295–1304.
18. Barrett M, Burchmore R, Stich A, Lazzari J, Frasch A, Cazzulo J, Krishna S. The trypanosomiases. Lancet 2003; 362:1469–1480.
19. Davies C. Leishmaniasis: new approaches to disease control. Br Med J 2003; 326:377–382.
20. Bruschi F, Murrell K. New aspects of human trichinellosis: the impact of new Trichinella species. Postgrad Med J 2002; 78:15–22.
21. Geerts S, de Borchgrave J, Dorny P, Brandt J. Trichenellosis: old facts and new developments. Verhandelingen-Koninklijke Academie voor Geneeskunde van Belgie 2002; 64:233–234.
22. De N, Murrell K, Cong le D, Cam P, Chau le V, Toan N, Dalsgaard A. The food-borne trematode zoonoses of Vietnam. Southeast Asian J Trop Med Pub Health 2003; 34(suppl 1):12–34.
23. Chomel B. Control and prevention of emerging zoonoses. J Vet Educ 2003; 30:145–147.
24. Anantaphruti M. Parasitic contaminants in food. Southeast J Trop Med Pub Health 2001; 32(suppl 2):218–228.
25. Ludwig W, Kraus F, Allwinn H, Doerr H, Preiser W. Viral Zoonoses—a threat under control? Intervirology 2003; 46:71–78.

2

Symptoms and Signs in Tropical Medicine

SHANU GUPTA

University of Southampton,
Southampton, U.K.

D. G. JAMES

York Terrace East Regents Park,
London, U.K.

OM P. SHARMA

Keck School of Medicine, University of
    Southern California,
Los Angeles, California, U.S.A.

I. Introduction

During our years in medical school, we were trained in the art of observation and the importance of accurate and thorough history taking. Indeed, these remain the building blocks on which the differential diagnosis is based and, such as, they bear repeating (1). The training is, perhaps, required more in tropical medicine than any other medical specialty. Clinical acumen is acutely and urgently needed when modern laboratory and radiological facilities are neither affordable nor available.

What follows re-emphasizes the methods to be pursued in analyzing and assessing patients with tropical pulmonary disease. It consists of three parts:

1. Questioning the patient about his or her medical history
2. Performing the physical examination of the respiratory system and
3. Examining the extra-pulmonary signs and symptoms

Once a strong clinical framework is constructed, its further development and refinement depend on the clinical experience, power of observation, and systematic reading of the medical literature. Good physicians continue to learn throughout their careers; it is the most essential element of a physician's development. As Cowper said, "Knowledge to become wisdom needs experience."

II. Medical History

Our era of high technology has profoundly altered our practice of medicine. Technologic advances have bestowed on the clinician a heady capacity to diagnose and control human illness. It is our contention, however, that this machine-generated hubris has cost us dearly. The physician, in striking a Faustian bargain, has traded away the art of observation and power of reasoning. We have become extremely versatile in chasing a single abnormal laboratory test. We have at our fingertips numerous, often exotic, explanations for a solitary biochemical aberration, but we find ourselves unable to comprehend the significance of the information to the patient as a whole. An accurate, relevant history is an arduous but important initial step in solving clinical problems; it establishes the tone for the patient–doctor relationship. If properly conducted, the dialogue engenders trust, confidence, and cooperation between two parties. The absolute must in this tableau is that the patient should be allowed to relate the story freely and in his or her own words. The physician should interject appropriately and should ask leading questions so that the discourse does not become verbose, misleading, and one-sided (2).

In most instances, an adequate medical history can be obtained in a fairly short time. As a student, one is taught to approach the diagnosis in a pre-established linear fashion. Take a history, examine the patient, look at the blood tests, analyze the chest X-ray, CT and MRI films, and so on. By the end of the process, perhaps the diagnosis will become clear. An experienced clinician, however, takes a different route. The clinician considers the presenting feature (e.g., cough, dyspnea, chest pain, hemoptysis, or fever) and then makes a mental note of such things as age, sex, place of origin, travels, occupation, hobbies, and habits and comes up with a list of possible diagnoses based on these "prior probabilities." It is crucial to understand that similar sets of "prior probabilities" for a presenting complaint will produce different diagnostic possibilities in patients from dissimilar backgrounds, for example, fever, cough, and erythema nodosum in a 23-year-old Irish woman from Dublin point to sarcoidosis; whereas, the similar constellation of clinical features in a 23-year-old woman from Bakersfield, California, indicates coccidioidomycosis; and the same features in 23-year-old woman from Norwalk, Connecticut, may suggest Lyme disease. Thus, knowledge not only of medical science but also of epidemiology and geography is invaluable for developing a reasonably accurate diagnostic list that is conducive to performing the focused physical examination and securing appropriate laboratory tests with minimal loss of money and time. In the example given above, for the patient from

Dublin, serum angiotensin converting estimation and a chest radiograph will be most useful; for the woman from Bakersfield, California, skin and serological test for coccidioidomycosis will nail the diagnosis; and for the patient from Norwalk, Connecticut, serological test for Lyme antibody is all that will be required. To observe and process seemingly unrelated scattered facts and develop a cogent diagnostic list requires experience (3).

A. Past History

The physician should enquire whether the patient ever had a chest roentgenogram. An old chest radiograph often provides invaluable information. A history of chicken pox extends a clue to a chest radiograph taken late in life showing military calcification. Generalized or localized (right middle lobe syndrome) bronchiectasis in adult years may be traced to episodes of severe respiratory infections or tuberculous pneumonia in childhood. Recurrent pneumonias in the same segment or lobe of the lung may be due to a sequestered lung or a localized obstruction due to a foreign body, whereas, in hypogammaglobulinemia and Kartagener's syndrome pulmonary infections are generalized.

B. Family History

The routine practice of asking a patient who has pulmonary symptoms whether a family member or friend has had tuberculosis or any infectious disease is not sufficient. We should always consider the possibility that a patient with chronic lung disease may have been born with an inherited defect, because all genetic defects do not necessarily become manifest in childhood. In a young adult with cough and dyspnea and a family history of emphysema, one must think about alpha-1 anti-trypsin deficiency. Hereditary hemorrhagic telangiectasia (Osler–Rendu–Weber syndrome) is a familial disorder inherited as an autosomal dominant. Telangiectasia are superficial and diffuse and may involve the lips, fingers, rest of the face, neck, distal limbs, and upper trunk, in order of frequency. The gastrointestinal tract and the lungs are commonly involved. Epistaxis, hemoptysis, hematemesis, and melena may develop. In a few patients, the pulmonary involvement may appear on a chest roentgenogram as an asymptomatic nodule (4). Sterility in an adult male patient with chronic lung disease or recurrent lung infections may be a clue to genetic lung disease, cystic fibrosis, immobile cilia syndrome, Young's syndrome, carboxymethylase deficiency, and hypogammaglobulinemia (Table 1) (5).

C. Occupational History

In the practice of tropical pulmonary medicine, the occupational history is extremely helpful. Paradoxically, it is either obtained poorly or not at all.

Table 1 Inherited Disorders with Recurrent Pulmonary Infections

Features	Cystic fibrosis	Immotile cilia syndrome	Young's syndrome	Protein-carboxyl methylase deficiency	Hypogammaglobulinemia
Pulmonary infections	Common	Common	Common	??	Common
Cilium/sperm structure	Normal	Abnormal	Normal	Normal	Normal
Vas and epididymus	Normal	Normal	Obstructed by secretions	Normal	Normal
Semen examination	Azoospermia	Immotile sperm	Azoospermia	Immotile sperm	Normal
Pancreas	Abnormal	Normal	Normal	Normal	Normal
Sweat test	Abnormal	Normal	Normal	Normal	Normal

Secure the occupational history in a chronological order from the time the patient left school and obtained his or her first job (part- or full-time), since certain substances may continue to exert their effect a long time after the person has discontinued contact with the particular agent. Asbestos is an excellent example of this delayed response that can occur in tropical as well as temperate climates. Ask the patient the name of their trade, the actual task done, the process employed, the tools used, the chemical substances handled, and the type of protective or preventive devices used.

Hypersensitivity pneumonitis or extrinsic allergic alveolitis develops in response to a variety of inhaled organic allergens. Accidental exposures to oxides of nitrogen, oxides of silver, chlorine, phosgene, and cadmium can produce lung damage. Certain other occupational exposures (e.g., zinc, lead chromates, radioactive substances, nickel) also predispose workers to the development of lung cancer (Table 2). Farmers and their families who work in confined areas with large animals, particularly swine, develop chronic respiratory symptoms and decline in the lung function. Sheepherders live in close proximity with dogs and sheep and are likely to develop hydatid disease. Butchers and dairy workers are candidates for catching brucellosis. Sewer crews can get leptospirosis (6).

D. Place of Birth and Travels

Significant information can be obtained from the history of birth and travels in countries where certain diseases are endemic (Table 3) (7). The return of a large number of military personnel from Far Eastern countries serves to focus attention on parasitic diseases, such as paragonimiasis, filariasis, strongyloides, and bacterial infections like melioidosis. Similarly, soldiers and army support staff returning from the Middle East and gulf countries may contract brucellosis, cutaneous leishmaniasis, and schistosomiasis. Visceral leishmaniasis (Kala-azar) and dermal leishmaniasis (Delhi boil) are endemic in India. Amebiasis is common in Mexico, Puerto Rico and other Caribbean islands, Russia, and South America. Tropical eosinophilia, an important cause of pulmonary infiltration with eosinophilia (PIE) syndrome, is a disease of Asian-Indians, while immigrants from the Mediterranean basin, Australia, New Zealand, and the Middle East may harbor hydatid disease. Familial Mediterranean fever may present as fever and joint pains in the Italians, Greeks, Cypriots, and in certain Middle Eastern races, whereas in the Africans similar presentation would make one think of sickle-cell disease. There are more than 200 million carriers of the sickle-cell trait worldwide, and sickle-cell disease is the most prevalent inherited disorder of Africans and African-Americans. There is substitution of glutamic acid by valine in the beta subunits of the hemoglobin molecule, and upon exposure to low oxygen tension mutant hemoglobin S becomes less soluble and aggregates into large polymers. The

Table 2 Common Causes of Hypersensitivity Pneumonitis

Condition	Antigen
Fungal causes	
Farmer's lung	Thermophilic actinomycetes
Air conditioner lung	Thermophilic actinomycetes
Bagassosis	Thermophilic actinomycetes
Mushroom picker's lung	Thermophilic actinomycetes
Maltworker's lung	*Aspergillus clavatus*
Cheese washer's lung	*Penicillium casei*
Sequoiosis	*Aurebasidium pullulans*
Maple bark stripper's disease	*Cryptostroma corticale*
Woodworker's disease	*C. corticale*
Suberosis	*Penicillium frequentans*
Paprika splitter's lung	Mucor
Dry rot lung	*Merulius lacrymans*
"Dog house disease"	*Aspergillus versicolor*
Lycoperdonosis	*Lycoperdon* sp.
Spatlese lung	*Botyris cinerea*
Animal causes	
Bird fancier's lung	Avian protein, blood
Rat handler's lung	Rat protein
Wheat weevil disease	Wheat weevil
Furrier's lung	Animal fur
Pituitary snuff taker's lung	Ox and pork protein
Chemical causes	
Isocynate lung	TDI, MDI
Pauli's reagent lung	Pauli's reagent
Hard metal disease	Cobalt
Cromolyn sodium lung	Cromolyn sodium
Bacterial causes	
Washing powder lung	*Bacillus subtilis* enzymes
B. subtilis alveolitis	*B. subtilis*
Bacillus sereus alveolitis	*B. sereus*
Uncertain causes	
Sauna lung	Lake water (?)
New Guinea lung	Hut thatch?
Ramin lung	Ramin wood
Insecticide lung	Pyrethrum (?)

resulting destroyed erythrocyte leads to hemolysis and vaso-occlusion. The pulmonary manifestation may be acute or chronic (Table 4), due to acute lung injury progressing towards acute respiratory distress syndrome, microvascular thrombosis and tissue infarction, release of inflammatory mediators, and interaction of sickle red cells with leucocytes (8–10).

Table 3 Geographical Distribution of Tropical Diseases

Worldwide	Brucellosis
	Giardiasis
	Hepatitis
	Legionellosis
	Leptosporiasis
	Listeriosis
	Malaria
	Rabies
	Tuberculosis
	Typhoid fever
Africa	Cholera
	Dengue
	Leishmaniasis
Sub-Saharan	Filiriasis
	Ebola
	Marburg hemorrhagic fever
	Lassa fever
	Malaria
	Schistosomiasis
	Trypanosomiasis
West and Central	Onchocerciasis
Central, Eastern, and Southern	Plague (*Yersinia pestis*)
	Typhus fever (*Rickettsia prowazekii*)
Tropical	Crimean Congo hemorrhagic fever
	Yellow fever
Asia	Cholera
South-East	Dengue
	Filariasis
	Crimean-Congo hemorrhagic fever
	Leishmaniasis
	Lyme disease
	Plague
	Schistosomiasis
	Typhus fever
Europe	
Mediterranean	Brucellosis
	Leishmaniasis
Central	Crimean Congo hemorrhagic fever
	Lyme disease
	Tick-borne encephalitis
North America	Lyme disease
South and Central America	Cholera
	Dengue
	Onchocerciasis

(*Continued*)

Table 3 Geographical Distribution of Tropical Diseases (*Continued*)

South and Central America (*contd.*)	Viral hemorrhagic fevers
	Leishmaniasis
	Plague (*Y. pestis*)
	Schistosomiasis
	Trypanosomiasis (Chagas' disease)
	Typhus fever (*R. prowazekii*)
	Yellow fever

E. Hobbies and Habits

Smoking history should be clear and detailed and should include the age at which the patient started smoking and the total number of cigarettes smoked. Patients should be asked about the use of intravenous drug abuse (talc

Table 4 Sickle Cell Disease

Pulmonary disease	Acute	Chronic
Interstitial lung disease	Pulmonary infiltrates correlate with neurological disease	Extent and severity of infiltrates correlate with number of previous acute attacks
Thromboembolism	Frequent	Frequent
Fat embolism	Lipid-laden macrophages in BAL preceding bone pain, fall in Hb and platelets	Leads to multifactorial pulmonary hypertension
Infection	Difficulty to diagnose Chlamydia, Mycoplasma, virus, Legionella, RSV	Lung scarring due to frequent previous acute infections
Airway hyperactivity	Common	Less obvious
Nocturnal O_2 desaturation	Associated with painful crises and obstructed sleep apnea	Frequent may lead to cor pulmonale
Pulmonary hypertension	Early	Associated with exercise intolerance and heart failure
Investigation	CBC; chest X-ray; sputum, blood, BAL cultures; bronchoscopy; ABG	Lung function and ABG, echocardiography, cardiac catheterization
Treatment	Vaccinations: Flu % Pneumovac; appropriate antibiotics, hydroxyurea, corticosteroids; blood transfusion; inhaled nitric oxide	Inhaled nitric oxide, prostacyclin and prostaglandin analogues, long-term O_2, calcium channel blockers, surgery

granulomatosis and ritalin-induced vasculitis) and the use of nose drops (lipoid pneumonia). They should be questioned about contacts with pigeons, parakeets, parrots (pigeon breeders' disease, ornithosis/psittacosis, cryptoco ccosis); dogs, cats, and rabbits (toxoplasmosis, tularemia, toxocariasis, asthma, cat scratch disease).

F. Drug-Induced Lung Disease

When a pulmonary illness appears in a patient who has another illness or illnesses [AIDS (acquired immuno deficiency symdrome); neoplastic diseases, particularly hematologic malignancies; diabetes mellitus; hypertension; cystic fibrosis] and has been receiving many drugs, the possibility of an adverse drug reaction must be considered. The spectrum of drug-induced lung disease ranges from an asymptomatic pulmonary infiltrate to fatal respiratory failure (Table 5).

G. Spread of Pulmonary Tuberculosis

The recent resurgence of tuberculosis in patients with AIDS and other immunological deficiencies forces us to remember that there is a tendency among patients undergoing gastrectomies and other extensive abdominal procedures to develop reactivation of tuberculosis. All tuberculin reactors undergoing the above surgical operations should receive preventive therapy with isoniazid and rifampin. Persons who have undergone gastrectomy absorb rifampin and isoniazid well (11).

III. Examination of the Chest

Next comes the physical examination of the respiratory system. The examination should be carried out gently and in a relaxed and pleasant atmosphere. The patient should not be forced to undergo any inconvenient or embarrassing procedures or put into any difficult postures or positions. The time-honored order of observation (inspection), palpation, percussion, and auscultation should be adhered to.

A. General Contours

Kyphosis and scoliosis are common in the tropics and may be either developmental or acquired, related to poor nutrition, tuberculosis, or trauma. If gross, they may give rise to severe impairment of lung function, cor pulmonale, and ventilatory failure. A funnel-shaped depression (pectus excavatum) of the sternum may occur in varying degrees. A deep depression may displace the heart to the left and lead to the erroneous diagnosis of heart failure. Unilateral flattening of the chest is seen in long-standing pulmonary or pleural tuberculosis. In advanced tuberculosis, one or both apices are often contracted, and a hollowing is produced above or below the clavicles. Although palpation and

Table 5 Drugs That Cause Pulmonary Reaction

Drug type	Generic
Antibiotics	Nitrofurantoin
	Sulfonamides
	Penicillins
	Cephalosporins
	Tetracycline
Anti-inflammatory	Salicylates, colchicine
	Penicillamine
	Gold
	Corticosteroids
Antiarrhythmic	Amidarone
	Procainamide, tocainide
	Propranolol
	Hydralazine
Anticancer (chemotherapeutic) agents	Bleomycin, busulfan
	Methotrexate, melphalan
	Cyclophosphamide, chlorambucil
	Cytosine arabinoside
	Vinblastine
	Nitrosourea
	Mitomycin C
Addictive drugs	Heroin, cocaine, methadone
All others	Tocolytics, talc
	Dilantin, methysergide
	Lymphangiographic dyes
	Radiation, oxygen, blood transfusion
	Hydrochlothiazide
	Cromolyn sodium

percussion are of limited value, they ascertain the limits of the lung resonance, the state of the pleura and the chest wall, and diaphragmatic movements. The adventitious sounds may arise in the lungs or pleura. Fine crepitations are present at the apices in tuberculosis and at the bases in pulmonary edema. Coarse crepitations are present in bronchitis, bronchiectasis, lung abscess, pulmonary edema, and interstitial fibrosis.

IV. Extrapulmonary Signs Helpful in Diagnosing Tropical Lung Disease

Because of our intense involvement with our specialty, we often fail to recognize the importance of signs and symptoms related to other organ systems. In this section, we will relate some of the common and uncommon constellations of signs and symptoms related to tropical lung disease. The liberal use of anecdotes and eponyms is designed to facilitate learning. Furthermore, we believe that eponyms add a human touch to the art of medicine.

A. Fever

This is one of the most common, most frustrating, and, paradoxically, one of the most helpful diagnostic signs in tropical medicine. In some cases, the pattern of fever establishes the diagnosis. There are three principal types of fever (Table 6) (12). When fever does not fluctuate more than about a degree and a half (Fahrenheit) during the 24 hours, but at no time becomes normal, it is called continued and is seen in enteric fever with or without pneumonitis. When the daily fluctuations exceed 2°, it is described as remittent and is often seen in tuberculosis. When fever is only present for several hours during the day it is intermittent. In *Plasmodium malariae* infection, the quartan fever (2-day gap) is virtually diagnostic. The dengue fever pattern is characterized as "saddle-back." In brucellosis, the fever waxes and wanes in a cycle lasting 2–4 weeks. This undulating pattern is also seen in leishmaniasis and various relapsing fevers.

B. Impaired Learning, Impaired Growth, and "Backwardness"

Parasitic worm infestations affect 2 billion persons and may particularly cause insidious effects on growth and development. Chronic infection impairs growth, learning, and school attendance. Eradication treatment is cheap, but extremely important. The World Health Organization and the World Bank have a large-scale plan to deworm 75% of school-age children; by 2010 this means treating a population of 398 million children. Sadly, many of these children are dismissed as just "backward" or "chesty children." The chest physician should recognize and treat these multisystem infections before it is too late (Table 7) (13).

C. Skin

(a) *Erythema nodosum*: This sign consists of painful red nodules that occur mainly on the shins. This dermatological curiosity has been the subject of intensive investigation by clinicians, dermatologists, and immunologists. It is an important, albeit, nonspecific, manifestation of many pulmonary diseases (Table 8).

(b) *Lupus vulgaris*: During the last years, the incidence of cutaneous tuberculosis has dramatically declined in the developed countries, but the disease remains common in the tropics. There is no established classification of skin tuberculosis. Lupus vulgaris is the most common of the skin tuberculosis lesions. It occurs after a primary infection and affects women three times more commonly than men. It consists of reddish brown, flat plaques with

Table 6 Types of Fever

Fever	Definition	Differential
Continuous	Temperature fluctuates $<1.5°F$ in 24 hours (but at no times normal)	• Enteric fever • Typhus • Pneumococcal pneumonia • Brucellosis
Remittent	Temperature fluctuates $>2°F$	• Tuberculosis • Sinusitis • Bronchial pneumonia • Viral infections • Rheumatic fever
Intermittent	Fever only for a few hours a day	• Malaria (quartan pattern of *Plasmodium malariae*) • Dengue ("saddle-back") • Brucellosis • Leishmaniasis
Recurrent	Regular, periodic episodes of fever interrupted by one or several days without fever	• *Borrelia* spp. • Visceral leishmaniasis • Trypanosomiasis • Filariasis
Undulating	Long rise, or fall, to normal temperatures, respectively, over a period of weeks, and periods without fever	• Burcellosis
Fever with chills	Rapid rise in fever to high levels associated with severe muscular contractions	• Septicemia • Bacterial endocarditis • Pneumonia • Allergic reactions • Transfusion incidents
Acute	<14 days duration	+Anemia • Malaria • Babesiosis • Bartonellosis • Infection in patient with Sickle-cell anemia Thalassaemia G-6-PD deficiency
Chronic	>14 days duration	+Leucocytosis • Deep abscess • Amebic liver abscess • Cholangitis +Eosinophilia • *Schistosoma mansoni* • *Schistosoma japonicum*

(*Continued*)

Table 6   Types of Fever (*Continued*)

Fever	Definition	Differential
Chronic (*contd.*)		• *Fasciola hepatica* • Lymphangitis exacerbations secondary to microfilariae • Viscera larvae migrans +Neutropenia • Malaria • Disseminated tuberculosis • Visceral leishmaniasis • Brucellosis • HIV infection +Normal white blood cell count • Localized TB • Brucellosis • Secondary syphilis • Trypanosomiasis • Toxoplasmosis • Subacute bacterial endocarditis • Systemic lupus erythematosus • Chronic meningococcal septicemia • Melioidosis +Variable white blood cell count • Tumor • Drug reactions

yellowish brown nodules located on the face, neck, arms, and legs in descending order of frequency. It heals in one area and expands in the other. Ulceration and scarring are characteristic features. The biopsy specimen shows epithelioid granulomas, and the tuberculin test is almost always positive.

(c) *Primary inoculation*: The lesion begins as a small papule or nodule that eventually ulcerates. The ulcer is shallow and has a granular base studded with miliary abscesses or necrotic membrane deposits. These ulcers are typically ragged and have undermined edges. Tuberculosis chancre should be considered a diagnostic possibility in any person with a chronic, painless ulcer and a history of contact with tuberculosis. The diagnosis can be made by demonstrating acid-fast bacilli in the pus or in the biopsy specimen.

(d) *Cutaneous ulcers*: It occurs in about 60% of the patients with tularemia. The ulcer may be single or multiple; the site reflects the source of

Table 7 Common Helminthic Infections in Childhood Causing Insidious Impaired Growth or Learning or "Backwardness"

Helminth	Age (yr)	Clinical features	Treatment
Trichuris (whipworm)	5–10	Protein malnutrition, dysentery, growth retardation, anemia	Mebendazole
Ascaris lumbricoides	5–10		Mebendazole
Schistosoma	10–14	Portal hypertension, periportal fibrosis, pulmonary hypertension, nephritis	Praziquantal
Hookworm (*Necator americanus* and *Ancylostoma duodenale*)	20–25	Iron deficiency anemia and cognitive defects	Mebendazole

infection. Ulcers in the upper extremity are usually associated with exposure to rabbits, possums, cats, and squirrels, whereas lesions on the legs are related to ticks and deerflies bites. Other lesions in tularemia include erythema nodosum, erythema multiforme, diffuse maculopapular rash.

(e) *Lupus pernio*: It is a chronic, bluish granulomatous infiltration of the nose, cheeks, ears, and sometimes lips and chin. The nasal mucosa is frequently involved. Occasionally, the nasal septum may be destroyed. Lupus pernio is seen in women with chronic sarcoidosis and is associated with

Table 8 Diseases Associated with Erythema Nodosum

Condition	Chest X-ray abnormality
Tuberculosis	Unilateral hilar adenopathy, patchy infiltrate
Histoplasmosis	Unilateral or bilateral hilar adenopathy, infiltrate
Brucellosis	Hilar adenopathy, infiltrate, pleural effusion
Coccidioidomycosis	Hilar adenopathy, patchy infiltrate
Psittacosis pneumonia	Parenchymal infiltrate
Behcet's disease	Interstitial infiltrate, arterial aneurysms
Sarcoidosis	Bilateral hilar adenopathy
Drugs (contraceptives, sulfa)	Patchy infiltrate
Streptococcal pneumonia	Patchy infiltrate, consolidation
Leprosy	Normal chest X-ray

interstitial and fibrotic lung disease, chronic uveitis, and bone lesions. In the tropics, leprosy, tuberculosis, syphilis, dermal leishmaniasis, rhinoscleroma, rhinohyma, leishmaniasis, and yaws may produce similar lesions. Wegener's granulomatosis and amiodarone can give rise to skin changes that may be mistaken for lupus pernio.

(f) *Skin plaques*: Chronic, purplish or discolored, elevated skin patches occurring on the limbs, trunk, and buttocks are common in many tropical and subtropical countries. In sarcoidosis these plaques are characteristically symmetrical, but in leprosy and fungal and parasitic infestations they may be single or randomly distributed.

(g) *Subcutaneous nodules*: Calabar swellings (from calabar beans) are about the size of half a goose egg, painless, though somewhat hot, nonpitting subcutaneous nodules seen in endemic areas for Loa loa. This filarial worm is widely distributed in West Africa, particularly in the Cameroons. The parasite is also found in the southern Sudan and Congo. Calabar swellings are transient, but recur at regular intervals, for many years after the patient has returned to Europe or the United States. *Onchocerca volvulus*, another filarial causes subcutaneous fibrous tumors, the size of a pea to that of a pigeon's egg. The regions of the body most frequently affected are those in which the peripheral lymphatics converge. Thus, the tumors are usually found in the axilla, the popliteal space, above the elbow, the suboccisubpital area, and in the intercostal spaces. In sarcoidosis, similar lesions constitute the Darrier–Roussey syndrome. *Trypanosoma cruzi* may cause subcutaneous swelling on the face known as Romana's sign (14,15).

(h) *Kaposi's sarcoma*: In 1872, Moricz Kaposi described the idiopathic pigmented sarcoma of the skin characterized by slowly progressive violaceous nodules composed of proliferating cells that resembled endothelial cells. There are three variants of Kaposi's sarcoma (KS). The first type of KS occurs principally in men of Italian and central European Jewish ancestry. The peak incidence of onset is in the sixth and seventh decades of life. The lesion starts as a dark blue or purplish lesion on the feet and legs. Pulmonary and visceral dissemination is rare.

The second type occurs in western Africa. This histologically similar neoplasm has a different clinical presentation. It affects younger persons, the peak incidence is in the third decade, the course is fulminant, and visceral involvement is common. The lymph nodes are the most frequently involved organs.

The third type of KS is extremely aggressive and has appeared in increasing numbers since 1982. It affects primarily young individuals with acquired immune deficiency syndrome (AIDS). The respiratory tract is frequently involved, and visceral dissemination is common. Hemoptysis occurs in the patients with endobronchial lesions. The chest roentgenographic features are diffuse interstitial nodulation, hilar and mediastinal adenopathy, and pleural effusion. About two-thirds of the patients show

Table 9 Important Lung–Eye Links

Chest X-ray appearance	Ocular examination	Possible systemic disorder
Infiltration + cavity	Uveitis, retinal vasculitis, choroidal tubercles	Tuberculosis, syphilis
Aneurysms, infarction	Uveitis, hypopyon, retinal vein occlusion	Behçet's disease
Cavity, infiltration	Scleritis, photophobia	Wegener's granulomatosis
Infiltrate	Conjunctivitis, scleritis, uveitis	Mycoplasma pneumonia
Infiltrate, hilar adenopathy, pleural effusion	Uveitis	Brucellosis
Hilar adenopathy	Uveitis, lacrimal gland enlargement, optic nerve involvement	Sarcoidosis
Pneumonic infiltrate	Conjunctivitis, photophobia	Tularemia
Pulmonary infiltrate	Lacrimal gland enlargement, conjunctivitis, swollen eye-lid Romana' sign	Chagas' disease
Pneumonia, pleural effusion, cavity	Uveitis, hypopyon	Paragonimiasis

typical bronchial wall lesions consisting of pinkish, red flat lesions that bleed easily on pressure. Pulmonary KS is a cause of significant mortality in these patients.

D. Occulopulmonary Syndromes

The lungs act in close harmony with other systems of the body including the eyes, and examination of the eyes is an integral part of the diagnostic plan to investigate pulmonary disease. The alert pulmonologist learns to recognize the lung–eye linkups for their diagnostic value and also for devising an appropriate therapeutic plan (Table 9).

V. Sarcoidosis

Sarcoidosis is now diagnosed in the tropical countries with increasing frequency. Uveitis occurs in about one-fourth of patients with this disease. It is most frequent in the 20–40-year age group and occurs twice as often in women. The most common lesion is iridocyclitis (anterior uveitis) followed by posterior uveitis accompanied by characteristic fundal lesions, periphlebitis, granulomas in the choroids, and neovascularization. Conjunctival follicles and lacrimal gland involvement are common but rarely produce symptoms. Optic nerve involvement may cause acute visual loss in a syndrome similar to demyelinating and tropical nutritional neuritis or chronic progressive visual loss associated with thickened optic nerves.

VI. Heerfordt–Waldenstrom Syndrome

It is characterized by uveitis, parotid enlargement, cranial nerve palsies (especially the seventh nerve), fever, hyperalgesia, meningism, papilloedema, and chest radiographic changes. The differential diagnosis of parotid enlargement in the tropics is wide (Table 10) (16).

A. Lofgren's Syndrome

The late Sven Lofgren of Stockholm delineated the association of erythema nodosum, bilateral hilar adenopathy, acute iritis, and acute parotitis. The syndrome is self-limiting and carries a good prognosis with ultimate resolution of sarcoidosis.

B. Behcet's Disease

It is also called the Silk Road disease. The pathologic process in Behcet's disease is vasculitis, particularly involving the veins, with deposition of antigen–antibody complexes. The typical features of Behcet's uveitis are severe anterior uveitis, often producing hypopyon, and posterior uveitis with retinal branch vein occlusion. Hemoptysis results when the pulmonary vasculature is involved (17).

C. Brucellosis

Patients with brucellosis have a multisystem disease with fever, malaise, chills night sweats, pneumonitis, pleural effusion, and joint pains. Ocular lesions

Table 10 Causes of Parotid Enlargement

Unilateral	Bilateral
Sialdenitis	Sarcoidosis
Sialosis	Sjogren's syndrome
Tuberculosis	Drugs: iodides
Cat-scratch disease	Melkersson–Rosenthal Syndrome
Lymphoma	Melioidosis
Actinomycosis	Sialadenitis
Melioidosis	Malnutrition Toxoplasmosis

generally develop after the acute phase and consist variably of iridocyclitis, keratitis, choroiditis, and optic neuritis.

D. Tuberculosis

Choroidal tubercles are found in patients with miliary tuberculosis. However, uveitis and retinal vasculitis is sometimes seen in patients who have recently been in contact with tuberculosis and who have a positive tuberculin test, but no other signs or evidence of active acid-fast infection. Frequently these patients are from the Asian continent. The characteristic retinal picture is one of occlusive venous vasculitis with dilated veins, retinal hemorrhages, and exudates and swollen optic discs. These patients progress to the development of new vessels with vitreous hemorrhage.

VII. Clubbing of the Fingers and Pulmonary Osteoarthropathy

Clubbing, a fingernail deformity, was first described by Hippocrates. When associated with periostitis and arthritis the syndrome is called hypertrophic pulmonary osteoarthropathy (HPO). HPO is associated with many pulmonary and extra-pulmonary states, and the idiopathic or familial form of HPO has also been described. In the tropical countries, clubbing and HPO most commonly occur in patients with bronchiectasis, lung abscess, and lung gangrene. Today, however, most cases are found in association with lung cancer, cystic fibrosis, and idiopathic pulmonary fibrosis. Other intrathoracic diseases associated with HPO include congenital lung disease, pleural and mediastinal neoplasms, and mesothelioma. The signs and symptoms of HPO regardless of the cause are similar. In patients who have arthritis associated with HPO, the large distal joints and big joints of the knees and ankles are involved. Less commonly, the small joints of the hands, wrists, and elbow are affected. The distribution is bilateral and symmetrical. The neighboring joints are red, tender, swollen, and painful. Clubbing is also bilateral with all digits being simultaneously affected. Clubbing may first appear in the thumb and the index finger. It starts at the base of the nail, with loss of nail angle, softening of the nail bed, and increases in the curvature of the nail. In periostitis, diffuse bone pain and tenderness of the shafts of long bones are found. A thickening of the periosteum is seen on X-ray films.

A. Lymphadenopathy and Tropical Medicine

Lymph node enlargement is a common feature of most tropical illnesses. The enlargement is sometimes noticed by the patient because of its acute and dramatic onset; at other times they are discovered by a physician on a routine examination, and, occasionally, one has to perform a systemic search for lymphatic enlargement. There are many illnesses that selectively involve the lymph nodes (Table 11).

Table 11 Some Causes of Lymphadenopathy with Tropical Lung Disease

Location of lymphadenopathy	Diseases
Suboccipital	Bacterial infections of the scalp
	Syphilis
	Viral infections
Cervical	Tuberculosis
	Brucellosis
	Tularemia, plague
	Lymphoma, Burkitt's lymphoma
	Trypanosomiasis
Supraclavicular	Tuberculosis
	Lymphoma
	Histoplasmosis, coccidioidomycosis
	Brucellosis, tularemia
	Trypanomiasis
Axillary	Cat scratch disease
	Carcinoma breast, lymphoma, melanoma
Epitrochlear	Syphilis
	Sarcoidosis
	Lymphoma
Inguinal	Syphilis
	Brucellosis
	Filariasis
	Trypanosomiasis
	Trauma
Generalized	Infections: HIV, infectious
	mononucleosis
	Leptospirosis
	Bartonellosis
	Lymphoma, leukemia,
	Trypanosomiasis
	Plague, tularemia

B. Splenomegaly

There is probably no sign in clinical medicine that so consistently captures the imagination of a clinician as does splenomegaly, particularly in the practice of tropical medicine. One of the most embarrassing experiences for an internist or a specialist is to be informed by a radiologist colleague that a large spleen is present, on an abdominal film or CT films, in a patient whose abdominal examination had been cursory. Superficial as well as deep palpation over the left abdominal half, the turning of the patient onto the right side, and the use of a firm examining table all contribute to the efficient examination of an enlarged spleen. The following causes of splenic enlargement need to

Table 12 Splenic Enlargement in Tropical Illness

Infectious	Infiltrative	Congestive	Hyperplastic
Malaria	Sarcoidosis	Portal hypertension	Sickle cell anemia
Parasites (schistosomiasis, leishmaniasis, echinococcosis)	Gaucher's disease	Banti's syndrome	Policythemia vera
Miliary tuberculosis	Lymphomas	Portal vein thrombosis	Mediterranean anemia
Brucellosis	Amyloidosis	Splenicveinthrombosis	Macroglobulinemia
Histoplasmosis	Leukemias		Tropical splenomegaly
Psittacosis	Berylliosis		Felty syndrome
Typhoid fever	Systemic lupus erythematosis		
Bacterial endocarditis			
Infectious mononucleosis			

be remembered when confronted with this clinical feature in a patient with suspected tropical lung disease (Table 12).

VIII. Conclusion

With a keen rise in adventurous international travel, it is becoming increasingly important to recognize diseases of the tropics. In an age of technological advancement in the medical arena, this account relates the ongoing importance of obtaining a thorough history on a background of comprehensive medical knowledge in the field of tropical medicine.

As has already been highlighted, geographical epidemiology and careful history, combined with signs and symptoms of pulmonary and extra-pulmonary pathology can guide the physician as to the cause. Once a cause is suspected, investigated, and confirmed, a treatment regimen may be initiated. Treatment for the various tropical diseases is readily available and alleviates disabling illness as well as preventing adverse sequelae.

In summary, this is a short account emphasizing the multitudinous signs and symptoms of tropical disease. It is our hope that health professionals, medical students, general practitioners, and pulmonologists may find it useful.

References

1. Sharma OP. Symptoms and signs in pulmonary medicine: old observations and new interpretations. Dis Month 1995; 41:581–638.
2. Bird B. Talking with patients. Am Pract 1955; 6:2705.
3. Bondi E, Margolis D, Lazarus D. Disorders of subcutaneous tissue. In: Freedberg IM, Eisen AM, Wolff K, Austen KF, Goldsmith LA, Katz ST, Fitzpatrick TB, eds. Dermatology in General Medicine. New York, USA: McGraw-Hill, 1999:1284–1286.
4. Fuchizaki U, Miyamori H, Kitagawa S, Kaneko S, Kobayashi K. Hereditary haemorrhagic telangiectasia (Rendu–Osler–Weber disease). Lancet 2003; 362:1490–1494.
5. Marwah O, Sharma O. Bronchiectasis. How to identify, treat, and prevent. Postgrad Med 1995; 97:149–159.
6. Sharma O. Hypersensitivity pneumonitis. Dis Month 1991; 37:411–470.
7. http://www.who.int/health-topics/. Cited October 25, 2003.
8. Johnson C, Verdegem T. Pulmonary complications of sickle cell disease. Semin Respir Med 1988; 9:287–296.
9. Siddiqui AK, Ahmed S. Pulmonary manifestations of sickle cell disease. Postgrad Med J 2003; 79:384–390.
10. Emburey SH, Vichinsky EP. Sickle cell disease. In: Hoffman R, Benz JR Jr, Shaltil SJ, et al. Haematology: Basic Principles and Practice. 3rd ed. Philadelphia: Churchill Livingstone, 2000:510–540.
11. George J, Zumla A. Advances in the management of tuberculosis: clinical trials and beyond. Curr Opin Pulm Med 2000; 6:193–197.
12. Spira AM. Assessment of travellers who return home ill. Lancet 2003; 361:1459–1469.
13. Awasthi S, Bundy D, Savioli L. Helminthic infections. Br Med J 2003; 327:433–435.
14. Sharma O. Selected pulmonary cutaneous syndromes. Semin Respir Med 1988; 9:239–246.
15. Barrett M, Burchmore R, Stich A, Lazzari J, Frasch A, Cazzulo J, Krishna S. The trypanosomiases. Lancet 2003; 362:1469–1480.
16. James DG, Sharma OP. Parotid gland sarcoidosis. Sarcoidosis Vasculitis Diffuse Lung Dis 2000; 17:27–32.
17. Erkan F. Pulmonary involvement in Behcet's disease. Curr Opin Pulm Med 1999; 5:314–318.

3

Tropical Pulmonary Radiology

ELI TUMBA TSHIBWABWA,
SAT SOMERS, and EDGAR JAN

Department of Radiology,
  McMaster University Medical Centre,
Hamilton, Ontario, Canada

JONATHAN L. RICHENBERG

Department of Radiology,
  The Royal Sussex County Hospital,
Brighton, U.K.

ZELENA-ANNE AZIZ

Department of Radiology,
  King's College Hospital,
London, U.K.

I. Introduction

This chapter describes the radiological findings of the more common conditions that affect the thorax in the tropics. Inevitably, the bulk of the discussion focuses on infectious diseases. The first part of this chapter considers the broader issues of imaging services in the tropics; the second part concentrates on the radiology of infectious and other disease states.

II. Imaging Services in the Tropics

In North America and elsewhere in the developed world, high-quality and timely imaging is taken for granted. Unfortunately, in the often-impoverished regions in the tropics, modern, dependable imaging is a scarce luxury. A hostile topography and climate exacerbate the differential. Many areas are remote and sparsely populated such that in many tropical countries, resources are often concentrated in a few urbanized areas (1–4). Clinicians who care for patients with pulmonary symptoms in the tropics must frequently accept suboptimal (or even no) imaging, or send their patients long distances. How can tropical lung radiology services be optimized?

The key to delivering a workable lung radiology service within the tropics is to match provision to demand. Imaging should be geared up for the investigation and treatment of infection (e.g., percutaneous image-guided empyema drainage). Plain radiography and ultrasound must form the core of any realistic imaging service (1,2,4,5). Whenever possible, equipment should be cheap and portable yet reliable and durable. Small machines may be used in field hospitals with rapid transmission of the images to large yet remote hospitals, where interpretation is possible. Tele-radiology is coming of age, and is well established in parts of Scandinavia that are sparsely populated and isolated, especially in winter.

With respect to ultrasonography, there are several high-quality yet compact and affordable units developed in the ironically high-tech world of North American intensive care units that would function admirably in the intensive environments experienced in a tropical hospital. Ultrasound provides a relatively cheap real-time method for guiding interventional procedures. Aspirates may provide samples from which organisms can be isolated so that valuable antibiotics can be husbanded and used only where appropriate. Computed Tomography (CT) plays a limited role and is found only in major centers. Currently, major South African cities have hospitals that provide such high-tech lung imaging to patients from the neighboring countries and even from as far as central and eastern Africa, where the few existing CT scanners cannot cope with the patient load.

III. Disease Profile of Lung Imaging in the Tropics

Climatic conditions in the tropics are such that pathogenic organisms, their vectors, and intermediate hosts thrive (6). Infectious diseases are a common cause of pulmonary disease in these areas. Sporadic infections in North America are endemic in the tropics. Tuberculosis (TB) is rife in many of the poorer communities in the world and the radiographic findings are so common as to be regarded as normal. The radiography of TB is all the more complex in the tropics because of the high coincidence of sarcoidosis in many regions. To make matters still more difficult, the classical findings of TB on chest radiographs may not be seen in the immunosuppressed patient. The specter of HIV and AIDS is ever present in the tropics. Other pulmonary infections, which are rare in the developed world yet commonplace in the tropics, include the parasitic infections of *Echinococcus* (hydatid), amebiasis, *Strongyloides*, paragonimiasis, and melioidosis.

Lung tumors, although prevalent, do not have the same relative importance as in the developed world, both because of the differing economic factors and the high incidence of infectious lung disease. Their imaging features are comparable to the findings in temperate regions, except to note that the patients may present later so that the radiographic findings are at the same time more florid (Figs. 1–5). Such an end-stage disease phenomenon is true for many lung conditions in the tropics: patients delay seeking medical advice due to poverty, traditional beliefs, limited access to health facilities or because they cannot afford to be sick. The radiology of pneumoconioses is not peculiar to the tropics, and there are many worthy reviews of the radiological evaluations of coal, tin, and gold miners. The discussion that follows is limited almost exclusively to the infectious diseases that ravage the lungs of many people in the tropics. By refining the content in this way, the essence of the differences between tropical and temperate lung radiology may be captured.

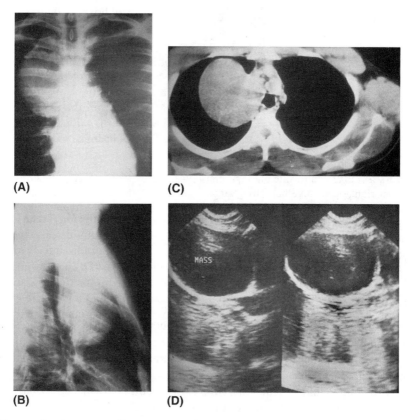

(A)

(C)

(B)

(D)

Figure 1   Posteroanterior (**A**) and lateral (**B**) chest radiographs and CT scan (**C**) and ultrasound (**D**) of a huge bronchogenic cyst in the upper lobe of the right lung.

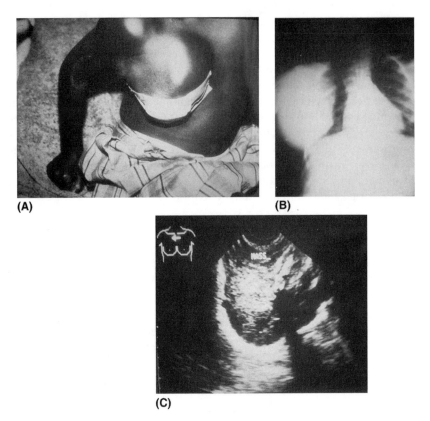

(A)   (B)

(C)

Figure 2 Black and white photograph of a 41-year-old patient (**A**) with a biopsy-proven right-sided huge non-Hodgkin's lymphoma of the chest wall. Chest radiograph (**B**) and ultrasound (**C**) demonstrate features of the well-circumscribed soft tissue mass. *Source*: Courtesy of Prof. M. Kawooya and Z. Muyinda, MD, Makerere University, Kampala, Uganda.

IV. Pulmonary Tuberculosis

TB has adapted to the tropics admirably: unknown in sub-Saharan Africa before the 19th century, by the 1950s infection due to *Mycobacterium tuberculosis* could be found in up to 50% of the adult population. Subsequently, socioeconomic changes, rapid urbanization, and the HIV epidemic have resulted in a 300–400% increase in TB cases in sub-Saharan Africa (7).

In young children, the tuberculin skin reaction may be depressed, and the chest radiograph becomes critical in making the diagnosis (8,9). While no single pulmonary radiological change is pathognomonic of TB, certain changes are associated with proven cases. Most children in both the Nigerian and the South African study had multiple pulmonary tuberculous lesions

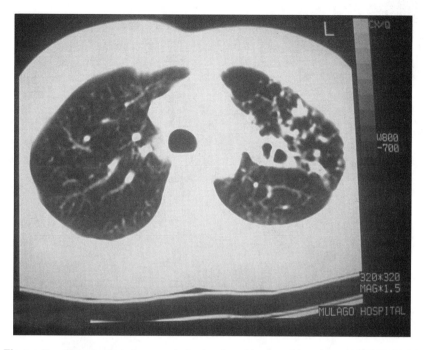

Figure 3 Chronic *Pseudomonas* infection in a 31-year-old patient with AIDS. CT scan through the lungs demonstrates dilated bronchi with adjacent inflammation in the upper part of the lingula. Sputum smear and culture were positive for *Pseudomonas*; CD_4 level was 30 cells/mm^3.

(compare with data from developed countries). This type of disease is probably caused by a combination of late presentation and the effect of malnutrition on their response (8,10).

Primary TB may manifest radiographically in five major ways: parenchymal consolidation, atelectasis, lymphadenopathy, pleural effusions, and miliary disease. The most frequent lesion seen in children in a Nigerian study of chest radiographs was mediastinal lymphadenopathy (79%), with right-sided involvement being more common (8). In a South African study that looked at children with advanced TB when they had their first radiograph, the incidence of lymphadenopathy was lower (43%) (9).

Overall, the frequency of lymphadenopathy seems to be lower than that seen in the West and may be related to the fact that children from less affluent countries are malnourished and present at a later stage of disease (11). Segmental lesions that consist of consolidation, collapse, and patchy inflammatory change are seen in more than two-thirds of cases (8,9), with the right lung, particularly the right lower lobe, being most frequently involved. Leung et al. (11) also found that right-sided changes were more

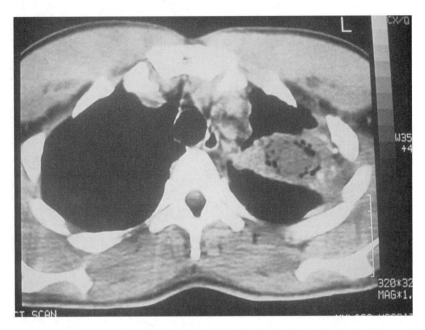

Figure 4   Aspergilloma. CT scan through the lungs depicts a fungus ball in an old tuberculous cavity.

common, although they did not observe a particular zonal predominance. The strong predilection of the right lobe (Fig. 6) as the site of parenchymal change would support the contention that the initial infection favors the right lung (9).

Pleural effusions, usually right sided, are seen in 12%, but hardly ever as the sole radiological manifestation (8). Miliary nodulation (10%) usually occurs in children younger than 5 years old (1,8). In two-thirds of the cases, it is associated with bronchogenic disease, segmental consolidation, or effusion. Miliary disease on the chest radiograph (Fig. 7) must be considered TB and treated empirically, not least because other causes including histoplasmosis, coccidiomycosis, fibrocystic disease, and hemosiderosis are rare in the tropics.

Cavitation, which is usually a feature of postprimary TB, is seen in 5–13% of cases (8,9). These features are more common in the younger age group and often indicate extrapulmonary TB. Calcification is seen in older children and is related either to the primary focus or to mediastinal lymphadenopathy. Calcification is not an indication of inactive disease.

V. Tuberculosis and HIV

The impact of the HIV epidemic on the incidence of TB is most evident in sub-Saharan Africa, where for the 10-year period from 1990 to 1999,

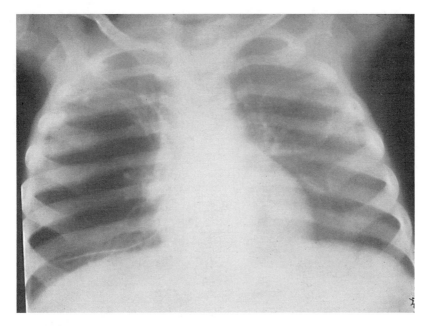

Figure 5 Chest radiograph of "measles" pneumonia demonstrates respiratory complications consisting of pneumothorax and bullae attributed to *Staphylococci* in a child with measles seen at the University Teaching Hospital, Lusaka, Zambia. Measles seems to be one of the most important causes of child mortality in the tropics.

15 million incident cases of TB were expected. Of these cases, 3.9 million (25%) were attributable to HIV infection. The number of new cases of TB per year in this region is forecast to double by the end of the decade (1).

Several studies have documented the modifying effect of HIV on TB and have compared the radiographic features of pulmonary TB in HIV-positive with HIV-negative patients (12–16). The general consensus is that patients with HIV are more likely to exhibit the radiographic features of primary TB. These manifestations (Table 1) include mediastinal and hilar lymphadenopathy, pleural effusions, middle and lower lung infiltrates, and miliary dissemination, with less cavitation being described. The typical radiographic appearances in HIV-negative individuals are usually that of postprimary TB, namely, cavitation, calcification, and upper lobe fibrotic changes. Although the features of dual HIV and TB infection are character-istic of primary tuberculosis, in most of these patients the disease is thought to be caused by reactivation as a result of cellular immunodeficiency. These patients behave as immunonaive individuals and develop a "childhood" pattern of tuberculosis (13).

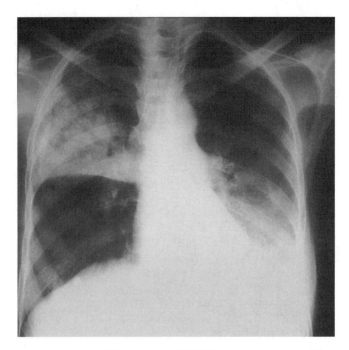

Figure 6   Chest radiograph in a 25-year-old HIV-negative patient with sputum that tested positive for acid-fast bacilli (AFB) reveals tuberculous segmental consolidation in the right upper and left lower lobes and ipsilateral right hilar adenopathy. This pattern supports the contention that the initial tuberculosis infection favors the right lung.

Atypical mycobacterial infection is rare in Africa despite its presence in the environment (7). Even in patients with AIDS, *Mycobacterium avium-intracellulare* has been infrequently isolated, which is in contrast to the North American experience (17). It has been postulated that the reason for the low prevalence is that diseases caused by *M. avium-intracellulare* occur late in the course of HIV-related immunosuppression after the occurrence of more virulent species.

VI. Pulmonary Complications in HIV Infection

Several studies from different countries in Africa have investigated HIV-positive patients who present with symptoms of bronchopulmonary disease (18–21). The findings have highlighted several points regarding the pulmonary manifestations of HIV-positive patients in this region.

  1.   TB is the most frequently encountered pulmonary complication that occurs in 23% and 49% of cases. Pulmonary infection by

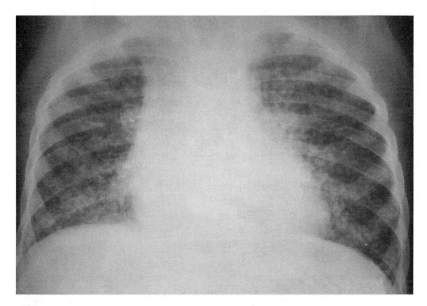

Figure 7 Miliary tuberculosis. Diffuse miliary nodules with hilar and mediastinal adenopathy are seen bilaterally on the chest radiograph in this 3-year-old patient.

atypical mycobacteria, *M. avium-intracellulare,* is rare. Mahomed et al. (21) suggest, however, that with increasing length of survival of HIV-infected patients in Africa, this infection will be found to be part of the spectrum as in the rest of the world.

2. Infection with *Pneumocystis carinii* is less common in African patients in contrast to AIDS patients in North America and Europe. Some researchers have attributed the lower prevalence rate to the fact that African patients with HIV infection die of diseases caused by more virulent organisms than *P. carinii* (e.g., *M. tuberculosis*) before *P. carinii* pneumonia can develop. There is, however, regional variation in the incidence of *P. carinii* pneumonia infection within the tropics [up to 40% in a cohort from Zimbabwe (20)], and *P. carinii* pneumonia is ignored when reading a chest radiograph of a patient in jeopardy. The problem is that several radiographic patterns have been documented, and they are usually nonspecific. Fine reticulonodular shadowing has been identified as being a strong independent predictor of *P. carinii* pneumonia (20,21). Other radiographic findings include alveolar or air space consolidation, lobar disease, and cystic lesions that result in pneumothorax. Some patients with *P. carinii* pneumonia may have a normal chest radiograph. The impression of other groups is that although *P. carinii* pneumonia occurs in Africa

Table 1 Chest Radiograph Patterns in Tuberculosis Seen in the Tropics in HIV-Positive and HIV-Negative Patients

	Radiographic pattern	HIV positive (%)	HIV negative (%)
Batungwanayo et al. (13)	Mediastinal and/or hilar adenopathy	30	0
	Pleural effusion	43	9
	Upper lobe infiltrate	16	55
	Cavitation	39	91
	Miliary disease	25	9
Pozniak et al. (14)	Mediastinal and/or hilar adenopathy	31	16
	Pleural effusion	26	13
	Upper lobe infiltrate	43	67
	Cavitation	40	64
Awil et al. (12)	Mediastinal and/or hilar adenopathy	26	6
	Pleural effusion	23	11
	Pneumonic infiltrate	46	26
	Cavitation	18	57
	Miliary disease	7	0
Saks and Posner (15)	Mediastinal and/or hilar adenopathy	50	8
	Pleural effusion	38	20
	Miliary disease	8	0
	Cavitation	38	82
	Atelectasis	31	82
Tshibwabwa et al. (16)	Mediastinal and/or hilar adenopathy	26	13
	Pleural effusion	16	6.8
	Miliary disease	9.8	5
	Cavitation	33	78
	Atelectasis	12	24

(Fig. 8), in a continent where diagnostic facilities are generally unavailable, pneumocystis is unlikely to be a relevant diagnosis (19).

3. Bacterial infection is common and is often found in association with other diseases. *Streptococcus pneumonia*, *Staphylococcus aureus*, *Nocardia*, *Klebsiella*, and *Haemophilus influenzae* are among the most common pathogens isolated (Fig. 9).

4. Fungal infections are rare, in most studies they appear infrequently. A study conducted by Batungwanayo et al. (13) reported pulmonary *Cryptococcus* in 13% of patients. The chest radiographic patterns

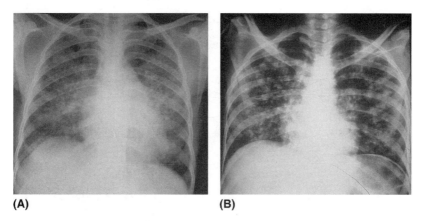

(A) **(B)**

Figure 8 *Pneumocystis carinii* pneumonia. (**A**) Chest radiograph in a 27-year-old patient with AIDS depicts bilateral, coarse reticulonodular infiltrates predominantly in the parahilar middle zone of both lungs. On both sides, the pulmonary lesions radiate out from the hilar regions. Bronchoalveolar lavage (BAL) was positive for *P. carinii* pneumonia. (**B**) Chest radiograph in 39-year-old patient with AIDS demonstrates extensive and fairly symmetrical alveolar nodules throughout the lungs. The apices are relatively spared. The pulmonary lesions resolved after 30 days of treatment with trimethoprim and sulfamethoxazole (TMP/SMX) for *P. carinii* pneumonia.

associated with cryptococcal pneumonitis include alveolar shadowing, interstitial infiltrates, miliary pattern, hilar adenopathy (Fig. 10); even a normal chest radiograph also seems to be the most common pulmonary fungal infection. *Aspergillosis* also seems to be the most common pulmonary fungal infection in the authors' experience of East and Central African setting (Fig. 11).

5. Inevitably, where laboratory and diagnostic services are limited, nonspecific pneumonitis is a common diagnosis (range: 19.4–38%).

VII. Kaposi's Sarcoma

Kaposi's sarcoma has been reported to occur fairly commonly in older patients in Central Africa, and the endemic variety, which is not HIV related, is a slowly progressive tumor that presents with chronic lymphoedema of the limbs in association with cutaneous and subcutaneous plaques and nodules (14). In patients with AIDS, the tumor is more aggressive, often multicentric, and progresses more rapidly than the endemic variety; bronchopulmonary lesions are common. The incidence of Kaposi's sarcoma in HIV-positive individuals who present with pulmonary disease is in the range of 6–16% (18). The radiographic features of Kaposi's sarcoma are essentially indistinguishable from opportunistic infections and include

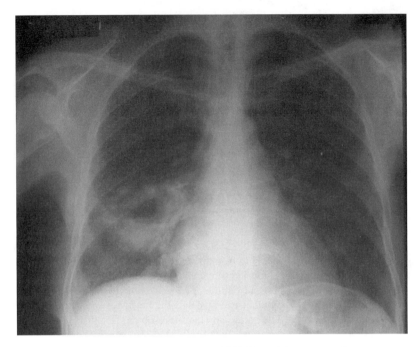

Figure 9 Chest radiograph in a 30-year-old HIV-positive patient demonstrates an abscess cavity containing fluid level in the mid lobe of the right lung. Note smooth wall and absence of adjacent air space consolidation. No ipsilateral adenopathy is evident. Sputum smear and culture were positive for *Klebsiella* pneumonia.

alveolar, interstitial, mixed alveolar-interstitial, and nodular patterns, with the nodular pattern being the most common. Clinical and bronchoscopic findings are central to the diagnosis (Figs. 12 and 13).

VIII. Amebiasis

Amebiasis is the third leading parasitic cause of death in the world. The disease is endemic in Mexico, the western part of South America, South Africa, Egypt, India, and Southeast Asia. Approximately 500 million people are infected with *Entamoeba histolytica*.

Amebic colitis and liver abscess are the most common intestinal and extraintestinal manifestations of *E. histolytica* infection. Pleuropulmonary complications occur almost exclusively in individuals with a liver abscess, with a reported incidence of between 4% and 14%. Thoracic disease may involve the pleura, lung parenchyma, or pericardium (22). Rupture of an amebic liver abscess into the pleural cavity leads to an amebic empyema, and subsequent rupture into the lung may produce an abscess or an area

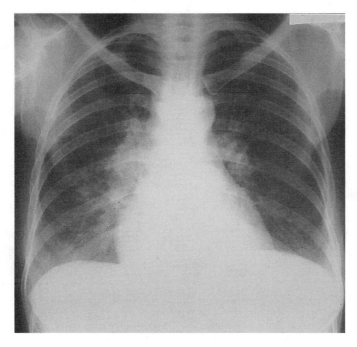

Figure 10 Chest radiograph of a 26-year-old patient with AIDS with proven cryptococcal infection depicts extensive right hilar and mediastinal adenopathy and presence of parahilar air space consolidation. The CD_4 level was 41 cells/mm^3.

of consolidation. Other pleuropulmonary complications include right-sided sympathetic effusions and basilar atelectasis. Bronchohepatic fistula is an unusual and distinctive problem characterized by expectoration of sputum that may resemble anchovy paste. Left hepatic abscesses occasionally produce left-sided pleuropulmonary complications and may result in lethal ruptures into the pericardium.

Amebic invasion of the thorax has also been reported to occur by way of the lymphatics from beneath the diaphragm. The occasional lung abscesses that occur with or without associated demonstrable amebic liver abscess have been attributed to embolization from a diseased liver or colon via the portal system or hepatic veins, the valveless paravertebral veins, the inferior vena cava, and through the thoracic duct and subclavian vein.

The radiographic features of pleuropulmonary amebiasis are not specific for the disease, but in conjunction with the history, a physical examination may suggest the diagnosis (Fig. 14). Elevation of the right hemidiaphragm is a frequent finding, occurring in about 50% of patients with amebic liver abscess. Other features include areas of consolidation adjacent to the diaphragm, which may contain a cavity; occasionally a pulmonary

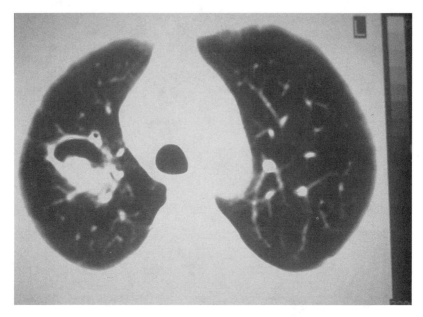

Figure 11 Aspergillosis infection in a 22-year-old patient with AIDS. CT scan through the lungs reveals a right upper lobe irregular thick-walled cavity with a crescent of air and internal soft tissue mass. The CD_4 level was 31 cells/mm^3.

abscess may be seen distant from the liver and indicates hematogenous dissemination (22). Pleural effusions seen on chest radiograph may be massive (29%) or small and produce only blunting of the right costophrenic angle (20%). Ultrasound of the pleural space (and image-guided aspiration) provides a cheap and reliable means of making the diagnosis (Fig. 15).

IX. Hydatid Disease

Hydatid disease is a worldwide zoonosis produced by the larval stage of the *Echinococcus* tapeworm. Humans may become intermediate hosts through contact with a definitive host (usually a domesticated dog) or ingestion of contaminated water or vegetables. In humans, the liver is involved in ~75% of cases, the lung in 15%, and other anatomic locations in 10% (23).

Most cysts in the lung are acquired in childhood, remain asymptomatic for many years, and are discovered incidentally on "routine" chest radiographs. The typical hydatid cyst on chest radiographs is a well-defined homogenous nodule more than 3 cm in diameter, although they may vary from 1 to 20 cm (Fig. 16). Centrally located cysts are usually round, although more peripheral cysts may be oval or polycyclic (24). Cysts are

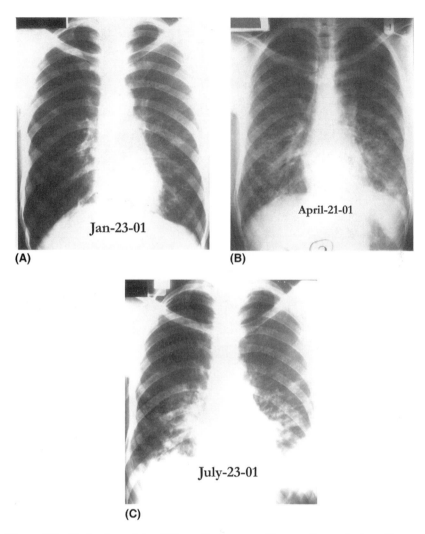

Figure 12 Endemic variety of Kaposi's sarcoma. Chest radiographs in a 25-year-old patient with grade IV-B Kaposi's sarcoma depict progression of shadows from **(A)** increased bronchovascular shadows to **(B)** reticulolinear, and finally **(C)** a faint nodular pattern predominantly in both lung bases. *Source*: Courtesy of Prof. M. Kawooya, Makerere University, Kampala, Uganda, and E. Katongole Mbidde, MD, Uganda Cancer Institute, Kampala, Uganda.

multiple in 30% of cases, bilateral in 20%, and located in the lower lobes in 60%. Calcification in pulmonary cysts is extremely rare (0.7% of cases) (25), although it may be a feature of pericardial, pleural, and mediastinal cysts (26,27).

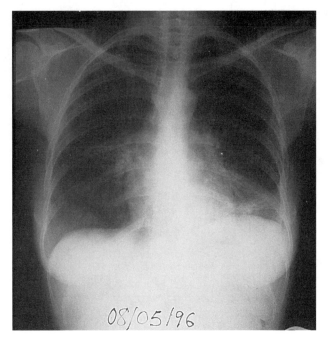

Figure 13 Kaposi's sarcoma pulmonary involvement. Chest radiograph depicts interstitial infiltrates consistent with interlobular septal thickening in a 28-year-old patient with AIDS with mucocutaneous Kaposi's sarcoma. This nodular thickening radiates from both hila towards the lower lobes. Airspace consolidation and segmental atelectasis in the left lower lobe are evident.

A closed cyst is indistinguishable from other large nodular lesions within the lung on chest radiograph (28). When cyst growth produces erosions in the bronchioles, air may be introduced between the pericyst and the ectocyst (laminated membrane). This manifests as a thin radiolucency in the upper part of the cyst and is known as the crescent sign or meniscus sign (23–25). This sign, however, is not specific for hydatid disease and is seen in cavities containing a fungus ball or tumor. If more air enters this space, the parasitic membranes (endocyst) collapse further, and an air–fluid level is seen. When it has completely collapsed, the crumpled endocyst floats freely in the cyst fluid, which is the water lily sign (24,25). von Sinner et al. (26) have outlined several newer radiological signs of hydatid disease on ultrasound, CT, and Magnetic Resonance Imaging (MRI), which are summarized in Table 2. In some cases, in which the signs such as the "serpent" and "spin" signs are characteristic, a confirmed diagnosis of *Echinococcus* may be possible.

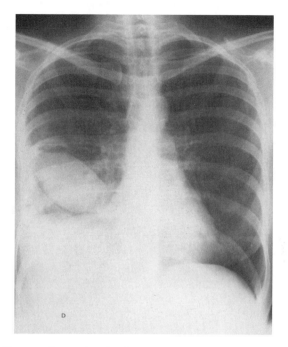

Figure 14 Chest radiograph of a 35-year-old patient demonstrates an amebic empyema tracking in the right oblique fissure. There is elevation of the right dome diaphragm. This particular patient had an amebic abscess of the liver that ruptured through into the pleural cavity.

X. Pulmonary Strongyloides

Strongyloides stercoralis is a small nematode endemic in tropical and subtropical regions. The ova of the female nematode hatch into rhabditi-form (nonmigratory) larvae that are capable of maturing into noninfectious adults or molting into filariform (infective) larvae. Initial invasion occurs when the patient's skin is exposed to contaminated soil or feces. The filari-form larvae penetrate the dermis and migrate through the venous system to the lungs, ascend the trachea, are swallowed into the digestive tract, and infect the small intestine mucosa. Most larvae penetrate the glandular epithelium into the intestinal lumen and are excreted as feces. Some larvae, however, re-enter the blood stream and migrate through the lungs without a soil cycle. This ability for autoinfection means that infestation can be lifelong and extremely heavy; massive autoinfection leads to disseminated strongyloidiasis, the hyperinfection syndrome, which results in severe pulmonary disease (29,30).

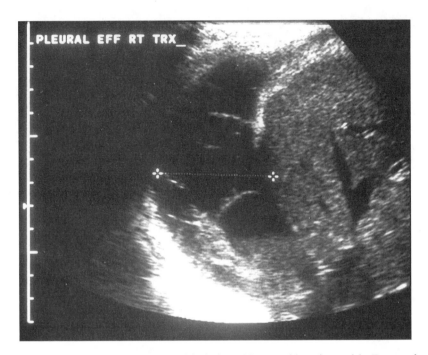

Figure 15 Pleuropulmonary amebiasis in a 27-year-old patient with *Entamoeba histolytica* intestinal manifestation. Subcostal abdominal ultrasound demonstrates a large loculated pleural effusion with internal echoic debris. No associated demonstrable amebic liver abscess was evident. Ultrasound-guided aspiration reveals characteristic chocolate-brown pus.

The primary migratory phase of the parasite through the lung results in the larvae piercing the pulmonary capillaries and entering the alveolar ducts. During this transit from the vascular bed to the respiratory tree, variable degrees of hemorrhage and edema result along with desquamation of epithelial cells and the migration of macrophages and inflammatory cells towards the parasites producing ill-defined, patchy homogenous consolidation or, less frequently, fine miliary nodulation on chest radiographs. In patients with pre-existing chronic lung disease, the progress of the filariform larvae's primary migration through the lungs is retarded by excessive bronchial secretions or inflammation, which causes a moderate to severe pulmonary strongyloidiasis. This infection may produce segmental or even lobar opacities. Pulmonary opacities can be chronic, and serial radiographs may show migration of the opacities through the lungs.

The pulmonary manifestations of the hyperinfection syndrome include severe bronchospasm, extensive pneumonia, pulmonary hemorrhage, and the development of the adult respiratory distress syndrome.

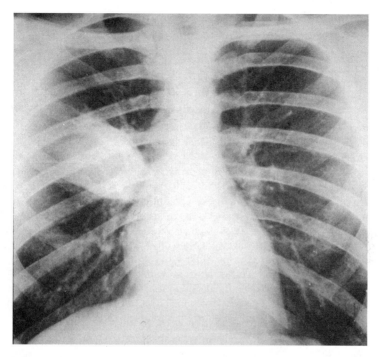

Figure 16 Pulmonary hydatid disease. Chest radiograph in a 40-year-old patient demonstrates a well-demarcated homogenous mass consistent with an unruptured hydatid cyst in the right upper lobe. *Source*: Courtesy of the Department of Radiology, McMaster University, Hamilton, Ontario, Canada.

Pleural effusions are seen (40%) (29) more frequently in patients with heavy *Strongyloides* infection. Secondary infections from bacteria or fungi are common and are significantly associated with the development of shock lung. Pulmonary cavitation and abscess formation may occur, and these suggest superimposed bacterial infection.

XI. Paragonimiasis

Paragonimiasis is an infestation caused by the trematode parasite *Paragonimus*. The lungs are primarily affected, although central nervous system involvement does occur (31). The radiographic features are not specific and are easily confused with those of pulmonary TB. There is a high rate of a normal chest radiograph in confirmed cases of paragonimiasis: 12.8% from a study in India (32) and 20% from a Nigerian study (31). The most common radiographic feature is multiple areas of patchy shadowing of low density with indistinct margins. There is no lobar or segmental

Table 2 Summary of the Radiological Signs of Hydatid Disease Seen on Ultrasound, CT or MRI

Radiological sign	Diagnostic characteristics
Rim sign	The presence of a low-signal intensity rim separating the parasitic cyst from the patient's tissue assumed to represent the pericyst. More conspicuous if it is contiguous to the thoracic wall and less so if it is bordering lung parenchyma
Serpent sign	The "snake" appearance on ultrasound, CT, and MRI that results from collapse of parasitic membranes
Spin or whirl sign	Collapsed parasitic membranes on MRI may have a twirled and twisted appearance
Cyst wall sign	Cyst wall can be visualized on ultrasound, CT, and MRI
Ring enhancement sign	Ring enhancement of the pericyst following contrast, which occurs mainly in infected cysts due to hypervascularization of the pericyst. On CT and MRI, the ring enhancement is similar to that of an abscess.
Halo sign	A dense halo sign may be seen surrounding pulmonary hydatid cysts in CT and MRI. It is caused by allergic or inflammatory infiltrates or atelectatic lung.

Source: From von Sinner WN, Rifai A, Te Strake L, Siek J. Magnetic resonance imaging of thoracic hydatid disease. Acta Radiol 1990; 31:59–62.

preponderance, but the midzones are commonly affected with shadowing that extends from the perihilar regions to the periphery. Occasionally, cystic areas develop eccentrically within the areas of opacity; these have smooth outlines and have been likened to "bubbles" that develop within the shadow (31). Linear streaky shadows are seen less often (2.6%) (32). Other features include pleural reaction or thickening (28%), with pleural effusion seen in 10%. Although none of the radiographic features are pathognomonic, a combination of the above appearances should alert the radiologist to the diagnosis in a patient from an endemic area who presents with typical blood-stained, rusty, or chocolate-colored sputum (Fig. 17).

XII. Melioidosis

Melioidosis is endemic in Southeast Asia. The organism is a gram-negative bacillus, *Pseudomonas pseudomallei*, that infects humans via contaminated soil or dust that enters the respiratory or alimentary tract or enters through a skin wound (33). The bacteria may remain quiescent in an infected person for long periods and then become reactivated causing clinical symptoms (34,35). Clinically, melioidosis may manifest in four different ways (33).

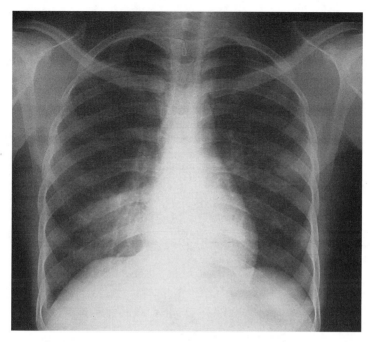

Figure 17 Paragonimiasis. Chest radiograph in this 35-year-old patient from the Congo who presented with cough and brown sputum demonstrates bilateral infiltrates with subtle foci of lucency, which suggest cavitation. Sputum was negative for AFB but positive for paragonimiasis. Complete regression of both lesions was evident on follow-up after therapy with praziquantel.

- Patients with the acute form present with fever and chills, and without antibiotics there is usually rapid progression to overwhelming septicemia. A diffuse pneumonitis develops accompanied by multiple liver, spleen, and subcutaneous abscesses. Acute respiratory distress syndrome is a common sequela. The most common radiographic appearance in the acute form is the presence of multiple, small irregular densities that range in size from 4 to 10 mm, which can simulate disseminated tuberculosis. These nodules may coalesce, which results in segmental or lobar consolidation. Pleural effusion or empyema is seen, but hilar adenopathy is rare.
- The subacute form begins with a prodromal period, which eventually presents with chest pain, low-grade fever, and weight loss. Chest radiograph (Fig. 18) normally reveals a lobar infiltrate, usually within the upper lobe, and often shows cavitation.
- In subclinical melioidosis, the patient is asymptomatic, although serologic test results are positive. Most infected persons fall into this category (36). The radiographic appearances mimic those of

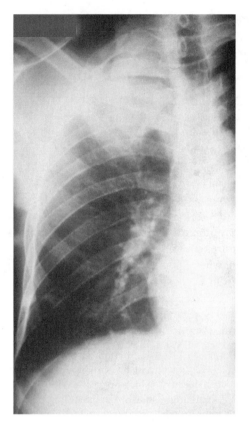

Figure 18 Pulmonary melioidosis. Chest radiograph in a 36-year-old non-autochthonous patient with chronic cough demonstrates a right upper lobe air space consolidation. The pulmonary lesions resemble those of TB reactivation. Sputum for AFB and TB cultures tested negative. This particular patient from Southeast Asia was seen with the disease during his visit in the Congo on business. *Pseudomonas pseudomallei* were obtained from culture and sputum. *Source*: Courtesy of Pierre-Anatole Matusila, MD, Kinshasa, Congo.

   TB with an upper lobe infiltrate and cavity formation. These
   patients are at risk of developing an acute exacerbation.
 • Chronic melioidosis is usually extrapulmonary, in which skin
   lesions or osteomyelitis represent the primary site of infection.

   The most important factor involved in establishing the diagnosis of
melioidosis is a high index of suspicion, and the diagnosis should be enter-
tained in patients with a febrile illness and a localized suppurative process
in an endemic area (37).

XIII. Severe Acute Respiratory Syndrome (SARS)

A new tropical disease has recently emerged near the beginning of the 21st century. Severe acute respiratory syndrome (SARS), identified as a coronavirus, originated from southern China and infected over 8000 people from 29 different countries, including tropical areas in South East Asia, and claimed 774 lives between November 1, 2002 to July 31, 2003 (38). Patients present with symptoms consisting of cough, fever, chills, myalgia, shortness of breath, and diarrhea. SARS is spread by droplet infection, however, the virus has also been isolated in the stool and urine (39). Radiology plays an important role in the diagnosis, monitoring of treatment response, and the follow-up of patients during the convalescent period (39).

Early in the disease, the chest radiograph may show only a peripheral opacity, which may range from ground-glass to consolidation in appearance. A particular area to examine is the paraspinal region behind the heart, which is frequently where lung lesions are detected on high-resolution computed tomography in suspected SARS patients with normal radiographs (40). In the more advanced cases, there is widespread opacification, which may be ground-glass or consolidative affecting large areas with the presence of air-bronchograms (Fig. 19). The lower zones tend to be affected first and

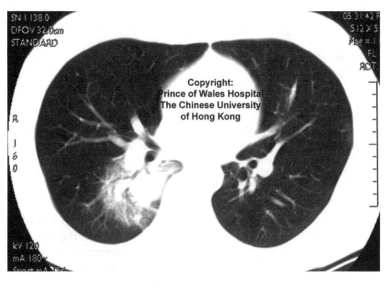

Figure 19   SARS. HRCT thorax performed on day 3 after onset of symptoms. Ill-defined consolidation with air-bronchogram in apical segment of right lower lobe. *Source*: Courtesy of Dr. Gregory Antonio, Dr. Anil Ahuja, and Dr. Grace Mak, the Department of Diagnostic Radiology and Organ Imaging, Chinese University of Hong Kong.

are not uncommonly bilateral. Parenchymal scarring may develop during the recovery period (39). Calcification, cavitation, pleural effusion, or lymphadenopathy are not features of this disease (40).

XIV. Conclusion

A high-quality chest radiograph and a timely, accurate report are often impossible in the tropics. Rational matching of service to need, enthusiasm, commitment, and exploitation of information technology all go some way toward enabling patients with pulmonary disease to be imaged. The radiological findings will reflect the high preponderance of infectious disease. TB, HIV, and TB modified by HIV may be "routine" features in some parts of the tropics. Elsewhere, infestation with ameba, hydatid, strongyloides, paragonimiasis, and melioidosis accounts for radiographic signs. SARS is a reminder that tropical diseases are not necessarily exclusive to the tropics. The key is to have these conditions firmly in mind when reading tropical radiographs and be aware that the pattern of disease may be different between the patient from the tropics and the more familiar patient from downtown New York.

References

1. Richenberg JL, Tshibwabwa ET. Radiology and imaging services in the tropics. In: Cook GC, Zumla A, eds. Manson's Tropical Diseases. 21st ed. London: WB Saunders, 2003:509–513.
2. Mindel S. Role of imager in a developing world. Lancet 1997; I:426–429.
3. Schandorf C, Ketteh GK. Analysis of the status of X-ray diagnosis in Ghana. Br J Radiol 1998; 71:1040–1048.
4. Tshibwabwa ET, Mwaba P, Bogle-Taylor J, Zumla A. Four-year study of abdominal ultrasound in 900 Central African adults with AIDS referred for diagnostic imaging. Abdom Imaging 2000; 25:290–296.
5. Kurjak K, Kos M. Ultrasound screening for fetal anomalies in developing countries: wish or reality? Ann NY Acad Sci 1998; 847:233–237.
6. Bovornkitti S. Tropical pulmonary diseases. Respirology 1996; 1:11–21.
7. Pallangyo KJ. Clinical features of tuberculosis among adults in sub-Saharan Africa in the 21st century. Scand J Infect Dis 2001; 33:488–493.
8. Aderele WI. Radiological patterns of pulmonary tuberculosis in Nigerian children. Tubercle Lung Dis 1980; 61:157–163.
9. Freiman I, Geefhuysen J, Solomon A. The radiological presentation of pulmonary tuberculosis in children. S Afr Med J 1975; 49:1703–1707.
10. Mbala L, Mashako M, Kashongwe M. Childhood tuberculosis in a rural tropical area: risk factors. Trop Doct 2002; 32:119–120.
11. Leung AN, Muller NL, Pineda PR, Fitzgerald JM. Primary tuberculosis in children: radiographic manifestations. Radiology 1992; 182:87–91.

12. Awil PO, Bowlin SJ, Daniel TM. Radiology of pulmonary tuberculosis and human immunodeficiency virus infection in Gulu, Uganda. Eur Respir J 1997; 10:615–618.

13. Batungwanayo J, Taelman H, Dhote R, Bogaerts J, Allen S, van de Perre P. Pulmonary tuberculosis in Kigali, Rwanda: impact of human immunodeficiency virus infection on clinical and radiographic presentation. Ann Rev Respir Dis 1992; 146:53–56.

14. Pozniak AL, Latif AS, Neill P, Houston S, Chen K, Robertson V. Pulmonary Kaposi's sarcoma in Africa. Thorax 1992; 47:770–773.

15. Saks AM, Posner R. Tuberculosis in HIV positive patients in South Africa: a comparative radiological study with HIV negative patients. Clin Radiol 1992; 46:387–390.

16. Tshibwabwa ET, Mwinga A, Pobee JOM, Zumla A. Radiological features of pulmonary tuberculosis in 963 HIV-infected adults at three Central African hospitals. Clin Radiol 1997; 52:837–841.

17. O'Keefe EA, Wood R. AIDS in Africa. Scand J Gastroenterol 1996; 31: 147–152.

18. Tshibwabwa E. Pulmonary radiological features of AIDS in the tropics. In: Zumla A, Johnson M, Miller M, eds. AIDS and Respiratory Medicine. 1st ed. London: Chapman & Hall Medical, 1997:59–69.

19. Abouya YL, Beaumel A, Lucas J, Dago-Akribi A, Coulibaly G, N'Datz M, Konan JB, Vapi A, De Cock Km. *Pneumocystis carinii* pneumonia: an uncommon cause of death in African patients with acquired immunodeficiency syndrome. Am Rev Respir Dis 1992; 145:617–620.

20. Malin AS, Gwanzura LKZ, Klein S, Robertson VJ, Musvaire P, Mason PR. *Pneumocystis carinii* pneumonia in Zimbabwe. Lancet 1995; 346:1258–1261.

21. Mahomed AG, Murray J, Klepman S, Richards G, Feldman C, Levy NT, Smith C, Kallenbach J. *Pneumocystis carinii* pneumonia in HIV infected patients from South Africa. East Afr Med J 1999; 76:80–84.

22. Whittaker LR. Pulmonary amoebic disease. In: Cockshott P, Middlemiss H, eds. Clinical Radiology in the Tropics. 1st ed. Edinburgh, London and New York, 1979:167–168.

23. Beggs I. The radiology of hydatid disease. Am J Roentgenol 1995; 145: 639–648.

24. Balikian JB, Mudarris FF. Hydatid disease of the lungs: a roentgenologic study of 50 cases. Am J Roentgenol 1974; 122:692–707.

25. Jerray M, Benzarti M, Garrouche A, Klabi N, Hayouni A. Hydatid disease of the lungs: study of 386 cases. Am Rev Respir Dis 1992; 146:185–189.

26. von Sinner WN, Rifai A, Te Strake L, Siek J. Magnetic resonance imaging of thoracic hydatid disease. Acta Radiol 1990; 31:59–62.

27. von Sinner WN. New diagnostic signs in hydatid disease: radiography, ultrasound, CT and MRI correlated to pathology. Eur J Radiol 1991; 12:150–159.

28. Lewall DB, McCorkell SJ. Rupture of echinococcal cysts: diagnosis, classification, and clinical implications. Am J Roentgenol 1996; 146:391–394.

29. Woodring JH, Halfhill H, Reed JC. Pulmonary strongyloidiasis: clinical and imaging features. Am J Roentgenol 1994; 162:537–542.

30. Woodring JH, Halfhill H, Berger R, Reed JC, Moser N. Clinical and imaging features of pulmonary strongyloidiasis. South Med J 1996; 89:10–19.
31. Ogakwu M, Nwokolo C. Radiological findings in pulmonary paragonimiasis as seen in Nigeria: a review based on one hundred cases. Br J Radiol 1973; 46:699–705.
32. Singh TS, Muttum SS, Razaque MA. Pulmonary paragonimiasis: clinical features, diagnosis and treatment of 39 cases in Manipur. Trans Roy Soc Trop Med Hyg 1986; 80:967–971.
33. Reeder MM, Palmer PE. Acute tropical pneumonias. Semin Roentgenol 1980; 15:35–49.
34. Sharma OP, Maheshwari A. Lung diseases in the tropics. Part 1: tropical granulomatous disorders of the lung: diagnosis and management. Tubercle Lung Dis 1993; 74:295–304.
35. Sharma OP, Maheshwari A. Lung diseases in the tropics. Part 2: common tropical lung diseases: diagnosis and management. Tubercle Lung Dis 1993; 74:359–370.
36. Leelarasamee A, Bovornkitti S. Melioidosis: review and update. Rev Infect Dis 1989; 11:413–423.
37. Koponen MA, Zlock D, Palmer DL, Merlin TL. Melioidosis: forgotten, but not gone. Arch Intern Med 1991; 151:605–608.
38. WHO Communicable Disease Surveillance and Response. Cumulative number of reported probable cases of severe acute respiratory syndrome (SARS) from Nov 1, 2002 to July 31, 2003. Published online at http://www.who.int/csr/sars/country/table2003 09 23/en/ on September 26, 2003.
39. Goh JS, Tsou IY, Kaw GJ. Severe acute respiratory syndrome (SARS): imaging findings during the acute and recovery phases of disease. J Thorac Imaging 2003; 18:195–199.
40. Wong KT, Antonio GE, Hui DSC, Lee N, Yuen EHY, Wu A, Leung CB, Rainer TH, Cameron P, Chung SSC, Sung JJY, Ahuja AT. Radiological appearances of severe acute respiratory syndrome. J Hong Kong Coll Radiol 2003; 6:4–6.

4

Recent Advances in the Immunology of the Respiratory Tract

CHAIM OSCAR JACOB

Department of Medicine, Keck School of Medicine, University of Southern California, Los Angeles, California, U.S.A.

The lung and airways are mucosal surfaces that are common sites for infections (1). Although respiratory tract infections are a major cause of morbidity and mortality worldwide (2), the tropics have certain unique characteristics that have specific influence on the practice of pulmonary medicine in these regions (3,4). First, the high-temperature and high-humidity climate and the general state of socio-economic underdevelopment in many of the countries within the tropics provide an ideal environment for the thriving of pathogenic microorganisms, their vectors, and intermediate hosts. Second, the cultural and educational background of many of the people living in the tropics exposes them to pathogens and when infected, they readily become reservoirs for or carriers of these infectious organisms (3). Also, people affected with tropical infections often already have a general immunoincompetence (often caused by malnutrition or other diseases) that reduces the effectiveness of their response to otherwise mild infections. Especially, the human immunodeficiency virus (HIV) pandemic is causing a large spectrum of opportunistic infections with devastating effects particularly in these regions of the world (4). Furthermore, many of the particular tropical parasitic infections induce inadequate immunity and as a matter of fact the scientific community has invested much less time and effort toward the understanding and controlling of these diseases. Ultimately, the adverse socio-economic conditions of the underdeveloped countries impede attempts to eradicate or control these tropical diseases.

In the following, my plan is to provide the reader with an overview of recent developments in research on immunity of the lung and the respiratory tract. Detailed knowledge of the immune mechanisms and pathways will improve the understanding of respiratory physiology and pathology and potentially lead to novel diagnostics and therapies. I hope that the advances in the immunology of the respiratory tract will be realized promptly and implemented toward the control of tropical pulmonary diseases.

I. The Mucosal Immune System

In contrast to the systemic immune system, the mucosal surfaces of the respiratory system, digestive system, and the urinogenital tract are constantly and directly exposed to the external environment, resulting in their encounter with a vast quantity of antigenic, mitogenic, and toxic stimuli. The respiratory pathway is especially prone to exposure to microorganisms and other potential allergenic substances due to the exchange of oxygen and carbon dioxide that requires the constant ventilation of a large volume of external air that may contain pathogens. Furthermore, the digestive tract shares the pharynx with the airways, opening another possibility for the uptake of microorganisms and food antigens into the respiratory tract. The estimated antigenic load presented to the mucosal immune system in a single day is far greater than the total antigenic exposure of the systemic immune system in the lifetime of the organism (5).

As far as it is understood to date, the mucosal immune system has several basic functions: (1) barrier against penetration of microorganisms and immunogenic components into the circulation and thus into the inner environment of the organism; (2) suppressing immune responses, a function dubbed "oral or mucosal tolerance"; (3) immunoregulatory function through maintenance of what may be called "mucosal homeostasis"; and (4) promoting immune responses against harmful pathogens.

It should be emphasized that the mucosal immune system is different from its systemic counterpart in that suppressing immunity rather than promoting immune response might be viewed as a more prominent function (6). Other characteristic features of mucosal immunity include an extensive innate defense system, capability to generate antimicrobial molecules, unique ways of antigen presentation, and the existence of lymphocyte populations, which differ from blood lymphocytes either in their origin, phenotype, repertoire, or cytokine secretion profile (5,6).

The respiratory tract uses mechanical, chemical, and cellular strategies to protect the host against the potential constituents of its mucosal surface. Usually, pathogens are cleared from the respiratory tract without inflammation or disturbance of the local function or structure. In case the first-line host-defense system fails to clear the microorganism, secondary inflammatory reactions are activated. Cystic fibrosis, associated with overwhelming respiratory infections, represents a classical example of the serious consequences of impaired host defense. Paradoxically, excess and/or uncontrolled host defenses and inflammatory responses contribute to pulmonary pathology such as in asthma or COPD.

The mucosal surfaces are covered mostly with single-layered epithelium, which functions as a physical and functional barrier. The mucosal surface of the respiratory system [estimated as $80 \, m^2$ in humans (5)] changes along the airways. The proximal part of respiratory tract mucosal surface in the nostrils and oropharynx is lined by stratified squamous epithelium. From the nasal turbinates and upper trachea down to the respiratory bronchioles the lining is a pseudostratified ciliated epithelium interspersed with goblet cells capable of producing mucous. The walls of the larger airways contain glands composed of two secretory cell types: the serous and the mucous cells. The epithelial layer becomes less stratified and thinner in the distal parts of the airways. The epithelium of the distal airways, the bronchioles, consists mainly of ciliated and Clara cells. The terminal air sacs and the alveoli are lined by a single layer of flattened epithelial cells (pneumocytes of type I and II). In addition to cells lining the airways and alveoli, other cells of the immune system contribute to host defense, including alveolar macrophage, neutrophil, eosinophil, dendritic cell (DC), mast cell, natural killer cell, and lymphocytes (7).

For didactic purposes, it is practical to subdivide the mucosal immune system into inductive sites in which antigen uptake and processing takes place and effector sites at which engagement of lymphocytes, granulocytes, and mast cells occur (7). The main points of entry of luminal antigen into the mucosal-associated lymphoreticular tissue (MALT) are its inductive sites, the Peyer's patches in the gut-associated lymphoreticular tissue (GALT), the nasal-associated lymphoreticular tissue (NALT), and the tonsils in the upper respiratory tract.

MALT consists of an organized tissue represented by lymphoid follicles and of lymphocytes dispersed throughout the epithelium or lymphocytes dispersed under the epithelium within the lamina propria. The organized lymphoid tissue is covered by an epithelial layer, which differs from the epithelium covering other parts of the mucosa by containing unique membranous epithelial cells called M cells. These M cells have on their basolateral surface a specialized site equipped with adhesive molecules through which it interacts with intraepithelial lymphocytes. The M cells are capable of absorbing particular antigens and transferring them from the lumen into the follicles very efficiently. The importance of lymphocyte–epithelial cell interaction for maintenance of M cell function is exemplified by the demonstration that interaction of epithelial cells with T and B lymphocytes induces epithelial cells to differentiate into M cells (8). The lymphoid tissue in the NALT and the tonsils share structural features with the Payer's patches such as M cells and are composed of loose networks in which lymphocytes, DCs, and macrophages are embedded. Organized lymphoid tissue in the form of lymphoid follicles is found in the bronchus-associated lymphoid tissue (BALT) only in infants; in adults it is found only under pathological conditions. The immune system of the upper airways differs from the BALT also in the predominance of IgA in the upper airway's secretion, while in the alveoli IgG predominate.

Following induction in the MALT, mature lymphocytes leave the inductive sites and migrate to the effectors sites such as the lamina propria and the lung. Two types of immunological outcomes are generated by the MALT (9). One result is the development of B cells capable of producing immunoglobulins (Ig) that can reach the draining lymph nodes and other mucosal tissues where they differentiate to specific Ig producing plasma cells. A second outcome is the activation and differentiation of T-cells into subtypes capable of producing different cytokines and undertaking various physiological functions. T-cell activation and differentiation requires at least two separate signals. The first signal is produced via the T-cell receptor/CD3 complex after its interaction with the major histocompatibility complex (MHC) class I or class II molecules and antigen on the surface of an APC. The second signal is created by costimulatory or accessory molecules found on the surface of the APC that interact with their specific ligands on T-cells. The interactions of CD28 with B7-1 or B7-2, OX40 with OX40L, ICOS with B7H are examples of such second signals (9).

The basic defense mechanism of mucosal surfaces is the innate (nonspecific) immunity involving processes that protect the host immediately after exposure to microorganisms. By contrast, adaptive immunity, which is believed to be the more central part of the systemic immune system, has a much slower onset (days, weeks) and the nature of the response tends to be more antigen-specific and clonal. Recently, it became evident that the innate immune system also plays a direct role in the activation and orientation of the subsequent adaptive immune response.

II. TLRs

At the forefront of the innate immune system, a set of cell-surface receptors called pattern recognition receptors (PRRs) have been characterized (10–12). These receptors are capable of recognizing conserved pathogen-associated molecular patterns (PAMPs) common to entire classes of microorganisms such as lipopolysacharides (LPS), CpG containing bacterial or viral DNA and peptidoglycans (Table 1). The PAMPs are essential for microbial survival and therefore are evolutionarily conserved, which makes them good targets for innate immune recognition. Following the demonstration in the fruit fly *Drosophila melanogaster* that Toll receptors carry important immune functions, 10 to 11 homologues, the Toll-like receptors (TLRs), were found in human and mouse, respectively (12,13). Human TLR10 does not have an ortholog in the mouse genome, whereas mouse TLR11 and TLR12 are absent from the human genome. Mammalian TLRs have been shown to play a critical role in cellular activation by a variety of microbial molecules (reviewed in Ref. 14) such as LPS (TLR4), peptidoglycan (TLR2), flagellin (TLR5), dsRNA (TLR3), and unmethylated CpG DNA motifs (TLR9) (Table 1). The importance of TLRs to host defense in humans is exemplified by the identification of polymorphisms in the genes encoding human TLR4 and TLR2. These mutations result in hypoactive or inactive receptors and are associated with increased sensitivity to different infectious agents (15–18). Toll-like receptors are type I transmembrane proteins characterized by an extracellular domain composed of amino-terminal leucine-rich repeats (LRRs) flanked by characteristic cysteine clusters on the C-terminal (CF motif) side of LRRs (in mammals), and a 150-amino-acid intracytoplasmic domain-designated TIR, which they share with members of the interleukin-1 receptor (IL-1R) family and plant disease resistance (R) genes. The TIR (Toll/IL-1R/R) domains have been found

Table 1 Activation of TLRs by Microorganismal PAMPs

PAMP	Pathogen	PRR
Triacylated lipoprotein	Most bacteria	TLR1/TLR2
Diacylated lipoprotein	Bacteria, mycoplasma	TLR2/TLR6
Peptidoglycan	Most bacteria	TLR2/TLR6
Double-standed RNA	Viruses	TLR3
LPS	Most gram negative bacteria	TLR4/CD14
Flagellin	Flagellated bacteria	TLR5
Low molecular imidazoqui-noline compounds		TLR7
Unmethylated double stranded DNA	Bacteria, some viruses (MCMV)	TLR9
Lipoarabinomannan	Mycobacteria	TLR2, MBL
Heat shock proteins	Most bacteria	TLR2/TLR4
Low calcium response protein (LorV)	Gram negative Yersinia bateria	TLR1/CD14
19 kDa lipoprotein	Mycobacterium tuberculosis	TLR2
Zymosan	Yeast cell wall product	TLR2

in many proteins involved in development and innate immunity in both animals and plants (14 and references therein).

TLRs are expressed in monocytes and dendritic cells (13), but also in a variety of other cells, including epithelial cells. For example, human trachiobronchial epithelial cells express TLR 1–6 with TLR2 being most abundantly expressed (19).

Some TLRs have been shown to form heterodimers, thus expanding their recognition spectrum. This is best exemplified by TLR2, which is activated by microbial molecules such as peptidoglycans. When TLR2 is associated with TLR1 to form a heterodimer, it can mediate response to triacylated bacterial lipopeptides such as Pam3CSK4 or OspA. On the other hand, when TLR2 is associated with TLR6, it can mediate recognition of diacylated mycobacterial lipopeptides such as MALP-2 (14). TLRs can also associate with non-TLR accessory molecules to mediate recognition and response to microbial molecular patterns. For example, TLR4 requires association with the 25 kDa molecule MD-2 to reach the plasma membrane and interact with LPS (20). Cell activation of TLR4 by LPS requires also the GPI-anchored coreceptor CD14 (14).

In addition to microbial molecules, TLRs have been reported to be activated by endogenous components such as heat-shock proteins (21), or extracellular matrix proteins like proteoglycans, hyaluronic acid, and fibronectin (22,23). Directly relevant to lung immunology, TLRs can be activated by β-defensins (24) and by surfactant protein-A (25). These results raise the intriguing possibility that not only by molecules derived from foreign microorganisms but also by those from the damaged self may activate TLRs. This may enable the innate immune system to distinguish between harmless commensal and infectious microorganisms that generate tissue damage.

The TLRs are signaling receptors, which upon stimulation activate transcription factors such as NF-κB and AP1, and mitogen-activated protein (MAP) kinases that lead to the production of cytokines, such as TNFα and IL-6, and upregulation of the costimulatory molecules CD80 and CD86 on DCs (26). Furthermore, TLR3 and TLR4 can activate the transcription factor IRF3 and induce production of the cytokine IFN-β (27,28).

More recent studies have shown that TLRs participate in the induction and/or direction of the adaptive immune response. Thus, in MyD88-deficient mice it was demonstrated (29) that TLRs are necessary for inducing T_H1 polarized responses, but not T_H2 responses. (MyD88 is a cytoplasmic protein that is recruited to the TLRs after stimulation and functions as an adaptor between receptors of the TLR family and downstream signaling kinases.) Likewise, MyD88-deficient mice develop a polarized, nonprotective T_H2 response when infected by the intracellular parasite *Leishmania major*, instead of the T_H1 response that results in protection of genetically resistant wild-type mice (29). On the other hand, Bottomly's group reported that LPS signaling through TLR4 is necessary to induce both T_H1 and T_H2 responses in a mouse model of allergic sensitization to inhaled antigen. Furthermore, the type of adaptive response induced depends on the dose of LPS used. Low doses of LPS trigger a T_H2 response in this model, whereas inhalation of high doses of LPS results in T_H1 responses (30). These results point to a possible role of TLRs in inflammatory diseases such as allergic asthma.

In addition to TLRs capability to control activation of T_H cells by upregulating costimulatory molecules on APCs, they are also involved in blocking T regulatory (T_R) cells. Pasare and Medzhitov (31) have demonstrated in a recent publication that microbial induction of the TLR pathway induces secretion of cytokines, especially IL-6 that blocks the suppressive effect of T_R cells allowing activation of pathogen-specific adaptive immune responses.

III. T_H1 vs. T_H2

$CD4^+$ helper T-cells (T_H) are classified as T_H0 cells, capable of producing a wide range of cytokines, and T_H1 or T_H2 polarized cells. T_H1 and T_H2 cells secrete a narrow nonoverlapping range of cytokines that tend to have mutually antagonistic biological activities. T_H1 cells secrete IL-2, IFNγ and TNFβ and can induce delayed-type hypersensitivity reactions. T_H2 polarized cells secrete IL-4, IL-5, IL-6, IL-10, and IL-13 but no IL-2 or IFNγ. Some of these cytokines play an important role in controlling T_H1 or T_H2 development. IL-12 and to a lesser degree IL-18 are responsible for the generation of Th1 subsets. It is believed that the role of IL-18 is indirect by upregulatin of IL-12 receptor β2 chain on T-cells and by the transcription factor AP-1–dependent transactivation of the IFNγ promoter (32,33). T_H2 differentiation is regulated primarily by IL-4 and to a lesser extent by IL-13. There are some evidences to suggest that in certain conditions IL-13 can force T_H2 development in an IL-4–independent fashion (34). The original in vivo source of these master cytokines has been a matter of debate (35). It seems that different types of DCs may be the source of the cytokines responsible for T_H1/T_H2 polarization. Splenic $CD8a^+$ DCs tend to elicit T_H1 responses, while $CD8a^-$ DCs favor T_H2 responses (35). Even though both subtypes of DCs can be found in the mucosal immune system, antigen-activated DCs from Peyer's patches preferentially induce T_H2 type rather than T_H1 immune responses (36,37). Similar bias toward induction of T_H2 responses has been shown for DCs from the respiratory tract (38,39). In humans, as in mice, monocyte-derived myeloid DCs have been shown to induce preferentially T_H1 responses whereas plasmacytoid DCs favor T_H2 responses (35). The signaling pathways in T lymphocytes differentiating toward a T_H1 or a T_H2 have been clarified to a great extent in the last several years [reviewed in Ref. (9)]. IL-12 induces T_H1 differentiation via activation of STAT4 and consecutive induction of IFNγ. Another master transcription factor for T_H1 cells is T-bet, which is activated following STAT1 induction by IFNγ (40). On the other hand, IL-4 induces T_H2 cytokine production in mucosal T-cells by activating STAT6 followed by the activation of the transcription factor GATA3 (41). GATA3 can exert also a STAT6-independent autoactivation, creating a feedback pathway that stabilizes the T_H2 commitment (42).

The discovery of T_H1 and T_H2 subtypes of T-cells in the 1980s provided a useful conceptual framework for understanding immunity to infectious diseases (43). It predicted that immunity to intracellular pathogens was preferentially mediated by T_H1 cells, which activate macrophages and promote B-cells to secrete complement-fixing and virus-neutralizing IgG_{2a} antibodies. Indeed, many pathogen molecules such as *Escherichia coli* LPS (44), CpG motifs in bacterial DNA (45), flagelin (46), and viral ds RNA (47) have been shown to bind TLRs and stimulate IL-12 production by innate immune cells such as DCs and direct the induction of T_H1 immune responses. On the other hand, the paradigm predicted that immunity to extracellular pathogens was mediated to a greater extent by T_H2 cells, which provide helper activity for antibody production, especially IgG_1, IgE, and IgA. Thus, pathogen-derived molecules such as yeast hyphae (48), helminth components (49), and cholera toxin (50) have been shown to activate DCs that drives the differentiation of naïve T-cells to the T_H2 phenotype.

However, the same effector mechanisms that can protect the host from microorganisms can also induce immune-mediated pathology if not properly regulated. Thus, proper regulation of these processes is an essential part of the immune response to pathogens. To limit collateral damage, the T_H1/T_H2 model incorporates mechanisms of reciprocal regulation by cytokines secreted by the other subtype or possibly through IL-10 secreted by T_H2 and some T_H1 cells, via a negative feedback loop. However, evidence is accumulating in the last several years to suggest that functionally distinct subpopulations of T_R cells are involved in the control of the T-helper subtypes. These new findings suggest that the T_H1/T_H2 paradigm needs to be re-evaluated and fine tuned for our understanding of T-cell responses during infection.

IV. T-Regulatory Cells

T-regulatory (T_R) cells are a small subset of $CD4^+$ T-cells, which express the CD25 marker, and suppress T-cell activation. T_R cells are involved in the control of a number of immune-related pathologies such as autoimmunity, graft rejection, and inflammatory bowel disease. The CD4 T_R subset is a heterogeneous population. Although a complete characterization of all the different $CD4^+$ T_R cell populations is still lacking, several subsets have been identified (51,52). Naturally occurring T_R cells (so called because they can be isolated from unmanipulated mice), constitute 5–10% of peripheral CD4 T lymphocytes present in healthy individuals. These cells are $CD4^+$ $CD25^+$ and express CTLA-4. They proliferate poorly upon TCR stimulation in vitro and their growth is dependent on IL-2. In addition to the naturally occurring T_R cells, several induced populations of T-lymphocytes such as anergic cells, T_R1 cells, and T_H3 cells that inhibit the activation of other T-cells have been described (51,52).

Anergic T-cells are defined as T-cells that do not proliferate or produce IL-2 upon antigen restimulation (53). Some anergic T cell clones are able to suppress T-cell responses both in vitro and in vivo by a mechanism involving modification of antigen-presenting cell (APC) function (54,55). T-cells that have been made anergic in vivo display high levels of IL-10 production (56). Another population of T-cells that exhibit regulatory activity is T_R1 cells. Repetitive stimulation of naïve $CD4^+$ cells in vitro, in the presence of exogenous IL-10, leads to the generation of T_R1 cells that produce high levels of IL-10 and are able to inhibit both T_H1 and T_H2 responses in vivo (57,58). Beside IL-10, interferon-α has been also shown to promote the generation and expansion of human T_R1 cells in vitro (59). Lastly, T_H3 cells are induced following oral administration of antigen and secrete predominantly TGFβ, a potent immune suppressive cytokine, and a switch factor for IgA production (51). T_H3 cells have been shown to inhibit autoimmune pathology in a number of animal models including EAE, diabetes, and colitis (60).

Towards the elucidation of T_R cell biology on the molecular level, the Foxp3 transcriptional factor was identified as a master regulator that promotes T_R cell differentiation (61). Using a retroviral transduction vector, Hori et al. (61) demonstrated that ectopic expression of *Foxp3* converted naïve $CD4^+CD25^-$ T-cells into cells with the phenotypic and functional characteristics of T_R cells. Most importantly, the Foxp3-transduced T-cells were able to inhibit autoimmune gastritis and inflammatory bowel disease in murine models in vivo. Furthermore, Foxp3-deficient mice have no $CD4^+CD25^+$ T_R cells (62) and develop a spectrum of autoimmune and inflammatory disorders similar to the phenotype observed in rodents lacking $CD4^+CD25^+$ T_R cells.

The failure of the host to clear certain pathogens and the development of chronic infections in the face of proper innate immune mechanisms, detectable T_H1, and antibody responses have been difficult to rationalize under contemporary views of the roles of the immune system. Persistence of infections, such as those caused by HIV and hepatitis C virus, have been explained either on the basis of an imbalance in the T_H1/T_H2 response or a failure to mount a protective immune response. However, suppression of the protective immune response by anti-inflammatory cytokines or cells induced directly or indirectly by the pathogen might provide a more plausible explanation for the chronic infections caused by certain parasites, bacteria, and viruses (63,64). Indeed, recent studies suggest that pathogen recognition by innate immune receptors may not be stimulatory. Thus, molecules derived from some bacterial pathogens can inhibit APC activation, resulting in suppression of immunity (62). Both IL-10 and nonactivated APCs may enhance the development of pathogen-specific T_R cells, which have been shown in a number of different types of infections (65–67). Studies on the immune response to *Bordatella pertussis* exemplify this notion: *B. pertussis* is a gram-negative bacterium that causes the respiratory disease, whooping cough, in children. Recovery from infection is associated with development of pathogen-specific T_H1 response in children and susceptible mice (68,69). Further evidence of the protective role of T_H1 cells in the process is suggested by the fact that adoptively transferred T_H1 cells from convalescent mice confer protection (69) and IFNγ-receptor knock out mice develop lethal disseminating infection (70). Athymic or SCID mice fail to clear the infection, but the bacteria do not disseminate from the lung (69), suggesting that innate responses may prevent bacterial dissemination before the development of adaptive immunity. However, induction of T_H1 and IgG responses are suppressed during the acute stage of infection (64). Indeed investigators from the Mills' group have shown that *B. pertussis* filamentous hemagglutinin (FHA) specific Tr1 clones are induced at the mucosal surface of the respiratory tract of infected mice (65). The Tr1 clones secreted high levels of IL-10, but not IL-4 or IFNγ, and suppressed T_H1 responses against *B. pertussis* or an unrelated pathogen (65). Furthermore, FHA inhibited IL-12 and stimulated IL-10 production by DCs, and these DCs directed naive T-cells into the regulatory subtype. In addition, TLR4 is involved in this pathogenic process by activating innate IL-10 production in response to *B pertussis*, which both directly and by promoting IL-10 producing T_R1 cells inhibit the T_H1 response (70). Thus, the TLR activation and the induction of T_R1 cells may represent an evasion strategy by the pathogen to subvert protective T_H1 responses.

V. IgA

IgA represents the most prominent antibody class at mucosal surfaces (71) and the second prevalent antibody class in human serum. In fact, more IgA is produced daily than all other isotypes combined (66 mg/kg/day) (71). This abundance warrants further study and, although scientific interest has increased over the years, the biological role of IgA is still not fully understood.

Presumably the isotype switching of B lymphocytes to IgA-producing cells occurs in mucosal inductive sites, while IgA production by plasma cells occurs in mucosal effector sites. Neither T_H1- nor T_H2-type cytokines contribute significantly to the switching of B cells to surface IgA-positive cells. This process requires TGF-β (5). Also cell–cell interaction at the mucosal inductive sites between local DC, T and B lymphocytes are important for the differentiation of B cells into IgA-producing cells. Thus, activated T-cells and DC from Peyer's patches are more effective in switching $sIgM^+sIgA^-$ producing cells than are T and DC cells derived from the spleen (5).

In human serum, IgA is predominantly monomeric and constitutes 15–20% of the total amount of Igs, whereas at mucosal sites IgA in the form of secretory IgA (SIgA) represents the principal antibody class. Two subclasses termed IgA1 and IgA2 have been defined that differ by the presence or absence of a 13-amino-acid hinge region (71). This region, exclusively present in IgA1, has many O-linked glycosylation sites and is a target for at least two families of IgA1 bacterial proteases, expression of which has been linked to pathogenicity. IgA2 is not susceptible to proteolysis by such proteases and bears two additional N-linked carbohydrate chains. The assembly of SIgA is complex and involves the polymeric Ig receptor (pIgR) (72). At the mucosal surface, IgA is expressed with an adjoining peptide, termed the J-chain, which stimulates dimerization (71,72). The pIgR synthesized in the epithelial cell is transported to the basolateral surface where it binds its ligand, dimeric IgA, or some larger polymer of IgA (collectively called pIgA) and then undergoes transcytosis. Having reached the apical membrane of the epithelial cell, its extracellular, ligand-binding domain is cleaved off. The remainder of pIgR that binds covalently to pIgA is called the secretory component (SC), and the SC–pIgA complex is referred to as SIgA (72). Interestingly, pIgR without pIgA can also undergo transcytosis leading to the release of free SC (72) into the lumenal secretions.

Until recently, the only role attributed to the SC has been to protect SIgA from proteolytic degradation. However, in a mouse model of respiratory infection by *Shigella flexneri*, it has been shown that the protective capacity of pIgA is enhanced on association to SC (73). The identical stability of SIgA and pIgA in the respiratory tract environment cannot simply explain this effect. Rather, SC is involved in establishing local interactions with bronchial mucus that results in the peculiar localization of the SIgA molecule, as compared to pIgA distributed randomly in lung tissue. This differential distribution of the two forms of antibody influences the number and localization of bacteria within the infected tissue, and therefore accounts for the difference observed in the respective protective capacities of SIgA and pIgA. Furthermore, in vitro deglycosylation of SC with *N*-endoglycosidase H before association with pIgA abrogates the capacity of SC to anchor the reconstituted SIgA molecule to mucus, and results in a level of protection comparable to pIgA alone (73). Thus, SC is directly involved in the SIgA function in vivo by permitting, through its carbohydrate residues, the appropriate localization of the antibody and, in turn, the exclusion of pathogens from the mucosal surfaces.

Notwithstanding SC's susceptibility to proteolytic degradation in vivo, free SC found in mucosal secretions may also function as a nonspecific microbial scavenger. Thus, it has been shown that free SC contributes to reduce the effects of *Clostridium difficile* toxin A on hamster brush border membranes (74) and limits infection by enterotoxigenic *E. coli* (75) through binding to fimbrial colonization factors.

SIgA is considered the primary mediator of immunity in mucosal areas through several proposed mechanisms: First, SIgA is a hydrophilic, negatively charged molecule because of the predominance of hydrophilic amino acids in the Fc region of IgA, and abundant glycosylation of both IgA and SC. As such, SIgA can surround microorganisms with a "hydrophilic shell" and prevent bacterial penetration. Other mechanisms include its ability to agglutinate microbes, interfere with bacterial motility by interacting with their flagella, and neutralize the action of bacterial products such as enzymes and toxins. Lastly, it has been suggested that IgA can neutralize viruses intracellularly. While antibodies usually do not protect against intracellular pathogens, IgA can intersect virus particles and interfere with virus replication or assembly when in transit through an infected epithelial cell (76,77). IgA–virus complexes might subsequently be excreted into the lumen.

On a precautionary note, it should be kept in mind that only very few IgA-deficient subjects exhibit serious health complications (71), suggesting that there are still many open questions concerning the role of IgA in immunity.

In addition, it should be noted that SIgA is not the predominant antibody in all secretions. Some mucosal secretions in humans also contain IgG such as in the lung alveoli. It has been proposed that in the airway mucosa exudation occur not only in injured but also in mildly inflamed tissues leading to external transfer of IgG in a passive fashion. It remains largely unknown how IgG crosses the epithelial barrier to function at mucosal surfaces.

VI. Collectins: Surfactant Proteins A and D and MBL

The immune defense of the lung involves the pulmonary surfactant, a complex mixture of lipids, phospholipids, and proteins important for normal respiratory function [reviewed recently in Ref. (78)]. Two of the surfactant proteins, (SP)-A and SP-D, belong to a family of mammalian lectins called collectins that are involved in innate immunity.

Beside the two surfactant proteins, there is an additional collectin involved in respiratory defense, the mannan or mannose-binding lectin (MBL). The collectins are very large, oligomeric glycoproteins, each composed of identical or very similar polypeptides. Each polypeptide has a characteristic four-domain structure: an N-terminal cysteine-rich portion, followed by a collagen-like sequence, an α-helical coiled coil region, and a C-type lectin domain at the C-terminus. The full-size native collectin molecule is assembled by polymerization of groups of three polypeptide chains to form a single subunit and by linking multiple subunits through disulfide bonding into oligomers. The extent of oligomerization of these subunits is variable, particularly for SP-A, but the accepted major oligomer of human collectin consists of six subunits (18 polypeptides) for SP-A and MBL and four subunits for SP-D. The oligomerization is important for high-avidity binding and pattern recognition (79).

SP-A and SP-D are synthesized by alveolar type II and Clara cells in the lung (78) and are most abundant in lung surfactant. SP-D is also found on mucosal surfaces outside the lung (78). A major biological role of the collectins is to selectively recognize microorganisms entering the lung by binding to patterns of carbohydrate arrays on microbial surfaces, and enhance their phagocytosis/clearance by opsonization or agglutination. It has been reported recently that SP-A and SP-D have also a direct antimicrobial and antifungal activity by enhancing cell-membrane permeability in *E. coli*. and *Histoplasma capsulatum* (80,81).

Although the full spectrum of in vivo targets of SP-A and SP-D is not known, a growing number of respiratory pathogens to which they bind have been identified. These include gram-negative bacteria (*E. coli, Pseudomonas aeruginosa, Klebsiella pneumonia, Haemophilus influenzae*), gram-positive bacteria (Group A and group B *Streptococcus*), mycobacteria (*Mycobacterium tuberculosis, Mycoplasma pulmonis*), viruses (Influenza A, Cytomegalovirus), and fungi (*Pneumocystis carinii, Aspergillus fumigatus*) (78). In addition to binding respiratory pathogens, the collectins also bind allergenic particles, including house dust-mite extracts and pollen-grain granules (78).

As with any other component of the immune system, the outcome of the binding of microorganisms by the collectins may not always be beneficial to the host. Hence, there may be damaging consequences such as increased infection as with cytomegalovirus or increase uptake of mycobacteria. Then again, collectins may modulate immune responses to pathogens by regulating cytokine production at pulmonary infection sites. It is known that alveolar macrophages recruit additional phagocytic cells to the site of pulmonary infections through the release of cytokines. This task requires a careful control to ensure a correct balance of inflammatory cells, since they have the potential to damage lung tissue. SP-A is capable of reducing the extent of cytokine release following pulmonary infections as exemplified by SP-A knockout mice, which show increased cytokine production after challenge by a number of pathogens (82).

Recent evidence suggests a critical role for surfactant-associated collectins in modulating asthma and allergic disease. Thus, the degree of polymerization of SP-A has been shown to be lower in some allergy patients than in healthy individuals (78). Also, SP-A decreases the proliferative response of dust-mite allergen and phytohemagglutinin-stimulated lymphocytes from children with stable asthma (83). SP-A and SP-D are able to directly inhibit allergen-induced histamine (84) and lymphocyte proliferation (83). SP-D seems to be involved also in the advanced stages of asthmatic disease characterized by airway remodeling. This remodeling leads to the production of goblet cells at the expense of Clara cells. Goblet cells have been shown to produce SP-D in a murine model of asthma (85).

Rather then viewing goblet cell hyperplasia as solely a pathological process (the conventional model), these findings imply that these cells may have an anti-inflammatory and immunomodulatory role. Further, SP-A and SP-D have been identified as being involved in the clearance of apoptotic cells in the lung. Mice made deficient in SP-D show increased number of apoptotic cells in their airway and spontaneously develop emphysema and pulmonary fibrosis (86). These observations substantiate the likelihood that SP-D functions to decrease pathological airway remodeling in chronic asthma.

MBL has a quaternary structure and target-binding specificities similar to SP-A, but functionally it is the only collectin able to activate the complement system. Similarly to SP-A and SP-D, the oligomerization of MBL allows high avidity binding to carbohydrate ligands due to the multiple lectin domains present. Smaller MBL oligomers with lower degree of polymerization bind less-avidly to carbohydrate surfaces and are defective in activating complement (87).

The primary source of MBL is the liver and is most abundant in blood but is present in most body fluids, such as in buccal cavity and upper airway secretions and saliva. Serum levels of MBL are variable in human ranging from 0 to 3 µg/mL (88). Interestingly, at least 5% of the population is deficient or have extremely low levels of the protein (88). The health consequences of MBL deficiency are not understood as yet. Neither are the concentration and biochemical forms of MBL present in the airways known at present.

MBL can trigger activation of complement, resulting in deposition of C3b/iC3b on targets and stimulation of phagocytic uptake via the C3 receptors, CR1, CR3, and CR4 (78). The complement system is a major mediator of innate-immune defenses involved in inflammation, opsonization, and lysis. As the concentrations of complement proteins are very low in body fluids other than blood plasma, it remains unclear whether complement activation by MBL has an important role in the respiratory tract.

VII. Host Defense Molecules

The epithelial fluid lining all mucosal surfaces such as the airway secretion contain specific families of defense molecules that constitute an essential part of the innate mucosal defense system. Interestingly, this aspect of the immune system is only rudimentarily covered, if at all, by most current immunology textbooks.

It is estimated that lysozyme and lactoferrin are the most abundant antimicrobial protein of airway secretions, at $\sim$0.1–1 mg/mL (89). Secretory leukoprotease inhibitor (SLPI) is about 10-fold less abundant (89). The concentrations of neutrophil and epithelial defensins in respiratory fluid are highly variable with levels estimated between hundreds of nanograms to tens of micrograms/mL with significant increase in their concentration during inflammation (90).

Lysozyme, a 14 kDa antimicrobial polypeptide, is a component of both phagocytic and secretory granules of neutrophils and is also produced by monocytes, macrophages, and epithelial cells. Lysozyme is an enzyme directed against the β 1→4 glycosidic bond between *N*-acetylglucosamine and *N*-acetylmuramic acid residues that make up peptidoglycan, the cell wall material of bacteria. Lysozyme is highly effective against many grampositive species, for example, *Bacillus megaterium*, *Micrococcus lysodeicticus*, and many streptococci, but ineffective against Gram-negative bacteria (91).

Lactoferrin is an 80 kDa, iron-binding protein that is highly abundant in the specific granules of human neutrophils and in epithelial secretions. Lactoferrin inhibits microbial growth by sequestering iron essential for microbial respiration (92).

Secretory leukoprotease inhibitor (SLPI) is a 12 kDa nonglycosylated polypeptide consisting of two similar domains. The N-terminal domain has modest antimicrobial activity in vitro against both gram-negative and grampositive bacteria (93). The C-terminal domain acts as an effective inhibitor of neutrophil elastase and may also be involved in intracellular regulation of responses to lipopolysaccharide (94).

A. Antimicrobial Peptides: Defensins and Cathelicidins

Defensins are 3–5 kDa cationic peptides with a characteristic three-dimensional structure and with six conserved cysteine residues that form three disulfide bonds (90). On the basis of the position of the cysteine residues and the disulfide bond-pairing pattern, defensins have been divided into two main families, the α- and β-defensins. In humans, both families are encoded by a cluster of genes on chromosome 8, suggesting that all defensins evolved from a common ancestral gene (95). Defensins are synthesized as prepropeptides and are post-translationally processed into mature, active peptides. The microbicidal activity of defensins is believed to be mediated via the formation of a microbial-selective, membrane-spanning pore, which leads to dissipation of electrochemical gradients and cell lysis (90). Three closely related α-defensins, human neutrophil peptides HNP-1, HNP-2, and HNP-3, are major components of the dense azurophil granules of neutrophils, and a fourth, HNP-4, is found in the same location but is much less abundant (89). Among the β-defensins HBD1 and HBD2 have been detected in airway surface fluid and saliva and are probably secreted by epithelial cells to operate at the mucosal surface (89). In in vitro testing, HBD1 and HBD2 are active against Gram-negative bacteria including *E. coli* and *P. aeruginosa*. HBD3 is expressed in the tonsils, oral cavity, and much less at the airway surfaces (89,90). HBD3 has potent antibacterial activity against Gram-positive bacteria including *S. aureus* (89).

In addition to their bactericidal function, a number of recent studies have demonstrated the ability of defensins to act as chemoattractants for dendritic cells, monocytes, and T-cells (96). Hence, HBD1 and HBD2 are chemotactic for immature DCs and memory T-cells via interaction with the chemokine receptor CCR6 (90). Another defensin, the epithelial β-defensin MBD2 has been shown to act as an endogenous ligand for TLR4, to induce maturation of DCs (90). By these activities, the defensins may provide an additional link between the mucosal innate defense system and adaptive immunity.

Cathelicidins (97) are members of a large family of mammalian polypeptides with a conserved N-terminal precursor cathelin domain, containing typically about 100 amino acid residues, and a highly heterogeneous cationic C-terminal peptide (10–40 amino acid residues). The mature cathelicidin peptide is generated after extracellular proteolytic cleavage that frees the C-terminal peptide from the cathelin precursor domain. Mature cathelicidins show a wide spectrum of antimicrobial activity and, more recently, some of them have also been found to exert other biological activities [reviewed recently in Ref. (97)].

While there are 11 cathelicidins genes in cattle and eight genes in sheep, the sole known human cathelicidin gene, mapped to chromosome 3, has been named hCAP18, FALL39/LL37, or LL37 (97). Its abundance in neutrophils-specific granules appears to be about one-third of that of lysozyme or lactoferrin, the two major proteins of specific granules. Exemplifying the overlap of phagocytic, adaptive immunity and epithelial host defenses, the mRNA for the human cathelicidin was also found in the testis, in inflamed keratinocytes, in other squamous epithelia, in human airway epithelia, and a large variety of immune cells including NK, γδT-cells, B-cells, monocytes, and mast cells in addition to neutrophils.

In vitro, the human cathelicidin LL-37 displayed both LPS binding and broad-spectrum microbicidal activities (97,98). It also inhibits LPS-induced cellular responses, such as release of TNF-α, nitric oxide, and tissue factor. Expression of LL-37 gene in mouse airways reduced bacterial load and decreased inflammatory response in *P. aeruginosa*-infected mice (99). Furthermore overexpression of LL-37 in a human bronchial xenograft model of cystic fibrosis restored the deficient antimicrobial activity (98), demonstrating that LL-37 maintains biological activity in the airways.

LL-37 has chemotactic effects in vitro, inducing selective migration of human peripheral blood monocytes, neutrophils, and CD4 T-cells but not DCs (97). The chemotactic activity of LL-37 is mediated by binding to formyl peptide receptor-like 1 (FPRL1) (100). Using the same functional receptor FPRL1, LL-37 induces Ca^{2+} flux in monocytes (98). In mast cells, LL-37 induces histamine release and intracellular Ca^{2+} mobilization (97).

It should be emphasized that until recently the only biological function attributed to these peptide molecules was limited to their direct antimicrobial activity. The subsequent findings that various defensins and cathelicidin peptides can also interact with host cells and trigger a variety of activities unrelated to direct microbial killing has challenged our perception of these molecules. Rather then viewing these peptides as first-line effectors of innate immunity, the paradigm is shifting to a much more complex interactive picture involving the orchestration of inflammatory and immune responses, and participation in the cross-talk between innate and adaptive immunity.

As a final point, the close functional and evolutionary relationship between the antimicrobial peptides, discussed above, and bona fide immunoregulatory molecules is further illustrated by some chemokines such as CCL28.

Chemokines are known to play essential roles in innate and adaptive immunity by regulating migration and activation of leukocytes via transmembrane G protein-coupled receptors (101). In humans, more than 45 members and 18 functional receptors have been identified (101). According to the arrangement of the conserved amino-terminal cysteine residues, the chemokines are classified into four subfamilies: CXC, CC, C, and CX3C (101). Based on the classification of these four subfamilies, a systematic nomenclature system of the chemokine ligands has been formulated recently (102). Except for the two transmembrane-type chemokines, CX3CL1 and CXCL16, chemokines are small (8–14 kDa), mostly cationic polypeptides with two to three intramolecular disulfide bonds (101,102). CCL28 (also called mucosa-associated epithelial chemokine) is a recently described CC chemokine signaling via the chemokine receptors CCR10 and CCR3 (103). CCL28 is expressed at high levels in the salivary glands, respiratory tract, and distal colon and is produced by the epithelial cells in these tissues. CCL28 displays a chemoattractant function for immune cells expressing the chemokine receptors CCR10 (such as some memory T-cells) and CCR3 (such as eosinophils in peripheral human blood). Recent work in a mouse mucosal tissue has demonstrated that CCL28 exerts a potent, salt-sensitive antimicrobial activity against a broad spectrum of microbes including *Candida albicans*, gram-negative and gram-positive bacteria (104). Thus, CCL28 may represent the first chemokine that not only attracts immune cells into certain mucosal tissues but functions also as a potent antimicrobial factor when secreted by epithelial cells at these mucosal surfaces (104).

VIII. Malnutrition and Immune Response

Nutritional status is an important factor contributing to immune competence (Table 2) (105,106) and has specific relevance to the practice of medicine in the tropics (3,4). Malnutrition or undernourishment (either due to insufficient intake of calories or deficiency in specific nutrients) impairs the immune system. Impaired immune system increases the susceptibility to infections and also worsens and/or lengthens the course of the infection. Infectious diseases themselves might cause additional nutritional deficiency because of reduced intake or reduced absorption, such as in diseases causing diarrhea (4). This leads to what is sometimes called a vicious cycle, resulting in a poorer outcome than anticipated for the same infectious disease in a nutritionally balanced subject (Fig. 1). There is an additional loop in the cycle connecting infection and immune system, namely that certain infections can cause direct immunosuppression. Measles has long been known to suppress T-cell immune responses and predispose the patient to secondary infections, but HIV is the most decisive example of immunosuppression caused by an infectious agent. Some investigators have emphasized that not only can nutrition influence the immune response but also the immune response can, in turn, influence nutritional status. Hence, a variety of cytokines are released during an immune response to a pathogen. Some of these cytokines, for example, IL-1, IL-6, and TNFα have been shown to influence nutrient absorption and metabolism. Since most of these experiments have been carried out in somewhat artificial in vitro systems, and because the lack of direct explanatory evidence to ascribe the nutritional consequences to a certain cytokine or group of cytokines, I remain somewhat skeptical about the relevance of this "nutrition–immune system" loop to practical medicine.

   During the 1990s, the role of deficiency in essential dietary components such as vitamins and minerals in host response to infections became widely recognized (105). For instance, multiple field studies of vitamin A supplementation in various populations around the world demonstrated a marked decrease in overall infant and childhood mortality and morbidity.

Table 2 Examples of Nutrient Deficiency Effect on Immune System

Nutrient deficiency	Immunological outcome	
	Decrease in	Increase in
Food restriction (human)	Immune competence at <60% of body weight $CD4^+/CD8^+$ ratio plasma complement	Circulating B cell circulation Abs
Calorie restriction (mice, rats)	Tumor virus expression and malignancy prokuferation of autoreactive B1 cells TH_1 cytokins and IL-6, TNFα, TGF-β	T-cell proliferation
Protein and protein-energy deficiency (human)	Humoral and cell-mediated parameters	Oxidative stress
Protein deficiency (mice)	DTH circulating IgG macrophage function tissue repair	TH_2 oxidative stress splenic regulatory T cells
Arginine and glutamine deficiency (human)	Immune competence T cell development	
Nucleic acid restriction (human)	NK activity DTH, IL-s production T cell proliferation	
Vitamin A deficiency	TH_2 response mucus secreting cells	TH_1 reponse keratinization of epithelial cells
Vitamin E deficiency	$CD4^+/CD8^+$ ratio	Oxidative stress lipid peroxidation and damage to all membranes
Selenium deficiency	Glutathione peroxidase IL-2 R expression CTL, NK and macrophage activity	Oxidative stress neutrophile adherence mutation rate and pathogenesis of several viruses
Iron deficiency	DTH, CTL, macrophage and neutrophile activity TH_1 cells (but not TH_2 cells) proliferation malaria infection	

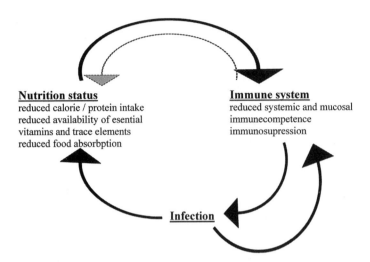

Figure 1 Malnutrition immune system infection cycle. *Source*: Adapted from Ref. 4.

With the exception of measles, it has been considerably difficult to show that the improvement in the survival of these children was specifically attributable to an effect on susceptibility or immune response to specific infections. However, as discussed by Gerald Keusch (107), there are other plausible explanations that have not been considered and tested. For example, vitamin A deficiency might cause keratinization of the respiratory epithelium, leading to reduced mucus production and diminished competence to clear bacterial pathogens (105) (Table 2).

IX. Immune Evasion Mechanisms

Finally, I would like to bring to the forefront a salient notion I only hinted at throughout this discussion. I am referring to the notion that many, if not most infectious microorganisms, have developed sophisticated evasion mechanisms to escape immune elimination. From this perspective the mammalian immune system, especially its adaptive arm, seems to be ineffective, or to use Peter Parham's phrase "the immune system seems to fight today's threats with the solutions of past problems" (108). I would like to illustrate this predicament using *Mycobacterium tuberculosis* as a case in point, highly relevant to tropical pulmonary medicine.

The bacterial pathogen, *M. tuberculosis* is responsible for over 2 million deaths annually (109). It is believed that approximately 10% of those infected will ever develop active disease (110). Thus, it is estimated that the bacterium manages to persist in a latent state, but is alive in immunocompetent hosts of about one-third of the world population (109). The bacterium actually lives within the macrophage, the cell whose function is to eliminate such microorganisms. Recent advances have clarified the various immune evasion strategies used by *M. tuberculosis*. A major antimicrobial mechanism available for activated macrophages is the nitric oxide synthase 2 (NOS2)-dependent pathway, which generates nitric oxide and related reactive nitrogen intermediates (RNIs) from L-arginine. *M. tuberculosis* has developed multiple mechanisms to evade the toxicity of RNIs such as the genes NoxR1, NoxR3, and AhpC, which confer RNI resistance (110 and references therein).

Another effective antimicrobial mechanism is the delivery of phagocytized bacteria to the lysosomal compartment, where hydrolytic enzymes will kill the bacteria optimally at acidic pH. It has been demonstrated that *M. tuberculosis* is capable of excluding vacuolar H^+-ATP from the phagosome, thereby avoiding the hostile acidic intraphagosomal environment (111). The fusion of pathogen-containing phagosomes with lysosomes is a highly regulated process (dubbed phagosomal maturation), which involves interaction with various endocytic vacuoles. The bacterium is capable of arresting the maturation process at various stages such as when the two GTPases, Rab5 and Rab7, are recruited (112). Hence, a virulence factor, mannosylated lipoarabinomannan (ManLAM), a glycolipid from *M. tuberculosis* is able to attenuate the activity of PI-3K kinase and to inhibit the recruitment of early endosomal autoanitgen1 (EEA1) (113). Also *M. tuberculosis* can interfere in the maturation process by inhibiting Ca^{2+} signaling via downregulation of calmodulin-dependent signal transduction (114,115). Fratti et al. (116) have recently shown that mycobacterial ManLAM can also interfere with the recruitment of syntaxin 6, a protein belonging to the soluble *N*-ethylmaleimide-sensitive factor attachment protein receptor (SNARE) family that participates in vesicular trafficking between the trans-Golgi and the phagosome. The mycobacterium can inhibit phagosome maturation also by modifying cellubrevin, another SNARE protein that is involved in phagosomal maturation (117). Lastly, *M. tuberculosis* can prevent phagosomal maturation through interaction with the host protein tryptophan aspartate-rich coat protein (TACO), which is necessary for phagolysosomal fusion (110,118).

The adaptive arm of the immune response to microorganisms such as *M. tuberculosis* involves a strong $CD4^+$ T-cell response with the production of effective cytokines. This complex procedure is initiated by mycobacterial antigen processing within APC (macrophages and dendritic cells), and presentation of these processed peptide antigens bound to MHC class II molecules on the surface of the APC. Work in many laboratories has demonstrated that *M. tuberculosis* can modulate antigen presentation at various stages [reviewed in Ref. (110)]. Thus, class II MHC expression on APC was reduced by at least two separate mechanisms: inhibition of the transcription of these molecules and their intracellular sequestration

(119,120) and inhibition of IFNγ signaling and consequently the prevention of IFNγ-induced upregulation of MHC molecules on activated APCs (121). Also because of the various effects of the pathogen on intracellular trafficking as discussed earlier, the intracellular processing of mycobacterial antigen is impaired (110). An important mycobacterial component responsible for these activities was identified as a 19 kDa lipoprotein, which acts through the host TLR2 (122,123) (Table 1).

It is noteworthy that mycobacterial peptide-MHC class II complexes are formed also in the infected phagosome (124). Thus, phagosomes can be isolated from infected cells and used as a resource of MHC class II-peptide complexes to stimulate mycobacterial antigen-specific T-cell hybridoma. In an elegant experiment, Ramachandra et al. (124) have observed that phagosomes infected with live *M. tuberculosis* have much fewer MHC class II-peptide complexes than phagosomes containing heat-killed *M. tuberculosis*, suggesting that live bacilli inhibited antigen processing within the infected phagosome. This may be the first demonstration that inhibition of antigen processing may represent an immune evasion mechanism that happens early in the infection while the 19 kDa lipoprotein-mediated inhibition of antigen processing and presentation may be relevant during the chronic infection stages (110).

Tumor necrosis factor (TNFα), one of the major cytokine products of macrophages, plays a crucial role in the immunity to *M. tuberculosis* (110,125). Thus, TNFα blockade in mice with chronic tuberculosis induces accelerated mortality and enhanced inflammatory reaction reflected in increased cellularity in the granulomatous lesions in the lung. Significantly, the bacterial burden in the TNFα neutralized mice peaked at 107 CFU per lung (a level of bacterial burden not expected to be lethal to these mice), suggesting that the severe inflammatory process associated with the blockage of TNFα contributed to the worsening of the prognosis (126). Recently, TNF neutralization became an important therapeutic modality in rheumatoid arthritis and Crohn's disease (127). A major side effect of anti-TNF therapy is the enhanced risks for developing tuberculosis. The data accumulation on such patients suggests that tuberculosis associated with TNF blockade is mostly the result of reactivation of latent infection (128). Further, examination of tissue obtained via open lung biopsy from a patient with anti-TNF-associated tuberculosis revealed no granuloma in the lesions, supporting the notion that TNF plays an important role in maintaining the integrity of granulomas in human tubercular infections (128). Thus, the role of TNFα in *M. tuberculosis* infection can be viewed as a protective modality relevant to its ability to regulate the formation of granulomas and preventing the dissemination of the infection; on the other hand, TNFα can be also viewed as causing the immunopathology of tuberculosis.

In a recent publication Shimono et al. (129) demonstrate that a strain of *M. tuberculosis* disrupted in the *mce1* operon (shown previously to contain a virulence factor involved in helping the pathogen invade cells) was unable to enter a stable persistent state of infection characterized by the formation of multiple well-defined granulomas in mouse lungs. Instead, the mutant continued to replicate and killed the mice. Granulomas had not formed properly in the lungs infected with the mutant strain but rather showed diffused and aberrant inflammatory cell migration. In addition, mouse macrophages infected in vitro with the mutant strain showed reduced capability to produce nitric oxide, TNFα, and induce a T_H1 response (129). However, they were not defective in promoting T_H2 response. The hypervirulence of the mutant strain may have resulted from its inability to stimulate an immune response that would otherwise induce organized granuloma formation and control the infection without killing the organism. The *mce1* operon of *M. tuberculosis* may be involved in modulating the host inflammatory response in such a way that the bacterium can enter a persistent state without being eliminated or causing active disease in the host. The lesson to be learned is that the immune response observed in wild-type *M. tuberculosis*, typified by the lung granuloma shield, not only protects the host from the pathogen, but also protects the bacteria from the host's other immune cells and potential strategies that may have otherwise killed the bacteria. In effect, the investigators have disrupted genes of the pathogen associated with persistent infection and meanwhile unmasked the pathogen's full virulence potential. The *M. tuberculosis mce1* operon may have evolved to "fine-tune" the host immune response to the bacillus' advantage to establish latent infection without causing active disease in the host (129).

X. Conclusion

The picture painted here is a complex one. It is clear that the fact that an immune response develops does not necessary mean that the host will be protected and disease free. Neither does exposure nor infection by a microorganism inevitably cause a state of disease in the host. Rather, both the immune system and the pathogen may prefer developing strategies of coexistence with each other. The inherent flaws of the mammalian immune system do not imply that we will never succeed in developing effective means of protecting ourselves from exceedingly evasive microorganisms. Rather, the lesson to be learned is that our immune system and the microorganisms can both be manipulated using available sophisticated molecular technologies toward our own goals. Thus, the prerequisite to being able to intervene successfully toward developing clinical strategies that do work is a detailed understanding of the immune mechanisms and gaining much more insight into the complexities of host–pathogen interaction.

References

1. Kyd JM, Foxwell AR, Cripps AW. Mucosal immunity in the lung and upper airway. Vaccine 2001; 19:2527–2533.
2. Message SD, Johnston SL. Host defense function of the airway epithelium in health and disease: clinical background. J Leukoc Biol 2004; 75:5–17.
3. Bovornkitti S. Tropical pulmonary diseases. Respiratology 1996; 1:11–21.
4. Zumla AI, James DG. Immunologic aspects of tropical lung disease. Clin Chest Med 2002; 2:283–308.
5. Tlaskalova-Hogenova H, Tuckova L, Lodinova-Zadnikova R, Stepankova R, Cukrowska B, Funda DP, Striz I, Kozakova H, Trebichavsky I, Sokol D, Rehakova Z, Sinkora J, Fundova P, Horakova D, Jelinkova L, Sanchez D. Mucosal immunity: its role in defense and allergy. Int Arch Allergy Immunol 2002; 128:77–89.
6. Mayer L. Mucosal immunity. Pediatrics 2003; 111:1595–1600.
7. van Ginkel FW, Nguyen HH, McGhee JR. Vaccines for mucosal immunity to combat emerging infectious diseases. Emerg Infect Dis 2000; 6:123–132.
8. Kerneis S, Bogdanova A, Kraehenbuhl JP, Pringault E. Conversion by Peyer's patch lymphocytes of human enterocytes into M cells that transport bacteria. Science 1997; 277:949–952.
9. Neurath MF, Finotto S, Glimcher LH. The role of Th1/Th2 polarization in mucosal immunity. Nat Med 2002; 8:567–573.
10. Medzhitov R, Janeway C J Jr. Advances in immunology: innate immunity. N Engl J Med 2000; 343:338–344.
11. Gordon S. Pattern recognition receptors: doubling up for the innate immune response. Cell 2002; 111:927–930.
12. Beutler B. Innate immunity: an overview. Mol Immunol 2004; 40:845–859.
13. Beutler B, Rehli M. Evolution of the TIR, tolls and TLRs: functional inferences from computational biology. Curr Top Microbiol Immunol 2002; 270:1–21.
14. Imler JL, Zheng L. Biology of Toll receptors: lessons from insects and mammals. J Leukoc Biol 2004; 75:18–26.
15. Arbour NC, Lorenz E, Schutte BC, Zabner J, Kline JN, Jones M, Frees K, Watt JL, Schwartz DA. TLR4 mutations are associated with endotoxin hyporesponsiveness in humans. Nat Genet 2000; 25:187–191.
16. Lorenz E, Mira JP, Cornish KL, Arbour NC, Schwartz DA. A novel polymorphism in the toll-like receptor 2 gene and its potential association with staphylococcal infection. Infect Immun 2000; 68:6398–6401.
17. Kiechl S, Lorenz E, Reindl M, Wiedermann CJ, Oberhollenzer F, Bonora E, Willeit J, Schwartz DA. Toll-like receptor 4 polymorphisms and atherogenesis. N Engl J Med 2002; 347:185–192.
18. Bochud PY, Hawn TR, Aderem A. Cutting edge: a Toll-like receptor 2 polymorphism that is associated with lepromatous leprosy is unable to mediate mycobacterial signaling. J Immunol 2003; 170:3451–3454.
19. Becker MN, Diamond G, Verghese MW, Randell SH. CD14-dependent lipopolysaccharide-induced beta-defensin-2 expression in human tracheobronchial epithelium. J Biol Chem 2000; 275:29,731–29,736.

20. Nagai Y, Akashi S, Nagafuku M, Ogata M, Iwakura Y, Akira S, Kitamura T, Kosugi A, Kimoto M, Miyake K. Essential role of MD-2 in LPS responsiveness and TLR4 distribution. Nat Immunol 2002; 3:667–672.

21. Vabulas RM, Wagner H, Schild H. Heat shock proteins as ligands of toll-like receptors. Curr Top Microbiol Immunol 2002; 270:169–184.

22. Okamura Y, Watari M, Jerud ES, Young DW, Ishizaka ST, Rose J, Chow JC, Strauss JF. The extra domain A of fibronectin activates Toll-like receptor 4. J Biol Chem 2001; 76:10,229–10,233.

23. Termeer C, Benedix F, Sleeman J, Fieber C, Voith U, Ahrens T, Miyake K, Freudenberg M, Galanos C, Simon JC. Oligosaccharides of Hyaluronan activate dendritic cells via toll-like receptor 4. J Exp Med 2002; 195:99–111.

24. Biragyn A, Ruffini PA, Leifer CA, Klyushnenkova E, Shakhov A, Chertov O, Shirakawa AK, Farber JM, Segal DM, Oppenheim JJ, Kwak LW. Toll-like receptor 4-dependent activation of dendritic cells by beta-defensin 2. Science 2002; 298:1025–1029.

25. Guillot L, Balloy V, McCormack FX, Golenbock DT, Chignard M, Si-Tahar M. Cutting edge: the immunostimulatory activity of the lung surfactant protein-A involves Toll-like receptor 4. J Immunol 2002; 168:5989–5992.

26. Medzhitov R. Toll-like receptors and innate immunity. Nat Rev Immunol 2001; 1:135–145.

27. Doyle S, Vaidya S, O'Connell R, Dadgostar H, Dempsey P, Wu T, Rao G, Sun R, Haberland M, Modlin R, Cheng G. IRF3 mediates a TLR3/TLR4-specific antiviral gene program. Immunity 2002; 17:251–263.

28. Kawai T, Takeuchi O, Fujita T, Inoue J, Muhlradt PF, Sato S, Hoshino K, Akira S. Lipopolysaccharide stimulates the MyD88-independent pathway and results in activation of IFN-regulatory factor 3 and the expression of a subset of lipopolysaccharide-inducible genes. J Immunol 2001; 167:5887–5894.

29. Muraille E, De Trez C, Brait M, De Baetselier P, Leo O, Carlier Y. Genetically resistant mice lacking MyD88-adapter protein display a high susceptibility to Leishmania major infection associated with a polarized Th2 response. J Immunol 2003; 170:4237–4241.

30. Eisenbarth SC, Piggott DA, Huleatt JW, Visintin I, Herrick CA, Bottomly K. Lipopolysaccharide-enhanced, toll-like receptor 4-dependent T helper cell type 2 responses to inhaled antigen. J Exp Med 2002; 196:1645–1651.

31. Pasare C, Medzhitov R. Toll pathway-dependent blockade of CD4 + CD25+ T cell-mediated suppression by dendritic cells. Science 2003; 299:1033–1036.

32. Dinerello CA. Interleukin-18, a proinflammatory cytokine. Eur Cytokine Netw 2000; 11:483–486.

33. Barbulescu K, Becker C, Schlaak JF, Schmitt E, Meyer zum Buschenfelde KH, Neurath MF. IL-12 and IL-18 differentially regulate the transcriptional activity of the human IFN-gamma promoter in primary CD4+ T lymphocytes. J Immunol 1998; 160:3642–3647.

34. Wills-Karp M. Interleukin-13 in asthma pathogenesis. Curr Allergy Asthma Rep 2004; 4:123–131.

35. Pulendran B, Bancherau J, Maraskovsky E, Maliszewski C. Modulating the immune response with dendritic cells and their growth factors. Trends Immunol 2001; 22:41–47.

36. Iwasaki A, Kelsall BL. Freshly isolated Peyer's patch, but not spleen, dendritic cells produce interleukin 10 and induce the differentiation of T helper type 2 cells. J Exp Med 1999; 190(2):229–239.

37. Iwasaki A, Kelsall BL. Unique functions of CD11b+, CD8 alpha+, and double-negative Peyer's patch dendritic cells. J Immunol 2001; 166:4884–4890.

38. Stumbles PA, Thomas JA, Pimm CL, Lee PT, Venaille TJ, Proksch S, Holt PG. Resting respiratory tract dendritic cells preferentially stimulate T helper cell type 2 (Th2) responses and require obligatory cytokine signals for induction of Th1 immunity. J Exp Med 1998; 188:2019–2031.

39. Holt PG, Stumbles PA. Characterization of dendritic cell populations in the respiratory tract. J Aerosol Med 2000; 13:361–367.

40. Szabo SJ, Sullivan BM, Stemmann C, Satoskar AR, Sleckman BP, Glimcher LH. Distinct effects of T-bet in TH1 lineage commitment and IFN-gamma production in CD4 and CD8 T-cells. Science 2002; 29:338–342.

41. Kurata H, Lee HJ, O'Garra A, Arai N. Ectopic expression of activated Stat6 induces the expression of Th2-specific cytokines and transcription factors in developing Th1 cells. Immunity 1999; 11:677–688.

42. Ouyang W, Lohning M, Gao Z, Assenmacher M, Ranganath S, Radbruch A, Murphy KM. Stat6-independent GATA-3 autoactivation directs IL-4-independent Th2 development and commitment. Immunity 2000; 12:27–37.

43. Coffman RL, Mosmann TR. CD4+ T-cell subsets: regulation of differentiation and function. Res Immunol 1991; 142:7–9.

44. Poltorak A, He X, Smirnova I, Liu MY, Van Huffel C, Du X, Birdwell D, Alejos E, Silva M, Galanos C, Freudenberg M, Ricciardi-Castagnoli P, Layton B, Beutler B. Defective LPS signaling in C3H/HeJ and C57BL/10ScCr mice: mutations in Tlr4 gene. Science 1998; 282:2085–2088.

45. Hemmi H, Takeuchi O, Kawai T, Kaisho T, Sato S, Sanjo H, Matsumoto M, Hoshino K, Wagner H, Takeda K, Akira S. A Toll-like receptor recognizes bacterial DNA. Nature 2000; 408:740–745.

46. Hayashi F, Smith KD, Ozinsky A, Hawn TR, Yi EC, Goodlett DR, Eng JK, Akira S, Underhill DM, Aderem A. The innate immune response to bacterial flagellin is mediated by Toll-like receptor 5. Nature 2001; 410:1099–1103.

47. Alexopoulou L, Holt AC, Medzhitov R, Flavell RA. Recognition of double-stranded RNA and activation of NF-kappaB by Toll-like receptor 3. Nature 2001; 413:732–738.

48. d'Ostiani CF, Del Sero G, Bacci A, Montagnoli C, Spreca A, Mencacci A, Ricciardi-Castagnoli P, Romani L. Dendritic cells discriminate between yeasts and hyphae of the fungus *Candida albicans*. Implications for initiation of T helper cell immunity in vitro and in vivo. J Exp Med 2000; 191:1661–1674.

49. Whelan M, Harnett MM, Houston KM, Patel V, Harnett W, Rigley KP. A filarial nematode-secreted product signals dendritic cells to acquire a phenotype that drives development of Th2 cells. J Immunol 2000; 164:6453–6460.

50. Gagliardi MC, Sallusto F, Marinaro M, Langenkamp A, Lanzavecchia A, De Magistris MT. Cholera toxin induces maturation of human dendritic cells and licences them for Th2 priming. Eur J Immunol 2000; 30:2394–2403.

51. Read S, Powrie F. CD4(+) regulatory T-cells. Curr Opin Immunol 2001; 13:644–649.

52. Maloy KJ, Powrie F. Regulatory T-cells in the control of immune pathology. Nat Immunol 2001; 2:816–822.
53. Jenkins MK, Schwartz RH. Antigen presentation by chemically modified splenocytes induces antigen-specific T cell unresponsiveness in vitro and in vivo. J Exp Med 1987; 165:302–319.
54. Chai JG, Bartok I, Chandler P, Vendetti S, Antoniou A, Dyson J, Lechler R. Anergic T-cells act as suppressor cells in vitro and in vivo. Eur J Immunol 1999; 29:686–692.
55. Vendetti S, Chai JG, Dyson J, Simpson E, Lombardi G, Lechler R. Anergic T-cells inhibit the antigen-presenting function of dendritic cells. J Immunol 2000; 165:1175–1181.
56. Buer J, Lanoue A, Franzke A, Garcia C, von Boehmer H, Sarukhan A. Interleukin 10 secretion and impaired effector function of major histocompatibility complex class II-restricted T-cells anergized in vivo. J Exp Med 1998; 187:177–183.
57. Groux H, O'Garra A, Bigler M, Rouleau M, Antonenko S, de Vries JE, Roncarolo MG. A CD4+ T-cell subset inhibits antigen-specific T-cell responses and prevents colitis. Nature 1997; 389:737–742.
58. Cottrez F, Hurst SD, Coffman RL, Groux H. T regulatory cells 1 inhibit a Th2-specific response in vivo. J Immunol 2000; 165:4848–4853.
59. Levings MK, Sangregorio R, Galbiati F, Squadrone S, de Waal Malefyt R, Roncarolo MG. IFN-alpha and IL-10 induce the differentiation of human type 1 T regulatory cells. J Immunol 2001; 166:5530–5539.
60. Faria AM, Weiner HL. Oral tolerance: mechanisms and therapeutic applications. Adv Immunol 1999; 73:153–264.
61. Hori S, Nomura T, Sakaguchi S. Control of regulatory T cell development by the transcription factor Foxp3. Science 2003; 299:1057–1061.
62. Powrie F, Maloy KJ. Regulating the regulators. Science 2003; 299:1030–1031.
63. Mills KH, McGuirk P. Pathogen-specific regulatory T-cells provoke a shift in the Th1/Th2 paradigm in immunity to infectious diseases. Trends Immunol 2002; 23:450–455.
64. Mills KH, McGuirk P. Antigen-specific regulatory T-cells—their induction and role in infection. Semin Immunol 2004; 16:107–117.
65. McGuirk P, McCann C, Mills KH. Pathogen-specific T regulatory 1 cells induced in the respiratory tract by a bacterial molecule that stimulates interleukin 10 production by dendritic cells: a novel strategy for evasion of protective T helper type 1 responses by *Bordetella pertussis*. J Exp Med 2002; 195:221–231.
66. Kullberg MC, Jankovic D, Gorelick PL, Caspar P, Letterio JJ, Cheever AW, Sher A. Bacteria-triggered CD4(+) T regulatory cells suppress *Helicobacter hepaticus*-induced colitis. J Exp Med 2002; 196:505–515.
67. Belkaid Y, Piccirillo CA, Mendez S, Shevach EM, Sacks DL. CD4+CD25+ regulatory T-cells control leishmania major persistence and immunity. Nature 2002; 420:502–507.
68. Ryan M, Murphy G, Gothefors L, Nilsson L, Storsaeter J, Mills KH. *Bordetella pertussis* respiratory infection in children is associated with preferential activation of type 1 T helper cells. J Infect Dis 1997; 175:1246–1250.

69. Mills KH, Barnard A, Watkins J, Redhead K. Cell-mediated immunity to *Bordetella pertussis*: role of Th1 cells in bacterial clearance in a murine respiratory infection model. Infect Immun 1993; 61:399–410.

70. Higgins SC, Lavelle EC, McCann C, Keogh B, McNeela E, Byrne P, O'Gorman B, Jarnicki A, McGuirk P, Mills KH. Toll-like receptor 4-mediated innate IL-10 activates antigen-specific regulatory T-cells and confers resistance to *Bordetella pertussis* by inhibiting inflammatory pathology. J Immunol 2003; 171:3119–3127.

71. van Egmond M, Damen CA, van Spriel AB, Vidarsson G, van Garderen E, van de Winkel JG. IgA and the IgA Fc receptor. Trends Immunol 2001; 22:205–211.

72. Phalipon A, Corthesy B. Novel functions of the polymeric Ig receptor: well beyond transport of immunoglobulins. Trends Immunol 2003; 24:55–58.

73. Phalipon A, Cardona A, Kraehenbuhl JP, Edelman L, Sansonetti PJ, Corthesy B. Secretory component: a new role in secretory IgA-mediated immune exclusion in vivo. Immunity 2002; 17:107–115.

74. Dallas SD, Rolfe RD. Binding of *Clostridium difficile* toxin A to human milk secretory component. J Med Microbiol 1998; 47:879–888.

75. de Oliveira IR, de Araujo AN, Bao SN, Giugliano LG. Binding of lactoferrin and free secretory component to enterotoxigenic *Escherichia coli*. FEMS Microbiol Lett 2001; 203:29–33.

76. Burns JW, Siadat-Pajouh M, Krishnaney AA, Greenberg HB. Protective effect of rotavirus VP6-specific IgA monoclonal antibodies that lack neutralizing activity. Science 1996; 272:104–107.

77. Bomsel M, Heyman M, Hocini H, Lagaye S, Belec L, Dupont C, Desgranges C. Intracellular neutralization of HIV transcytosis across tight epithelial barriers by anti-HIV envelope protein dIgA or IgM. Immunity 1998; 9:277–287.

78. Hickling TP, Clark H, Malhotra R, Sim RB. Collectins and their role in lung immunity. J Leukoc Biol 2004; 75:27–33.

79. Haagsman HP. Structural and functional aspects of the collectin SP-A. Immunobiology 2002; 205:476–489.

80. Wu H, Kuzmenko A, Wan S, Schaffer L, Weiss A, Fisher JH, Kim KS, McCormack FX. Surfactant proteins A and D inhibit the growth of Gram-negative bacteria by increasing membrane permeability. J Clin Invest 2003; 111:1589–1602.

81. McCormack FX, Gibbons R, Ward SR, Kuzmenko A, Wu H, Deepe GS Jr. Macrophage-independent fungicidal action of the pulmonary collectins. J Biol Chem 2003; 278:36,250–36,256.

82. Crouch E, Wright JR. Surfactant proteins a and d and pulmonary host defense. Annu Rev Physiol 2001; 63:521–554.

83. Wang JY, Shieh CC, You PF, Lei HY, Reid KB. Inhibitory effect of pulmonary surfactant proteins A and D on allergen-induced lymphocyte proliferation and histamine release in children with asthma. Am J Respir Crit Care Med 1998; 158:510–518.

84. Madan T, Kishore U, Shah A, Eggleton P, Strong P, Wang JY, Aggrawal SS, Sarma PU, Reid KB. Lung surfactant proteins A and D can inhibit specific IgE binding to the allergens of *Aspergillus fumigatus* and block allergen-induced

histamine release from human basophils. Clin Exp Immunol 1997; 110: 241–249.

85. Rogers DF. Airway goblet cell hyperplasia in asthma: hypersecretory and anti-inflammatory? Clin Exp Allergy 2002; 32:1124–1147

86. Clark H, Palaniyar N, Strong P, Edmondson J, Hawgood S, Reid KB. Surfactant protein D reduces alveolar macrophage apoptosis in vivo. J Immunol 2002; 169:2892–2899.

87. Chen CB, Wallis R. Stoichiometry of complexes between mannose-binding protein and its associated serine proteases. Defining functional units for complement activation. J Biol Chem 2001; 276:25,894–25,902.

88. Presanis JS, Kojima M, Sim RB. Biochemistry and genetics of mannan-binding lectin (MBL). Biochem Soc Trans 2003; 31:748–752.

89. Ganz T. Antimicrobial polypeptides. J Leukoc Biol 2004; 75:34–38.

90. Ganz T. Defensins: antimicrobial peptides of innate immunity. Nat Rev Immunol 2003; 3:710–720.

91. Ellison RT, Giehl TJ. Killing of gram-negative bacteria by lactoferrin and lysozyme. J Clin Invest 1991; 88:1080–1091.

92. Arnold RR, Cole MF, McGhee JR. A bactericidal effect for human lactoferrin. Science 1977; 197:263–265.

93. Hiemstra PS, Maassen RJ, Stolk J, Heinzel-Wieland R, Steffens GJ, Dijkman JH. Antibacterial activity of antileukoprotease. Infect Immun 1996; 64:4520–4524.

94. Zhu J, Nathan C, Ding A. Suppression of macrophage responses to bacterial lipopolysaccharide by a non-secretory form of secretory leukocyte protease inhibitor. Biochim Biophys Acta 1999; 1451:219–223.

95. Liu L, Zhao C, Heng HH, Ganz T. The human beta-defensin-1 and alpha-defensins are encoded by adjacent genes: two peptide families with differing disulfide topology share a common ancestry. Genomics 1997; 43:316–320.

96. Yang D, Chertov O, Bykovskaia SN, Chen Q, Buffo MJ, Shogan J, Anderson M, Schroder JM, Wang JM, Howard OM, Oppenheim JJ. Beta-defensins: linking innate and adaptive immunity through dendritic and T cell CCR6. Science 1999; 286:525–528.

97. Zanetti M. Cathelicidins, multifunctional peptides of the innate immunity. J Leukoc Biol 2004; 75:39–48.

98. Yang D, Chertov O, Oppenheim JJ. Participation of mammalian defensins and cathelicidins in anti-microbial immunity: receptors and activities of human defensins and cathelicidin (LL-37). J Leukoc Biol 2001; 9:691–697.

99. Bals R, Weiner DJ, Moscioni AD, Meegalla RL, Wilson JM. Augmentation of innate host defense by expression of a cathelicidin antimicrobial peptide. Infect Immun 1999; 67:6084–6089.

100. Le Y, Murphy PM, Wang JM. Formyl-peptide receptors revisited. Trends Immunol 2002; 23:541–548.

101. Yoshie O, Imai T, Nomiyama H. Chemokines in immunity. Adv Immunol 2001; 78:57–110.

102. Rossi D, Zlotnik A. The biology of chemokines and their receptors. Annu Rev Immunol 2000; 18:217–242.

103. Pan J, Kunkel EJ, Gosslar U, Lazarus N, Langdon P, Broadwell K, Vierra MA, Genovese MC, Butcher EC, Soler D. A novel chemokine ligand for CCR10 and CCR3 expressed by epithelial cells in mucosal tissues. J Immunol 2000; 165: 2943–2949.

104. Hieshima K, Ohtani H, Shibano M, Izawa D, Nakayama T, Kawasaki Y, Shiba F, Shiota M, Katou F, Saito T, Yoshie O. CCL28 has dual roles in mucosal immunity as a chemokine with broad-spectrum antimicrobial activity. J Immunol 2003; 170:1452–1461.

105. Field CJ, Johnson IR, Schley PD. Nutrients and their role in host resistance to infection. J Leukoc Biol 2002; 71:16–32.

106. Gershwin ME, Borchers AT, Keen CL. Phenotypic and functional considerations in the evaluation of immunity in nutritionally compromised hosts. J Infect Dis 2000; 182(suppl 1):S108–S114.

107. Keusch GT. The history of nutrition: malnutrition, infection and immunity. J Nutr 2003; 133:336S–340S.

108. Parham P. Some savage cuts in defence. Nature 1990; 344:709–710.

109. Dye C, Scheele S, Dolin P, Pathania V, Raviglione MC. Consensus statement. Global burden of tuberculosis: estimated incidence, prevalence, and mortality by country. WHO Global Surveillance and Monitoring Project. JAMA 1999; 282:677–686.

110. Chan J, Flynn J. The immunological aspects of latency in tuberculosis. Clin Immunol 2004; 110:2–12.

111. Sturgill-Koszycki S, Schlesinger PH, Chakraborty P, Haddix PL, Collins HL, Fok AK, Allen D, Gluck SL, Heuser J, Russell DG. Lack of acidification in *Mycobacterium* phagosomes produced by exclusion of the vesicular proton-ATPase. Science 1994; 263:678–681.

112. Vergne I, Chua J, Deretic V. *Mycobacterium tuberculosis* phagosome maturation arrest: selective targeting of PI3P-dependent membrane trafficking. Traffic 2003; 4:600–606.

113. Simonsen A, Lippe R, Christoforidis S, Gaullier JM, Brech A, Callaghan J, Toh BH, Murphy C, Zerial M, Stenmark H. EEA1 links PI(3)K function to Rab5 regulation of endosome fusion. Nature 1998; 394:494–498.

114. Malik ZA, Denning GM, Kusner DJ. Inhibition of Ca^{2+} signaling by *Mycobacterium tuberculosis* is associated with reduced phagosom–lysosome fusion and increased survival within human macrophages. J Exp Med 2000; 191:287–302.

115. Malik ZA, Iyer SS, Kusner DJ. *Mycobacterium tuberculosis* phagosomes exhibit altered calmodulin-dependent signal transduction: contribution to inhibition of phagosome–lysosome fusion and intracellular survival in human macrophages. J Immunol 2001; 166:3392–3401.

116. Fratti RA, Chua J, Vergne I, Deretic V. *Mycobacterium tuberculosis* glycosylated phosphatidylinositol causes phagosome maturation arrest. Proc Natl Acad Sci USA 2003; 100(9):5437–5442.

117. Fratti RA, Chua J, Deretic V. Cellubrevin alterations and *Mycobacterium tuberculosis* phagosome maturation arrest. J Biol Chem 2002; 277:17, 320–17,326.

118. Ferrari G, Langen H, Naito M, Pieters JA. Coat protein on phagosomes involved in the intracellular survival of mycobacteria. Cell 1999; 97:435–447.
119. Wojciechowski W, Desanctis J, Skamene E, Radzioch D. Attenuation of MHC Class II expression in macrophages infected with *Mycobacterium bovis* bacillus Calmette–Guerin involves class II transactivator and depends on Nramp1 gene. J Immunol 1999; 163:2688–2696.
120. Hmama Z, Gabathuler R, Jefferies WA, Dejong G, Reiner NE. Attenuation of HLA-DR expression by mononuclear phagocytes infected with *Mycobacterium tuberculosis* is related to intracellular sequestration of immature Class II heterodimers. J Immunol 1998; 161:4882–4893.
121. Ting L-M, Kim AC, Cattamanchi A, Ernst JD. *Mycobacterium tuberculosis* inhibits IFN-γ transcriptional responses without inhibiting activation of STAT1. J Immunol 1999; 163:3898–3906.
122. Noss EH, Tai RK, Sellati TJ, Radolf JD, Belisle J, Golenbock DT, Boom WH, Harding CV. Toll-like receptor 2-dependent inhibition of macrophage class II MHC expression and antigen processing by 19-kDa lipoprotein of *Mycobacterium tuberculosis*. J Immunol 2001; 167:910–918.
123. Pai RK, Convery M, Hamilton TA, Boom WH, Harding CV. Inhibition of IFN-gamma-induced class II transactivator expression by a 19-kDa lipoprotein from *Mycobacterium tuberculosis*: a potential mechanism for immune evasion. J Immunol 2003; 171:175–184.
124. Ramachandra L, Noss E, Boom WH, Harding CV. Processing of *Mycobacterium tuberculosis* antigen 85B involves intraphagosomal formation of peptide-major histocompatibility complex II complexes and is inhibited by live bacilli that decrease phagosome maturation. J Exp Med 2001; 194:1421–1432.
125. Smith S, Liggitt D, Jeromsky E, Tan X, Skerrett SJ, Wilson CB. Local role for tumor necrosis factor alpha in the pulmonary inflammatory response to *Mycobacterium tuberculosis* infection. Infect Immun 2002; 70:2082–2089.
126. Mohan VP, Scanga CA, Yu K, Scott HM, Tanaka KE, Tsang E, Tsai MC, Flynn JL, Chan J. Tumor necrosis factor-α is required to prevent reactivation and limit pathology in latent murine tuberculosis. Infect Immun 2001; 69:1847–1855.
127. Shanahan JC, St. Clair EW. Tumor necrosis factor-α blockade: a novel therapy for rheumatic disease. Clin Immunol 2002; 103:231–242.
128. Keane J, Gershon S, Wise RP, Mirabile-Levens E, Kasznica J, Schwieterman WD, Siegel JN, Braun MM. Tuberculosis associated with infliximab, a tumor necrosis factor α-neutralizing agent. N Engl J Med 2001; 345:1098–1104.
129. Shimono N, Morici L, Casali N, Cantrell S, Sidders B, Ehrt S, Riley LW. Hypervirulent mutant of *Mycobacterium tuberculosis* resulting from disruption of the *mce1* operon. Proc Natl Acad Sci USA 2003; 100:15,918–15,923.

5

Bronchoscopy: Diagnostic and Interventional Approach in Tropical Pulmonary Diseases

CARLA R. LAMB

Interventional Pulmonary Medicine,
  Pulmonary and Critical Care
  Department, Lahey Clinic Tufts
  University
Burlington, Massachusetts, U.S.A.

EDITH R. LEDERMAN

Head of Clinical Medicine, Parasitic Disease
  Program, US Naval Medicine Research
  Unit 2,
Jakarta, Indonesia

NANCY F. CRUM

Division of Infectious Disease Medicine,
  Naval Medical Center,
San Diego, California, U.S.A.

Pulmonary diseases both infectious and environmental are particularly common within the tropics generally defined as Central and South America, sub-Saharan Africa, South and Southeast Asia. These diseases are responsible for 20–40% of outpatient medical visits and hospital admissions (1). The rising population of HIV-infected individuals with associated opportunistic infections and tuberculosis accounts for a large portion of pulmonary infection in these regions. The spectrum of pulmonary diseases once found only in the tropical and subtropical arenas now are emerging in both North America and Europe due to the breadth of international travel and a rising immigrant population. Table 1 lists a number of the infectious and noninfectious pulmonary diseases encountered in tropical regions.

This chapter is meant to guide the clinician specifically in the practical application of bronchoscopy (if readily available) as a complementary procedure for diagnosis and possibly intervention when the airways may be more directly involved due to a tropical pulmonary illness. Table 1 includes notations by the diseases where bronchoscopy may have a role. More importantly, the limitations of bronchoscopy will be discussed based on

The information presented herein is the opinion of the authors and no way reflects the opinions, views, or endorsements of the U.S. Navy.

Table 1 Tropical Pulmonary Diseases

Bacterial
Tuberculosis[a]
Nocardiosis[a]
Meliodiosis[a]
Q fever
Brucellosis
Leptospirosis
Typical pathogens[a]: Streptococcus, Hemophilus, Moraxella, Staphylococcus,
   Mycoplasma, Chlamydia
Fungal
Cryptococcus[a]
Histoplasmosis[a]
Coccidioidomycosis[a]
Paracoccidioidomycosis
Penicilliosis
Aspergillosis[a]
Pneumocystic carinii[a]
Parasites
Paragonimiasis[a]
Amebiasis[a]
Echinococcosis[a]
Filariasis[a]
Strongyloidiasis[a]
Ascariasis[a]
Toxoplasmosis[a]
Hookworm[a]
Gnathostomiasis
Syngamosis[a]
Sparganosis
Schistosomiasis
Malaria
Other
Loffler's syndrome (associated with round worms/hookworms)[a]
Tropical pulmonary eosinophilia (associated with filarial parasites)[a]
Dust-induced pulmonary diseases[a]

[a]Bronchoscopy may have a role in diagnosis.

the practicality and availability of the necessary personnel, equipment, and
laboratory processing to render specimen collection and evaluation. Clearly,
such resources are limited in rural areas and sputum specimens are
obtained without bronchoscopy. Serum specimens and other body fluids
may offer the most practical means to obtain a diagnosis.

I. Tuberculosis

Mycobacterium tuberculosis infects one-third of the world's population and is
the leading cause of death (2 million annually) due to an infectious disease.
The distribution is worldwide with resurgence particularly in areas where
HIV is pandemic (2). Rates of tuberculosis occur disproportionately in
developing countries with 95% of cases and 98% of deaths in these areas.
Diagnosis is confirmed by sputum examination with acid-fast positive bacilli
exhibiting characteristic serpentine cording. Typically 10,000 organisms per
mL of sputum are necessary for smear positivity. Pulmonary specimens
acquired by bronchoscopy including washings, brushings, and transbronchial lung biopsy will render the diagnosis of tuberculosis 58–96% (average
rate of 72%) (3–6). An incidence of tuberculosis was 8.3% in a series
of 1734 patients who underwent bronchoscopy with bronchial cultures.

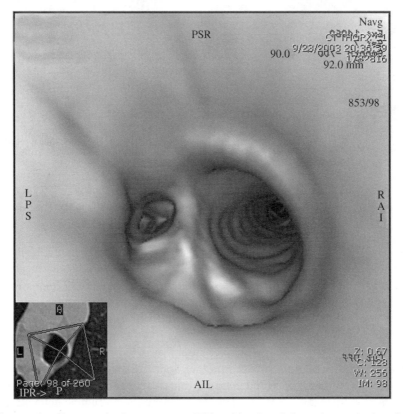

Figure 1 Computerized tomogram (CT) with virtual bronchoscopic imaging
demonstrates the left mainstem stenosis secondary to primary tuberculosis infection.

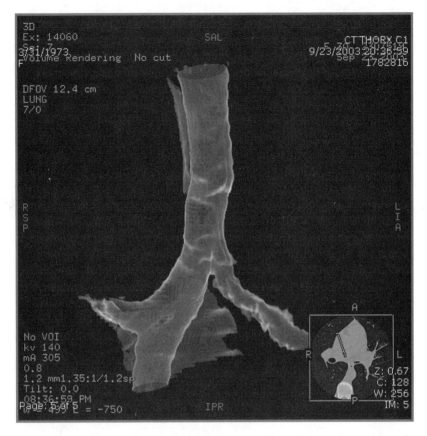

Figure 2 CT reconstruction of airway images allows for precise preprocedure planning with accurate measurements of both length and diameter of the stenotic region of the left mainstem.

Among those with identified tuberculosis, a positive bronchial culture was obtained in 82.6%. The positive bronchial culture was the only means of diagnosis in 44% (7). Some studies note that the utilization of higher doses of topical lidocaine, may have inhibited growth of the organism, thereby reducing the diagnostic yield (8). There have been mixed reviews on the added diagnostic benefits to bronchoscopic lung biopsy. While one report demonstrated that bronchoscopic biopsy was positive in only 16% of patients with infection proven by other specimen cultures, another study reported in 50 patients with positive cultures, that bronchial brushings significantly increased diagnostic yield when compared to bronchial washings alone. There was also a suggestion that bronchial lung biopsy increased immediate diagnosis due to identification of caseating granulomas (9,10).

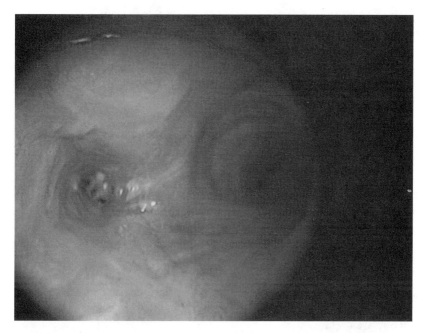

Figure 3   Left mainstem bronchial stenosis as seen through the rigid bronchoscope.

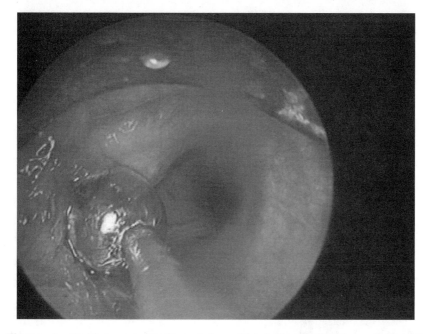

Figure 4   Rigid bronchoscopy and bronchial balloon dilatation of the left mainstem stenosis to restore the bronchial diameter and optimize the airway.

Bronchoscopy certainly increases the yield of culture diagnosis when the patient is unable to produce an adequate sputum specimen.

The broad spectrum of the bronchoscopic appearance of tuberculosis may include: normal mucosa, mucosal and submucosal granulomas, ulcerative mucosa, endobronchial polyps, tracheobronchial stenosis, and transbronchial lymphnode erosion (11–13). A number of these findings can present as airway compromise with wheezing and airway obstruction. Although less common, it is the delayed development of tracheal or bronchial stenosis despite appropriate medical therapy that requires more definitive intervention as the patient may be significantly symptomatic. Surgical resection is generally the standard approach to this problem. The patient may require a lobectomy with sleeve resection or pneumonectomy depending on the extent and location of the stenotic region. If the patient cannot undergo a surgical procedure secondary to limited pulmonary function or other comorbidities, an alternative strategy of serial balloon dilation and airway stenting can be utilized (14). Our institution employs CT scan imaging with virtual airway imaging and reconstruction to assess the extent of stenosis to allow for preprocedural planning. This is followed by rigid bronchoscopy with sequential balloon dilation and a silicone stent (Figs. 1–5).

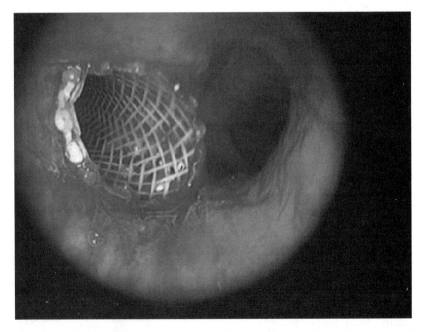

Figure 5   Silicone stent placement of the left mainstem bronchus with an optimally patent airway.

II. Melioidosis

Melioidosis due to the gram-negative bacteria, *Burkholderia pseudomallei* (formerly, *Pseudomonas pseudomallei*), causes both acute and unresolving upper lobe predominant granulomatous pneumonia acquired in Southeast Asia (especially Northeast Thailand) or Australia. This infection may lie dormant for many years and reactivate under periods of immune compromise. Late infections are most common among HIV-infected patients (14). Endobronchial lesions are rare and generally resolve with appropriate antibiotic therapy (15). Tuberculosis, malignancy, and the endemic mycoses are in the differential diagnosis. Bronchoscopy may serve two purposes in the evaluation of melioidosis: bronchoscopy washings for adequate culture of the organism and washings, brushings, and biopsy to more definitively rule out malignancy (16,17). There is one case report of an infection with B. pseudomallei occuring in an individual without a significant travel history. It was later discovered the infection occurred due to a poorly disinfected bronchoscope (18).

III. Q Fever

Coxiella burnetti is a gram-negative coccobacillus endemic worldwide with variable incidence rates among regions. Humans are infected by inhaling contaminated aerosols from zoonotic reservoirs; those working with animals such as farmers, veterinarians, and abattoir workers have the highest risk. One-half of patients will have pneumonia, although only 28% have cough (19). Lower lobe or pleural-based infiltrates are most commonly seen. Rarely pseudotumors may occur and bronchoscopy may not be helpful in establishing this diagnosis (20). While bronchoscopy with biopsy may sometimes demonstrate the organism within alveolar macrophages, the diagnosis is most often made with serologic assays.

IV. Brucellosis

Brucella melitensis has a worldwide distribution with significant rates of infection in Middle Eastern and Mediterranean countries. Humans acquire the disease from animal reservoirs by ingestion, inhalation, or through cutaneous contact (21). Although inhalation of contaminated aerosols is a known route of infection, primary pneumonia does not occur (22). Most pulmonary manifestations occur after ingestion of the organism with subsequent bacteremia and lung involvement. Cough is noted in 17–38% of adults. Less frequently, pulmonary findings include pleuritic chest pain and crackles. Miliary disease, nodules, air space opacities, adenopathy, and pleural disease can be seen (23). The organism has been isolated from sputum; however, there is no clear role for bronchoscopy. The diagnosis is usually established by blood culture or serology.

V. Leptospirosis

A spirochetal infection caused by *Leptospira interrogans,* which infects humans through skin or mucous membrane contact with contaminated water or soil. Classic disease manifestations include fever myalgias and conjunctival suffusion. Pulmonary involvement occurs in 20–70% and is usually due to vasculitis of the pulmonary capillaries resulting in hemorrhage (24). While most cases of hemorrhage are mild and self-limited, massive hemoptysis and respiratory failure are described and associated with Weil's syndrome of renal and hepatic dysfunction. Radiographic findings include a patchy alveolar infiltrate with increased lung markings (24). The diagnosis is made by serology. There is no clear role for bronchoscopy in actual diagnosis of the organism, but rather in identifying the extent and location of the pulmonary hemorrhage.

VI. Cryptococcosis

Cryptococcus neoformans is a fungal disease acquired by inhalation (Fig. 6). The organism is commonly found in pigeon droppings and in geographic areas that support growth of the red river gum tree (i.e., sub-Saharan Africa, Southern California). The most common disease manifestations are pulmonary infections and meningitis. Most pulmonary lesions are asymptomatic and are discovered incidentally. The relative lack of symptoms is due to the poor inflammatory response to the pathogen as a result of its antiphagocytic polysaccharide capsule (25). Most pulmonary infections spontaneously resolve in the immunocompetent host. The diagnosis is established by culture or by visualizing the organism on histopathology with silver, mucicarmine, or PAS stains (26). Of note, *Cryptococcus* may colonize in the respiratory tract of patients with underlying pulmonary disorders; thus, isolation alone may not represent disease (27). Bronchoscopy with bronchoalveolar lavage and biopsies are useful for diagnosis (28–30). When yeast forms are found in BAL or sputum that is suggestive of *Cryptococcus*, the cryptococcal antigen assessment on that specimen may allow for a rapid confirmation of the pathogen. Rarely, endobronchial lesions mimic malignancy and bronchoscopic biopsies assist in distinguishing the two (31). Serology (cryptococcal antigen test) is very sensitive and specific for the diagnosis.

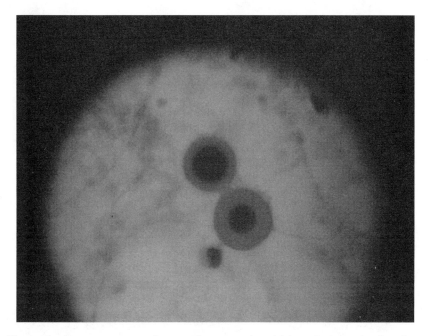

Figure 6 *Cryptococcus neoformans* demonstrating thick encapsulated cell wall.

VII. Histoplasmosis

Histoplasmosis is a common pulmonary fungal infection with a broad spectrum of pulmonary manifestations. This ranges from acute pneumonia, miliary disease, extensive calcific nodularity, and fibrosing mediastinitis. The role of bronchoscopy as a complementary diagnostic aid has been reported in a group of 469 patients with histoplasmosis, the diagnosis was established in 71 patients. Bronchoscopy was the only diagnostic method in 11% of those patients (3,32).

VIII. Coccidioidomycosis

Coccidioides immitis is a fungal infection with numerous clinical presentations. It occurs by inhalation of arthroconidia and often manifests as pneumonia. Endotracheal and endobronchial disease with or without airway obstruction has rarely been reported (33–40). Often with treatment the airway involvement will resolve; however, if there is extensive mucosal involvement and or endobronchial polyps in a patient with risk factors for refractory disease (immunocompromised, African American), then an interventional pulmonary approach may be necessary to preserve a patent airway until a full response to therapy has occurred (Fig. 7). These photos

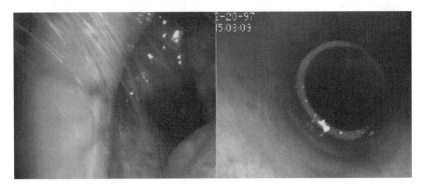

Figure 7 (*Left*) Endotracheal coccidioidomycosis with nodular infiltration and narrowing of the trachea. (*Right*) Patent trachea following silicone stent placement. *Source*: Photos courtesy of Dr. James Harrell, University of San Diego Medical Center, Interventional Pulmonology, San Diego, CA, U.S.A.

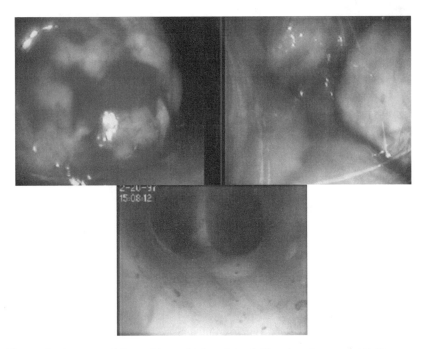

Figure 8 Extensive bilateral bronchial nodular infiltration from coccidioidomycosis. Upper photos demonstrate left and right mainstem bronchi with near occlusion. Bottom photo demonstrates Y silicone stent placement and patent airways. *Source*: Photos courtesy of Dr. James Harrell, University of San Diego Medical Center, Interventional Pulmonology, San Diego, CA, U.S.A.

demonstrate a patient who was in the miliary and was exposed to a significant "load" of coccidioidomycosis while digging a foxhole. The patient was an African American and presented with acute respiratory distress and stridor. The diagnosis was made after intubation with bronchoscopic biopsies revealing cocciodiodomycosis spherules and a positive culture. Despite amphotericin B therapy, the patient required a Y-silicone tracheobronchial stent placed via rigid bronchoscopy for airway protection (Fig. 8). This intervention provided a secure airway, allowed safe extubation and completion of several months of intravenous antifungal therapy. At the time of follow-up, both the CT scan and bronchoscopic inspection demonstrating complete resolution of the endobronchial abnormalities, the stent was removed with rigid bronchoscopy.

IX. *Pneumocystis carinii*

PCP is a common cause of severe pneumonia among immunocompromised patients worldwide. It was initially characterized as a protozoa, but further genetic studies indicated that it is a fungus. Its recently assigned new name is now *P. jiroveci.* The epidemiology of this infection has rapidly changed with the HIV epidemic. The clinical presentation includes fever, dry cough, dyspnea, and hypoxemia. Diagnosis was established by open lung biopsy until the 1980s (27). Bronchoscopy with bronchoalveolar lavage is now the diagnostic procedure of choice if induced sputum is unrevealing. Bronchoscopic specimens have a sensitivity of 55–97% (27,41). Both silver stains and direct fluorescent antibody are useful for detection of the organism in respiratory specimens. A cell count with differential of the bronchoalveolar lavage specimen is predictive of a higher morbidity and mortality when the neutrophils present are greater than 5% (42). For patients receiving pentamidine, a higher yield of organisms occurs in the upper lobes due to the poor deposition of the drug in these areas. Transbronchial biopsy may be utilized when the diagnosis is in question if the BAL is negative and the patient is not responding to empiric therapy, but this is not routinely advocated due to the risk of pneumothorax (27).

X. Paragonimiasis

Paragonimus westermani (the lung fluke) and other less common species are trematodes that may accidentally infect humans after ingestion of contaminated raw crustaceans or the flesh of wild boars (43). The disease occurs throughout the world, especially in Asia (Korea, Japan, and the Philippines), Africa (Nigeria), and South America (44). The disease is rare in the United States, but has been described with *P. kellicotti* and *P. westermani* (45,46). The worm leaves the intestine and migrates through the peritoneal space into the pleural space with the formation of an effusion. The adult worm then enters the lung parenchyma with resultant pneumonitis, pneumonia, or bronchiectasis. Cysts form in these areas and contain both living and dead worms. Pulmonary symptoms typically occur a mean of 6 months after infection (47). Fever, cough, and hemoptysis may occur with necrotic tissue resembling "iron filings" appearing in the sputum as cysts rupture. This disease is often mistaken for tuberculosis (48). Pleural manifestations include hydropneumothoraces. Radiographically, patchy airspace consolidations appearing as "cotton wool" lesions are typical (47,49). The diagnosis is established by identifying eggs in the sputum, pleural fluid, or stool. The sensitivity of multiple sputum samples is 54–89%, with most experts recommending collection of six or more samples (49). Bronchoscopy has been successful in making the diagnosis and identifying secondary complications such as bronchial stenosis (43,48,50,51). Bronchoscopy is more sensitive than routine sputum specimens for the detection of ova. Postbronchoscopy sputum samples have a higher yield of organism recovery due to presumably the dislodging of ova during the bronchial washings (43). ELISA is available for the serologic diagnosis.

XI. Amebiasis

Entamoeba histolytica infects approximately 10% of the world's population and is the third leading parasitic cause of death worldwide (52,53). The disease is most prevalent in areas of poor hygiene and sanitation. It is acquired via the fecal–oral route and the organisms reside in the colonic wall. Ninety percent of cases are asymptomatic, while 10% have invasive colitis. Dissemination to other organs, particularly the right lower lobe of the liver, lungs, or CNS, occurs in 2–20% of symptomatic cases (54). Pleuropulmonary amebiasis almost always occurs in association with liver abscess. Those with liver abscess will have pulmonary involvement in 7–20% of cases (53,55). Cough is a predominant feature while pleurisy, anchovy paste sputum production due to rupture into a bronchus, wheezing, and hemoptysis are less common (52). Lung abscess occurs due to direct transdiaphragmatic contamination from a hepatic abscess or by hematogenous spread (55). Most patients with pulmonary disease have negative stool examinations for cysts or trophozoites. Sputum demonstrates trophozoites in nearly 30% of cases in one report, whereas, the sensitivity of pleural fluid is less than 10% (56). Serologic diagnosis with ELISA is useful.

XII. Echinococcosis

Echinococcus is a cestode parasitic infection due to *Echinococcus granulosus*, which causes cystic hydatid disease. The disease is found in Africa, Asia,

South America, Australia, Central Europe, and Mediterranean countries (57). Humans are incidental hosts through accidental ingestion of eggs, usually among those with close contact to dogs or sheep. The eggs penetrate the intestinal wall gaining access to the circulation and lymphatics, which then lead to deposition in the liver (65%) and/or lungs (25%). Most cases are asymptomatic and are recognized incidentally on routing radiographic imaging (58). Symptoms may result from mechanical compression seen in bronchial tree rupture (50). The diagnosis may be established by finding protoscolices, hooklets, or membranes in the sputum or bronchial washings (58–61). The presence of a whitish-yellow membrane during bronchoscopy is suggestive (62). Bronchoscopy has been shown to be diagnostic and may prevent the need for more invasive procedures (62). In a study of 100 cases, bronchoscopy was found to show pathological changes in 70% of those undergoing the procedure (63). Rare complications such as the formation of a bronchobiliary fistula may be confirmed by bronchoscopy (64). Serology is positive in approximately one-half of cases with solitary pulmonary cysts; however, in the presence of a ruptured lesion into the bronchial tree or hepatic system the sensitivity of serology is as high as 90% (61).

XIII. Filariasis

Filariasis is a mosquito-borne nematode due to *Wuchereria bancrofti* or *Brugia malayi* endemic to Southeast Asia, Africa, and South America. Infection occurs by a mosquito bite. Clinical syndromes include tropical pulmonary eosinophilia (TPE), which is suggested by cough and wheezing with a nocturnal predominance. Diffuse miliary radiographic changes and a marked eosinophilia (>3000 cells/mm^3) are often present (65). The pathogenesis is thought to be due to immune hyper-responsiveness to the microfilarial stage of the infection. Diagnosis is difficult as microfilariae are seldom detected in the peripheral blood with TPE. Confirmation of the diagnosis may be established by visualizing the microfilariae on bronchial brushing or lung biopsy (66). They will enhance with routine BAL stains such as the Papanicolaou. The affected airways may appear edematous and hyperemic on bronchoscopy (67). A positive filarial antibody test is suggestive of the diagnosis.

XIV. Strongyloidiasis

Strongyloides stercoralis is a nematode infection with a worldwide distribution with endemicity in tropical and subtropical areas. Africa has prevalence rates of 10–50%, while in the United States the highest rates are found in the southeastern states where up to 4% are infected (68). Infection may persist for decades. Humans are infected through skin penetration

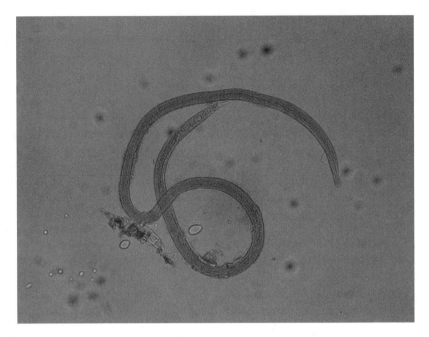

Figure 9 *Strongyloides stercoralis.*

by filariform larvae during contact with contaminated soil. The larvae spread hematogenously to the lungs following migration up the airway to the gastrointestinal tract. Acute infection, hyperinfection, and disseminated disease may involve the lungs, pleural space, and pericardium. Hypereosinophilia with pneumonia may occur during primary infection and may be confused with TPE; patients with strongyloidiasis may also have antibodies that cross-react with the filarial serologic test. Chronic infections may lead to cough, dyspnea, and wheezing, thereby simulating asthma (69). Hyperinfection occurs predominantly in immunocompromised or debilitated persons. Typically eosinophilia is absent in these cases. Diagnosis can be established by isolating adult or rhabditiform larvae in the respiratory samples, stools, and duodenal aspirates. The first step in diagnosis is stool examination, but the sensitivity is only 27–73% (68). An ELISA serology provides a presumptive diagnosis, but cross-reaction with other helminthic infections has been noted (70). The larvae, eggs, and adult worms can be noted in wet preparations, Gram stain, and Papanicolaou stain of sputum specimens (19). Bronchoalveolar lavage, bronchial brushings, and transbronchial biopsy have also been utilized for the diagnosis and in some cases, concomitantly diagnosed the underlying immunopromising condition of a pulmonary malignancy (71–74).

XV. Toxoplasmosis

Toxoplasma gondii is a coccidian parasite that can infect all mammals. Its definitive host is the feline. Although not all infection with this organism results in disease, those who are immunocompromised are most at risk for acute and disseminated manifestations. Pulmonary disease is generally only significant for the immunocompromised host. Once the oocysts are ingested, tissue invasion and dissemination of the parasite occurs. It is the tachyzoite form that can penetrate and infect nearly any type of host cell. Serologic tests such as an ELISA with IgM and IgG antibodies helps discern acute from past exposures. The clinical pulmonary syndrome in the immunosuppressed host is one of fever, cough, and dyspnea. An interstitial pneumonia, lobar consolidation, nodules, and cavities, with or without a pleural effusion, may be seen. Bronchoscopy with bronchoalveolar lavage and transbronchial biopsy may be extremely helpful due to the broad differential diagnosis of the clinical syndrome. The organisms seen in these specimens must then be distinguished from other intracellular organisms such as *Leishmania* (75).

XVI. Dirofilaria

Dirofilariasis occurs when the dog heartworm, *Dirofilaria immitis*, is transmitted via a mosquito bite to a human. Larvae may die in the skin, or hematogenously spread leading to embolization of pulmonary arterioles with resultant local thrombosis and granulomatous reaction. The resulting nodule or mass is 1–4 cm in diameter and uncalcified (76). It is generally asymptomatic and is usually diagnosed after resection of a pulmonary nodule by thoracotomy or video-assisted thoracotomy (77,78). There may be some role for transbronchial brush and biopsy, but these may be nondiagnostic due to sample size (76,79).

XVII. Syngamosis

Syngamosis, caused by the nematode *Syngamus laryngeus*, also known as the "gapeworm," is endemic to South America, the Caribbean, Korea, Thailand and the Philippines. This infection leads to chronic tracheobronchial infections in animals, particularly domestic fowl, but can occur in humans as well. Transmission to humans is not well understood nor is the lifecycle of the organism. Patients with syngamosis present with a chronic cough, wheezing, pleuritic chest pain, hemoptysis, fever, and weight loss. The parasites can easily be visualized and extracted by bronchoscopy as they reside attached to the respiratory mucosa of the trachea and bronchi (80). The ova may be visualized in bronchoscopy washings, sputum specimens, or stool samples (81). In addition to manual extraction of the worms, treatment with albendazole may be warranted (82). Worms may also be spontaneously expectorated.

XVIII. Malaria

Malaria caused by *Plasmodium falciparum*, among others, may have a number of pulmonary complications in 5–15% of cases including pulmonary edema, acute respiratory distress syndrome or secondary bacterial pneumonia (83). The diagnosis is made with Giemsa-stained blood smears with identification of the parasites. There is no known role for bronchoscopy among these cases.

XIX. Other Parasites

Migrating larval stages of schistosomiasis, *Ascaris*, or hookworm infection may cause respiratory symptoms, pulmonary infiltrates, and eosinophilia collectively described as Loffler's syndrome. *Ascaris lumbricoides* is a common helminthic parasite with a worldwide prevalence of 25% of the population; the most affected areas include Southeast Asia, Africa, and Central and South America in descending order (76). Ingestion of eggs results in the occurrence of larvae in the small intestine, which then hematogenously disseminate to the lungs. During this pulmonary phase of disease, patients develop migratory round appearing infiltrates that develop 10 days after egg ingestion and typically resolve within 7–10 days. The cause is due to an immune hypersensitivity response. Patients are generally asymptomatic, but may have cough, dyspnea, mild hemoptysis, or wheezing. *S. japonicum* can lead to chronic lung disease from ova deposition. Pulmonary disease during the intestinal phase is rare. Stool studies are typically negative during the pulmonary phase, as it takes 40 or more days for larvae in the lungs to produce eggs (76). Sputum or BAL specimens are useful in the diagnosis by demonstrating *Ascaris* larvae or *S. japonicum* ova (84).

Hookworms, *Ancyclostoma duodenale* and *Necator americanus*, have the same prevalence and route of infection as ascariasis. Migration through the lungs can cause Loffler's syndrome, but most cases are asymptomatic. Hookworm dermatitis is an important clue to the diagnosis. Patchy, transient infiltrates particularly in the hilar areas occur due to intra-alveolar hemorrhage caused by larvae migration (76). Like ascariasis, stool examination is not helpful. The diagnosis requires demonstration of larvae in respiratory or gastrointestinal secretions.

XX. Dust-Induced Interstitial Lung Disease in Tropical Environments

Although there is little published information on this entity, there are a number of diseases that bear mentioning. The inhalation of environmental dusts and associated diseases is of particular concern in India. Silicosis, in particular, is a predominant one due to the number of miners of silica, copper, mica, lead, and zinc, for example (85). Silicosis, asbestosis and coal workers' pneumoconiosis are probably the most recognized. The role of BAL with or without transbronchial lung biopsy may assist primarily by distinguishing these causes of interstitial lung diseases from infectious ones (85).

XXI. Conclusion

It is necessary for the pulmonary physician to be aware of the specific pulmonary diseases that are seen in the tropics and to also consider tropical diseases in those who have a travel history of visiting tropical regions. It is equally vital to know the bronchoscopic role or lack thereof in these diseases when trying to establish a definitive diagnosis. There is also a role for the interventional pulmonologist to preserve the airway of the patient with tracheobronchial involvement of a variety of these diseases by means of airway dilation and stenting as a bridge to more definitive therapy.

References

1. Reeder MM, Palmer PE. Acute Tropical Pneumonias. Seminars in Roentgenology, Vol XV, No 1 January 1980; 35–49.
2. Maartens G, Beyers N. Tuberculosis in the tropics. Clin Chest Med 2002; 23:341–350.
3. Cortese DA, Prakash UBS. Bronchoscopy in Pulmonary Infections. Chapter 14, Bronchoscopy. 188–189, 1994, Raven Press, Ltd.
4. Danek SJ, Bower JS. Diagnosis of pulmonary tuberculosis by flexible fiberoptic bronchoscopy. Am Rev Resp Dis 1979; 119:677–679.
5. WongthimS, Udompanich V, Linthongkul S, Sharoenlap P, Nuchprayoon C. Fiberoptic bronchoscopy in diagnosis of patients with suspected active pulmonary tuberculosis. J Med Assoc Thailand 1989; 72:154–159.
6. Baughman RP, Dohn MN, Loudon RG, Frame PT. Bronchoscopy with bronchoalveolar lavage in tuberculosis and fungal infections. Chest 1991; 99:92–97.
7. Ip M, Chau PY, So SY, Lam WK. The value of routine bronchial aspirate culture at fiberoptic bronchoscopy for the diagnosis of tuberculosis. Tubercle 1989; 70:281–285.

8. Jett JR, Cortese DA, Dines DE. The value of bronchoscopy in the diagnosis of mycobacterial disease. A five-year experience. Chest 1981; 80:575–578.
9. Stenson W, Aranda C, Bevelaque FA. Transbronchial biopsy culture in pulmonary tuberculosis. Chest 1983; 83:883–884.
10. Palenque E, Amor E, Bernaldo de-Quiros JC. Comparison of bronchial washing, brushing, and biopsy for diagnosis of pulmonary tuberculosis. Eur J Clin Microbiol 1987; 6:191–192.
11. Smith LS, Chillaci RF, Sarlin RF. Endobronchial tuberculosis. Serial Fiberop Bronchosc Nat Hist 1987; 91:644–647.
12. Albert RK, Petty TL. Endobronchial tuberculosis progressing to bronchial stenosis. Fiberoptic bronchoscopic manifestations. Chest 1976; 70:537–539.
13. Schwartz MS, Kahlstrom EJ, Hawkins DB. Airway obstruction secondary to tuberculosis lymph node erosion into the trachea: drainage via bronchoscopy. Otolaryngol Head Neck Surg 1988; 99:604–666.
14. Thummakul T, Wilde H, Tantawichien T. Melioidosis, an environmental and occupational hazard in Thailand. Mil Med 1999; 164:658–662.
15. Khoo KL, Cheng SC, Tan YK. Endobronchial mass in a patient with *Burkholderia pseudomallei* infection. Ann Acad Med (Sing) 2000; 29:108–109.
16. Bouvy JJ, Degener JE, Stinjen C, Gallee MP, van der Berg B. Septic melioidosis after a visit to Southeast Asia. Eur J Clin Microbiol 1986; 5:655–656.
17. Grosskopf S. An unusual cause of pneumonia. Austral Fam Phys 2000; 29: 552–553.
18. Markovitz A. Inoculation by bronchoscopy. West J Med 1979; 131:550.
19. Harris RA, Musher DM, Fainstein V, Young EJ, Clarridge J. Disseminated strongyloides. Diagnosis made by sputum examination. JAMA 1980; 244:65–66.
20. Lipton JH, Fong TC, Gill MJ, Burgess K, Elliott PD. Q fever inflammatory pseudotumor of the lung. Chest 1987; 92:756–757.
21. Sanford JP. Brucella pneumonia. Sem Resp Infect 1997; 12:24–27.
22. Buchanan TM, Faber LC, Feldman RA. Brucellosis in the United States, 1960–1972. an abattoir-associated disease Part 1. Clinical features and therapy. Medicine 1974; 53:403–413.
23. Patel PJ, Al-Suhaibani H, Al-Aska AK, Kolawole TM, Al-Kassimi FA. Chest radiograph in brucellosis. Clin Radiol 1988; 39:39–41.
24. Hill MK, Sanders CV. Leptospiral pneumonia. Sem Resp Infect 1997; 12: 44–49.
25. Sarosi GA. Cryptococcal pneumonia. Sem Resp Infect 1997; 12:50–53.
26. Gleason TH, Hammar SP, Barthas M, Kasprisin M, Bockus D. Cytological diagnosis of pulmonary cryptococcosis. Arch Pathol Lab Med 1980; 104:384–387.
27. Kroe DM, Kirsch CM, Jensen WA. Diagnostic strategies for *Pneumoncystis carinii* pneumonia. Sem Resp Infect 1997; 12:70–78.
28. Malabonga VM, Basti J, Kamholz SL. Utility of bronchoscopic sampling techniques for cryptococcal diseases in AIDS. Chest 1991; 99:370–372.
29. Sakowitz AJ, Sakowitz BH. Disseminated cryptococcosis. Diagnosis by fiberoptic bronchoscopy and biopsy. JAMA 1976; 236:2429–2430.
30. Whitaker D, Sterrett GF. *Cryptococcus neoformans*: a case diagnostically confirmed by transbronchial brush biopsy. Acta Cytol 1976; 20:105–107.

31. Mahida P, Morar R, Goolam Mahomed A, Song E, Tissandie JP, Feldman C. Cryptococcosis: an unusual cause of endobronchial obstruction. Eur Resp J 1996; 9:837–839.
32. Prechter GC, Prakash UBS. Bronchoscopy in the diagnosis of pulmonary histoplasmosis. Chest 1989; 95:1033–1036.
33. Winter B, Villaveces J, Spector M. Coccidioidomycosis accompanied by acute tracheal obstruction in a child. JAMA 1966; 195:125–128.
34. Ward PH, Berci G, Morledge D, Schwartz H. Coccidioidomycosis of the larynx in infants and adults. Ann Otolaryngol 1977; 86:655–660.
35. Beller TA, Mitchell DM, Sobonya RE, Barbee RA. Large airway obstruction secondary to endobronchial coccidioidomycosis. Am Rev Respir Dis 1979; 120:939–942.
36. Henley-Cohn J, Boles R, Weisberger E, Ballantyne J. Upper airway obstruction due to coccidioidomycosis. Laryngoscope 1979; 89:355–360.
37. Moskowitz PS, Sue JY, Gooding CA. Tracheal coccidioidomycosis causing upper airway obstruction in children. AJR Am J Roent 1982; 139:596–600.
38. Gardner S, Seilhemier D, Catlin F, Anderson DC, Hernried L. Subglottic coccidioidomycosis presenting with stridor. Pediatrics 1980; 66:623–625.
39. Wallace JM, Catanzaro A, Moser KM, Harrell JH. Flexible fiberoptic bronchoscopy for diagnosing pulmonary coccidoidomycosis. Am Rev Respir Dis 1981; 123:286–290.
40. Benitz WE, Bradley JS, Fee WJ, Loomie JC. Upper airway obstruction due to laryngeal coccidioidomycosis in a 5-year old child. Am J Otolaryngol 1983; 4:54–55.
41. Huang L, Hecht FM, Stansell JD, Montanti R, Hadley WK, Hopewell PC. Suspected *Pneumocystis carinii* pneumonia with a negative induced sputum examination. Is early bronchoscopy useful?. Am J Resp Crit Care Med 1995; 151:1866–1871.
42. Mason GR, Hashimoto CH, Dickman PS, Foutty LF, Cobb CJ. Prognostic implications of bronchoalveolar lavage neutrophilia in patients with *Pneumocystis carinii* pneumonia and AIDS. Am Rev Resp Dis 1989; 139:1336–1342.
43. Mukae H, Taniguchi H, Matsumoto N, Iiboshi H, Ashitani J, Matsukura S, Nawa Y. Clinicoradiologic features of pleuropulmonary *Paragonimus westermani* on Kyusu Island, Japan. Chest 2001; 120:51420.
44. Sharma OP. The man who loved drunken crabs. A case of pulmonary paragonimiasis. Chest 1989; 95:670–672.
45. Procop GW, Marty AM, Scheck DN, Mease DR, Maw GM. North American Parogonimiasis. Acta Cytol 2000; 44:75–80.
46. Scacewater R. Just another hemoptysis or a fluke?. Missouri Med 2001; 98:515–516.
47. Kagawa FT. Pulmonary paragonimiasis. Sem Resp Infect 1997; 12:1349–1358.
48. Beland JE, Boone J, Donevan RE, Mankiewicz E. Paragonimiasis (the lung fluke) and report of four cases. Am Rev Resp Dis 1969; 99:261–271.
49. Ogakwu M, Nwokolo C. Radiological findings in pulmonary paragonimiasis as seen in Nigeria: a review based on one hundred cases. Brit J Radiol 1973; 46:699–705.

50. Kilani T, Hammami SE. Pulmonary hydatid and other parasitic infections. Curr Opin Pulm Med 2002; 8:218–223.
51. Moon WK, Kim WS, Im JG, Kim IO, Yeon KM, Han MC. Pulmonary paragonimiasis simulating lung abscess in a 9-year old: CT findings. Pediatr Radiol 1993; 23:626–627.
52. Lyche KD, Jensen WA. Pleuropulmonary amebiasis. Sem Resp Infection 1991; 12:106–112.
53. Reed SL. Amebiasis: an update. Clin Infect Dis 1992; 14:385–393.
54. Bruckner DA. Amebiasis. Clin Microbiol Rev 1992; 5:356–369.
55. Kennedy D, Sharma OP. Hemoptysis in a 49 year old man. An unusual presentation of a sporadic disease. Chest 1990; 98:1275–1278.
56. Ochsner A, Debakey M. Pleuropulmonary complications of amebiasis. An analysis of 153 collected and 15 personal cases. J Thorac Surg 1939; 5:225.
57. van Lieshout L, de Jonge N, El-Masry NA, Mansour MM, Bassily S, Krijger FW, Deelder AM. Monitoring the efficacy of different doses of praziquantel by quantification of circulating antigens in serum and urine of schistosomiasis patients. Parastiol 1994; 108:519–526.
58. Vera-Alvarez J, Marigil-Gomez M, Abascal-Agorreta M. Echinococcus hooklets in sputum: sinus tract extension of a liver hydatid cyst to lung. Acta Cytol 1995; 39:1187–1189.
59. Allen AR, Fullmer CD. Primary diagnosis of pulmonary echinococcosis by the cytologic technique. Acta Cytol 1972; 16:212–216.
60. Oztek I, Baloglu H, Demirel D, Saygi A, Balkanli A, Arman B. Cytologic diagnosis of complicated pulmonary unilocular cystic hydatidosis. A study of 131 cases. Acta Cytol 1997; 41:1159–1166.
61. Oztek I, Baloglu H, Demirel D, Saygi A, Balkanli A, Arman B. Cytologic diagnosis of complicated pulmonary unilocular cystic hydatidosis. A study of 131 cases. Acta Cytol 1997; 41:1159–1166.
62. Tomb JA, Matossian RM. Diagnosis of pulmonary hydatidosis by sputum cytology. Johns Hopkins Med J 176; 139(suppl):38–40.
63. Saygi A, Oztek I, Guder M, Sungun F, Arman B. Value of fibreoptic bronchoscopy in the diagnosis of complicated pulmonary unilocular cystic hydatidosis. Eur Resp J 1997; 10:811–814.
64. Zapatero J, Madrigal L, Lago J, Baschwitz B, Perez E, Candelas J. Surgical treatment of thoracic hydatidosis. A review of 100 cases. Eur J Cardio-Thoracic Surg 1989; 3:436–440.
65. Uzun K, Ozbay B, Etlik O, Kotan C, Gencer M, Sakarya ME. Bronchobiliary fistula due to hydatid disease of the liver: a case report. Acta Chir Belg 2002; 102:207–209.
66. Ottesen EA, Nutman TB. Tropical pulmonary eosinophilia. Ann Rev Med 1992; 43:417–424.
67. Anupindi L, Sahoo R, Rao RV, Verghese G, Rao PV. Microfilariae in bronchial brushing cytology of symptomatic pulmonary lesions. Acta Cytol 1993; 37:397–399.
68. Prasad R, Goel MK, Mukerji PK, Agarwal PK. Microfilaria in bronchial aspirate. Ind J Chest Dis Allied Sci 1994; 36:223–225.

69. Wehner JH, Kirsch CM. Pulmonary manifestations of strongyloidiasis. Sem Resp Infect 1997; 12:122–129.
70. Nwokolo, C, Imohiosen EA. Strongyloidiasis of respiratory tract presenting as "asthma". Brit J Med 1973; 2:153–154.
71. Lindo JF, Conway DJ, Atkins NS, Bianco AE, Robinson RD, Bundy DA. Prospective evaluation of enzyme-linked immunosorbent assay and immunoblot methods for the diagnosis of endemic *Strongyloides stercoralis* infection. Am J Trop Med Hyg 1994; 51:175–179.
72. Rassiga AL, Lowry JL, Forman WB. Diffuse pulmonary infection due to *Strongyloides stercoralis*. JAMA 1974; 230:426–427.
73. Venizelos PC, Lopata M, Bardawil WA, Sharp JT. Respiratory failure due to *Strongyloides stercoralis* in a patient with a renal transplant. 1980; 78:104–106.
74. Williams J, Nunley D, Dralle W, Berk SL, Verghese A. Diagnosis of pulmonary strongyloides by bronchoalveolar lavage. Chest 1988; 94:643–644.
75. Gocek LA, Siekkinen PJ, Lankerani MR. Unsuspected strongyloides coexisting with adenocarcinoma of the lung. Acta Cytol 1985; 29:628–632.
76. Fishman's Pulmonary Diseases and Disorders, Alfred Fishman, Volume 1, third edition, 1998, McGraw Hill Co, Inc, 2391–2393.
77. Sarinas PSA, Chitkara RK. Ascariasis and hookworm. Sem Resp Infect 1997; 12:130–137.
78. Chitkara RK, Sarinas PS. Dirofilaria, visceral larva migrans, and tropical pulmonary eosinophilia. Sem Resp Infect 1997; 12:138–148.
79. Gomez-Merino E, Chiner E, Signes-Costa J, Arriero JM, Zaragozi MV, Onrubia JA, Mayol MJ. Pulmonary dirofilariasis mimicking lung cancer. Monaldi Arch Chest Dis 2002; 57:33–34.
80. Akaogi E, Ishibashi O, Mitsui K, Hori M, Ogata T. Pulmonary dirofilariasis cytologically mimicking lung cancer: a case report. Acta Cytol 1993; 37:531–534.
81. Birrell DJ, Moorhouse DE, Gardner MAH, May CS. Chronic cough and haemoptysis due to a nematode, "Syngamus laryngeus". Aust NZ J Med 1978; 8:168–170.
82. Leers WD, Sarin MK, Arthurs K. Syngamosis, an unusual cause of asthma: the first reported case in Canada. Can Med Assoc J 1985; 132:269–270.
83. Kim HY, Lee SM, Joo JE, Na MJ, Ahn MH, Min DY. Human syngamosis: the first case in Korea. Thorax 1998; 53:717–718.
84. Kemper CA. Pulmonary disease in selected protozoal infections. Sem Resp Infect 1997; 12:113–121.
85. Shimazu C, Pien FD, Parnell D. Bronchoscopic diagnosis of *Schistosoma japonicum* in a patient with hemoptysis. Resp Med 1991; 85:331–332.
86. Jindal SK, Aggarwal AN, Gupta D. Dust-induced interstitial lung disease in the tropics. Current Opin in Pulm Med 2001; 7(5):272–277.

6

Common Tropical Pneumonias: Diagnosis and Treatment

CARLOS M. LUNA and CARMEN FAURE

Division of Pulmonary Medicine, Hospital de Clinicas "Jose de San Martin," Universidad de Buenos Aires, Argentina

I. Introduction

Tropical climate (high temperature and humidity), but also social, economical, and cultural underdevelopment, expose people to common respiratory pathogens, and provide an ideal environment for some microorganisms, vectors, and intermediate hosts. Tropical pneumonia is defined in the present chapter as the presence of clues of parenchymal lung infection in patients who live or have traveled to, or lived in tropical zones. Due to international travels, physicians could face today in their daily practice, more often than in the past, common tropical pneumonias. History, physical exam, and complementary workout are precious tools for diagnosis that should be considered together with the geographical setting and the patient's lifestyle. Every year, millions of people travel abroad, exposing themselves to various diseases, they may return ill or become ill soon afterwards. Physicians should establish whether the disease is associated with the trip. Assessment should include geography and epidemiology.

A number of causes of pneumonia (tropical zoonoses, pulmonary complications of HIV/AIDS, malaria, typhoid fever, scrub typhus, dengue, leishmaniasis, leptospirosis, tuberculosis, mycosis, paragonimiasis, and meliodosis) are described in other chapters from this book and we refer the reader to those chapters. We will review tropical pneumonias due to common pathogens including Legionnaires' disease, community-acquired pneumonia (CAP) due to *Acinetobacter baumannii*, pneumonia due to common respiratory viruses, hanta pulmonary syndrome, Q fever, and severe acute respiratory syndrome (SARS). We will emphasize on the epidemiology, clinical presentation therapy, and prevention of those diseases in the tropical world area.

Exposition to microorganisms in tropical areas showed different patterns depending on if these infections were present in the tropics and not abroad (syphilis, appearing in Europe after Columbus' return), were not present in the tropics and arrived from abroad (small pox, introduced by the European conquerors), or were present but clinical or epidemiological characteristics were different in the tropical area (tuberculosis).

The explosive appearance of SARS in 2003 reminds us that new infectious diseases continue to emerge in the tropics and that the international public health community should take collaborative, powerful, and effective measures to protect the world population against them.

II. Legionnaires' Disease

Legionnaires' disease was first described after an outbreak of pneumonia due to *Legionella pneumophila* in people attending a convention of legionnaires in Philadelphia in 1977 (1). This etiology in community-acquired pneumonia has been recognized in the five inhabited continents of the world. There are few data on its incidence in most of the tropical countries where legionellosis is easily underdiagnosed, since the clinical manifestations are nonspecific, and specialized laboratory testing is required. This happens because of the combination of scarcity of health diagnostic resources available and a lack of interest to survey on the epidemiology in most of the countries from this world area (2,3). Travel-associated legionnaires' disease may occur and it is a concern among European countries because of morbidity among citizens of the European Union (4). Legionnaires' disease outbreaks have been reported with increased frequency among international travelers since the 1970s (5). An increasing trend of cases has been noticed since 1987. Countries in northern Europe whose tourist industries are rapidly expanding reported most of the cases associated with visits to warmer countries, especially in the older travelers who are more susceptible to infection with *Legionella* (6).

Legionella is an environmental pathogen that has found an ecologic niche in hot water supplies. Numerous studies have reported legionnaire's disease caused by *L. pneumophila* occurring in different water supplies (7). This pathogen is able to initiate a waterborne infection, the pathogen can be found in natural and treated water supplies. Water treatment technologies of standard quality have become inadequate to guarantee that water is free from this pathogen (8). This could be more serious in developing countries located in the tropical areas. Waters in marine and freshwater areas of Puerto Rico were analyzed for the presence of *Legionella* spp. by direct fluorescent antibody assay with guinea pig confirmation; several species, including *L. pneumophila*, were widely distributed among all sites and found in high densities in water collected in the rain forest from epiphytes in trees 9.25 m above the ground. *L. pneumophila* was the most abundant species at all sites, with average densities of 10^4/mL, very close to the range, which is potentially pathogenic for humans. Its density in sewage-contaminated coastal waters was the highest ever reported for marine habitats; density of *L. pneumophila* is positively correlated with concentrations of sulfates, phosphates, and pH. A survey of 88 fatal atypical pneumonia cases in Puerto Rico showed that 15% of the patients had *L. pneumophila* infections (9).

Outbreaks of *L. pneumophila* infection occur among travelers in camps, cruise ships, and hotels and represent about 15% of the reported cases of legionaries' disease (4,10–13). In one investigation of the source of infection in an outbreak happened in a cruise ship from New York to Bermuda, water samples from the ship, from sites on Bermuda, and from the ship's water source in New York City were cultured for legionellae and examined with PCR, identified 50 passengers with legionnaire's disease and that the exposure to whirlpool spas was the more probable source disease (odds ratio 16.2, 95% CI 2.8–351:7) (14).

A. Clinical Presentation

The initial reports of *Legionella* infection presented a picture of a severe pulmonary infection with extrapulmonary manifestations (15). In the first cases mortality was 21%, because *L. pneumophila* was unknown as a pathogen. Subsequent studies revealed *L. pneumophila* infection is not readily distinguishable from pneumonias caused by other organisms on the basis of clinical presentation. The incubation period is 2–10 days after exposure. Patients may experience prodromes as malaise, fever, chills. Ninety percent are febrile at presentation, respiratory failure requiring ventilatory support occurs in 15–50% of patients (16). Most of the patients with *L. pneumophila* infection have radiographic infiltrates on presentation. The initial infiltrate is alveolar and may appear segmental, lobar, patchy, or diffuse (3). Over the course of the first several days, the infiltrates tend to progress and involve additional lobes sometimes (Fig. 1A and B), this may occur after the institution of appropriate antibiotic therapy and does not necessarily indicate a therapeutic failure, but has been associated with an increased risk of mortality (17). Clearing of infiltrates tends to be slow. In the immunocompromised patients, cavity formation and pleural effusion are common (3).

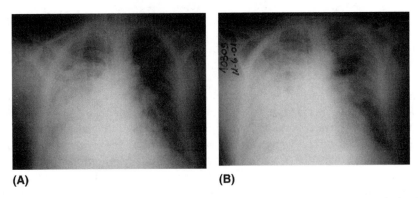

(A) **(B)**

Figure 1 (**A**) Initial chest X ray in a 56-year-old CPOD male who was admitted because of pneumonia. The patient was the employee in a building and was on charge of repairing the heater system taking contact with the water supply and with the spray of water coming from the water system. There are extensive bilateral infiltrates, ceftriaxone was instituted. (**B**) The second chest X ray obtained 24 hours later demonstrate a significant increase of density in both lungs, concomitant with a clinical deterioration. Mechanical ventilation was instituted and the diagnosis of *Legionella pneumophila* pneumonia was confirmed after the positivization of the immunochromatographic antigen in urine and the indirect immunofluorescence test in BAL fluid.

Specialized laboratory tests are the key for diagnosing this infection. Culture of the organism is the most important test, but needs to be done on selective media. Sensitivity of other tests, including direct fluorescent antibody, urinary antigen test, and serology, ranges between 25% and 90%. Fourfold conversion of antibody test (serology) and positivity of urinary antigen have a specificity of 100% (18).

B. Treatment

Newer macrolides (especially azithromycin) and quinolones (ciprofloxacin, levofloxacin, gatifloxacin, and moxifloxacin) are the antibiotics of choice for legionnaires' disease. The antibiotics are usually prescribed on admission, most of the cases before the confirmation of diagnosis, so the initial empirical antimicrobial therapy should include the just mentioned antibiotics by the initial time. Gastrointestinal dysfunction commonly seen in legionnaires' disease may compromise the absorption of oral antibiotics; thus, parenteral administration is prudent on admission. Duration of therapy is 10–14 days, longer duration could be appropriate for the immunosuppressed patients (3).

C. Prevention

The assessment for control measures against *Legionella* bacteria proliferation should be carried out in response to a cluster, but also on a regular basis, in order to prevent cases of disease. In one study, investigations and control measures were successful in preventing further cases in 31 out of 35 accommodation sites investigated (19). In legionnaire's disease linked to travel on a cruise ship, investigations confirmed the source to be the ship's water system and control measures were instituted that included pasteurization, super chlorination, and chlorine dioxide dosing. The Public Health Laboratory Service Communicable Disease Surveillance Centre identified three previous cases associated with the same ship's water system including one fatality (11).

III. Community-Acquired Pneumonia Due to *Acinetobacter baumannii*

Acinetobacter baumannii is an aerobic gram-negative nonfermenting bacillus, ubiquitous in soil and fresh water. This microorganism is a frequent skin commensal in healthy people (20), it is also a well-recognized pathogen of nosocomial pneumonia, particularly when there are conditions increasing the risk of appearance of multiresistant microorganisms (tracheal intubation, prolonged mechanical ventilation, and prior broad-spectrum antibiotic therapy) (21–23). Bacteria of the genus *Acinetobacter* have become increasingly important as nosocomial pathogens. They compromise at least 21 DNA groups identified by DNA–DNA hydrolyzation methods.

Community-acquired pneumonia due to *A. baumannii* (CAAP) is very unusual, there have been less than 100 cases reported in the literature, most of the cases were associated with underlying conditions producing debilitating illness and with a high mortality rate (about 50%) (24–30). It occurs predominantly in men, and is often associated with underlying conditions such as cigarette smoking, alcohol abuse, diabetes mellitus, and chronic pulmonary diseases (31).

Taking into account the previously mentioned epidemiologic characteristics, CAAP cases have been much more commonly reported in tropical areas, especially during the wet season. CAAP is considered a major cause of community-acquired pneumonia in tropical northern Australia, accounting for 10% of cases and 20% of deaths from bacteremic community-acquired pneumonia (25). The reason why CAAP is much more common in tropical areas may be that skin and pharyngeal carriage of *A. baumannii* is common in tropical environments but negligible in other geographic areas, being isolated from the skin of near 4% of people in Hong Kong during the hot humid season (32).

A. Clinical Presentation

In a retrospective study, chart, and radiographic reviews of all patients who were admitted to national Taiwan University Hospital from January 1993 to

August 1999 fulfilled the criteria for CAP and had isolate of *A. baumannii* from blood or pleural fluid at hospital admission. In 13 patients who were included, 85% acquired the infection during the warmer months of April to October, 92% had devastating course presenting with septic shock and respiratory failure, and 85% needed ventilatory support, and 46% had leukopenia. Lobar consolidation was found in 92% and pleural effusion was present in 31% of cases.

All patients had positive blood culture results, two (15%) had positive pleural effusion cultures, and nine patients (69%) had positive sputum cultures. The outcome was troublesome as 62% died (30). *A. baumannii* should be considered as a possible etiologic agent in community-acquired lobar pneumonia when patients with a fulminating course present during the warmer and more humid months of the year, and in young alcoholics.

Microbiological identification in blood or sputum can be difficult because of frequent misinterpretation and possible confusion with *Staphylococcus* spp. or *Haemophilus influenzae* or *Neisseriae*. A good sputum smear, defined as a gram stain smear of an adequate sputum specimen that comes from the lower respiratory tract and contains >25 leukocytes per high power (100×) field on microscopic examination, can help early diagnosis and treatment.

B. Treatment

Early antibiotic therapy is required because of the fulminant clinical course, with approximately 50% fatality rate (31). Antimicrobial susceptibility of *A. baumannii* when isolated as a causative microorganism of community-acquired pneumonia appears to be much better than for those strains isolated from patients with nosocomial infections. In one series, all the isolates were susceptible to imipenem; and around 70% were sensitive to both, aminoglycosides, fluoroquinolones, extended spectrum penicillins, and ceftazidime. Interestingly, all the isolates were resistant to aztreonam (30). Adequate initial empiric antimicrobial therapy appears to be essential, as happens with ventilator-associated pneumonia due to *A. baumannii* (23), a mortality rate of near 90% was observed in those patients who did not receive initial adequate antibiotic therapy, while it was 20% in those receiving initial adequate antibiotic therapy.

C. Prevention

There exist plenty of data about the prevention of nosocomial *A. baummanii* pneumonia but not of the community-acquired presentation. Community-acquired pneumonia should be suspected in patients living in some tropical areas during the hot wet season, if there are some antecedents like cigarette smoking, alcohol abuse, diabetes mellitus, or chronic pulmonary diseases; avoidance of such risk factors should be advisable for prevention. Suspected cases should be reported immediately to local public health authorities so that public health measures can be taken.

IV. Respiratory Viruses

The respiratory viruses implicated in lower respiratory tract infections include influenza viruses, respiratory syncytial virus (RSV), parainfluenza virus, and rinovirus. The commonest viruses associated with community-acquired pneumonia in adults are influenza viruses and RSV. The high density of populations and insufficient sanitary conditions increases the risk to acquire viral diseases in tropical areas (33). The etiology and pathology of viral and bacterial respiratory pathogens are similar in industrialized and developing countries (34,35). Several studies have evaluated the seasonal trends of viral respiratory tract infections in tropical countries. In temperate climbs, there are distinct seasonal peaks in the winter months. Despite the absence of a winter season in tropical countries, consistent seasons of infection, albeit less distinct, have been observed (36). With few exceptions, RSV and influenza infections have been observed mainly during the rainy seasons in Asian, African, and South American tropical countries (37).

Respiratory Syncytial Virus Infections

RSV originally recovered from a colony of chimpanzees with coryza and designated chimpanzee coryza agent has been known primarily as respiratory pathogens in young children. They are now recognized as important pathogens in adults as well. Adults infected with these viruses tend to have more variable and less distinctive clinical findings than children, and the viral cause of the infection is often unsuspected. The consistency of the annual outbreaks of these agents and the frequency of reinfection suggest that they impose a considerable, but ill-defined, disease burden throughout life. The increasing number of patients who receive intense immunosuppression after undergoing transplantation of bone marrow and solid organs has highlighted the role of RSV as a potential opportunistic pathogen (38).

RSV infections accounted for 72% of respiratory tract viral outbreaks in two large general hospitals in Singapore in one study performed between September 1990 and September 1994 (36). The RSV trends were associated with higher environmental temperature, lower relative humidity and higher maximal day-to-day temperature variation (6). This is confirmed by a study of the epidemiology of RSV infection in tropical and developing countries. RSV was found to be the most common cause of acute lower respiratory tract infections in children, with an average of 65% of cases requiring hospital treatment (39). Infection is seasonal, occurring most frequently in the cold season in areas with temperate and Mediterranean climates and in the wet season in tropical countries with seasonal rainfall (March–August). The etiologic factors were associated with environmental parameters such as temperature and humidity, thus accounting for the seasonal trends in disease outbreaks.

Influenza

Influenza is a major cause of annual epidemics and intermittent pandemics throughout the world. It continues to be a significant cause of illness in all age groups. The antigenic composition of the neuraminidase and hemagglutinin of the viral surface is different between different viral populations. There are three different hemagglutinins (H1, H2, and H3), additionally two neuraminidases (N1 and N2) have been described in human influenza A virus. The possibility of a new pandemic of influenza is related with the appearance of a new virus antigenically different to the three described in human beings (H1N1, H2N2, and H3N2). This so-called antigenical shift has been recently faced with the introduction of H5N1, an avian influenza virus type A, in Hong Kong. The close contact between humans and animals, especially pigs and birds in some tropical areas, is believed to potentiate transfer of new genetically reassorted influenza virus into the human population. In addition, domestic and migrating birds may also play a role in transferring new strains to humans. Reports of human cases of H5N1, during 1997, prompted the destruction of millions of chickens in Hong Kong and southern China. Influenza A H5N1 infection is characterized by fever, respiratory symptoms, and lymphopenia and carries a high risk of death (33–80%). Although the described cases of the infection appears to have been acquired directly from infected poultry, the potential exists for genetic reassortment with human influenza viruses and the evolution of human-to-human transmission (40). Two recent cases of influenza virus type A, H9N2 in Hong Kong highlight the potential of avian influenza strains to cause human illness and trigger a pandemic (41,42). This supports the theory of chronic avian infection among migrating birds in Asia as a reservoir for new influenza strains.

Travel-associated infections with influenza have been well documented. Clearly, outbreaks occur in large groups on cruises, airplanes, and tour groups associated with droplets spread by close contact within such groups. National influenza surveillance is undertaken by countries worldwide, and such surveillance can determine the spread of disease in tropical countries as well (43).

The increase combined with the short times taken to cross borders has allowed for the faster transmission of infectious diseases such as influenza for which travelers are the carriers of disease. Consistent seasonal variations were observed with influenza A virus (peaks in June, December–January), influenza and parainfluenza viruses represented 11% of cases in one study (36).

A. Clinical Presentation

RSV: Among children, RSV infection is the cause of 50–90% of hospitalizations for bronchiolitis, 5–40% of those for pneumonia, and 10–30% of those for tracheobronchitis (44). Primary RSV infections are rarely asymptomatic. Clinical manifestations of RSV infections in young adults are mainly limited to the upper respiratory tract. Nonproductive cough is commonly reported. Mild symptoms have been seen in the elderly with RSV infection. They tend to mimic those reported with influenza virus infection, with 50% having fever and 40% having lower respiratory tract symptoms. Up to 10% of patients will have pneumonia. Bacterial cultures are often positive in these pneumonia cases, so the role of RSV in causing the pneumonia is not totally clear (45).

Diagnosis of RSV relies on culture, immunofluorescent or EIA antigen detection, Reverse-transcriptase-polymerase chain reaction (RT-PCR), or serology. Culture, IFA and EIA techniques are far more sensitive in infants than in adults (46). Both IgM and IgG assays are available with mixed success. IgM assays are difficult to standardize and guarantee reliability.

Influenza: Diagnosis of influenza is usually made clinically once a local outbreak is documented. However, simultaneous influenza viruses type A and B may occur and other common respiratory viruses, such as RSV and rhinoviruses, can be isolated during epidemics. Specific diagnosis can be made using standard viral culture of nasopharyngeal washes, throat swabs, or sputum. Initial detection takes approximately 48 hours and an additional 3 to 6 days to make specific identification. New rapid diagnostic assays are becoming available. RT-PCR will detect noninfectious viruses and lead to rapid viral typing (47). Office-based rapid antigen detection kits are now available. Sensitivity and specificity range from 60% to 95% and 52% to 99%, respectively.

B. Treatment

RSV: Specific antiviral therapy with aerosolized ribavirin is less well studied in adults than in infants (48). Because the mortality rates in bone marrow transplant recipients is so high, use of ribavirin plus immunoglobulin treatment has been reported in several patients with some improved outcomes. Only controlled studies can answer the real utility of these antiviral agents for this infection.

Influenza: Antiviral medications for influenza (Table 1). Amantadine and rimantadine act by inhibiting uncoating of the influenza virion after the virus enters the host cell, they inhibit influenza type A but not type B strains. They must be taken daily throughout the period of exposure to prevent infection. Rimantadine differs from amantadine in having a lower risk of central nervous system side effects and less frequent dose adjustments with renal impairment. Resistance to these drugs may occur. Antiviral therapy has been expanded with the addition of the neuraminidase inhibitors (oseltamivir and zanamivir). These newer antivirals are active against both A and B strains. The cost of the neuraminidase inhibitors is higher and their safety profile and efficacy better than for amantadine and rimantadine. Both kinds of antivirals will shorten the duration of symptoms by 50% if given within 48 hours of the onset of illness.

C. Prevention

RSV: There is no vaccine available for RSV. Development of safe and effective RSV vaccines should be a priority, especially for use in high-risk adults.

Influenza: Prevention of influenza by annual vaccination using an inactivated vaccine against a mixture of two type A and one type B virus strains is recommendable. Vaccine formulations contain the inactivated strains that had been circulating during the previous epidemic and change frequently because of mutations in the hemagglutinin or neuraminidase antigens. The benefits of annual influenza vaccination have been tested in all age groups, although it is recommended only for the population at risk. Different studies demonstrate that it is cost effective and prevents serious complications and death.

Table 1 Comparison of the Different Antiviral Drugs Used to Treat and Prevent Influenza Virus Infection

Characteristic	Anti-M protein	Neuraminidase inhibitors
Drugs	Amantadine and rimantadine	Oseltamivir and zanamivir
Prophylaxis or treatment of influenza A	+++	+++
Prophylaxis or treatment of influenza B	No	+++
Oral absorption	Good	Good (oseltamivir)
Gastrointestinal adverse effects	++	+ (oseltamivir)
Bronchoconstriction (inhaled powder)	−−	+ (zanamivir)
Central nervous system effects	+++ amantadine	+
	++ rimantadine	
Resistance acquisition	++	+

V. Hanta Pulmonary Syndrome

Hantaviruses, transmitted from rodents to human beings, can cause the hantavirus pulmonary syndrome (HPS) described in 1993 in the southwestern United States (49–53). HPS was identified as a seemingly new human infectious disease caused by variants of hantaviruses: Sin Nombre virus, Bayou virus, New York virus, and Black Creek Canal virus. Like other tropical infectious diseases that can be found in other chapters in this book, HPS is one of the so-called zoonoses. HPS is primarily an infection of rodents that can be transmitted to man. According to the clinical outcome, this viral infection belongs to the group of viral zoonoses that produce hemorrhagic fever. Hemorrhagic fevers are rare in visitors of tropical areas.

This infectious disease has an influenza-like prodromal stage, but can progress to a catastrophic hemodynamic failure and pulmonary edema. In 1994, isolated cases of HPS were reported in Brazil, followed by nearly 20 cases in Paraguay, Bolivia, Argentina, and Uruguay (54). In 1995, an epidemic outbreak began in the southern part of Argentina and Chile (55). HPS is not essentially a tropical disease, but can appear in tropical areas (approximately 200 cases of this emergent disease were reported in Brazil until August 2002, with a 40% fatality rate) and is associated with the exposure to the virus that can occur during travels. A high index of suspicion, detailed investigation of the travel, and exposure history of the patient, and a basic understanding of the incubation periods and distributions of the various reservoirs of hemorrhagic fever viruses are imperative, as are prompt notification and laboratory confirmation (56).

At autopsy the lungs of patients with HPS are edematous. Hyaline membranes with little cellular debris are usually present. An interstitial in filtrate with mononuclear cells is present, but it is not common to find polymorphonuclear parenchymal infiltrate.

A. Clinical Presentation

The HPS induced by the *Sin Nombre* virus infection is characterized by an initial prodrome phase lasting 3 to 6 days, with fever, myalgias, malaise, and headache. Thereafter, respiratory symptoms and shock appear suddenly, pulmonary edema due to plasma extravasation, vascular volume is reduced and the hematocrit rises. Disseminated intravascular coagulation associated with thrombocytopenia is common and patients may die from bleeding. Mortality is greatest in the first 24 hours of this phase, pulmonary edema and shock last between 3 and 6 days. Patients who survive enter the diuretic phase of the illness and then enter in the convalescent phase that may last as long as 6 months.

All patients with HPS have abnormal chest radiographic findings including Kerley B lines, hiliar indistinctness, or peribronchial cuffing

(Fig. 2A), all of these indicating pulmonary interstitial edema. Later, with the worsening of the clinical picture, patients develop air space edema that usually begins in the dependent regions and then progresses outward (Fig. 2B). Pleural effusion is present in nearly all HPS patients (Fig. 2B).

Hematologic findings include thrombocytopenia, leukocytosis with left shift, and hemoconcentration with high hematocrit. Elevation of the alveolar–arterial oxygen gradient is common.

The diagnosis is confirmed by identification of antibodies to *Sin Nombre* virus antigens or by the detection of viral RNA in blood mononuclear cell preparation, using RT-PCR (57,58).

B. Therapy

During the last years, the outcome of HPS has improved; this better survival rate is attributable to a better recognition of the less severe cases and an improved medical management of those more severe. There is no specific medical therapy for this infection and therapeutic measures are entirely

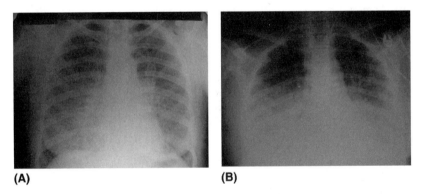

(A)   **(B)**

Figure 2   (A) Initial chest X ray in a 35-year-old previously healthy female who was admitted because of pneumonia and orthostatic hypotension. The female was an administrative employee and began with fever, malaise, and myalgia 2 days before admission. Pulse oximetry of the female was 85%, white blood cells count 6500, with only few scattered rales. Intravenous ceftriaxone + chlarytromycin was instituted. General condition of the female worsened and was admitted to the ICU. (B) After admission, mechanical ventilation was instituted and hypotension was managed with intravenous fluids. The second chest X ray obtained 10 hours later demonstrate dramatic changes while severe hypoxemia ensued (PaO2/FIO2 = 95). Hantavirus infection was confirmed by serology after 24 hours from admission. The female stayed on mechanical ventilation during 5 days with progressive improvement. The female had no known contact with the common epidemiological antecedent of hanta pulmonary syndrome, but probably acquired the infection 2 weeks before during a trip to a rural tourist resort 100 km away from Buenos Aires.

supportive, including vasoactive drugs and mechanical ventilation. The initial empiric therapy should include antimicrobials for severe community-acquired pneumonia, including coverage of *P. carinii* and other pathogens that could be present in the geographic area of concern (plague, leptospirosis, etc.).

The combination of severe capillary leak and myocardial insufficiency with shock mandate to treat these patients monitoring the oxygenation begin invasive mechanical ventilation when required, monitoring the cardiovascular function using a Swan–Ganz catheter maintaining a low wedge pressure (8–12 mmHg) and satisfactory cardiac index (>2.2 L/min/m^2). Some authors suggested that modification of the immune response using corticosteroids could be of benefit in this syndrome, but this has not been systematically demonstrated in clinical trials (59). Severe cardiac arrhythmias can occur, if these arrhythmias are associated with electromechanical dissociation they are accompanied by a poor outcome and aggressive therapy including extracorporeal membrane oxygenation (ECMO) could be recommended. Ribavirin has been used empirically taking into account that the family Bunyaviridae has been sensitive in vitro to this antibiotic. This effectivity has not been demonstrated in clinical trials up to this date (59,60).

C. Prevention

Infection in rodents does not cause disease but is believed to result in life-long carriage of virus with prolonged seeding in urine, feces, and saliva. Transmission to humans occurs via inhalation of aerosolized rodent excreta; consequently, rodents and their excreta must be avoided. Although there have not been documented cases of person-to-person transmission of the Sin Nombre virus, there is evidence from the South American variety of the virus (Andes virus) that suggest that it may be indeed transmissible (Fig. 3) and then respiratory isolation of cases should be recommended (61,62).

VI. Q Fever

Q fever is the other zoonosis that can produce community-acquired pneumonia and is not mentioned in other chapters of this book. Q fever is caused by *Coxiella burnetii*, an intracellular obligate bacterium. This spore-forming microorganism is a small gram-negative coccobacillus. The most common animal reservoirs are goats, cattle, sheep, cats, and occasionally dogs.

The animal Q fever is sometimes designated "coxiellosis." The organism reaches high concentrations in the placenta of infected animals. Aerosolization occurs at the time of parturition and infection follows inhalation of this aerosol. The acute disease varies in severity from minor to fatal, with the possibility of serious complications.

Pneumonia is one of three common clinical syndromes that result from the illness; the other two are nonspecific febrile illness and hepatitis. There is a chronic form of Q fever, almost always manifested as endocarditis but that

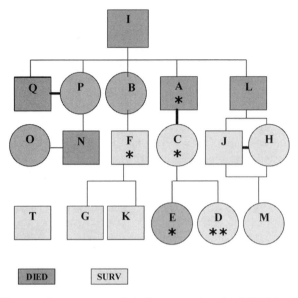

Figure 3 Cluster of cases occurred during an outbreak of HPS in the area of El Bolson in the south of Argentina (*Males = squares; females = circles*). Most of the cases have had different kind of contact between them (*thin lines*) or were spouses (*wide lines*) and lived in the geographic area of El Bolson, but there were some evidences that suggested that the South American variety of the virus responsible of this outbreak (Andes virus) could be also transmitted via person to person: five of the 16 cases occurred in physicians (*), and one of them (case D) (**) happened in one physician after her contact with another physician, who had HPS, while the physician was hospitalized critically ill in Buenos Aires (about 1500 km away from the endemic area). *Source*: From Refs. 61, 62.

occasionally could manifest itself as hepatitis, osteomyelitis, or endovascular infection.

The presentation can range from very mild pneumonia to severe pneumonia, requiring mechanical ventilation. Q fever was described in 1935 as an outbreak of febrile illness among abattoir workers in Brisbane, Australia (63). Since then, this infection has been shown to be present worldwide.

A. Clinical Presentation

In a clinical study carried out in the southern area of the Spanish Gran Canaria island, 59 Q fever cases were reported between 1998 and 2000; 65% happened from January to July; The commonest finding was elevation of hepatic enzymes (87.5%), only 7.5% of cases developed pneumonia (64). Other presentations included pneumonia and hepatitis (5%), arthritis

(2.5%), and acute glomerulonephritis (2.5%). Multiple round opacities are a common finding on chest radiography (65).

In pneumonia, the most frequent complains were cough, chest pain, and round opacities in chest radiography (64).

Symptoms of Q fever pneumonia include, headache, cough, pleuritic chest pain, myalgia, arthralgia, most patients are febrile. The spectrum of illness due to Q fever pneumonia ranges from very mild to very severe.

About 25% of patients with Q fever pneumonia have an elevated white blood cell count. Lymphopenia is common. Thrombocytopenia may be present in 10% of the patients at the time of presentation; however, thrombocytosis is not uncommon during the course of the illness. Occasionally, platelet counts of 1 million/mL are seen. A low serum sodium concentration may occur, usually as a result of inappropriate secretion of antidiuretic hormone. Mild alteration of liver function tests is not uncommon. Microscopic hematuria is present in about 50% of patients with Q fever pneumonia. A variety of autoantibodies have been described in acute Q fever, including antimitochondrial, anticardiolipin, and anti-smooth muscle antibodies. Although in cat-associated Q fever in Nova Scotia, Canada, multiple rounded opacities are a hallmark of Q fever pneumonia, in most instances, however, there is nothing distinctive about the radiographic appearance of Q fever pneumonia.

Diagnosis of Q fever is based on isolation of the agent in cell culture, its direct detection, namely by PCR, and serology. Detection of high phase II antibodies titles 1–3 weeks after the onset of symptoms and identification of IgM antibodies are indicative to acute infection. High phase I IgG antibody titles >800 as revealed by microimmunofluorescence offer evidence of chronic *C. burnetti* infection (65).

The indirect immunofluorescence antibody test is best. A fourfold or greater rise in antibody between acute and convalescent samples is diagnostic. In general, a 2-week interval between the acute and convalescent sample is sufficient. Diagnosis based on a single serum sample is not ideal; however, a phase II IgM titer of more than 1:64 or a phase II IgG titer of more than 1:256 is strong evidence of recent *C. burnetii* infection, using the indirect immunofluorescence assay (IFA) test (65). *C. burnetii* can be isolated in embryonated eggs or in tissue culture. Most laboratories are not able to work with *C. burnetii* because of its extreme infectiousness. The shell vial technique is useful for isolating *C. burnetii* and for determining antibiotic susceptibility. *C. burnetii* has been isolated from the blood of 15% of patients with Q fever pneumonia sampled prior to antibiotic therapy (using tissue culture in a shell vial technique) and during the first few days of disease, and in 50% of patients with Q fever endocarditis (65).

Polymerase chain reaction can be used to amplify *C. burnetii* DNA from tissue (65).

B. Treatment

For acute Q fever pneumonia, the treatment of choice is doxycycline
100 mg twice daily for 10 days. Alternative therapies are a fluoroquinolone
(particularly one of the newer respiratory fluoroquinolones) or a macrolide
plus rifampin. Susceptibility to macrolides is variable. In a real-time polymerase chain reaction assay using a murine macrophage cell line after 6
days of treatment, tetracycline, rifampin, and ampicillin significantly inhibited the replication of *C. burnetii*, while chloramphenicol and ciprofloxacin
did not (65).

C. Prevention

A combination of hygiene measures, natural immunizations produced by
exposition in the workplace, and vaccination constitute the major measures
of prophylaxis. Application of live vaccines, obtained on the basis of
attenuated and recombined strains (which have a full-scale set of specific
antigens) are recommended (66).

VII. SARS

In November 2002, the first case of what was to become known as the severe
acute respiratory syndrome (SARS) was identified in Guangdong province,
located below the Tropic of Cancer in China. The number of cases reported
in this original area and in surrounding places (geographically tropical) is
much higher than the cases reported in other world areas like Europe and
North America (Fig. 4). The dramatic spread of SARS appeared to herald
the onset of a new infectious disease that would become endemic worldwide.
However, almost as quickly as it spread, it was brought under control. Much
has been learned in the intervening time about SARS and its causative agent,
SARS-associated coronavirus (SARS-CoV).

After an incubation period of approximately 14 days, the illness has a
relatively insidious onset with uncommon upper respiratory tract symptoms
followed by lower respiratory tract symptoms worsening slowly but steadily
during the first 10 to 15 days. The viral load is initially low, reaches a peak
during the second week, and appears to be higher in patients with more
severe disease. In children, the viral load, the degree of infectivity, and the disease itself are apparently milder. This may explain why no transmission has
been identified from patients in whom symptoms have not yet developed
and why in most cases transmission has occurred in hospitals. There is a
heterogeneity in the risk of transmission; airplane flights in which infection
in one single passenger resulted in illness in more than 10% of the other
passengers, whereas no known disease was transmitted by four symptomatic
SARS passengers on another similar flight (67). In all the 2003 outbreaks, a

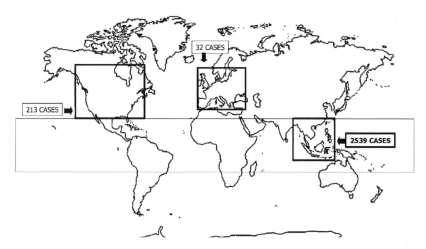

Figure 4 Planisphere showing the location of the cases of SARS reported during the 2003 epidemics in different world areas. It can be appreciated that there were 2539 cases in the tropical area of southeast Asia (mainly in the Guangdong province in China and surrounding places). These figures are in contrast with the 32 cases reported in Europe and the 213 cases reported in North America (United States and Canada).

minority of patients were associated with the majority of the transmitted cases, including cases that were transmitted despite the implementation of infection-control precautions (68).

For future outbreaks, the challenge is to be prepared for an early recognition. The reservoir for SARS-CoV may include humans in special settings as in hospitals, laboratories, and animals (68). It is unlikely that a human reservoir currently exists, as SARS-CoV has not spread from person to person at a rate that would allow its persistence in the general population, there is no evidence that the disease is infectious more than 10 days after the resolution of fever or that patients with SARS have chronic or relapsing infection that might result in the transmission of the virus to other people. Laboratories that continue to work with SARS-CoV are potential sources of infection; there have been few cases of SARS that resulted of a laboratory accident (69,70). It is vital when one is working with SARS-CoV to adhere to the biosafety guidelines established by the World Health Organization. Thus, animals represent the most important potential reservoir for disease. SARS-CoV–like viruses have been isolated from Himalayan palm civets found in a live-animal market in Guangdong province (71). But the findings to date are not sufficient to permit the identification of either the natural reservoir of SARS or the animal responsible for cross-species transmission to humans.

A. Clinical Presentation

Infected people present initially with fever, myalgia, malaise, and chills. Cough is a common finding, but other respiratory signs and symptoms appear later in the course of the illness. Upper respiratory track findings are not common, a watery diarrhea occurs in some cases. Initial laboratory findings lack any specificity and do not permit discrimination from other common causes of community-acquired pneumonia (72). Chest radiograph and/or CT scan are abnormal in most of the patients showing ground-glass opacities and focal consolidation as the commonest findings (73,74). One-third of patients improve and the resting two-thirds have persistent fever, increasing shortness of breath tachypnea, desaturation, and worsening of the physical signs and radiographic abnormalities. About 25% of the patients require admission to an intensive care unit and require mechanical ventilation. Those patients with worst outcome eventually develop severe respiratory failure, multiple organ failure, sepsis, or intercurrent medical illness (75).

SARS is a viral pneumonia that progresses rapidly. The initial manifestations do not permit its clinical differentiation from other acute community-acquired pneumonias. The occurrence of lower respiratory disease, in epidemiologically linked clusters of patients raises the level of suspicion but is not unique to SARS. Diseases such as influenza can cause similar outbreaks. The case definition of SARS has been refined over time. During a hospital outbreak in Hong Kong, an emergency-room study showed that the initial case definition of suspected SARS that was published by the WHO had a sensitivity of 26% and a specificity of 96% (76). Additional cases were uncovered through daily clinical and radiographic follow-up evaluation of epidemiologically linked patients who did not meet a sufficient number of criteria to satisfy the case definition. Given the lack of characteristic clinical features associated with SARS, the definition of cases had to rely heavily on the contact history of known patients (77).

B. Therapy

Patients with suspected SARS are initially treated empirically with broad-spectrum antibacterial drugs that are effective against other agents that acute community-acquired pneumonia to exclude these diagnoses. Before the causative agent was known, ribavirin was used by some as a broad-spectrum empirical antiviral agent for the treatment of patients with SARS (75,77,78). There are a number of potential targets for antiviral drugs in the replication cycle of SARS-CoV, including fusion inhibitors and protease inhibitors (79). The availability of the full genome sequence of the virus provides the basis for targeted strategies to develop antiviral drugs and vaccines.

Some patients have deterioration during the second week of illness in spite of a decreasing viral load, and it has been suggested that part of the damage to the lungs may be immunopathologic in nature (77). Some have reported that early therapy with regimens of high-dose methylprednisolone is useful in modulating the damage to the lungs, but no data from randomized, placebo-controlled trials are available to confirm a clinical benefit.

C. Prevention

Measures took by health authorities and the care providers to contain the spread of SARS included isolation of exposed people, restricting hospital visits, and adopting new infection-control procedures at all levels of the health care system. There may persist nosocomial transmission to patients and visitors.

VIII. Summary

L. pneumophila, *A. baumannii*, common respiratory viruses, hantavirus, *C. burnetti,* and SARS-CoV may produce pneumonia in people who live or have traveled to tropical zones. History, including geography and epidemiology, physical exam and complementary workout are precious tools for their diagnosis, therapy and prevention. Exposition to microorganisms in tropical areas may show different patterns.

L. pneumophila is able to initiate a waterborne infection and has been found in natural and treated water supplies in the tropics. Legionellosis is underdiagnosed in most of the tropical countries, because of the scarcity health diagnostic resources available and lack of specialized laboratory testing and of interest to survey on its epidemiology in the area.

CAP due to *A. baumannii* is unusual, most of the cases have been reported in tropical areas (in northern Australia, accounted of 10% of cases and 20% of deaths from bacteremic CAP), especially during wet season. It is associated with underlying conditions producing debilitating illness and has mortality rate of about 50%. Early adequate initial empiric antimicrobial therapy is essential.

High density of population and insufficient sanitary conditions increases the risk to acquire viral pneumonias due to influenza virus and RSV in the tropical area. Seasonal trends in tropical countries are different because of the absence of a winter season. Viral pneumonias are observed mainly during the rainy seasons in Asian, African, and South American tropical countries.

Hanta pulmonary syndrome can progress to a catastrophic hemodynamic failure and pulmonary edema. In 1994, isolated cases of HPS were reported in Brazil, followed by nearly 20 cases in Paraguay, Bolivia, Argentina, and Uruguay, and then an epidemic outbreak began in the southern part of Argentina and Chile. HPS can appear in tropical areas and is associated with the exposure to the virus that can occur during travels.

Q fever was described in 1935 as an outbreak of febrile illness among abattoir workers in Brisbane, Australia. Since then, this infection has been shown to be present worldwide.

The last common tropical pneumonia described was SARS. The explosive appearance of this disease in 2003 reminds us that new infectious diseases continue to emerge in the tropics and that the international public health community should take collaborative, powerful, and effective measures to protect world population against them.

A high index of suspicion, detailed investigation of travel, and exposure history of the patient, and a basic understanding of the incubation periods and distributions of the various pathogens that may produce common pneumonias in the tropics, are imperative for the diagnosis.

References

1. Fraser DW, Tsai TR, Orenstein W, Parkin WE, Beecham HJ, Sharrar RG, Harris J, Mallison GF, Martin SM, McDade JE, Shepard CC, Brachman PS. Legionaries' disease: description of an epidemic of pneumonia. N Engl J Med 1977; 297:1189–1196.
2. Luna CM. *Legionella pneumonia* an unusual fact in Argentina. Different epidemiology or marker of under-developement? Medicina (Buenos Aires) 1999; 59:311.
3. Murder RR, Yu VL. Legionella. In: Sarosi G, Glasroth J, Niederman MS, eds. Respiratory Infections. Philadelphia: Lippincott Williams & Wilkins, 2001: 413–423.
4. Jarraud S, Reyrolle M, Riffard S, Lo Presti F, Etienne J. Legionnaire's disease in travellers. Bull Soc Pathol Exot 1998; 91:486–489.
5. Lane CR, Joseph CA, Bartlett CR. European surveillance of travel associated legionnaire's disease 1996. Eurosurveillance 1998; 3:6–9.
6. Zuckerman JN. Imported tropical respiratory tract infections. Curr Opin Pulm Med 1999; 5:164–167.
7. Leclerc H, Schwartzbrod L, Dei-Cas E. Microbial agents associated with waterborne diseases. Crit Rev Microbiol 2002; 28:371–409.
8. States SJ, Conley LF, Kuchta JM, Oleck BM, Lipovich MJ, Wolford RS, Wadowsky RM, McNamara AM, Sykora JL, Keleti G, Yee RB. Survival and multiplication of *Legionella pneumophila* in municipal drinking water systems. Appl Environ Microbiol 1987; 53:979–986.
9. Ortiz-Roque CM, Hazen TC. Abundance and distribution of Legionellaceae in Puerto Rican waters. Appl Environ Microbiol 1987; 53:2231–2236.
10. Habib NA, Behrens RH. Respiratory infections in the traveler. Curr Opin Pulm Med 2000; 6:246–249.

11. Regan CM, McCann B, Syed Q, Christie P, Joseph C, Colligan J, McGaffin A. Outbreak of legionnaire's disease on a cruise ship: lessons for international surveillance and control. Commun Dis Pub Health 2003; 6:152–156.
12. Castellani Pastoris M, Lo Monaco R, Goldoni P, Mentore B, Balestra G, Ciceroni L, Visca P. Legionnaire's disease on a cruise ship linked to the water supply system: clinical and public health implications. Clin Infect Dis 1999; 28:33–38.
13. Guerrero IC, Filippone C. A cluster of legionnaire's disease in a community hospital—a clue to a larger epidemic. Infect Control Hosp Epidemiol 1996; 17:177–178.
14. Jernigan DB, Hofmann J, Cetron MS, Genese CA, Nuorti JP, Fields BS, Benson RF, Carter RJ, Edelstein PH, Guerrero IC, Paul SM, Lipman HB, Breiman R. Outbreak of legionnaire's disease among cruise ship passengers exposed to a contaminated whirlpool spa. Lancet 1996; 347:494–499.
15. Kirby BD, Snyder KM, Meyer RD, Finegold SM. Legionnaire's disease: report of sixty-five nosocomially acquired cases of review of the literature. Medicine (Baltimore) 1980; 59:188–205.
16. Woodhead MA, Macfarlane JT. Legionnaire's disease: a review of 79 community acquired cases in Nottingham. Thorax 1986; 41:635–640.
17. el-Ebiary M, Sarmiento X, Torres A, Nogue S, Mesalles E, Bodi M, Almirall J. Prognostic factors of severe Legionella pneumonia requiring admission to ICU. Am J Respir Crit Care Med 1997; 156:1467–1472.
18. Waterer GW, Baselski VS, Wunderink RG. Legionella and community-acquired pneumonia: a review of current diagnostic tests from a clinician's viewpoint. Am J Med 2001; 110:41–48.
19. Rota MC, Caporali MG, Massari M. European Guidelines for Control and Prevention of Travel Associated Legionnaire's Disease: the Italian experience. Euro Surveill 2004; 9. Epub ahead of print.
20. Rosenthal SL. Sources of *Pseudomonas* and *Acinetobacter* species found in human culture material. Am J Clin Pathol 1974; 62:807–811.
21. Glew RH, Moellering RC Jr, Kunz LJ. Infections with *Acinetobacter calcoaceticus* (*Herellea vaginicola*): clinical and laboratory studies. Medicine 1977; 56:79–97.
22. Forster DH, Daschner FD. *Acinetobacter* species as nosocomial pathogens. Eur J Clin Microbiol Infect Dis 1998; 17:73–77.
23. Luna CM, Vujacich P, Niederman MS, Vay C, Gherardi C, Matera J, Jolly EC. Impact of BAL data on the therapy and outcome of ventilator associated pneumonia. Chest 1997; 111:676–685.
24. Glick LM, Moran GP, Coleman JM, O'brien CF. Lobar pneumonia with bacteremia caused by *Bacterium anitratum*. Am J Med 1959; 27:183–186.
25. Anstey MN, Currie BJ, Withnall KM. Community-acquired *Acinetobacter pneumonia* in the northern territory of Australia. Clin Infect Dis 1992; 14:83–91.
26. Achar KN, Johny M, Achar MN, Menon NK. Community-acquired *Acinetobacter pneumonia* with survival. Postgrad Med J 1993; 69:934–937.
27. Bick JA, Semel JD. Fulminant community-acquired *Acinetobacter pneumonia* in a healthy woman. Clin Infect Dis 1993; 17:820–821.

28. Bilgic H, Akin ES, Tasan Y, Ekiz K, Seber O. A case of *Acinetobacter calcoaceticus* pneumonia. Thorax 1995; 50:315–316.

29. Yang CH, Chen KJ, Wang CK. Community-acquired *Acinetobacter pneumonia*: a case report. J Infect 1997; 35:316–318.

30. Chen M-Z, Hsueh P-R, Lee L-N, Yu C-J, Yang P-C, Luh K-T. Severe community-acquired pneumonia due to *Acinetobacter baumannii*. Chest 2001; 120: 1072–1077.

31. Drault JN, Herbland A, Kaidomar S, Mehdaoui H, Olive C, Jouanelle J. Community-acquired *Acinetobacter baummmanii* pneumonia. Ann Fr Anesth Reanim 2001; 20:795–798.

32. Chu YW, Leung CM, Houang ET, Ng KC, Leung CB, Leung NY, Cheng AF. Skin carriage of acinetobacters in Hong Kong. J Clin Microbiol 1999; 37:2962–2967.

33. Hufert FT, Schmitz H. Virus diseases in patients returning from the tropics. Ther Umsch 1994; 51:569–576.

34. Ehrengut W, Sarateanu DE, AgRhaly A, Koumare B, Simaga SY, Diallo D. Prevalence of antibodies against respiratory viruses in children of Koulikoro (Mali). Tropenmed Parasitol 1984; 35:119–122.

35. Goyenechea A, Bello M, Savon C, Masa AM, Roges G. Serologic study for determining the circulation of respiratory viruses in Havana City. Rev Cubana Med Trop 1992; 44:198–204.

36. Chew FT, Doraisingham S, Ling AE, Kumarasinghe G, Lee BW. Seasonal trends of viral respiratory tract infections in the tropics. Epidemiol Infect 1998; 121:121–128.

37. Shek LP, Lee BW. Epidemiology and seasonality of respiratory tract virus infections in the tropics. Paediatr Respir Rev 2003; 4:105–111.

38. Whimbey E, Ghosh S. Respiratory syncytial virus infections in immunocompromised adults. Curr Clin Top Infect Dis 2000; 20:232–255.

39. Weber MW, Mulholland EK, Greenwood BM. Respiratory syncytial virus infection in tropical and developing countries. Trop Med Int Health 1998; 3:268–280.

40. Hien TT, Liem NT, Dung NT, San LT, Mai PP, Chau NN, Suu PT, Dong VC, Mai LTQ, Thi NT, Khoa DB, Phat LP, Truong NT, Long HT, Tung CV, Giang LT, Tho ND, Nga LH, Tien NTK, San LH, Tuan, LV, Dolecek C, Thanh TT, de Jong M, Schultsz C, Cheng P, Lim W, Horby P, the World Health Organization International Avian Influenza Investigative Team, Farrar J. Avian influenza A (H5N1) in 10 patients in Vietnam. N Engl J Med 2004; 350(12):1179–1188.

41. Mase M, Imada T, Sanada Y, Etoh M, Sanada N, Tsukamoto K, Kawaoka Y, Yamaguchi S. Imported parakeets harbor H9N2 influenza A viruses that are genetically closely related to those transmitted to humans in Hong Kong. J Virol 2001; 75:3490–3494.

42. Peiris M, Yuen KY, Leung CW, Chan KH, Ip PL, Lai RW, Orr WK, Shortridge KF. Human infection with influenza H9N2. Lancet 1999; 354:916–917.

43. Lassalle C, Grizeau P, Isautier H, Bagnis O, Michault A, Zeller H. Epidemiological surveillance of grippe and dengue. Reunion, 1996. Bull Soc Pathol Exot 1998; 91:61–63.

44. Hall CB, McCarthy CA. Respiratory syncytial virus. In: Mandell GL, Dolin R, eds. Mandell, Douglas, and Bennett's Principles and Practice of Infectious Diseases, B.J. Philadelphia: Churchill Livingstone, 2000:1782–1801.
45. Greenberg SB. Respiratory viral infections in adults. Curr Opin Pulm Med 2002; 8:201–208.
46. Munoz FM, Galasso GJ, Gwaltney JM Jr, Hayden FG, Murphy B, Webster R, Wright P, Couch RB. Current research on influenza and other respiratory viruses: II international symposium. Antiviral Res 2000; 46:91–124.
47. Linde A. The importance of specific virus diagnosis and monitoring for antiviral treatment. Antiviral Res 2001; 51:81–94.
48. Dominguez KD, Mercier RC. Treatment of RSV pneumonia in adults: evidence of ribavirin effectivenss? Ann Pharmacother 1999; 33:739–741.
49. Hullinghorst RL, Steer A. Pathology of epidemic hemorrhagic fever. Ann Intern Med 1953; 38:77–101.
50. Kessler WH. Gross anatomic features found in 27 autopsies of epidemic hemorrhagic fever. Ann Intern Med 1953; 38:73–76.
51. Lukes KJ. The pathology of thirty-nine cases of epidemic hemorrhagic fever. Am J Med 1959, 1954; 16:639–650.
52. Duchin JS, Koster FT, Peters CJ, Simpson GL, Tempest B, Zaki SR, Ksiazek TG, Rollin PE, Nichol S, Umland ET, Moolenaar RL, Reef SE, Nolte KB, Gallaher MM, Butler JC, Breiman RF, for The Hantavirus Study Group. Hantavirus pulmonary syndrome: a clinical description of 17 patients with a newly recognized disease. N Engl J Med 1994; 330:949–955.
53. Hallin G, Simpson SQ, Crowell RE, James DS, Koster FT, Mertz GJ, Levy H. Cardiopulmonary manifestations of hantavirus pulmonary syndrome. Crit Care Med 1996; 24:252–258.
54. Weissenbacher MC, Cura E, Segura EL, Hortal M, Baek LJ, Chu YK, Lee HW. Serological evidence of human hantavirus infection in Argentina, Bolivia and Uruguay. Medicina (B Aires) 1996; 56:17–22.
55. Padula PJ, Colavecchia SB, Martinez VP, Gonzalez Della Valle MO, Edelstein A, Miguel SD, Russi J, Riquelme JM, Colucci N, Almiron M, Rabinovich RD. Hantavirus pulmonary syndrome outbreak in Argentina: molecular evidence for person-to-person transmission of Andes virus. Virology 1998; 241:323–330.
56. Bausch DG, Ksiazek TG. Viral hemorrhagic fevers including hantavirus pulmonary syndrome in the Americas. Clin Lab Med 2002; 22:981–1020.
57. Jenison S, Yamada T, Morris C, Anderson B, Torrez-Martinez N, Keller N, Hjelle B. Characterization of human antibody responses to four corners hantavirus infections among patients with hantavirus pulmonary syndrome. J Virol 1994; 68:3000–3006.
58. Hjelle B, Spiropoulou CF, Torrez-Martinez N, Morzunov S, Peters CJ, Nichol ST. Detection of Muerto Canyon virus RNA in peripheral blood mononuclear cells from patients with hantavirus pulmonary syndrome. J Infect Dis 1994; 170: 1013–1017.
59. Levy H. Hantavirus infection. In: Niederman MS, ed. Respiratory Infections, G.S.a.J.G. Philadelphia: Lippincott Williams and Wilkins, 2001:445–455.
60. Chapman LE, Mertz GJ, Peters CJ, Jolson HM, Khan AS, Ksiazek TG, Koster FT, Baum KF, Rollin PE, Pavia AT, Holman RC, Christenson JC,

Rubin PJ, Behrman RE, Bell LJ, Simpson GL, Sadek RF. Intravenous ribavirin for hantavirus pulmonary syndrome: safety and tolerance during 1 year of open-label experience. Ribavirin Study Group. Antivir Ther 1999; 4:211–219.

61. Padula PJ, Edelstein A, Miguel SD, Lopez NM, Rossi CM, Rabinovich RD. Epidemic outbreak of hantavirus pulmonary syndrome in Argentina. Molecular evidence of person to person transmission of Andes virus. Medicina (B Aires) 1998; 58(suppl 1):27–36.

62. Pinna DM, Martinez VP, Bellomo CM, Lopez C, Padula P. New epidemiologic and molecular evidence in favour of interhuman transmision for the Sout linaje of Andes hantavirus. Medicina (B Aires) 2004; 64:43–46.

63. Derrick EH. 'Q' fever, new fever entity: clinical features, diagnosis and laboratory investigation. Med J Aust 1937; 2:281–299.

64. Bolanos M, Santana OE, Perez-Arellano JL, Angel-Moreno A, Moreno G, Burgazzoli JL, Martin-Sanchez AM. Q fever in Gran Canaria: 40 new cases. Enferm Infect Microbiol Clin 2003; 21:20–23.

65. Marrie TJ. *Coxiella burnetti* pneumonia. Eur Respir J 2003; 21:713–719.

66. Hutson B, Deaker RA, Newland J. Vaccination of cattle workers at risk of Q fever on the north coast of New South Wales. Aust Fam Physician 2000; 29:708–709.

67. Olsen SJ, Chang HL, Cheung TY, Tang AF, Fisk TL, Ooi SP, Kuo HW, Jiang DD, Chen KT, Lando J, Hsu KH, Chen TJ, Dowell SF. Transmission of the severe acute respiratory syndrome on aircraft. N Engl J Med 2003; 349:2416–2422.

68. Low DE, McGeer A. SARS—one year later. N Engl J Med 2003; 349:2381–2382.

69. Normile D. Infectious diseases. Second lab accident fuels fears about SARS. Science 2004; 303:26.

70. Senior K. Recent Singapore SARS case a laboratory accident. Lancet Infect Dis 2003; 3:679.

71. Guan Y, Zheng BJ, He YQ, Liu XL, Zhuang ZX, Cheung CL, Luo SW, Li PH, Zhang LJ, Guan YJ, Butt KM, Wong KL, Chan KW, Lim W, Shortridge KF, Yuen KY, Peiris JS, Poon LL. Isolation and characterization of viruses related to the SARS coronavirus from animals in southern China. Science 2003; 302:276–278.

72. Muller MP, Tomllinson C, Marrie T. Discriminative ability of laboratory parameters in severe acute respiratory syndrome (SARS). In: 43rd ICAAC, Chicago, September 14–17, 2003.

73. Wong KT, Antonio GE, Hui DS, Lee N, Yuen EH, Wu A, Leung CB, Rainer TH, Cameron P, Chung SS, Sung JJ, Ahuja AT. Severe acute respiratory syndrome: radiographic appearances and pattern of progression in 138 patients. Radiology 2003; 228:401–406.

74. Wong KT, Antonio GE, Hui DS, Lee N, Yuen EH, Wu A, Leung CB, Rainer TH, Cameron P, Chung SS, Sung JJ, Ahuja AT. Thin section CT of severe acute respiratory syndrome. Evaluation of 73 patients exposed to or with the disease. Radiology 2003; 228:395–400.

75. Tsui PT, Kwok ML, Yuen H, Lai ST. Severe acute respiratory syndrome: clinical outcome and prognostic correlates. Emerg Infect Dis 2003; 9:1064–1069.

76. Rainer TH, Cameron PA, Smit D, Ong KL, Hung AN, Nin DC, Ahuja AT, Si LC, Sung JJ. Evaluation of WHO criteria for identifying patients with severe acute respiratory syndrome out of hospital: prospective observational study. BMJ 2003; 326:1354–1358.
77. Peiris JS, Yuen KY, Osterhaus AD, Stohr K. The severe acute respiratory syndrome. N Engl J Med 2003; 349:2431–2441.
78. Lee N, Hui D, Wu A, et al. A major outbreak of severe acute respiratory syndrome in Hong Kong. N Engl J Med 2003; 348:1986–1994.
79. Holmes KV, Enjuanes L. Virology: the SARS coronavirus: a postgenomic era. Science 2003; 300:1377–1378.

7

Pleural Effusions in the Tropics

ARUNABH TALWAR, SHRADDHA TONGIA, and ALAN M. FEIN

Division of Pulmonary and Critical Care Medicine, Department of Internal Medicine,
North Shore University Hospital,
Manhasset, New York, U.S.A.

The warm climate and general socioeconomic status in tropical countries provide an ideal environment for pathogenic organisms, their vectors and intermediate hosts to flourish. Tropical pulmonary infections are the leading cause of infection-attributable morbidity and mortality and many of them may present with significant pleural involvement.

In addition, international travel and changing immigration patterns have made tropical diseases part of the scope of medicine throughout the world (1). Each year millions of travelers visit tropical countries and many spend time in the areas where they are at risk for infectious diseases (2). Today, it is essential for any practicing physician to be aware of the common tropical lung diseases. Particularly, while evaluating pulmonary infections in a returned traveler, a thorough understanding of common organisms, their epidemiology, and their modes of presentation are required.

Pleural effusions may be seen more frequently in developing regions than in developed regions and the etiological spectrum is more varied (3). A common etiology is *Mycobacterium tuberculosis* either as pleural disease with or without pulmonary involvement (4). Parapneumonic effusions and empyema are common complications of pneumonia due to *S. pneumoniae*,

Streptococcus pyogenes, *S. aureus*, and *Klebsiella pneumonia*. However, other pathogens like parasitic protozoa and helminthes can also cause pleural disease syndromes unfamiliar to practicing physicians and may result in delay in diagnosis and management.

In addition, any syndrome associated with edema may also cause pleural effusion: cardiac failure, cirrhosis of the liver, hypoproteinemia, endomyocardial fibrosis, and neoplastic diseases should also be considered in the tropical settings. This review of the common tropical pleuropulmonary disorders is necessarily selective, primarily focusing on organisms causing pleural diseases specifically in the tropics, mainly tuberculous pleural effusions and parasitic pleural effusions.

I. Tuberculous Pleural Effusion

In the last two decades, there has been a significant rise in the prevalence of tuberculosis worldwide (5). Many factors have contributed to this increase including increase in aging population, the development of drug-resistant strains of *Mycobacterium tuberculosis* and the rising number of people with immunosuppression from HIV infection (6). Pleural tuberculosis is one of the most frequent extrapulmonary manifestations of tuberculosis (7).

A. Epidemiology

Tuberculous pleural effusion is a result of discharge of mycobacterial antigens into the pleural space. It may be a sequel to a primary infection 6–12 weeks prior or it may represent reactivation tuberculosis (8). In the past, tubercular pleural effusions were most commonly seen in children and young adults after a primary tuberculous infection. Lately, an upward shift in the age spectrum is seen and most effusions are now associated with reactivation disease and often occur in association with underlying pulmonary parenchymal disease (9).

B. Pathogenesis

Tuberculous pleural effusion occurs when a small subpleural focus of *M. tuberculosis* ruptures into the pleural space initiating an interaction between the bacilli and pleural mesothelial cells, macrophages and CD4+ T lymphocytes. The clinical syndrome is a reflection of an in situ delayed hypersensitivity reaction (10,11). Recent studies suggest a role for mesothelial cells in the pathogenesis of tubercular pleuritis (12). Mycobacterial antigens mediate chemokine expression in these cells and result in release of interleukins (IL1 to IL6) tumor necrosis factor-alpha (TNF-α), α and β chemokines. Alpha chemokine [IL8 and neutrophil activating protein (NAP-2)] are chemotactic for neutrophils and lymphocytes, while β chemokines [macrophage inflammatory protein-1 (MAP-1) and mononuclear chemoattractant protein-1 (MCP-l)] are chemotactic for monocytes and macrophages (13–16). The stimulated CD4 lymphocytes in the pleura produce interferon gamma (IFN-γ) (10) and this along with TNF-α help differentiate macrophages into epithelioid and giant cells leading to granuloma formation. Downregulating cytokines for this reaction seem to be transforming growth factor-β (TGF-β) and 1,25-dihydroxyvitamin D (17). TGF-β is an immunosuppressive cytokine and a potent modulator in tissue repair. It suppresses TNF-α and IFN-γ released by inflammatory cells. The levels of TGF-β are significantly elevated in tuberculous pleural effusion as compared to the nontuberculosis pleural effusion and may play an important role in regression of granulomatous inflammation and promotion of pleural fibrosis by stimulating mesothelial cells and fibroblasts (10).

Compared with peripheral blood, pleural fluid is enriched with T lymphocytes. The CD-4 (helper-inducer) to CD-8 (suppressor/cytotoxic) ratio is 3:4 in pleural fluid compared with 1:7 in blood (18). In fact, lymphocyte percentages above 85% are very suggestive of tuberculous pleuritis (19).

The intense inflammatory reaction obstructs the lymphatic pores in the parietal pleura, resulting in accumulation of protein and fluid in the pleural cavity (20,21). This is likely to be the primary pathogenic mechanism in tuberculous effusions.

C. Clinical Features

Most patients complain of pleuritic chest pain followed by nonproductive cough and dyspnea. Although tuberculosis is generally a chronic disease, tuberculous pleural effusion most often manifests as an acute illness. Infrequently, the onset may be less acute with mild chest pain, low-grade fever, cough, weight loss, and anorexia. Tuberculous pleural effusion is almost always unilateral and is usually small to moderate in size, although massive effusion can also occur. Loculation of an effusion prolongs the illness. In tropical countries, tuberculosis is a common cause of loculated effusion (22). Most patients with tuberculous pleuritis have a positive PPD (7), although up to 59% will be negative in AIDS patients (23,24).

D. Diagnosis

Radiologically, patients have a unilateral small to moderate size pleural effusion. The coexistence of associated pulmonary abnormalities on chest radiography is reported in 9–50% of cases (7,25). The diagnosis of tuberculosis pleural effusion depends upon the demonstration of acid-fast bacilli in the pleural fluid or pleural biopsy specimens or presence of caseous granulomas in the pleura.

Pleural Fluid Examination

Pleural fluid is typically straw-colored with a high protein content and with marked lymphocytosis (19). Lower protein content may be found in patients with acquired immunodeficiency syndrome (AIDS). The presence of a greater than 5% mesothelial cells and eosinophils in significant number (greater than 10%) provides a strong evidence against the diagnosis of tuberculosis (26). Pleural fluid pH is usually higher than 7.3 and pleural fluid glucose concentration is not significantly decreased (27). A larger volume of fluid removed during thoracentesis can enhance detection of the mycobacteria. The fluid can be centrifuged to enrich and concentrate the organism. The sensitivity of pleural fluid culture varies from 23% to 86% and sensitivity of needle pleural biopsy culture varies from 39% to 71% (26,27). The culture yield is same with conventional culture method and BACTEC^{TM} system, but is rapid with the latter technology (28). Bedside inoculation of pleural fluid provides more positive results than laboratory inoculation (28).

Polymerase chain reaction (PCR) can be utilized for diagnosis and also for determining the drug susceptibility (29). In pleural fluid, various investigators have reported disparate results with PCR (sensitivity 61–94% and specificity 78–100%) (30,31). However, until these tests are standardized they are still considered as investigative tools and further data are needed to establish its sensitivity and specificity.

Pleural Biopsy

The finding of nercotizing caseous granuloma in biopsy specimens is the most efficient test (51–87.8%) (9,26,27,32). The combined yield of direct acid-fast stains of pleural fluid and biopsy tissue coupled with mycobacterial culture exceeds 90% (32). The pleural biopsy procedure has potential disadvantages of pneumothorax and needle breakage. Moreover, patchy involvement of pleura may result in an inconclusive biopsy. Recently, ultrasound (US) -guided trucut needle biopsy and video-assisted thoracoscopic (VATS) pleural biopsy are being utilized to increase the sensitivity. These procedures allow detection of patchy pleural involvement, which resulted in inconclusive biopsy with the standard needle biopsy technique (33).

Enzymes and Cytokines

In recent years, there has been considerable effort to investigate the usefulness of diverse pleural fluid tests in the diagnosis of tuberculous pleuritis (34). However, in our opinion, only adenosine deaminase (ADA) and IFN-γ have shown diagnostic utility.

Adenosine deaminase (ADA) is the enzyme that downregulates the amount of toxic purines in lymphocytes by catalyzing the conversion of adenosine and deoxyadenosine into inosine and deoxyinosine, respectively. There are two isoenzymes of ADA: ADA1 composed of two dimers, ADA1c and ADA1m, is found in all cells; the cellular origin of ADA2 is uncertain although it is mainly found on monocytes and macrophages. The pleural fluid in tuberculous pleurisy primarily contain ADA2, whereas that of empyema contain ADA1 (25).

The pleural fluid adenosine deaminase is a good marker of pleural tuberculosis and is produced by monocytes (35). In different series, its sensitivity ranges from 90% to 100% (36–39). Almost all patients with tubercular pleuritis have an ADA level of above 40 U/L (21). The high diagnostic yield does not appear to decrease in HIV-positive patients (38). False-positive results can be seen in pyothorax, lung cancer, lymphoma, and pleural mesothelioma. False-negative ADA occurs when a tubercular pleurisy patient has either inadequate immune response or is in an early stage of the disease (40). A ratio of ADA1/ADA (cut off value 0.4) may also help improve sensitivity and specificity of the test (41).

Elevated pleural fluid IFN-γ can also be used as a marker for the diagnosis of tuberculosis (42). When a cut off value of 140 pg/mL is used, a sensitivity is 74–100% and specificity is 91–100% (42,43). The ratio of pleural fluid IFN-γ to serum IFN-γ is also significantly higher in tuberculous versus malignant effusions (44). False positives have been described in lymphomas and other malignancies. The test is however expensive and often requires special processing and delays diagnosis.

E. HIV and Tuberculosis Pleural Effusion

The incidence of extrapulmonary tuberculosis is about 50% in patients with AIDS, whereas, it is 10–15% in patients without HIV infection (45).

In HIV-positive patients, pleural effusion often is associated with disseminated disease than in contrast to HIV-negative patients. Anergy is more frequent in HIV-positive patients (47–59%) than HIV-negative (12–24%). In tuberculous effusions in HIV patients, there is a greater burden of bacilli in the pleural fluid due to the impaired host response; thereby resulting in higher yield of acid-fast bacilli in pleural tissue compared to HIV-negative patients (46). Hence, identification of mycobacteria in pleural fluid by direct staining as well as by pleural biopsy culture is greater in HIV-positive patients, but finding of granulomas are less frequent (47,48).

F. Treatment

There are multiple regimens effective in patients with TB pleurisy. The recent American Thoracic Society recommends a 6-month course of chemotherapy (three or four drugs for 2 months followed by two drugs for the next 4 months) has been found to be highly effective in patients with tuberculous pleural effusion (49). In general, an initial phase of rifampin, isoniazid, pyrazinamide, and ethambutol are administered daily for 2 months and is followed by isoniazid and rifampin for another 4 months.

Steroids have been proposed in the treatment in order to decrease pleural inflammation. Addition of steroids results in a quicker improvement in symptoms (fever, chest pain, anorexia) and resorption of pleural fluid, but steroids also risk dissemination. A recent Cochrane review of all the published trials concluded that there are insufficient data to support the use of steroids in pleural TB (50).

G. Complications of Tuberculosis Pleural Effusion

Residual pleural thickening occurs in more than half of the patients. The presence of residual pleural thickening is not affected by administration of antituberculosis drugs. It has been suggested that a therapeutic thoracentesis decreases the incidence of residual pleural thickening (51).

Empyema thoracis is a particularly disastrous complication seen in long neglected cases of pleural tuberculosis. It most often occurs due to rupture of a superficial tuberculosis cavity into the pleural space or occasionally due to rupture of a caseous paratracheal lymph node or paravertebral abscess into the pleural cavity. The patient has clinical features of pleural effusion, but is more toxic and has clubbing with intercostal tenderness. Rarely, empyema thoracis may manifest as a draining sinus tract (tuberculosis empyema necessitanes). Besides antituberculosis therapy, management includes intercostal chest tube drainage and antibiotics for superimposed infection. Conventional surgical procedures like decortication, rib resection, or thoracoplasty may still have to be performed for complete cure and relief of chronic drainage (52).

II. Pleural Effusion Secondary to Parasitic Infections

In the developing world, the magnitude of the parasitic infections is staggering and although lung pathology may not be the most common clinical presentation its presence results in a significant burden of illness (53). Many organisms classified as parasitic protozoa or helminthes may cause pulmonary disease. *Plasmodium falciparum* and *Entamoeba histolytica* infections are common protozoans associated with pulmonary involvement though the pleural involvement is usually seen with *E. histolytica*.

Helminthic parasites may cause pulmonary disease by at least three mechanisms: (1) during obligatory migration of the larva from the gut through the pulmonary capillaries to the alveoli and back to the gut (e.g., ascariasis, strongyloidiasis, and hookworm infections); (2) by passage through the pulmonary vasculature as part of a blood-borne stage of the parasite's life cycle (e.g., schistosomiasis, filariasis, trichinosis); and (3) by residence of the adult or cyst form in pulmonary tissue (e.g., paragonimiasis, echinococcosis).

Helminthic parasites are multicellular, metazoan organisms, and infections with a diversity of these organisms elicit eosinophilia and IgE production that are controlled by cytokines of Th2 lymphocyte (54). Although peripheral eosinophilia may provide a hematological clue to the presence of helminthic infection, sensitivity is below 100%. Increased IgE levels seem to correlate with the increasing levels of tissue invasion, probably due to the secretion of factors by parasites that stimulate IL-4. Total serum IgE declines after successful treatment.

Definite evidence of pulmonary involvement in parasitic infections requires demonstration of ova or larva in the sputum, bronchoalveolar lavage, pleural fluid or lung tissue, which is not always possible.

Thus, considerable emphasis is placed on serological tests and major advances have been made in diagnostic parasitic serology, particularly in enzyme-linked immunosorbent assay (ELISA) methods and the use of monoclonal antibodies (55).

The most frequent causes of parasitic pleural involvement are paragonimiasis, amebiasis, ecchinococcosis. Most of the parasitic effusions are associated with eosinophilic pleural effusions (EPE), which is defined as a pleural effusion that contains at least 10% eosinophils that may be caused by a variety of conditions (Table 1). In general, eosinophilic effusions account for 5–16% of exudative pleural effusions (56). Peripheral eosinophilia is more commonly present with helminthic infection. In contrast to infections with multicellular helminthic parasites, infections with single-celled protozoan parasites do not characteristically elicit blood or pleural eosinophilia. Parasitic infections must be considered in residents of or travelers to endemic areas. Stools should be evaluated for ova and parasites. Careful examination of cytologic preparation may reveal parasites (57) ova or echinococcal hooks (58). In some cases, ova may be found in the sputum but this is more common usually when parenchymal involvement is present (59). Serological tests for paragonimiasis, sparogonimiasis, toxocariasis, strnogyloidosis, and amebiasis may be the only diagnostic tool when parasites or ova cannot be found in the respiratory samples or stools. Bronchoscopy is rarely helpful in establishing the diagnosis of parasitic infections (60) but show evidence of eosinophilia in the bronchoalveolar lavage. Pleural biopsy has a limited role and only rarely a specific diagnosis of a parasitic infection can be established (61). In some cases, skin biopsy reveals parasites in cutaneous myasis (62), *Dranculossis medinensis* infection (63), or spargonosis (64).

A. Paragonimiasis

Paragonimiasis is a parasitic disease caused by the trematode *Paragonimus.* The pulmonary form is most commonly seen with *Paragonimus westermanni*

Table 1 Etiology of Eosinophilic Pleural Effusions

Blood/air in pleural space
  Chest trauma, hemothorax, pneumothorax, thoracotomy, thoracoscopy,
    pacemaker insertion, thoracentesis
Infection
  Bacterial, Q fever, *Mycoplasma pneumoniae*, viral, fungal, parasitic,
    actinomycosis, tuberculosis
Uremic pleuritis
Malignancy
  Metastatic carcinoma, malignant mesothelioma, malignant lymphoma
    multiple myeloma
Autoimmune disorders
  Rheumatoid arthritis, Churg–Strauss disease, sarcoidosis, systemic
    lupus erythematosus, eosinophilic fascitis
Drug reactions
  Nitrofurantoin, isotretinoin, glicazide, dantrolene, vitamin B6
    mesalamine, bromocriptine, propylthiouracil, fluoxetine, warfarin
  Pulmonary embolism
  Chronic eosinophilic pneumonia
  Acute eosinophilic pneumonia
  Loeffler's syndrome
  Hypereosinophilic syndrome
  Hodgkin's disease
  Benign asbestos pleural effusion
  Pancreatitis, pancreatic pseudocyst
  Subhepatic infection
Transudates
  Heart failure, cirrhosis
Idiopathic

and *Paragonimus miyazakii*. Paragonimiasis is a food-borne parasitic disease endemic in certain areas of east and southeast Asia (65).

Pathogenesis

Human infection occurs by ingestion of raw or incompletely cooked fresh water crabs or crayfish infected with the metacercaria (larval stage) of the worm (65). After ingestion, larvae enter the peritoneal cavity through the intestinal wall. They then migrate up and through the peritoneal cavity to the diaphragm, pleural space, and visceral pleura entering the lung.

In the lung, the larvae mature into adult lung flukes. The eggs produced by mature flukes are expectorated or swallowed and excreted in feces. In the water, eggs develop into ciliated miracidia that infect fresh water snails. Another larval form develops in the snails and is eventually released as cercariae that penetrate crayfish and crabs to complete the cycle (66).

Clinical Manifestations

In the early stages of the infection, patients present with abdominal pain, and or pleuritic chest pain, as the larvae penetrate the diaphragm and migrate within the pleural cavity. Cough, malaise, and chest pain may also develop with larval migration within the lung parenchyma. In the lung, they mature into adult forms that deposit eggs in the lung parenchyma leading to hemorrhage, necrosis that may present as bronchopneumonia, interstitial pneumonia, bronchitis, bronchiectasis, collapse, fibrosis, pleural thickening, or pleural effusions. Recurrent hemoptysis is a common complaint in late stages of the disease (67). The sputum typically has a characteristic chocolate color and is composed of a mixture of blood, inflammatory cells, and *Paragonimus* eggs.

Radiologic Findings

The appearance of the radiographs varies with the stage of the infection and the surrounding tissue reaction. The initial finding is patchy air-space consolidation due to hemorrhagic pneumonia caused by migrating larva. At this stage, pleural effusion or pneumothorax is frequently seen. As larvae mature into adults, cysts form around them, which is filled with hemorrhagic fluid, surrounded by pericystic airspace consolidation. It appears as a localized mass-like consolidation on radiographs. Cysts that communicate with adjacent bronchus appear as air cysts within the consolidated lung or as ring shadows. Pleural involvement is represented by pleural effusion (60%), hydropneumothorax (30%) and pleural thickening (10%) (68).

Diagnosis

The diagnosis should be suspected in a patient with history of exposure in an endemic area. It can be established by detecting eggs in the sputum, stool, and bronchoalveolar lavage or biopsy specimen, or a positive anti-*Paragonimus* antibody test. The levels of IgE and *P. westermanni* specific IgE and IgG immunoglobulins are elevated and higher in the pleural fluid than in the serum, suggesting that these antibodies are produced in the pleural space (69). ELISA is highly sensitive and specific in detecting antibodies and eggs are demonstrable in less than 50% of cases (70). Enzyme-linked immunosorbent assay and immunoblot serological tests may also be helpful (67). The pleural fluid is frequently eosinophilic and exudative with low glucose (<10 mg/dL), low pH (<7.10), and high LDH (> 1000 IU/L). The pleural fluid also shows presence of cholesterol crystals while the presence of ova is rare. Peripheral and pleural fluid eosinophilia is common (71,72). Increased IL-5 levels are present in the pleural fluid and correlate significantly with the percentage of eosinophils in both pleural effusions and peripheral blood (72,73).

Treatment

The treatment of choice is praziquantel 25-mg/kg-body weight three times a day for 3 days. Response to praziquantel can be followed by a downward trend in peripheral eosinophilia, cessation of egg passage in sputum or stool, improvement in chest radiograph, and decreasing antibody titer to *Paragonimus*. For heavy infections, a second course may be required. The alternative treatment is bithionel or niclofalan. Thoracotomy and decortication may be necessary when pleural surfaces are abnormally thickened and penetration of drugs into the pleural space is insufficient to eradicate infection (68).

B. Amebiasis

Amebiasis is an infection with the protozoan *E. histolytica* and is the third most common cause of death from parasitic diseases after malaria and schistosomiasis (74). It produces a spectrum of clinical illness ranging from dysentery to abscess of liver and other organs. Pleuropulmonary involvement is the most frequent complication of amebic liver abscess.

Pathogenesis

Human infection is caused by ingestion of *E. histolytica* cyst in fecally contaminated food and drink. Excystation occurs in the lumen of the small intestine. Trophozoites are formed, which adhere to the mucus and epithelial layers. Sometimes, active trophozoites burrow deep into the mucosal wall and form flask-shaped ulcers in the mucosa with narrow opening to the gut lumen. Trophozoites may enter the mesenteric veins, reach liver via portal circulation, occasionally they enter systemic circulation through the venules of middle and inferior rectal veins and vertebral veins and are deposited in different organs. The lung is the second most common extraintestinal site of amebic involvement after the liver.

Pleuropulmonary involvement, which is reported in 20–30% patients, is the most frequent complication of amebic liver abscess. Common clinical presentations include sterile sympathetic effusions, contiguous spread from the liver and rupture into the pleural space resulting in amebic empyema (75,76). Rarely, a hepatobronchial fistula may cause cough, productive of large amounts of necrotic material.

Clinical Manifestations

Pleuropulmonary involvement like amebic liver abscess occurs predominantly in men. The reported male:female ratio varies from 9:1 to 15:1 (77). Patients with sympathetic pleural effusion frequently experience pleuritic chest pain referred to the scapula or the shoulder. Most patients have a tender enlarged liver (78). It is common to hear pleural rub in patients with an amebic liver abscess extending to the pleura. Transdiaphragmatic rupture of hepatic abscess may present with dramatic onset of severe pain, respiratory distress, shock, and sometimes death may occur (79). The pleural effusion is frequently massive; the rupture into the right pleural space is seen in about 90% of patients. Hemoptysis is common; a brisk bout of hemoptysis followed by expectoration of anchovy sauce-like pus indicates that the pus is of liver origin. Hemoptysis due to pulmonary infarction may occur as a result of thromboembolism of the lung from the amebic liver abscess (80).

Diagnosis

The diagnosis should be suspected in all patients from endemic areas with right-sided pleural effusion. Neutrophilic leukocytosis was observed in 30%. Eosinophilia is usually not a feature. Serum alkaline phosphatase level is elevated in more than 75% of patients, whereas the level of transaminases are elevated in about 50% cases (81).

The roentgenogram of the chest may show elevation of the right dome of the diaphragm with or without the pleural effusion (82). Ultrasonography and computed tomography (CT) scanning can also demonstrate the hepatic abscess and the pleural effusion (83).

The pleural effusion is typically described as "chocolate sauce" or "anchovy paste" in appearance. A positive diagnosis can be established by demonstration of trophozoites in the pleural effusion but is seen in only 10% of patients (81,84). Several tests have been developed for the diagnosis of extraintestinal amebiasis including indirect hemagglutination test (IHA), ELISA, and the indirect fluorescent antibody test. The detection of IgM antibodies may be more useful in diagnosing acute cases because antibodies appear early and persist in the serum for a short period of time. The gel diffusion is positive in more than 95% of patients with acute invasive disease and reverts to negative after 6–12 months.

Treatment

Metronidazole is currently the drug of choice. Side effects include nausea, anorexia, metallic taste, dizziness, and a disulfuram-like reaction with alcohol. If the pleural effusion is large enough to cause respiratory distress, a therapeutic thoracentesis or tube thoracostomy may be performed. Bacterial superinfection, which is present in up to one-third of the patients with amebic empyema, responds to antibiotics therapy. In some of these cases, open drainage or decortication may be necessary. After successful treatment of invasive disease, patients should be considered for eradication of the intestinal phase of the disease with a luminal agent (85) like iodoquinol, diloxanide furoate, and paramomycin.

C. Echinococcosis (Hydatid Disease)

Human echinococcosis is caused by three species of the tapeworm (*Echinococcus granulosus*, *Echinococcus multilocularis*, and *Echinococcus vogeli*). *E. granulosus* is the most prevalent, producing cystic hydatid disease in about 90% of cases. *E. granulosus* is most commonly seen in sheep and cattle raising countries, particularly in the Middle East, Australia, New Zealand, South America, and Central Europe. The disease is particularly common in Lebanon and Greece. The liver (60–70%) and the lungs (20–30%) are the most frequently involved organs. Pulmonary disease, in particular, appears to be more common in younger individuals (86).

Pathogenesis

The definitive host for *E. granulosus* is the dog or wolf, while humans are the accidental hosts. When man ingests feces containing eggs, larvae emerge in the duodenum, enter the blood, and usually lodge in either the liver or the lung. The parasite grows and may be latent for 10–20 years before producing symptoms. The resulting symptoms depend upon the site, type, and rate of growth of the cystic lesions (87). While most patients are asymptomatic, some may occasionally expectorate the contents of the cyst, or develop symptoms due to compression of the surrounding structures. The cyst may erode into bronchi, mediastinum, or pleural cavity.

Clinical Manifestations

Pleural involvement usually can occur due to rupture of a pulmonary hydatid cyst; often simultaneous rupture into the pleural space and tracheobronchial tree is observed (88). Since the cyst is not fertile after rupture, pleural hydatidosis is rare (88). Rarely hepatic cyst rupture into the pleural space may occur. Occasionally, sympathetic pleural effusion may accompany a pulmonary or hepatic hydrated cyst (89).

Hepatic cyst rupture into the pleural space is associated with an acute illness characterized by chest pain, cough, respiratory distress, fever, and shock. In half of the cases, simultaneous rupture into the bronchial tree is manifested by expectoration of large quantities of cyst membranes and pus; pulmonary cyst rupture has a similar presentation (88). In addition, a bronchopleural fistula often produces a hydropneumothorax that may become secondarily infected.

Diagnosis

In endemic areas, the diagnosis is established utilizing the clinical picture, radiological findings, and serological tests (90). MRI, CT scan, and ultrasound reveal a solitary well-defined cyst with thick or thin walls. In up to 30% of cases, cysts may be multiple. In rupture of the cyst, usual findings include an elevated right hemidiaphragm, moderate right pleural effusion, right lower lobe pneumonitis, and hydropneumothorax (89,91–93). The definitive diagnosis of pleural echinococcosis is established by the demonstration of echinococcal scolices with hooklets in the pleural fluid stained by toluidine blue. In pleural tissue, a fibrinopurulent exudate with eosinophils is observed (58). Thoracentesis reveals turbid, yellow fluid with an abundance of polymorphonuclear cells and eosinophils. Casoni skin test and Weinberg complement fixation test are positive in about 70–75% of cases (88). Detection of antibody to specific echinococcal antigens by immunoblotting has the highest degree of specificity.

Treatment

Surgical excision of the cyst is the treatment of choice (94). An immediate thoracotomy is recommended for patients who have ruptured hepatic or pulmonary cyst into the pleural space. When a hepatic cyst has ruptured, the objectives of surgical treatment are to remove the parasite, to drain the hepatic and pleural cavity and re-expand the lungs. If the surgical procedure is delayed, a decortication may also be required (95). Patients with hydatid cysts should be treated with antiprotozoal therapy if all cysts cannot be removed or when rupture of a cyst has occurred. The treatment of choice is albendazole, 400 mg twice a day for at least 28 days (96).

D. Other Parasitic Infections

Pneumocystis pneumonia is the most common opportunistic pulmonary infection in patients with AIDS (97). It usually presents with diffuse bilateral interstitial infiltrates. There have been a few case reports of pleural effusion secondary to *Pneumocystis carinii* in patients with AIDS (98–100). All reported cases were receiving aerosolized pentamidine.

The pleural fluid is an exudate, with lactate dehydrogenase (LDH) more than 400 IU/L, the ratio of the pleural fluid to serum LDH is more than 1:0, pleural fluid protein level below 3.0 g/dL and the ratio of the pleural fluid to the serum protein less than 0.50 in all patients. The pleural fluid glucose and pH are not reduced.

In most cases, the diagnosis is established by visualization of *Pneumocystis* in pleural fluid stained with *Gomori methenamine* silver. It appears that *Pneumocystis* pleural disease is an anatomic extension of smoldering subpleural *Pneumocystis* pneumonia.

The treatment is the same as the treatment of pulmonary *Pneumocystis*, trimethoprim, and sulfamethoxazole 5 mg/kg with 25 mg/kg three times a day for a total of 21 days. The other main pleural complication of *P. carinii* is spontaneous pneumothorax requiring chest tube drainage.

Malaria is a major tropical disorder. Human malaria is caused by four species belonging to the genus *Plasmodium* (*Plasmodium vivax, P. falciparum,*

P. ovale, and *P. malariae*). The parasite is transmitted to humans following the bite of an infected female anopheline mosquito. The clinical picture varies and ranges from mild upper respiratory problems to severe and rapidly fatal pulmonary edema. Pleural effusions in malaria are rather uncommon (101,102). Pleural effusion is frequently found at autopsy in patients dying of pulmonary edema. The effusions probably have little clinical significance, since they are never large enough to compromise respiratory function seriously (103).

Other parasitic infections that have rarely been associated with pleural diseases include leishmaniasis (104), Loeffler's syndrome (105,106), lymphatic filariasis (61,107), sparaganosis (64), aniskiasis (108), hypodermiasis (62), *Strongyloides stercoralis* (60), *Trichomonas* (109), *Toxocara canis* (110), loiasis (57), and sporotrichosis (111), schistomiasis (112) and *Dracunculus medinensis* infection (63). Some parasites including pentastomids and mansonella sp. (113) can be found in pleura incidentally by radiographs or autopsy, but seldom if ever cause pleural disease (106).

III. Pleural Effusion Secondary to Fungal Infection

The occurrence of fungal infection is rising rapidly worldwide. The increase in the rate of fungal infections has been attributed mainly to the increasing use of broad-spectrum antibiotics, intravascular devices, and hyperalimentation, as well as secondary to increasing number of critically ill or immunocompromised patients in hospital populations (114). Candida and Torulopsis species are the most common pathogens in fungal empyema thoracis, accounting for 82% of the fungal isolates from pleural effusion, with *Candida albicans* representing 60% of all *Candida* species isolates (115,116). The common fungal infections involving the pleura are discussed below.

A. Histoplasmosis

Histoplasma capsulatum is a dimorphic fungus found in soil that is enriched by bird or bat droppings. The organism is found in both temperate and tropical climates worldwide with endemic areas concentrated along river valleys. Based on skin test surveys, prevalence among the general population in areas of Central and South America can be as high as 40%. While southeast Asian and African populations are also endemically affected, prevalence rates tend to be much lower (117). *Histoplasma capsulatum var duboisii* is a variant found only in Africa, mainly in Western and Central regions of the continent.

Infection with *H. capsulatum* rarely causes pleural effusions. When the pleural space is involved, exudative pleural effusions are present. The effusions are thought to result from visceral pleural inflammation and rupture of a peripheral granuloma is uncommon. Dissemination of histoplasmosis to the pleural space may occur hematogenously as well (118).

Histoplasmosis may resemble tuberculosis clinically. Disseminated histoplasmosis is an increasingly important opportunistic infection in patients with the acquired immunodeficiency syndrome (AIDS). There have been case reports of pleural effusion secondary to histoplasmosis in patients with AIDS (119). Patients usually have a subacute illness characterized by a low-grade fever, anorexia, malaise, and pleuritic chest pain.

Diagnosis

The chest radiograph usually reveals an infiltrate or a subpleural nodule in addition to the pleural effusion (120,121). Pleural fluid analysis reveals an exudate with relatively high protein content, containing predominantly lymphocytes. The pleural biopsy may reveal noncaseating granulomas. The diagnosis is made by culturing *H. capsulatum* from the pleural fluid, sputum, or biopsy material by routine fungal cultures or by demonstrating the organism in biopsy material.

Treatment

In normal host with acute histoplasmosis, pleural effusion is self-limited and usually resolves spontaneously over several weeks (122).

If patient is symptomatic and develops fibrosis, a decortication should be considered. On rare occasions, patients with parenchymal histoplasmosis may develop a bronchopleural fistula with the subsequent development of a loculated fungal empyema (123). Such patients should be treated with drainage and decortication and antifungal therapy (amphotericin B and itraconazole) (119,124).

B. Blastomycosis

Patients with blastomycosis may have signs and symptoms similar to those of tuberculous pleuritis. Pulmonary infection with *Blastomyces dermatitis* may result in pleural involvement, either effusion (2–15%) or pleural thickening (88%) (125).

Diagnosis

The diagnosis of blastomycosis should be considered in patients with a clinical picture suggestive of tuberculous pleuritis (126). The wide range of radiographic findings includes parenchymal disease, mass-like lesions, and pleural effusion. The pleural fluid is usually an exudate with predominantly small lymphocytes, although polymorphonuclear leukocytes may predominate. The pleural fluid glucose and LDH is normal. Microscopic examination of the pleural fluid sometimes reveals budding yeast typical of B. *dermatitis* (125). However, the usual method of diagnosis is culture, which takes 2–6 weeks. Pleural biopsy may reveal noncaseating granulomas. The complement fixation test is the most widely used test for the serologic diagnosis of blastomycosis; however, its clinical value is limited.

Treatment

Pleural blastomycosis should be treated with itraconazole 400 mg qd for 6 months or amphotericin B with a total dose of 2 g. Itraconazole is the treatment of choice for immunocompetent individuals and amphotericin is the drug of choice for immunocompromised hosts.

C. Cryptococcosis

Cryptococcus neoformans is a budding, encapsulated yeast found worldwide in bird droppings, decaying fruit, and soil. With the advent of AIDS, crypto-coccosis has become increasingly common. High prevalence is seen in areas of western Africa, Haiti, and Thailand (127). Cryptococcal infection rarely presents with pulmonary manifestations and even more rarely with pleural effusion. In most cases, the disease spreads outside the thorax, usually to the central nervous system. Pleural cryptococcosis has been reported to be associated with HIV infection (128), liver cirrhosis, and agammaglobu-linemia and appear to occur from extension of a subpleural pulmonary cryptococcal nodule into the pleural cavity. Patients with cryptococcal pneumonia may present with a wide spectrum of clinical findings ranging from asymptomatic patients to those with cough and dyspnea to severe pro-gressive pneumonia.

Diagnosis

The pleural fluid is a lymphocyte predominant exudative. Culture of fluid is positive in about half of the patients; in the others diagnosis is established by histological study, culture of lung tissue, or identification of cryptococcal antigen in serum or pleural fluid (129). Serum cryptococcal antigen is highly sensitive and specific. Bronchoalveolar lavage often shows organisms on direct smears and by culture. Wright-stained smears show much small yeast within macrophages with a large clear space around the organisms. A mucicarmine stain colors the carbohydrate capsule a bright crimson, con-firming the diagnosis. Pulmonary cryptococcosis in nonimmunosuppressed patients is a diagnosis often made by surgical biopsy. Surgical excision may be curative.

Treatment

Patients with pulmonary cryptococcosis should be treated with amphotericin B and/or fluconazole. Lifelong maintenance therapy with fluconazole is necessary in AIDS patients.

D. Coccidioidomycosis

Coccidioidomycosis is a multisystem disease caused by inhalation of the spores of *Coccidioides immitis*. The pleural disease occurs early in the disease accompanying acute primary coccidioidomycosis or when a coccidiodal cavity adjacent to the pleura ruptures to produce a hydropneumothorax (130). Pleural effusion may be present in 7–15% symptomatic cases with primary coccidioidomycosis (131). Patients are febrile and report pleuritic chest pain. The effusions are small and resolve in a few days. The chests radiograph reveals parenchymal infiltrates in addition to effusion in about 50% of patients. The cause of effusion may be rupture of a subpleural granuloma, or an immune complex pleuritis in response to coccidiodal antigen or contiguous spread of infection from lung.

Diagnosis

The pleural fluid is exudative with small lymphocytes. Peripheral eosinophilia is common but pleural fluid eosinophilia (<7% cases) is uncommon. Culture, serology, and/or skin testing establish the diagnosis. The cultures are positive for *Coccidioides immitis* in about 20% of the cases but culture of biopsy specimen is the most sensitive test, with yield approaching 100%. The pleural biopsy may reveal evidence of granulomas as well (131).

Treatment

Most patients with primary coccidioidomycosis and pleural effusion require no systemic therapy. Medical treatment is necessary with amphotericin B or the azoles (euconazole or itraconazole) if there is evidence of disseminated disease. Chronic effusions are seen in 3% of cases of chronic coccidioidomycosis. In some chronic cases, hydropneumothorax may follow the pleural from rupture of a chronic pulmonary lesion. These patients are acutely ill with systemic signs of toxicity. Such patients in addition to medical treatment require chest tube drainage or may even require surgical lung resection (132).

IV. Pleural Effusions Due to Viruses

Viral lower respiratory tract infection has been associated with pleural effusion. The incidence of pleural effusions in viral pneumonia is reported to be 2–9% of cases (133). When pleural effusions are specifically targeted with lateral decubitus chest views, 18% of cases with viral pneumonia revealed an effusion (134). Pleural effusions have also been reported due to other viral infections such as respiratory syncytial virus, influenza virus, measles after vaccination, viral hepatitis, lassa fever, and adenovirus infections (135,136). In general, these effusions are small, transient, and asymptomatic. They tend to resolve within 2 weeks and require no pleural space drainage. Measles pneumonia is encountered in tropical countries. Pneumothorax and pleural effusion can be seen in up to 4% of affected children (137). The diagnosis usually depends on clinical symptoms, isolation of the virus or the demonstration of a significant increase in the antibodies to the virus.

A. Hantavirus Infections

Hantaviruses are single-stranded, negative-sense RNA viruses that encompass 25 antigenically distinguishable viral species (138). They are enveloped virus particles, measuring 80–115 nm in diameter, and belong to the family *Bunyaviridae*. Hantavirus pulmonary syndrome (HPS), caused mainly by Sin Nombre virus, is primarily a lung infection; the kidneys and the skin are largely unaffected (139). Hantaviruses are transmitted by aerosols of rodent excreta, saliva, and urine. The most common mode of transmission is inhalation of dust or dried particles with dried saliva or waste products of an infected rodent (140).

The HPS is characterized by flu-like symptoms: fever, myalgias, headache, and cough. Other symptoms can include chills, abdominal pain, diarrhea, and malaise. Subsequent symptoms include coughing and shortness of breath, tachypnea, tachycardia, dizziness, arthralgia, sweating, and back or chest pain (141). The disease progresses rapidly; further symptoms can include thrombocytopenia, hypoxemia, and interstitial pulmonary edema. Eventually, the patient experiences hypotension, shock, and respiratory distress. The vast majority of patients with HPS have evidence of pleural effusions caused by the rare cardiac dysfunction, or alternatively may be due to the profound vascular leak. The pleural fluid can be a transudate in initial phase (representing cardiopulmonary dysfunction) or an exudative due to capillary leaks (142).

Diagnosis

Thrombocytopenia, increased immature granulocytes, and large immunoblastoid lymphocytes, accompanied by an elevated white blood cell count are commonly observed. The partial thromboplastin and prothrombin times are increased. The serum lactate, lactate dehydrogenase, aspartate aminotransferase, and alanine aminotransferase levels are elevated. IgG or IgM to *Hantavirus* strains Seoul, Hantaan, Puumala, Dobrava, and Sin

Nombre, may be detected serologically (143). Chest radiographs of HPS patients show diffuse interstitial pulmonary infiltrates, advancing to alveolar edema with severe bilateral involvement. Severe infections may have pulmonary secretions with a total protein ratio of edema fluid/serum greater than 80%.

Treatment

The patients usually need intensive cardiopulmonary support. Treatment with intravenous ribavirin or amantadine may be effective (144).

B. Dengue Fever

Dengue virus infection is the most common arthropod-borne disease worldwide with an increasing incidence in tropical and subtropical regions (145). Dengue viruses belong to the family of *Flaviviridae* and are transmitted by the bite of infected *Aedes* mosquitoes. Dengue virus infection frequently may remain asymptomatic or manifest as nonspecific viral infection. In severe cases dengue fever (DF), dengue hemorrhagic fever (DHF), and dengue shock syndrome (DSS) are characterized by high and often biphasic fever, malaise, frontal headache, retro-orbital pain, arthralgia with backache, myalgia, generalized lymphadenopathy, and a centrifugal macular or maculopapular rash. Laboratory abnormalities include a usually mild elevation of liver enzymes, thrombocytopenia, and abnormal coagulation (146).

The definition of DHF as established by the World Health Organization includes a dengue-like illness with hemoconcentration (hematocrit elevated by >20%), marked thrombocytopenia ($<100 \times 10^9$/L), and hemorrhagic manifestations such as petechiae, conjunctival and gingival bleeding, epistaxis, melena, hematuria, and a positive tourniquet test (147). Up to 30% of patients with DHF may progress to DSS as a consequence of increased vascular permeability leading to hypovolemia, hypotension with narrowing of the pulse pressure (<20 mmHg), and circulatory shock. Pleural effusions are common with DHF and are usually exudates (76) but can be transudates (148). The effusions are usually small and bilateral. The pathogenesis of the effusions appears to be a systemic increase in the permeability of capillaries induced by cytokines.

Diagnosis

Dengue disease can be verified by virus isolation, detection of viral RNA by reverse transcription polymerase chain reaction, or identification of dengue virus-specific antibodies. A greater than four-fold rise in hemagglutination inhibition, complement fixation, or neutralizing antibody titers provides laboratory confirmation of dengue infection.

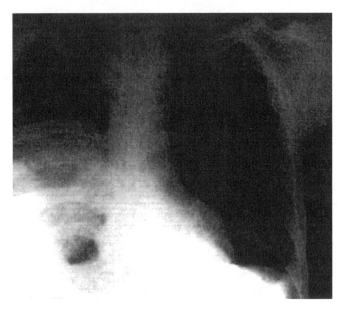

Figure 1 Pleural effusion roentgenogram of the chest.

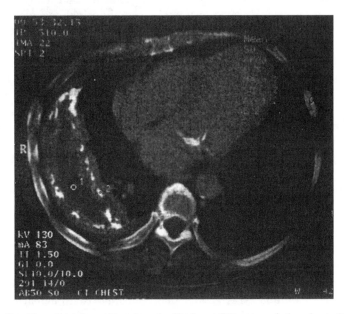

Figure 2 Chronic tubercular pleural effusion—CT scan of the chest. Note the calcifaction of the visceral and parietal pura.

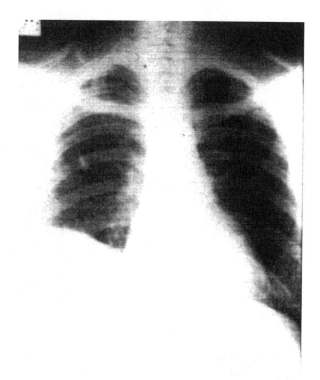

Figure 3 Roentgenogram of the chest of a patient with amebic liver abscess.

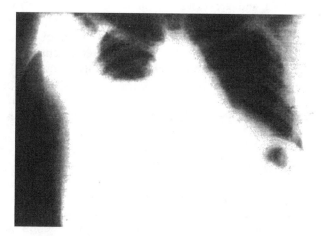

Figure 4 Roentgenogram of the chest of the same patient after 2 days with massive right pleural effusion due to rupture of the abscess in the right pleural cavity.

V. Atypical Infections

Actinomycosis mainly caused by *Actinomyces isrelii,* is characterized by formation of abscesses and multiple sinus tracts. The infection arises from endogenous sources such as infected gums of teeth. Pleural disease occurs in 50–80% of the cases (149). The pleural fluid is exudative with lymphocyte predominance. Sulfur granules in the pleural fluid are strongly suggestive of actinomycosis. The fluid should be gram stained to look for gram-positive long-branching filaments characteristic of actinomycosis and cultured anerobically. The drug of choice is penicillin 10–20 million units for 4–6 weeks, followed by 12 months of therapy with oral penicillin. Chest tube drainage is required if the fluid is an empyema (135).

Nocardiasis is usually caused by *Nocardia asteroids* and is considered an opportunistic infection most commonly seen in immunocompromised patients with AIDS, malignancies, or other chronic diseases. The lung is involved in 50% of the cases and pleural effusion is seen in 25–50% of cases (118).

The pleural fluid is an exudate. The pleural fluid cultures may or may not be positive for *N. asteroids.* When nocardia is not identified in pleura fluid, bronchoscopy can help provide the material for gram stain or for modified acid-fast stain. Sulfonamides are the drug of choice and duration should be at least 6 weeks and are frequently necessary for longer period of time. Surgical management is at times necessary for appropriate drainage of the pleural cavity (150).

Q fever is caused by the rickettsial agent *Coxiella burnetti* and acquired by inhalation of contaminated dust particles or by drinking unpasteurized milk. The clinical picture is similar to a primary atypical pneumonia including fever, cough, and myalgias. Pleural effusion are relatively common (10–35%) and are exudative in nature (151). The diagnosis is established by demonstrating a positive *C. burnetti* complement fixation reaction with increased titers from 2 weeks of onset of the symptoms (135). The treatment of choice is doxycycline or tetracycline.

Occasionally, other bacterial infections may also show involvement of the pleura including *Salmonella typhi* (152), melioidosis (153), leptospirosis (154), and brucellosis (155,156). The pleural effusions in brucella infections may be very similar to tuberculosis including increased ADA levels (157).

VI. Conclusion

The spectrum of pleural disease in tropical regions involves a vast gamut of infectious diseases and represents a considerable burden of illness. These pleuropulmonary infections are a significant cause of infection attributable morbidity and mortality, which is preventable if appropriate clinical and laboratory tools are in place to facilitate early detection of the pulmonary infections, identification of the pathogen involved, and institution of appropriate therapy. Consequently, there is still great scope of improvement in implementing potentially effective interventions to improve the outcome of pleural infectious diseases.

References

1. Petney TN. Environmental, cultural and social changes and their influence on parasite infections. Int J Parasitol 2001; 31(9):919–932.
2. Ryan ET, Kain KC. Health advice and immunizations for travelers. N Engl J Med 2000; 342(23):1716–1725.
3. Laughlin L. Clinical practice in the tropics. In: Strickland G, ed. Hunter's Tropical Medicine and Emerging Infectious Diseases. Philadelphia: W B Saunders, 2000:1–7.
4. Sinzobahamvya N, Bhakta HP. Pleural exudate in a tropical hospital. Eur Respir J 1989; 2(2):145–148.
5. Mehta JB, et al. Epidemiology of extrapulmonary tuberculosis. A comparative analysis with pre-AIDS era. Chest 1991; 99(5):1134–1138.
6. Goodman PC. Tuberculosis and AIDS. Radiol Clin North Am 1995; 33(4):707–717.
7. Seibert AF, et al. Tuberculous pleural effusion. Twenty-year experience. Chest 1991; 99(4):883–886.
8. Moudgil H, Sridhar G, Leitch AG. Reactivation disease: the commonest form of tuberculous pleural effusion in Edinburgh, 1980–1991. Respir Med 1994; 88(4):301–304.
9. Chan CH, et al. Clinical and pathological features of tuberculous pleural effusion and its long-term consequences. Respiration 1991; 58(3–4):171–175.
10. Maeda J, et al. Local production and localization of transforming growth factor-beta in tuberculous pleurisy. Clin Exp Immunol 1993; 92(1):32–38.
11. Condos R, et al. Local immune responses correlate with presentation and outcome in tuberculosis. Am J Respir Crit Care Med 1998; 157(3 Pt 1):729–735.
12. Perez-Rodriguez E, Jimenez Castro D. The use of adenosine deaminase and adenosine deaminase isoenzymes in the diagnosis of tuberculous pleuritis. Curr Opin Pulm Med 2000; 6(4):259–266.
13. Goodman RB, et al. Cytokine-stimulated human mesothelial cells produce chemotactic activity for neutrophils including NAP-1/IL-8. J Immunol 1992; 148(2):457–465.
14. Nasreen N, et al. Mycobacterium-induced transmesothelial migration of monocytes into pleural space: role of intercellular adhesion molecule-1 in tuberculous pleurisy. J Infect Dis 1999; 180(5):1616–1623.
15. Mohammed KA, et al. Mycobacterium-mediated chemokine expression in pleural mesothelial cells: role of C-C chemokines in tuberculous pleurisy. J Infect Dis 1998; 178(5):1450–1456.
16. Pace E, et al. Interleukin-8 induces lymphocyte chemotaxis into the pleural space. Role of pleural macrophages. Am J Respir Crit Care Med 1999; 159(5 Pt 1):1592–1599.

17. Barnes PF, et al. Transpleural gradient of 1,25-dihydroxyvitamin D in tuberculous pleuritis. J Clin Invest 1989; 83(5):1527–1532.
18. Ellner JJ, et al. The immunology of tuberculous pleurisy. Semin Respir Infect 1988; 3(4):335–342.
19. Sahn SA. State of the art. The pleura. Am Rev Respir Dis 1988; 138(1):184–234.
20. Leckie WJ, Tothill P. Albumin turnover in pleural effusions. Clin Sci 1965; 29(2):339–352.
21. Light RW. Pleural diseases. In: John JR, Barrett KB, Vassiliou JC, eds. Tuberculous Pleural Effusions. Philadelphia: Lippincott Williams and Wilkins, 2001:182–195.
22. Pasricha P, et al. Clinical and roentgenological profiles and etiological correlations of encysted pleural effusions. Respiration 1990; 57(1):40–44.
23. Epstein DM, et al. Tuberculous pleural effusions. Chest 1987; 91(1):106–109.
24. Relkin F, et al. Pleural tuberculosis and HIV infection. Chest 1994; 105(5): 1338–1341.
25. Ferrer J. Tuberculous pleural effusion and tuberculous empyema. Semin Respir Crit Care Med 2001; 22(6):637–646.
26. Ferrer J. Pleural tuberculosis. Eur Respir J 1997; 10(4):942–947.
27. Morehead RS. Tuberculosis of the pleura. South Med J 1998; 91(7):630–636.
28. Schluger NW, Rom WN. Current approaches to the diagnosis of active pulmonary tuberculosis. Am J Respir Crit Care Med 1994; 149(1):264–267.
29. Roth A, Schaberg T, Mauch H. Molecular diagnosis of tuberculosis: current clinical validity and future perspectives. Eur Respir J 1997; 10(8):1877–1891.
30. Querol JM, et al. Rapid diagnosis of pleural tuberculosis by polymerase chain reaction. Am J Respir Crit Care Med 1995; 152(6 Pt 1):1977–1981.
31. Villegas MV, Labrada LA, Saravia NG. Evaluation of polymerase chain reaction, adenosine deaminase, and interferon-gamma in pleural fluid for the differential diagnosis of pleural tuberculosis. Chest 2000; 118(5):1355–1364.
32. Valdes L, et al. Tuberculous pleurisy: a study of 254 patients. Arch Intern Med 1998; 158(18):2017–2021.
33. Blanc FX, et al. Diagnostic value of medical thoracoscopy in pleural disease: a 6-year retrospective study. Chest 2002; 121(5):1677–1683.
34. Chiang CS, et al. Neopterin, soluble interleukin-2 receptor and adenosine deaminase levels in pleural effusions. Respiration 1994; 61(3):150–154.
35. Villena V, et al. Rapid automated determination of adenosine deaminase and lysozyme for differentiating tuberculous and nontuberculous pleural effusions. Clin Chem 1996; 42(2):218–221.
36. Valdes L, et al. Value of adenosine deaminase in the diagnosis of tuberculous pleural effusions in young patients in a region of high prevalence of tuberculosis. Thorax 1995; 50(6):600–603.
37. Burgess LJ, et al. Use of adenosine deaminase as a diagnostic tool for tuberculous pleurisy. Thorax 1995; 50(6):672–674.
38. Riantawan P, et al. Diagnostic value of pleural fluid adenosine deaminase in tuberculous pleuritis with reference to HIV coinfection and a Bayesian analysis. Chest 1999; 116(1):97–103.

39. Banales JL, et al. Adenosine deaminase in the diagnosis of tuberculous pleural effusions. A report of 218 patients and review of the literature. Chest 1991; 99(2):355–357.

40. Echave-Sustaeta J, et al. False negatives of ADA in pleural tuberculosis. Ann Med Intern 1996; 13(11):562.

41. Perez-Rodriguez E, et al. ADA1/ADAp ratio in pleural tuberculosis: an excellent diagnostic parameter in pleural fluid. Respir Med 1999; 93(11): 816–821.

42. Villena V, et al. Interferon-gamma in 388 immunocompromised and immuno-competent patients for diagnosing pleural tuberculosis. Eur Respir J 1996; 9(12):2635–2639.

43. Valdes L, et al. Diagnosis of tuberculous pleurisy using the biologic para-meters adenosine deaminase, lysozyme, and interferon gamma. Chest 1993; 103(2):458–465.

44. Chen YM, et al. An analysis of cytokine status in the serum and effusions of patients with tuberculous and lung cancer. Lung Cancer 2001; 31(1):25–30.

45. Espinal MA, et al. Infectiousness of *Mycobacterium tuberculosis* in HIV-1-infected patients with tuberculosis: a prospective study. Lancet 2000; 355(9200):275–280.

46. Sharma SK, Ahluwalia G. HIV and tuberculosis. Indian J Chest Dis Allied Sci 2000; 42(2):77–81.

47. Richter C, et al. Clinical features of HIV-seropositive and HIV-seronegative patients with tuberculous pleural effusion in Dar es Salaam, Tanzania. Chest 1994; 106(5):1471–1475.

48. Kitinya JN, et al. Influence of HIV status on pathological changes in tubercu-lous pleuritis. Tuber Lung Dis 1994; 75(3):195–198.

49. Blumberg HM, et al. American Thoracic Society/Centers for Disease Control and Prevention/Infectious Diseases Society of America: treatment of tubercu-losis. Am J Respir Crit Care Med 2003; 167(4):603–662.

50. Matchaba PVJ. Steroids for treating tuberculous pleurisy (Cochrane Review). In: The Cochrane Library. Issue 1. Oxford: Update Software, 2001.

51. Barbas CS, et al. The relationship between pleural fluid findings and the devel-opment of pleural thickening in patients with pleural tuberculosis. Chest 1991; 100(5):1264–1267.

52. Gaensler EA. The surgery for pulmonary tuberculosis. Am Rev Respir Dis 1982; 125(3 Pt 2):73–84.

53. Mahmoud A. In: Lenfant C, ed. Parasitic Lung Diseases. New York: Mercel Dekker, Inc., 1997:v–vi.

54. Wilson RA. Immunity and immunoregulation in helminth infections. Curr Opin Immunol 1993; 5(4):538–547.

55. Singh B. Molecular methods for diagnosis and epidemiological studies of parasitic infections. Int J Parasitol 1997; 27(10):1135–1145.

56. Kalomenidis I, Light RW. Eosinophilic pleural effusions. Curr Opin Pulm Med 2003; 9(4):254–260.

57. Klion AD, et al. Pulmonary involvement in loiasis. Am Rev Respir Dis 1992; 145(4 Pt 1):961–963.

58. Jacobson ES. A case of secondary echinococcosis diagnosed by cytologic examination of pleural fluid and needle biopsy of pleura. Acta Cytol 1973; 17(1):76–79.
59. Johnson JR, et al. Paragonimiasis in the United States. A report of nine cases in Hmong immigrants. Chest 1982; 82(2):168–171.
60. Emad A. Exudative eosinophilic pleural effusion due to *Strongyloides stercoralis* in a diabetic man. South Med J 1999; 92(1):58–60.
61. Gupta K, et al. Microfilariae in association with other diseases. A report of six cases. Acta Cytol 2002; 46(4):776–778.
62. Uttamchandani RB, et al. Eosinophilic pleural effusion in cutaneous myiasis. South Med J 1989; 82(10):1288–1291.
63. Gentilini M, et al. A case of eosinophilic pleurisy due to *Dracunculus medinensis* infection. Trans R Soc Trop Med Hyg 1978; 72(5):540–541.
64. Ishii H, et al. A rare case of eosinophilic pleuritis due to sparganosis. Intern Med 2001; 40(8):783–785.
65. Yokogawa M. Paragonimus and paragonimiasis. Adv Parasitol 1965; 3: 99–158.
66. Minh VD, et al. Pleural paragonimiasis in a Southeast Asia refugee. Am Rev Respir Dis 1981; 124(2):186–188.
67. Blair D, Xu ZB, Agatsuma T. Paragonimiasis and the genus *Paragonimus*. Adv Parasitol 1999; 42:113–222.
68. Mukae H, et al. Clinicoradiologic features of pleuropulmonary *Paragonimus westermani* on Kyusyu Island, Japan. Chest 2001; 120(2):514–520.
69. Sharma OP. The man who loved drunken crabs. A case of pulmonary paragonimiasis. Chest 1989; 95(3):670–672.
70. Im JG, et al. Pleuropulmonary paragonimiasis: radiologic findings in 71 patients. AJR Am J Roentgenol 1992; 159(1):39–43.
71. Yee B, et al. Pulmonary paragonimiasis in Southeast Asians living in the central San Joaquin Valley. West J Med 1992; 156(4):423–425.
72. Yokogawa M, et al. Immunoglobulin E: raised levels in sera and pleural exudates of patients with paragonimiasis. Am J Trop Med Hyg 1976; 25(4): 581–586.
73. Taniguchi H, et al. Elevated IL-5 levels in pleural fluid of patients with *Paragonimiasis westermani*. Clin Exp Immunol 2001; 123(1):94–98.
74. Walsh JA. Problems in recognition and diagnosis of amebiasis: estimation of the global magnitude of morbidity and mortality. Rev Infect Dis 1986; 8(2):228–238.
75. Herrera-Llerandi R. Thoracic repercussions of amebiasis. J Thorac Cardiovasc Surg 1966; 52(3):361–375.
76. Avirutnan P, et al. Dengue virus infection of human endothelial cells leads to chemokine production, complement activation, and apoptosis. J Immunol 1998; 161(11):6338–6846.
77. Charoenratanakul S. Tropical infection and the lung. Monaldi Arch Chest Dis 1997; 52(4):376–379.
78. Cameron EW. The treatment of pleuropulmonary amebiasis with metronidazole. Chest 1978; 73(5):647–650.

79. Ibarra-Perez C. Thoracic complications of amebic abscess of the liver: report of 501 cases. Chest 1981; 79(6):672–677.

80. Thorsen S, et al. Extra-intestinal amebiasis: clinical presentation in a non-endemic setting. Scand J Infect Dis 1993; 25(6):747–750.

81. Lyche KD, Jensen WA. Pleuropulmonary amebiasis. Semin Respir Infect 1997; 12(2):106–112.

82. Fulton AJ, et al. Pulmonary complication of amoebic liver abscess. Austral Radiol 1982; 26(1):60–63.

83. Boultbee JE, et al. Experiences with grey scale ultrasonography in hepatic amoebiasis. Clin Radiol 1979; 30(6):683–689.

84. Kubitschek KR, et al. Amebiasis presenting as pleuropulmonary disease. West J Med 1985; 142(2):203–207.

85. Griffiths JK, WD. Protozoan Infections of the Thorax. New York: McGraw-Hill, 1998.

86. Ozcelik C, et al. Surgical treatment of pulmonary hydatidosis in children: experience in 92 patients. J Pediatr Surg 1994; 29(3):392–395.

87. Jerray M, et al. Hydatid disease of the lungs. Study of 386 cases. Am Rev Respir Dis 1992; 146(1):185–189.

88. Xanthakis DS, et al. Hydatid cyst of the liver with intrathoracic rupture. Thorax 1981; 36(7):497–501.

89. von Sinner W. Pleural complications of hydatid disease (*Echinococcus granulosus*). Rofo Fortschr Geb Rontgenstr Neuen Bildgeb Verfahr 1990; 152(6):718–722.

90. Wen H, New RR, Craig PS. Diagnosis and treatment of human hydatidosis. Br J Clin Pharmacol 1993; 35(6):565–574.

91. Balikian JP, Mudarris FF. Hydatid disease of the lungs. A roentgenologic study of 50 cases. Am J Roentgenol Radium Ther Nucl Med 1974; 122(4):692–707.

92. Balikian JP, Idriss IA, Dagher IK. Hydatid tension pneumothorax. Report of a case. J Med Liban 1974; 27(5):551–556.

93. Lewall DB, McCorkell SJ. Rupture of echinococcal cysts: diagnosis, classification, and clinical implications. AJR Am J Roentgenol 1986; 146(2): 391–394.

94. Cangir AK, et al. Surgical treatment of pulmonary hydatid cysts in children. J Pediatr Surg 2001; 36(6):917–920.

95. Skerrett SJ, PJ. Parasitic infections of the pleural space. Semin Respir Med 1992; 13:242–258.

96. Drugs for parasitic infections. Med Lett Drugs Ther 1998; 40(1017):1–12.

97. Stover DE, et al. Spectrum of pulmonary diseases associated with the acquired immune deficiency syndrome. Am J Med 1985; 78(3):429–437.

98. Balachandran I, Jones DB, Humphrey DM. A case of *Pneumocystis carinii* in pleural fluid with cytologic, histologic and ultrastructural documentation. Acta Cytol 1990; 34(4):486–490.

99. Mariuz P, et al. Pleural *Pneumocystis carinii* infection. Chest 1991; 99(3):774–776.

100. Horowitz ML, et al. *Pneumocystis carinii* pleural effusion. Pathogenesis and pleural fluid analysis. Am Rev Respir Dis 1993; 148(1):232–234.

101. Al-Ibrahim MS, Holzman RS. Bilateral pleural effusions with *Plasmodium falciparum* infection. Am J Trop Med Hyg 1975; 24(6 Pt 1):910–912.
102. Sirivichayakul C, et al. Pleural effusion in childhood falciparum malaria. Southeast Asian J Trop Med Pub Health 2000; 31(1):187–189.
103. Sharma OP, Maheshwari A. Lung diseases in the tropics. Part 2: common tropical lung diseases: diagnosis and management. Tuber Lung Dis 1993; 74(6):359–370.
104. Miller RF, et al. Pleural effusions in patients with AIDS. Sex Transm Infect 2000; 76(2):122–125.
105. Shibuya T. Eosinophilic response in parasitic diseases. Nippon Rinsho 1993; 51(3):825–831.
106. Roberts PP. Parasitic infections of the pleural space. Semin Respir Infect 1988; 3(4):362–382.
107. Milanez de Campos JR, et al. Human pulmonary dirofilariasis: analysis of 24 cases from Sao Paulo, Brazil. Chest 1997; 112(3):729–733.
108. Matsuoka H, et al. A case report of serologically diagnosed pulmonary anisakiasis with pleural effusion and multiple lesions. Am J Trop Med Hyg 1994; 51(6):819–822.
109. Walzer PD, Rutherford I, East R. Empyema with *Trichomonas* species. Am Rev Respir Dis 1978; 118(2):415–418.
110. Jeanfaivre T, et al. Pleural effusion and toxocariasis. Thorax 1996; 51(1): 106–107.
111. Morrissey R, Caso R. Pleural sporotrichosis. Chest 1983; 84(4):507.
112. Feldman C, et al. Diffuse interstitial pulmonary fibrosis and spontaneous pneumothorax associated with *Schistosoma haematobium* infestation of the lungs. A case report. South Afr Med J 1986; 69(2):138–139.
113. Bartoloni A, et al. *Mansonella ozzardi* infection in Bolivia: prevalence and clinical associations in the Chaco region. Am J Trop Med Hyg 1999; 61(5):830–833.
114. Horn R, et al. Fungemia in a cancer hospital: changing frequency, earlier onset, and results of therapy. Rev Infect Dis 1985; 7(5):646–655.
115. Ko SC, et al. Fungal empyema thoracis: an emerging clinical entity. Chest 2000; 117(6):1672–1678.
116. Chen KY, et al. Pulmonary fungal infection: emphasis on microbiological spectra, patient outcome, and prognostic factors. Chest 2001; 120(1):177–184.
117. Houston S. Tropical respiratory medicine. 3. Histoplasmosis and pulmonary involvement in the tropics. Thorax 1994; 49(6):598–601.
118. George RB, Penn RL, Kinasewitz GT. Mycobacterial, fungal, actinomycotic, and nocardial infections of the pleura. Clin Chest Med 1985; 6(1):63–75.
119. Marshall BC, et al. Histoplasmosis as a cause of pleural effusion in the acquired immunodeficiency syndrome. Am J Med Sci 1990; 300(2):98–101.
120. Brewer PL, JP. Himmelwright, pleural effusion due to infection with *Histoplasma capsulatum*. Chest 1970; 58(1):76–79.
121. Weissbluth M. Pleural effusion in histoplasmosis. J Pediatr 1976; 88(5): 894–895.

122. Schub HM, Spivey CG Jr, Baird GD. Pleural involvement in histoplasmosis. Am Rev Respir Dis 1966; 94(2):225–232.
123. Richardson JV, George RB. Bronchopleural fistula and lymphocytic empyema due to *Histoplasma capsulatum*. Chest 1997; 112(4):1130–1132.
124. Swinburne AJ, et al. Histoplasmoma, pleural fibrosis, and slowly enlarging pleural effusion in an asymptomatic patient. Am Rev Respir Dis 1987; 135(2):502–503.
125. Failla PJ, et al. Blastomycosis: pulmonary and pleural manifestations. South Med J 1995; 88(4):405–410.
126. Ibrahim TM, Edinol ST. Pleural effusion from blastomycetes in an adult Nigerian: a case report. Niger Postgrad Med J 2001; 8(3):148–149.
127. Daley CL. Tropical respiratory medicine. 1. Pulmonary infections in the tropics: impact of HIV infection. Thorax 1994; 49(4):370–378.
128. Chechani V, Kamholz SL. Pulmonary manifestations of disseminated cryptococcosis in patients with AIDS. Chest 1990; 98(5):1060–1066.
129. Davies SF, Sarosi GA. Fungal pulmonary complications. Clin Chest Med 1996; 17(4):725–744.
130. Batra P. Pulmonary coccidioidomycosis. J Thorac Imag 1992; 7(4):29–38.
131. Mortara L, Bayer AS. Fever, cough, pleuritic chest pain, and pleural fluid eosinophilia in a 30-year-old man. Chest 1994; 105(3):918–919.
132. Einstein HE, Chia JK, Meyer RD. Pulmonary infiltrate and pleural effusion in a diabetic man. Clin Infect Dis 1992; 14(4):955–960.
133. George RB, et al. Mycoplasma and adenovirus pneumonias. Comparison with other atypical pneumonias in a military population. Ann Intern Med 1966; 65(5):931–942.
134. Fine NL, Smith LR, Sheedy PF. Frequency of pleural effusions in mycoplasma and viral pneumonias. N Engl J Med 1970; 283(15):790–793.
135. Light RW. Pleural Diseases. 4th ed. Baltimore: Lippincott Williams and Wilkins, 2001.
136. Gross PA, Gerding DN. Pleural effusion associated with viral hepatitis. Gastroenterology 1971; 60(5):898–902.
137. Akamaguna AI, Odita JC. The radiological aspects of chest complication in childhood measles. Ann Trop Paediatr 1982; 2(3):129–132.
138. Clement JP. Hantavirus. Antiviral Res 2003; 57(1–2):121–127.
139. Botten J, et al. Persistent Sin Nombre virus infection in the deer mouse (*Peromyscus maniculatus*) model: sites of replication and strand-specific expression. J Virol 2003; 77(2):1540–1550.
140. Levy H, Simpson SQ. Hantavirus pulmonary syndrome. Am J Respir Crit Care Med 1994; 149(6):1710–1713.
141. Boone JD, et al. Infection dynamics of Sin Nombre virus after a widespread decline in host populations. Am J Trop Med Hyg 2002; 67(3):310–318.
142. Bustamante EA, Levy H, Simpson SQ. Pleural fluid characteristics in hantavirus pulmonary syndrome. Chest 1997; 112(4):1133–1136.
143. Hujakka H, et al. Diagnostic rapid tests for acute hantavirus infections: specific tests for Hantaan, Dobrava and Puumala viruses versus a hantavirus combination test. J Virol Meth 2003; 108(1):117–122.

144. Lednicky JA. Hantaviruses. a short review. Arch Pathol Lab Med 2003; 127(1):30–35.
145. Kautner I, Robinson MJ, Kuhnle U. Dengue virus infection: epidemiology, pathogenesis, clinical presentation, diagnosis, and prevention. J Pediatr 1997; 131(4):516–524.
146. Rigau-Perez JG, et al. Dengue and dengue haemorrhagic fever. Lancet 1998; 352(9132):971–977.
147. Ramirez-Ronda CH, Garcia CD. Dengue in the Western Hemisphere. Infect Dis Clin North Am 1994; 8(1):107–128.
148. Laferl H. Pleural effusion and ascites on return from Pakistan. Lancet 1997; 350(9084):1072.
149. Fife TD, Finegold SM, Grennan T. Pericardial actinomycosis: case report and review. Rev Infect Dis 1991; 13(1):120–126.
150. Conant EF, Wechsler RJ. Actinomycosis and nocardiosis of the lung. J Thorac Imag 1992; 7(4):75–84.
151. Esteban C, et al. Increased adenosine deaminase activity in Q fever pneumonia with pleural effusion. Chest 1994; 105(2):648.
152. Hovette P, et al. Pleuropulmonary manifestations of salmonellosis. Med Trop (Mars) 1998; 58(4):403–407.
153. Chong VF, Fan YF. The radiology of melioidosis. Austral Radiol 1996; 40(3):244–249.
154. Matos ED, et al. Chest radiograph abnormalities in patients hospitalized with leptospirosis in the city of Salvador, Bahia, Brazil. Braz J Infect Dis 2001; 5(2):73–77.
155. Papiris SA, et al. Brucella haemorrhagic pleural effusion. Eur Respir J 1994; 7(7):1369–1370.
156. Sahn SA. Pleural effusions in the atypical pneumonias. Semin Respir Infect 1988; 3(4):322–334.
157. Dikensoy O, et al. Increased pleural fluid adenosine deaminase in brucellosis is difficult to differentiate from tuberculosis. Respiration 2002; 69(6): 556–559.

8

Tropical Granulomas: Diagnosis

VIOLETA MIHAILOVIC-VUCINIC

Medical School, University of Belgrade,
Serbia and Institute of Pulmonary Diseases,
University Clinical Center,
Belgrade, Serbia

OM P. SHARMA

Keck School of Medicine, University of
Southern California,
Los Angeles, California, U.S.A.

A granuloma is a focal collection of inflammatory cells that include mononuclear cells, macrophages, and giant cells along with a number of lymphocytes, plasma cells, and fibroblasts. Granulomatous reactions may be classified functionally into two major categories (1). The first group consists of lesions characterized by delayed-type hypersensitivity, antigen-specific response. These granulomas have a high rate of cell turnover, are very active lesions, and are seen in tuberculosis, sarcoidosis, hypersensitivity pneumonitis, and schistosomiasis. The second type is a foreign body granuloma that lacks an antigen-specific response and often is an inactive, minimally destructive lesion. These low-turnover granulomas are seen in berylliosis, where the offending agent is inanimate and inert. The composition of the causative irritant and its degradability and immunogenecity are decisive factors in the development of a granuloma (2).

I. Morphology of Granuloma

Granulomas are dynamic entities going through evolutionary and involutionary phases of cell proliferation and death that are probably regulated by localized cell–cell interactions. The mature granuloma is caused by an influx of hematogenous mononuclear phagocytes and their local proliferation, maturation, and activation (3).

A. Epithelioid Cells

These are derived from macrophages, and are large mononuclear cells about 20 μm in diameter. The maturation of macrophages is influenced by many stimuli such as immune complexes, phagocytic burden, membrane perturbants such as phorbol esters, arachidonate metabolites, and specific activators such as lymphokines, chemotactic factors, and interferons (4). Epithelioid cells are round or oval in shape and may be of two types: one with abundant granular endoplasmic reticulum and mitochondria, the other with predominant vacuoles containing pale fibrillar material. They are poorly phagocytic, but actively pinocytic, with strong microbicidal activity (5). They possess avid secretory properties that have been confirmed by immunocytochemical localization of products such as angiotensin converting enzymes (6).

B. Giant Cells

These are formed by the fusion of macrophages or epithelioid cells and may be up to 300 μm in diameter and contain as many as 30 nuclei. Fusion takes place either as a result of secretion of specific lymphokines or membrane events associated with attempts by mononuclear cells to phagocytoze large particles. The two mechanisms may act synergistically. Fusion initially results in a heterokaryon with randomly scattered nuclei that later redistribute by a microtubule-dependent mechanism to form a peripheral ring (7). Foreign body and Langhans' giant cells are poorly phagocytic and their function is uncertain.

C. Inclusion Bodies

Both epithelioid cells and giant cells may contain curious, calcium-rich, star-shaped, or conchoid inclusion bodies—Schaumann, asteroid, and residual bodies—all of which are nonspecific and nondiagnostic. They represent the end products of active metabolism and secretion. Inclusion bodies are found in tuberculosis, syphilis, sarcoidosis, chronic beryllium lung disease, Crohn's disease, and extrinsic allergic alveolitis (8).

D. Lymphocytes

Granulomas often contain lymphocytes of both T and B types. T lymphocytes usually form a peripheral rim, whereas B cells are found within the granuloma and can be identified by immunofluorescence tests. Immunoperoxidase techniques to analyze lymphocytes and identify various patterns have been used. Granulomas form an effective cell-mediated response, as in tuberculoid leprosy, sarcoidosis, and tuberculosis. These granulomas demonstrate a high number of helper cells within epithelioid cell aggregates and a surrounding rim of suppressor cells. Granulomas from poor cell-mediated response, as in lepromatous leprosy, granuloma annulare, and rhinoscleroma, show a near equal number of helper and suppressor phenotypes evenly distributed throughout the granuloma (9). In general, T-helper cells are involved in the maintenance of a granuloma. CD-4+ T-helper cells, necessary for the development of granulomas, are further classified into functional types, Th1 and Th2. Th1 cells participate in a delayed-type response through the production of interleukin-2, interferon-gamma, and tumor necrosis factor-alpha; TH2 cells make IL-4, IL-3, and IL-10, which are important for the development of B cells and eosinophilia. There is a reciprocal relationship between TH1 and TH2 lymphokine expression. Granulomas of sarcoidosis and tuberculoid leprosy make large quantities of TH1-type lymphokines and less of TH2 type; whereas, granuloma that synthesize predominantly Th2 cytokines make small amounts of Th1 type. Cyclosporin A, a potent T-cell suppressor, can completely inhibit granuloma formation.

II. Function of Granuloma

The basic function of a granuloma is to keep the offending agent subdued and, eventually to destroy it. In doing so, the granuloma disturbs the traffic of circulating immune reactor cells within the lymphoid organs and other tissues. This could contribute the peripheral depression of delayed-type hypersensitivity commonly observed in granulomatous disorders. Macrophages, which are not very phagocytic, are highly active secretory cells capable of releasing a variety of potent enzymes including lysozyme, angiotensin converting enzyme (ACE), plasminogen activator, collagenase, elastase, and 1, 25-dihydroxy D3 (10). Many of these enzymes are capable of lysing extracellular fibrin, collagen, and elastin. Plasmin activates enzymatic cascade generating mediators of inflammation.

III. Immunological Events at the Site of Granuloma

Granuloma formation is an expression of a series of complex inflammatory events. Most studies analyzing the immunopathogenesis of granuloma formation have been performed in tuberculosis, leprosy, sarcoidosis, and hypersensitivity pneumonitis. Evidence has accumulated in recent years to show that cytokines, such as interleukin-1 (IL-1), migration inhibition factor, and chemotactic factors play an important role in the initiation and maintenance of granulomatous inflammation (11). In hypersensitivity and foreign body granuloma models, IL-1, but not IL-2 activity is detected that correlates with activity and size of granulomas. Natural killer (NK) cell cytolytic activity is suppressed in active pulmonary granulomatous inflammation.

Gallium (^{67}Ga) lung scans during active granuloma formation demonstrate the presence of a large number of activated alveolar macrophages in the lung parenchyma. These activated macrophages process and present antigen to lymphocytes. The macrophages release IL-1 that serves as a maturational signal and augments T-cell proliferation. The helper T cells produce IL-2, which is nonantigen-specific. Under its influence, the responding cell acquires IL-2 receptors, proliferates, and differentiates into an effector cell. Lymphocytes from the lung also produce gamma-interferon, a chemotactic factor for circulating monocytes, and other lymphokines, including migration inhibition factor. These chemical mediators provide cells for the continuing maintenance of granulomas (12).

IV. Causes of Lung Granulomas

There are numerous causes of pulmonary granulomas. Some of these are well known, others are only partially identified, and still others are barely understood and difficult to identify. Certain granulomatous lung diseases are limited to the tropics or are more common there than in temperate regions because of the tremendous variations in the epidemiological factors that determine the distribution, prevalence, incidence, and endemicity of disease. The causative agents range from live replicating intracellular organisms (bacteria, mycobacteria, viruses, fungi) to nonreplicating metazoans (helminths) to inanimate substances (metals, chemical agents) and organic antigens.

V. Differential Diagnosis

A careful history and physical examination are mandatory. The points discussed below should be emphasized.

A. Location and Travels

In India, the most common case of pulmonary granuloma is tuberculosis, whereas in Egypt and North Africa schistosomiasis should be included in the differential diagnosis. Brucellosis is a common granulomatous disease in the Middle East. Granulomas in association with visceral leishmaniasis should be considered in residents of almost every developing country. In sharp contrast to the tropics, coccidioidomycosis and sarcoidosis head the list in California; whereas, histoplasmosis is the frequent culprit in the mid-western United States. Thus, it is absolutely essential to obtain a thorough history of the patient's residence and recent travels.

B. Occupational History

Brucellosis is an occupational hazard of veterinary surgeons, laboratory personnel, and abbatoir workers. In Kuwait, brucellosis is a major health hazard among sheep and camel herders, most of whom drink raw milk and have close contact with animals. Farmer's lung disease is caused by antigenic products of thermophilic actinomyces (*Microplolypora faeni*). The causative agent is not histologically detectable, but a positive history of exposure is of diagnostic value, since it might lead one to estimate levels of circulating precipitins against the antigen. Chronic beryllium disease, although rare, continues to be a hazard because the metal is being used increasingly in a variety of industries, especially ceramics and metallurgy.

C. Hobbies

Pigeon breeder's disease, parakeet lung, talc granulomatosis, mushroom picker's lung, and many others are acquired while the individual indulges in an apparently harmless pursuit of pleasure. Intravenous drug abuse involving injection of talc-containing drugs intended for oral use is known to cause granulomatous inflammation in the lung. This habit is usually the result of a shortage of available heroin. Granulomas due to coccidiodes may occur in individuals indulging in such activities as unearthing Indian relics and rock hunting. A careful social history including hobbies and habits may, therefore, provide invaluable clues to determining the cause of some pulmonary granulomas diseases.

D. Family History

If more than one member of the family is ill, the answer might lie in the home environment. The incidence of tuberculosis diminishes as social and economic conditions improve. Poor housing with associated overcrowding increases the risk of massive infection or reinfection if one of the occupants has infectious tuberculosis. Leprosy has long been considered to occur only after exposure to a human case. The most important mode of spread of *Mycobacterium leprae* being by droplets from the sneezes of lepromatous patients with heavily infected nasal mucus membrane. However, evidence has been accumulating that this conventional view is wrong and that an environmental nonhuman source is critical to some *M. leprae* infections. Recent observations with monoclonal antibodies have shown that phenolic glycolipid I antigen, unique to the *M. leprae* cell wall, is found in soil.

E. Physical Examination

Sarcoidosis, leprosy, fungal diseases, and tuberculosis are multisystem disorders. The patient should be examined carefully for ocular lesions, dermatological changes, joint involvement, peripheral lymphadenopathy, splenomegaly, and neurological involvement. Remittent fever, splenomegaly, and hepatomegaly in a chronically ill patient may suggest visceral leishmaniasis.

F. Chest Roentgenographic Features

In pulmonary tuberculosis, the chest roentgenogram may show unilateral hilar adenopathy, miliary infiltration, and an upper lobe infiltrate with or without a cavity. In sarcoidosis, bilateral hilar adenopathy occurs in more than 50% of the patients. The X-ray findings in beryllium lung disease are nonspecific. In the early stages, there is a general haziness, or ground glass appearance throughout both lungs. As the disease progresses, however, bronchovascular and hilar shadows increase. Reticulation may be observed in some cases, primarily in the upper lung regions, with evidence of over expansion at the bases. Thus, an ability to recognize a few radiographic patterns goes a long way in evaluating a patient with a lung granuloma (Table 1).

G. Histological Findings

Recognition of typical features of a granuloma, special stains [Acid Fast Bacilli (AFB), fungi], culture of tissue, and examination of tissue under a polarizing light microscope considerably narrow the diagnostic possibilities.

Table 1 Common Chest Radiographic Patterns

Features	TB	Sarcoidosis	HP	CBD	WG
Hilar adenopathy	Unilateral	Bilateral	Absent	Rare	Absent
Pulmonary infiltrate	Upper lung fields, may be miliary	Mid and lower lung fields	Upper lung fields, may be diffuse	Diffuse	Patchy, nodular
Cavity formation	Common	Uncommon	Absent	Absent	Common
Mediastinal adenopathy	May occur	Uncommon	Absent	Absent	Absent
Pleural effusion	Common	Uncommon	Absent	Absent	Rare
Large nodules	May occur	May occur	Absent	Absent	Common

Abbreviations: TB, tuberculosis; HP, hypersensitivity pneumonitis; CBD, chronic beryllium disease; WG, Wegener's granulomatosis.

Caseation is characteristic of the mycobacterium-induced granulomas, whereas the sarcoid or beryllium-induced granulomas practically never undergo caseation. The histological picture of hypersensitivity granulomas, however, is seldom specific and cannot be independently used as a diagnostic tool for the identification of specific diseases.

H. Skin Tests

The Kveim–Siltzbach skin test is most helpful in differentiating sarcoidosis from all other granulomatous disorders. However, not only is the antigen not generally available but there is also a lack of standardized preparations. Tuberculin, histoplasmin, and coccidioidin skin tests have minor but important roles. There are no skin tests for hypersensitivity pneumonitis. In general, skin tests play only a limited role in diagnosing granulomatous diseases.

I. Laboratory Tests

A determination of the serum and bronchoalveolar lavage fluid (BALF) angiotensin converting enzyme (ACE) may be useful in establishing the diagnosis of sarcoidosis. The serum level of ACE (SACE) is thought to reflect the granulomatous load in the body, and is elevated in up to 80% of patients with sarcoidosis. SACE levels fall with resolution of granulomata and can prove useful in monitoring the course of the disease. SACE levels are nonspecific, however, and may be elevated in many diseases (Table 2). Even so, elevated SACE levels associated with hypercalcemia strongly suggests sarcoidosis. This combination, however may also occur in Hodgkin's disease and miliary tuberculosis. Both agglutinating and complement-fixing antibody titers may be used in the diagnosis of brucellosis. Titers may persist at low levels for months or years, especially in patients with chronic infections. There is a problem of cross-reaction with *Francisella tularensis*, *Yersinia enterolitica*, and other organisms. Serological titers are important in the

Table 2 Conditions Associated with Elevated Serum ACE Level

Likely to be confused with sarcoidosis	Not likely to be confused with sarcoidosis
Asbestosis	Coccidioidomycosis
Berylliosis	Diabetes mellitus
Granulomatous hepatitis	Idiopathic respiratory disease syndrome
Hypersensitivity pneumonitis	Gaucher's disease
Lymphoma	Inflammatory bowel disease
Miliary tuberculosis	Pulmonary neoplasm
Primary biliary cirrhosis	Leprosy
Silicosis	Liver cirrhosis

diagnosis of brucellosis, because the organisms are fastidious and require special media for optimal recovery from blood. The only abnormal laboratory findings in chronic infections with schistosoma may be peripheral eosinophilia and a mild increase of serum globulins, especially IgG. The sedimentation rate and C-reactive protein levels are not helpful in the evaluation of pulmonary granulomas.

The differential diagnosis of granulomatous disorders demands a synthesis of information provided by the clinician, the radiologist, the microbiologist, and the pathologist. Some of the conditions commonly encountered are discussed in the next sections.

VI. Mycobacterial Infections

A. Tuberculosis

There are more documented tuberculosis cases in the world today than have ever been recorded before, and with many third-world countries documenting high resistance rates to single and multiple drugs, it has become a major health problem worldwide. The tuberculous granulomas are usually characterized by central caseous necrosis, but in miliary tuberculosis noncaseating granulomas are more common. Hypercalcemia and elevated SACE levels may occur in miliary tuberculosis. Acid-fast stains and culture of body fluids or biopsied tissues are needed to confirm the diagnosis. Many laboratories use a flurochrome staining procedure with auramine O as the stain. This requires a fluorescent microscope for examination but is much faster because the slide can be scanned at a lower magnification (13–15).

B. Leprosy

This chronic infectious disease is caused by *Mycobacterium leprae*, an organism with suspected high infectivity but low pathogenicity and with a preference for growth in cool areas of the body. The disease is endemic in most of the tropical and warm, temperate countries of the world including Southeastern Asia, Africa, and South America. Incidence and prevalence figures are inaccurate because of the limited resource for health care in the areas most affected, and the stigma attached to the diagnosis. The conventional view regarding the mode of spread of *M. leprae*, including prolonged close contact and transmission by nasal droplet, is being strongly challenged. The granulomas in tuberculoid leprosy have little or no caseation. *M. leprae* bacilli are scanty or altogether absent and cannot be cultured or transmitted to usual laboratory animals. Systemic infections develop in thymectomized or irradiated mice, in nude mice, and in about 50% or normal nine banded armadillos. The latter are the main source of leprosy bacilli used for research. Elevated SACE levels may be noted in the leprosy patients. Leprosy may mimic other diseases involving the skin and peripheral nerves. The diagnosis is established by clinical evidence of the disease and biopsy. The lepromin test is usually positive in tuberculoid leprosy (TT) and negative in lepromatous leprosy (LL). Recent studies based on detection of *M. leprae*-specific phenolic glycolipid I give rise to the possibility of a serodiagnositic test for leprosy in the future. In terms of pulmonary function in leprosy, there is evidence of universal hyporesponsiveness in lepromatous leprosy, which is attributed to autonomic system involvement (16–18).

VII. Fungal Diseases

A. Bronchocentric Granulomatous

This is a necrotizing granulomatous disease of the lung centered principally around bronchi and bronchioles. Clinical manifestations include fever, cough, chest pain, and malaise. Most patients (50%) have a history of chronic asthma. Some patients have multiple allergies. Positive skin tests and serum precipitins to *Aspergillus* and isolation of *Aspergillus* from sputum cultures from several patients have been observed. Chest radiographic studies may reveal involvement of a single lobe or multiple lobes, with unilateral or bilateral involvement. Other radiological manifestations include multiple small or large nodules, consolidation, infarction patterns, and collapse (mucus plugging). Bronchograms may reveal segmental obstruction. The pathogenesis of bronchocentric granulomatiosis in asthmatic patients is likely to be related to hypersensitivity against Aspergillus antigens. The cause in nonasthmatic patients is not known (19,20).

B. Histoplasmosis

This granulomatous infection is acquired by inhalation. It has been reported from over 50 countries, including Africa, Southeast Asia, Mexico, and South America, with the first case being recognized in Panama in 1905. In the United States, the Mid-western portion of the county is the area of highest endemicity. Histoplasmosis may resemble sarcoidosis clinically, pathologically, and radiologically. Histoplasma granulomas tend to be round, are often microscopically solitary, and if, multiple, usually contain one dominant lesion. They are generally surrounded by sclerosing fibrosis and often contain calcium. Since the standard hematoxylin and eosin stain is inadequate, special stains such as silver and periodic acid-Schiff (PAS) may be necessary to visualize the organism in tissue sections. Although important in epidemiological studies, the histoplasmin skin test is not often helpful diagnostically and has the disadvantage of occasionally boosting a subsequent complement fixation titer. Serum complement fixation, immunodiffusion, and radioimmunoassay may be needed for accurate diagnosis (21,22).

VIII. Parasitic Diseases

A. Protozoa Leishmaniasis

Visceral leishmaniasis (kala azar) is a disease characterized by a long incubation period and a chronic course, remittent fever, leucopenia, anemia, and enlargement of the spleen and liver. The Mediterranean type is prevalent in the Mediterranean and Red Sea littorals, Sudan, Asian Russia, and Arabia, whereas the Indian type is prevalent in parts of India and Burma bordering the Bay of Bengal. The parasites, known as Leishman-Donovan bodies, are found in the cytoplasm of reticuloendothelial cells or free in the blood plasma. Transmission is either by the bite of the female sandfly, *Phlebotomus* spp. or transfusion of infected blood. Pulmonary involvement is usually characterized by signs and symptoms of bronchitis or bronchopneumonia. There is usually an increase in gammaglobulins, mainly IgG. The diagnosis depends on appropriate history, clinical evidence of splenomegaly, hepatomegaly, progressive granulocytopenia, and profound anemia. With the increase in incidence of human immunodeficiency virus (HIV) infections in Africa and other tropical countries, kala azar is emerging as an important opportunistic infection in the patients with the acquired immunodeficiency syndrome (AIDS). A sero-diagnostic assay for visceral leishmaniasis using monoclonal antibodies is now available (23–25).

B. Metazoa

Nematodes

Parasitic helminthes are common in almost all developing countries due to the prevailing sanitary conditions. Migration of a helminth through the lung may induce foreign-body-type cellular reactions with subsequent granuloma formation. Metazoan tissue parasites such as *Trichinella spiralis* larva and others are too large to be phagocytosed, but can secrete various antigens that are probably ingested by pinocytosis by the surrounding macrophages. The slow degradability of metazoans and the continuous antigenic stimuli emanating from them ensure that conditions for granuloma formation are fulfilled. Refractile structures representing fragments of the helminth may be seen in the center of the granuloma on lung biopsy. Patients may present with a visceral larva migrans syndrome, asthmatic symptoms, and eosinophilia. The nematodes causing pulmonary granulomas include *Ascaris lumbricoides, Toxocara canis, Capillaria aerophilia*, and others. Eosinophilia may be absent at the onset of respiratory symptoms. Compounding the diagnostic dilemma, stool samples may be negative for ova and parasites (26).

Tropical Pulmonary Eosinophilia

This disease is found mostly in India, Southeast Asia, and the South Pacific islands and should be considered in all patients with eosinophilia and miliary pulmonary infiltrates who give the appropriate history (Vijayan: Tropical eosinophilia).

C. Trematodes: Schistosomiasis

Schistosoma mansoni has a wide geographical distribution including Africa, the eastern Mediterranean, South America, and the West Indies. The disease is mainly due to eggs deposited in host tissue by the adult female worms, which induce inflammatory and fibrotic lesions in the host organs, including the intestines, liver, and lungs. Pulmonary hypertension and cor pulmonale induced by pulmonary arteritis as a result of *S. mansoni* egg deposition are well documented in the literature. Such pathological effects are due to collateral circulation in patients with liver fibrosis and portal hypertension, which provide direct access of eggs to the lungs. The *S. mansoni* egg granuloma is a T-cell-mediated, delayed-type hypersensitivity granuloma.

Pulmonary hypertension and cor pulmonale are less common with *Schistosoma japonicum* or *Schistosoma hematobium* infection. Diagnosis and assessment of morbidity are based on clinical features, stool egg count, and other laboratory findings (Schwartz: Schistosomiasis).

IX. Bacterial Disease

A. Brucellosis

This is a zoonotic infection caused by bacteria of the genus *Brucella*. It is an acute or chronic illness manifested principally by chills, relapses of fever, weakness, and vague aches and pains. In the United States, brucellosis is rare and is largely an occupational hazard of slaughterhouse workers and veterinarians. It is common in the Far East, Kuwait and other Gulf countries, South America, Mexico, and the Mediterranean region. This disease can be caused by any of the four species, each usually confined to its major animal host: *B. melitensis* to goats, *B. suis* to hogs, *B. abortus* to cattle, and *B. canis* to dogs (Chapter 1: Pulmonary Zoonoses).

B. Tularemia

Francisella (Pasturella) *tularensis* is a small gram-negative coccobacillus spread by contact with infected sheep. Tularemia is an occupational hazard of sheep-herders, trappers, and butchers. Tularemia may present in different ways depending upon the site of inoculation, but the most common clinical features are local ulcer formation and regional lymphadenopathy in association with symptoms of systemic febrile illness. Host defense mechanisms are not fully understood. However, immunity is associated with the appearance of delayed hypersensitivity to tularemia skin antigen. Septicemic tularemia usually causes miliary microabscesses in the liver, spleen, and lungs. With healing, these abscesses organize and granulomas may occur. There are many pathological similarities between tularemia and tuberculosis. On microscopic examination, mononuclear cells are prominent in the lesions and some may undergo caseous necrosis. Various degrees of organization, occasionally with giant cells present, occur with healing. Granulomatous pleuritis may be confused with tuberculous pleuritis. Because the organism is fastidious and highly infective, serological responses are usually used for diagnosis (27,28).

X. Granulomatous Diseases of Unknown Cause

These are a group of chronic granulomatous lung diseases in which no causative agents have been found.

A. Sarcoidosis

This granulomatous disorder of unknown cause has a worldwide distribution. Although it is much less frequent in tropical Africa, India, and Southeast Asia, the frequency of sarcoidosis in the central mountainous district of Japan is high. It most commonly affects young adults and presents most frequently with bilateral hilar adenopathy, pulmonary infiltration, and skin or eye lesions. It can involve almost any organ system in various combinations, giving rise to many clinical syndromes embracing all branches of medicine. Immunological features include depression of delayed-type hypersensitivity, suggesting impaired cell-mediated immunity, and elevated or abnormal immunoglobulins. Alveolar macrophages from sarcoidosis patients are HLA-DR/DS+, can present a variety of antigens to autologous blood T-cells, can spontaneously secrete IL-1 immune interferon and fibronectin, and display C3b and Fc membrane receptors. The diagnosis depends on the evidence of multisystem involvement, typical chest roentgenographic findings, and the presence of noncaseating granulomata in a tissue biopsy specimen. Elevated SACE and calcium levels are helpful (29,30).

B. Wegener's Granulomatosis

This disease, first described in the 1930s, is an organ-specific necrotizing granulomatous vasculitis involving principally the lungs, upper respiratory tract, and kidneys. The presentation may be generalized, with involvement of the nose, lungs, and kidneys, or limited to only the lungs. Common presenting symptoms include nasal crusting and bleeding. A long history of sinusitis or rhinitis may precede discovery of lung or renal involvement. Pulmonary symptoms include cough, hemoptysis, and chest pain. Renal symptoms, when present, usually occur after the onset of respiratory symptoms. Constitutional symptoms such as low-grade fever, weight loss, and malaise are more common in the presence of respiratory symptoms. The skin may be involved with maculopapular or ulcerative lesions. Neurological involvement may be present in up to 25% of patients with systemic Wegener's granulomatosis. The disease is presumed to be a manifestation of the delayed hypersensitivity response to an as yet unidentified antigen. Because patients with Wegener's' granulomatosis sometimes respond to treatment with trimethoprim-sulfamethoxazole, it is possible that the causative agent for the disease may be an as yet unidentified infectious agent. The predilection of the granulomatous inflammations to occur in the vessel wall has not been explained. The detection of circulating immune complexes in certain patients could indicate that the granulogenic agents are the large complexes that lodge in the vessel walls and are ingested by macrophages initiating the granulomatous process. However, complex formation may be secondary to the delayed hypersensitivity response induced by a granulomagenic agent (31–33).

C. Pulmonary Allergic Granulomatosis

Churg and Strauss described in 1951 a series of patients with asthma, eosinophillia, and vascular lesions similar to the type seen in polyarteritis nodosa. The disease may be organized into three distinct phases. The prodromal or allergic phase is characterized by asthma with or without associated allergic rhinitis. Peripheral blood eosinophilia, eosinophilic tissue infiltrates, and/or eosinophilic gastroenteritis characterize the second phase. Systemic vasculitis characterizes the third phase. The chest radiographic pattern is nonspecific, typically revealing transient patchy infiltrates, massive bilateral nodular infiltrates without evidence of cavitation, or an interstitial pattern.

The cause of the illness is unknown. The diagnosis is made by history of asthma, eosinophilia, elevated IgE levels, and histological features of necrotizing vasculitis associated with tissue infiltration by eosinophils, and extravascular granulomas (34,35).

D. Lymphomatoid Granulomatosis

This disease, first described in 1972, is characterized by pulmonary lymphoreticular infiltrates that are angiocentric and angiodestructive. Pulmonary symptoms are common and include cough, dyspnea, and chest pain. Constitutional symptoms are frequent; dermatological and neurological involvement is common. Chest radiographs usually reveal bilateral nodular infiltrates that are frequently peripheral and may be mistaken for metastatic tumors. Other possible radiological features include cavitation, indistinct lesions resembling pneumonia, and lesions that change in configuration and size. Approximately 10% of pulmonary disease, initially diagnosed as lymphomatoid granulomatosis, may eventually manifest as malignant lymphoma. Pulmonary involvement is the major cause of death, although a significant number of patients die from central nervous system involvement (36).

E. Crohn's Regional Enteritis

Intestinal involvement in sarcoidosis is extremely rare, and most reports are probably examples of Crohn's granulomatosis enteritis. Both disorders may be associated with erythema nodosum and iritis, and the histology is similar. Furthermore, bronchoalveolar lavage reveals similar alveolitis in both conditions. There are, however, many differences so the two conditions have not been frequent sources of confusion (37).

F. Primary Biliary Cirrhosis

Both primary biliary cirrhosis and chronic active hepatitis may be associated with respiratory disease. Primary biliary cirrhosis (PBC) occurs in women aged 30–50 years with mild jaundice, pruritus, xanthelasma, and granulomas alongside bile ducts. The hallmark of PBC is the presence of serum mitochondrial antibodies, which are almost always present. Chronic active hepatitis is associated with cryptogenic fibrosing alveolitis and this is particularly noted in persons who are HLA B8; DR 3.

G. Whipple's Disease

Whipple's disease affects middle-aged white males, presenting with polyarthritis, diarrhea, weight loss, and fever. They may have cough, dyspnea, and pleurisy. The affected organs are infiltrated with numerous macrophages containing PAS-positive, diastase-resistant glycoprotein, and electron microscopy reveals rod-shaped bacteria called *Trophyrema whippeli*. It is a cause of the shrinking lung syndrome, which may be evident in chest X rays and by respiratory symptoms. Occasionally, granuloma formation also occurs in Whipple's disease causing confusion in the differential diagnosis with sarcoidosis (38).

H. Behçet's Disease

The characteristic features of this syndrome are oro-genital ulceration, uveitis, erythema nodosum, and thrombophlebitis. It is particularly common in young adults with HLA-B51 and HLA-DRW52. The intrathoracic component is of pulmonary infarction, pleurisy, pericarditis, and superior venacaval syndrome. The physician should always stroke the patient's skin, for dermatographia is a very common physical sign in this disease (Chapter 17).

XI. Hypersensitivity Pneumonitides

This group of pulmonary disorders includes several diseases such as farmer's lung, mushroom worker's lung, malt worker's lung, maple bark disease, bird fancier's lung, and others. They are initiated in nonatopic subjects by inhalation of organic dust leading to chronic alveolar inflammation, interstitial infiltration, granuloma formation, and fibrosis. Spores of thermophilic actinomycetes, avian serum proteins in bird droppings, or powdered pituitary hormones inhaled by patients with diabetes insipidus can serve as offending agents. Repeated inhalation of the agents induces sensitization in a certain percentage of exposed individuals. Histopathological changes of the lung during the acute stage are characterized by infiltration of lymphocytes, macrophages, and plasma cells into the walls of the alveoli and the alveolar space, thickening of the alveolar septae, and appearance of noncaseating granulomas with epitheliod and giant cells. In the chronic stage, lymphocytic infiltration persists and interstitial fibrosis is pronounced. Although an immune cause has been implicated in the disease, the types of hypersensitivity reactions participating in the reactions are not clearly known.

The presence of high levels of precipitins in persons exposed to *M. faeni*, the organism causing farmer's lung, was though to indicate that antigen–antibody complexes may be responsible, but no correlation has been found between the presence or absence of precipitins and symptoms of the disease. The presence of epithelioid-cell containing granulomas is indicative of a delayed-type hypersensitivity reaction. Examination of BALF from chronically ill patients revealed that the number of T lymphocytes was considerably elevated over that found in the circulation. There appears to be no difference in the ratio of T4/T8 in asymptomatic or symptomatic pigeon breeders. It is interesting that T8 lymphocytes are the predominant phenotype of T cell in either group. Hypersensitivity pneumonitis should be suspected when a person regularly exposed to a heavy concentration of organic dusts complains, a few hours after re-exposure to the same dust, of general malaise, dry cough, and dyspnea without wheeze. If not detected early, and further exposure to the dust hazard is permitted, the symptoms continue and become very severe in some cases. At this stage, the patient may be febrile, cyanosed, and dyspneic at rest. A chest radiograph may show diffuse micronodular shadowing. Spirometry usually reveals a restrictive ventilatory defect without airflow obstruction, but a mixed restrictive–obstructive picture may be present. Diagnosis is confirmed serologically by a positive precipitin test and, if necessary, by a positive provocation test. Inhalation of the relevant aerosolized antigen is followed 3–6 hours later by fever, and a drop in FVC, often with recurrence of the symptoms (39).

XII. Oro-Facial Granulomatosis (Melkersson–Rosenthal Syndrome)

This is a rare granulomatous disorder of the mouth and adjacent tissues, involving the oral mucosa, gum, lips, tongue, pharynx, eyelids and skin of the face. Occasionally, facial palsy and trigeminal neuralgia occur. This clinical picture is mistaken for sarcoidosis. However, the patients with this disorder do not have chest X-ray changes or uveitis; the Kveim test is negative and serum angiotensin converting enzymes level normal (40) (Table 3).

XIII. Blau's Syndrome

Edward Blau, a Wisconsin pediatrician, first described a familial multisystem granulomatous inflammation that may readily be confused with childhood sarcoidosis because it presents with iridocyclitis, posterior uveitis, granulomatous skin lesions, arthritis, and elevated serum angiotensin-converting enzyme level. Family transmission is supposed to be autosomal dominant (41) (Table 4).

XIV. Beryllosis

The inhalation of beryllium dusts, salts, or fumes is associated with two types of pulmonary disease: an acute chemical pneumonitis caused by short

Table 3 A Comparison of Sarcoidosis and Oro-Facial Granulomatosis

Features	Sarcoidosis	Oro-facial granulomatosis
Sex distribution	Equal	Equal
Age (yr)	20–50	3–60
Swelling of lips	Not a feature	Typical feature
Buccal mucosa edema	No	Frequent
Gum hyperplasia	Absent	Present
Fissured tongue	No	Yes
Facial palsy	4%	13%
Ocular lesions	Yes	No
Chest X-ray	Abnormal	Normal
Hypercalcemia	13%	Absent
Serum ACE	Raised	Normal
Oral biopsy	May show granulomas	Shows granulomas

Table 4 A Comparison of Blau's Syndrome and Sarcoidosis

Features	Blau's syndrome	Sarcoidosis
Age group (yr)	Children	20–50
Arthritis	Yes	Yes
Panuveitis	Yes	Yes
Skin lesions	Yes	Yes
Lung lesions	No	Yes
Hypercalcemia	No	Yes
Familial	Yes	Yes
Autosomal transmission	Dominant	Recessive
Histology	Granuloma	Granuloma
Electron microscopy	Comma, worm-like bodies	Not typical
HLA association	DR2/4	HLA-B8/13, A1, Cw7 DR3
Serum ACE level	Normal	Raised

Abbreviation: ACE, angiotensin converting enzyme level.

exposures to high concentrations, and a chronic interstitial granulomatous lung disease caused by lower levels of exposure over a prolonged period. The natural source for beryllium, beryl ore, is mined in India, the Soviet Union, parts of Europe, and the United States. Modern uses for beryllium are found in the nuclear, electronics, and aerospace industry. Because of the widespread use of beryllium and its salt in industry, the incidence of chronic, dermal, and pulmonary berylliosis has sharply increased. The major organ affected by beryllium is the lung.

The acute pneumonitis is caused by direct injury of the lung by beryllium, whereas the chronic pulmonary disease is associated with an alveolitis characterized by a diffuse accumulation of lymphocytes and mononuclear phagocytes in the alveolar structures and noncaseating granulomas. Beryllium is thought to act as a class II restricted antigen, stimulating local proliferation and accumulation in the lung of beryllium-specific CD4+ (helper/ inducer) cells. The onset of symptoms may appear long after the initial exposure. These include progressive dyspnea, chronic nonproductive cough, weight loss, fatigue, and other symptoms. The chest X-ray may show a mottled appearance in both lungs with hilar adenopathy. On histological examination, chronic interstitial pneumonitis and noncaseating granulomas are present with epitheliod and giant cells, making it difficult to differentiate from sarcoid granulomas. At the later stage, fibrosis may be pronounced, with development of cor pulmonale. A mild exposure to beryllium may result in reversion of inflammation and healing without much residual disease, but higher intensities of exposure may cause permanent, severe disease. The diagnosis depends on a history of exposure, the presence of beryllium in tissues and body fluids, and pathological findings (42,43).

XV. Drug-Induced Pulmonary Granulomas

The drugs that are known to be associated with the production or induction of pulmonary granuloma are mineral oil, disodium cromoglycate, magnesium trisilcate (talc), methotrexate, and bacillus Calmette-Guerin (BCG). Aspirated oil is the most common cause of drug-induced granulomas. Abnormalities range from an asymptomatic solitary pulmonary nodule to diffuse disease. On aspiration, the oils are emulsified and engulfed by macrophages. Eventually, a fibrosis or a granulomatous reaction, which is usually a localized reaction, occurs. Pulmonary granulomas due to inhalation of cromolyn sodium in powder form are rare. There is only one case report of a postulated, tissue-proven cromolyn-induced diffuse pulmonary granulomatous reaction. Magnesium trisilicate, which is used as an excipient or bonding agent in the manufacture of methadone, methylphenidate, dextropropoxyphene, and amphetamine pills, may incite a granulomatous reaction in the pulmonary interstitium, arteries, and arterioles. Intravenous injection of talc-containing drugs intended for oral use may incite granulomatious inflammation and fibrosis surrounding the talc particles in the pulmonary interstitium in addition to causing emphysema. BCG, which is used extensively as a vaccination against *Mycobacterium tuberculosis* infection, and more recently as a stimulant of the body's immune system to treat prevention of various metastatic malignant diseases, has also been described to cause pulmonary granulomas. Methotrexate (MTX) is widely used for the treatment of a variety of tumors as well as for non-neoplastic conditions. Pneumonitis associated with this drug is well described, although the mechanism of lung injury is not known. The clinical presentation with fever and eosinophilia, the occasional findings of granuloma and multinucleated giant cells in pathological specimens, and the dramatic improvement in some patients following corticosteroid therapy suggest an immunological pathogenesis. The presence of increased BALF phenotypic helper/suppressor T cells in the patients with MTX pneumonitis suggests an immunologically mediated injury rather than a direct toxic effect of this drug (44).

XVI. Local Sarcoid (Granuloma) Reaction

It is well known that "sarcoid reaction" or "sarcoid-like" granulomas may be found in regional lymph nodes draining a carcinoma or a lymphoma. Granulomas have also been found amongst the tumor cells at the site of the primary neoplasm or lymphoma. This local reaction should not be

Table 5 A Comparison Between Local Sarcoid Reaction and Multisystem Sarcoidosis

Features	Local sarcoid reaction	Multisystem sarcoidosis
Age (yr)	Any	20–50
Chest X-ray	Usually normal	Abnormal
Delayed-type reaction	Normal	Depressed
Hypergammaglobulinemia	Absent	Present in about 30%
Hypercalcemia	Usually absent	Present in 13%
Kveim–Siltzbach test	Negative	Positive
Serum ACE level	Normal	Elevated in 60%
Histology	Granuloma	Granuloma
Organs involved	Single	Many

Abbreviation: ACE, angiotensin converting enzyme.

confused with systemic sarcoidosis or any other systemic granulomatous disease (Table 5).

XVII. Conclusion

International travel, student exchanges, and changing immigration patterns are steadily transforming tuberculosis and other granulomatous lung diseases in the United States and other developed countries. It is imperative that the clinician be aware of the increasing prevalence of illness previously regarded as "exotic." The definitive diagnosis of the cause of pulmonary granulomas is important. Mycobacterial, fungal, parasitic, and other infections must be differentiated and distinguished from a variety of noninfectious granulomatous lesions, since therapy is significantly different and, if inappropriate, may not only be ineffective but also, in many eases, deleterious.

References

1. Myrvik Q. Immunopathology of pulmonary granulomas. Adv Exp Med Biol 1982; 155:649–657.
2. Boros D. Granulomatous inflammation. Prog Allergy 1978; 24:184–243.
3. Ando M, Dannenberg A, Shima K. I Macrophage accumulation, division, maturation, and digestive and microbicidal capacities in tuberculous lesions. II Rate at which mononuclear cells enter and divide in primary BCG lesions and those of re-infection. J Immunol 1972; 109:8–19.
4. Adams J, Hamilton T. The cell biology of macrophage activation. Annu Rev Immunol 1984; 2:283–318.

5. Papadimitriou J, Spector W. The origin, properties and fate of epithelioid cells. J Pathol 1981; 105:187–203.
6. Adams J, Gacad M, Singer F, Sharma O. Production of 1,25-dihydroxyvitamin D3 by pulmonary alveolar macrophages from patients with sarcoidosis. Ann New York Acad Sci 1986; 465:587–594.
7. Chambers T. Multinucleate giant cells. J Pathol 1978; 126:125–148.
8. Jones-Williams W, Erasmus D, James V, Davies T. The fine structure of sarcoid and tuberculous granulomas. Postgrad Med 1970; 46:496–500.
9. Modlin R, Hofman f, Meyers R, Sharma O, Taylor C, Rea T. In situ demonstration of T lymphocytes subsets in granulomatous inflammation: leprosy, rhinoscleroma, and sarcoidosis. Clin Exp Immunol 1983; 51:430–438.
10. Weinstock J. The significance of angiotensin 1 converting enzyme in granulomatous inflammation. Sarcoidosis 1986; 3:19–26.
11. Yoshida T. Role of lymphokines in the induction and maintenance of the granuloma. In: Boros DL, Yoshida T, eds. Basic and Clinical Aspects of Granulomatus Diseases. New York: Elsevier, North-Holland, 1980:81–94.
12. Agostini C, Semenzato G. Biology and immunology of the granuloma. In: Geraint James D, Zumla A, eds. The Granulomatous Disorders. Cambridge, U.K.: Cambridge University Press, 1999:3–17.
13. Maartens G, Beyers N. Tuberculosis in the tropics. Clin Chest Med 2002; 23:341–359.
14. Zumla A, Grange J. Non-tuberculosis mycobacterial infections. Clin Chest Med 2002; 23:369–376.
15. Slotar D, Escalante P, Jones. Pulmonary manifestation of HIV/AIDS in the tropics. Clin Chest Med 2002; 23:355–367.
16. Jindal S, Dattatreya R, Kumar B, Kaur S. Airway hyporesponsive in leprosy—a clinical model of chronic pulmonary denervation, antithetic to asthma [abstr]. Chest 1989; 92:249S.
17. Blake L, Web B, Lary C, et al. Environmental non human source of leprosy. Rev Infect Dis 1987; 9:562–577.
18. Lieberman J, Rea T. Serum angiotensin-converting enzyme in leprosy and coccidioidomycosis. Ann Intern Med 1977; 87:423–425.
19. Brooker A, Sharma O. Bronchocentric granulomatosis and adult respiratory distress syndrome. Br J Dis Chest 1982; 76:189–193.
20. Katzenstein A, Carrington C, Liebow A. Lymphomatoid granulomatosis: a clinicopathologic study of 152 cases. Cancer 1979; 43:360–373.
21. Goodwin R, Des Prez R. State of art: histoplasmosis. Am Rev Respir Dis 1978; 117:929–956.
22. Houston S. Tropical respiratory medicine. Histoplasmosis and pulmonary involvement in the tropics. Thorax 1994; 49:598–601.
23. Baker R, Chiodoni P, Kaye P. Leishmaniasis. In: Geraint James D, Zumla A, eds. The Granulomatous Disorders. Cambridge, U.K.: Cambridge University Press, 1999:212–234.
24. Bogadon C, Rollinghoff M. The immune response to leishmania: mechanisms of parasitic control and evaluation. Int J Parasitol 1998; 28(1):51–66.
25. Mosser D, Britingham A. Leishmania, macrophages and complement: a tale of subversion and exploitation. Parasitology 1997; 115:9–23.

26. Cook G. Helminth-induced granulomatous disease. In: James DG, Zumla A, eds. The Granulomatous Disorders. Cambridge, UK: Cambridge University Press, 1999:205–211.
27. Bevanger L, Maeland J, Naess A. Agglutination and antibodies to *Francisella tularensis* outer membrane antigen in early diagnosis of the disease during an outbreak of tularemia. J Clin Microbiol 1988; 26:433–437.
28. Feldman K, Enscore R, Lathrop S, et al. An outbreak of primary pneumonic tularemia on and diffuse lung disease. N Engl J Med 2001; 345:1601–1606.
29. Hunnighake G, Costable U, Ando M, et al. ATS/ERS/WASOG statement on sarcoidosis. Sarcoidosis Vasculitis Diffuse Lung Dis 1999; 16:149–173.
30. Sharma O. Sarcoidosis: Clinical Management. London: Butterworth, 1984.
31. Travis W. Pathology of pulmonary granulomatous vasculitis. Sarcoidosis Vasculitis Diffuse Lung Dis 1996; 13:14–27.
32. Kallenberg C, Tervaert J. New treatments of ANCA-associated vasculitis. Sarcoidosis Vasculitis Diffuse Lung Dis 2000; 17:125–129.
33. DeRemee R. Wegener's granulomatosis. Curr Opin Pulm Med 1995; 1: 363–367.
34. Churg J, Strauss L. Allergic granulomatosis, allergic angiitis and periarteritis nodosa. Am J Pathol 1951; 27:277–301.
35. Chumbley L, Harrison F, DeRemee R. Allergic granulomatosis and angiitis: report and analysis of 30 cases. Mayo Clin Proc 1977; 52:427–484.
36. Koss M, Hochholzer L, Langloss J, Wehunt W, Lazarus A, Nichols P. Lymphomatoid granulomatosis: a clinicopathologic study of 42 patients. Pathology 1986; 18:282–288.
37. James D. Differential diagnosis of multisystem sarcoidosis. Sarcoidosis 1987; 4:1–7.
38. Fenollar F, Raoult D. Whipple's disease. Curr Gastroenterol Rep 2003; 5: 379–385.
39. Ando M, Suga M, Kohrogi H. A new look at hypersensitivity pneumonitis. Curr Opin Pulm Med 1999; 5:299–304.
40. James D. Mimics of sarcoidosis: oro-facial granulomatosis (Melkersson–Rosenthal syndrome). Sarcoidosis 1991; 8:84–85.
41. James D. A comparison of Blau's syndrome and sarcoidosis. Sarcoidosis 1994; 11:100–110.
42. Rossman M, Kern J, Elias J. Proliferative response of bronchoalveolar lymphocytes to beryllium. Ann Intern Med 1988; 108:687–693.
43. Infante P, Newman L. Beryllium exposure and chronic beryllium disease. Lancet 2004; 363:415–416.
44. Limper A, Rosenow E III. Drug induced interstitial lung disease. Curr Opin Pulm Med 1996; 2:396–404.

9

Immunopathogenesis and Treatment of Eosinophilic Lung Diseases in the Tropics

V. K. VIJAYAN

Vallabhbhai Patel Chest Institute, University of Delhi,
Delhi, India

I. Introduction

Pulmonary disease affecting the major airways and/or parenchyma associated with either blood and/or tissue eosinophilia is termed as eosinophilic lung disease. The first four cases with minimal respiratory symptoms, fleeting pulmonary infiltrates in chest X rays and peripheral blood eosinophilia were described by Loffler (1) in 1932 and he thought that it was caused by a variety of antigens. Zumla and James (2) stated that it was Muller who, after ingesting *Ascaris* ova and producing respiratory disease similar to that described by Loffler, attributed the syndrome to the pulmonary phase of ascariasis. Reeder and Goodrich (3) termed this condition as pulmonary infiltrate with eosinophilia (PIE) syndrome. Crofton et al. (4) classified PIE syndrome into five groups based on clinical manifestations: simple pulmonary eosinophilia (Loffler's syndrome), prolonged pulmonary eosinophilia, pulmonary eosinophilia with asthma, tropical eosinophilia, and polyarteritis nodosa. Leibow and Carrington (5) subsequently added chronic eosinophilic pneumonia to the classification. Based on the observation that eosinophils are an integral and consistent part of the lung inflammation, Allen and Davis (6) classified eosinophilic lung disease into 10 entities: simple pulmonary eosinophilia, chronic eosinophilic pneumonia, acute eosinophilic pneumonia, Churg–Strauss syndrome, idiopathic hypereosinophilic syndrome, asthma, allergic bronchopulmonary aspergillosis, bronchocentric granulomatosis, certain parasitic infections and certain drug reactions. Savani and Sharma (7) classified eosinophilic lung diseases into two subgroups: (i) intrinsic (primary, cryptogenic) in which the cause is not known and (ii) extrinsic (secondary) in which the cause is known. Although all types of eosinophilic lung diseases are encountered in the tropics as in other parts of the world, the diseases that are particularly prevalent in the tropics are due to parasitic infestations and certain infections. The important diseases that can cause eosinophilic lung diseases in the tropics are listed in Table 1.

Normally, eosinophils constitute 1–3% of peripheral-blood leukocytes and the absolute number is up to 350 cells per cubic millimeter (8). Eosinophils are produced in the bone marrow from pleuri-potential stem cells. The development of eosinophils is regulated by three cytokines: interleukin-3 (IL-3), IL-5, and granulocyte-macrophage colony stimulating factor (GM-CSF) (8). Interleukin-5 is responsible for the selective differentiation of eosinophils and stimulates the release of eosinophils from the bone marrow into the peripheral circulation (9,10). P-selection, an adhesion molecule present on the endothelium, helps the eosinophils to roll on the endothelial

Table 1 Eosinophilic Lung Diseases in the Tropics

---

1. Parasite-induced eosinophilic lung diseases
   (a) Nematodes
       (i) Pulmonary ascariasis
       (ii) Pulmonary ancylostomiasis
       (iii) Pulmonary strongyloidiasis
       (iv) Tropical pulmonary eosinophilia
       (v) Visceral larva migrans
       (vi) Pulmonary trichinellosis
   (b) Trematodes
       (i) Pulmonary schistosomiasis
       (ii) Pulmonary paragonimiasis
   (c) Cestodes
       (i) Pulmonary hydatid cyst
2. Bacteria-induced eosinophilic lung diseases
   (a) Pulmonary tuberculosis
   (b) Pulmonary brucellosis
3. Fungus-induced eosinophilic lung diseases
   (a) Pulmonary coccidiodomycosis
   (b) Pulmonary cryptococcosis
   (c) Pulmonary histoplasmosis
   (d) Allergic bronchopulmonary mycoses (ABPM)

---

cells (11). Eosinophils adhere to the endothelium of vessels by means of adhesion molecules present on endothelial cells and their corresponding ligands on eosinophils (12). Resting eosinophils normally express β_1 and β_2 integrins on their surface. Firm adherence of eosinophils to the endothelium occurs when β_2 integrins interact with intercellular adhesion molecule-1 (ICAM-I) and β_1 integrins interact with vascular-cell adhesion molecule-1 (VCAM-1) (8). Eosinophils are then attracted to the tissue by chemotactic factors such as leukotriene B_4, platelet-activating factor, interleukins (particularly IL-16), and various chemokines (13). The chemokines, eotaxin-1 and eotaxin-2, are specifically responsible for migration of eosinophils to the tissues (14).

In vitro experiments have demonstrated that eosinophils can survive in the tissues for at least 12 to 14 days in the presence of IL-3, IL-5, and GM-CSF (15). The eosinophil granules contain a crystalloid core composed of major basic protein (MBP) and a matrix composed of eosinophil cationic protein (ECP), eosinophil-derived neurotoxin (EDN), and eosinophil peroxidase (EPO). Eosinophils on activation release these toxic proteins, which have cytotoxic effects on respiratory epithelium and parasites (16–18). Eosinophils can also produce their own chemoattractants: RANTES (regulated upon activation normal T cell expressed and secreted), eotaxin, and platelet-activating factor (8). These chemoattractants facilitate the migration of eosinophils to the sites of inflammation. Eosinophils also generate lipid mediators: leukotriene C_4, leukotriene D_4, and leukotriene E_4, and these are slow-reacting substances of anaphylaxes, which increase vascular permeability and smooth muscle contraction (19).

Eosinophilia is the characteristic host immune response in patients with helminthic infections. Cytokines produced by CD4 helper T cells play an important role in parasitic diseases. The CD4 helper T cells exist in specialized subsets (Th-0, Th-1, Th-2) performing distinct functions by producing distinct sets of cytokines (20). CD4 Th-1 cells produce cytokines (IL-2, IFN-γ, and TNF-β) that activate phagocytes to destroy the infectious agents especially intracellular pathogens. CD4 Th-2 cells secrete IL-4 and IL-5 and these cytokines are essential for production of immunoglobulin E (IgE) and eosinophils. Th-0 cells show combined production of Th-1- and Th-2-type cytokines. Helminths induce the differentiation of helper T cells into Th-2 cells (21–23). The cytokines (IL-4 and IL-5) produced by Th-2 cells induce IgE and eosinophil-mediated destruction of the pathogens. It is not clear whether the Th-2-derived responses (IgE productions, eosinophilia, and mastocytosis) are important in the protective immune response to the parasite or are responsible for immune-mediated pathology or both.

IL-5 has been found to be particularly important in mediating the selective eosinophilia in filarial and other helminthic infections (24). It has also been reported that both IL-5 and eosinophils are required for the induction of airway hyper-responsiveness (AHR) by filarial helminths (25). Epidemiological studies carried out in areas endemic to *S. mansoni* and *S. haematobium* infections had shown that individuals resistant to reinfection after chemotherapy were those with high IgE (26) and elevated eosinophils (27), suggesting the involvement of Th-2-type responses in resistance to reinfection. Studies have also demonstrated that resistance to reinfection in schistosomiasis correlates not only with IL-5 but also with IFN-γ (28). In filariasis, individuals harboring high worm burdens show profound antigen-specific T-cell hyporesponsiveness and release low levels of IL-5 and IFN-γ compared to uninfected but exposed subjects (29). Reduction of worm burden by chemotherapy in filariasis is associated with increased cell proliferation and IFN-γ production, but IL-4 is unaffected (30). These studies involving schistosomiasis and filariasis suggest that both Th-1 and Th-2 cells play a role in the pathogenesis of helminthic infections.

II. Pulmonary Ascariasis

Ascaris lumbricoides is the most common intestinal helminthic infection (31). It has been estimated that 25% (approximately more than 1.5 billion people) of the world population is infected and the infection is most prevalent in tropical countries (32,33). *Ascaris lumbricoides* is the largest nematode infection of man. The adult worm is 15–40 cm long and resides in the jejunum and middle ileum of the intestine. The female worms can lay up to 240,000 eggs per day. Fertilized eggs are shorter and wider than unfertilized eggs. Both fertilized and unfertilized eggs are passed in the feces and released in the soil (34).

A. Life Cycle

The fertilized eggs embryonate within 2–4 weeks and become infectious depending on the environmental conditions (moist, warm, and shaded soil). These embryonated eggs can remain viable in the soil up to 17 months. Infection occurs through soil contamination of hands or food with eggs and then swallowed. The eggs hatch into larvae in the small intestine. These first-stage larvae molt into second-stage larvae in the lumen of the small intestine. The second-stage larvae penetrate the wall of the intestine and travel via capillaries and lymphatics to the hepatic circulation and to the right side of the heart and then reach the lungs. The second-stage larvae molt twice more in the alveoli to produce third- and fourth-stage larvae. The fourth-stage larvae are formed 14 days after ingestion, travel up to the trachea, and are then swallowed to reach the small intestine. It takes approximately 10 days for the fourth-stage larvae to reach the small intestine from the lung. The eggs are produced 10–25 days after initial ingestion. Adult worms live approximately 1–2 years in the intestine.

B. Immunopathogenesis

The mechanical trauma due to adult worms and migrating larvae is one of the factors responsible for the pathophysiologic consequences of *Ascaris* infection. Even a single worm can cause considerable morbidity, e.g., biliary obstruction can result when a worm migrates into the common bile duct (35). The migrating larvae can induce granuloma formation with eosinophils, neutrophils, and macrophages. In the lung, the larvae produce a hypersensitivity reaction. This may result in peribronchial inflammation, increased mucus production in the bronchi and bronchospasm. In addition to peripheral blood and tissue eosinophilia, *Ascaris* infection produces both specific and polyclonal IgE (36). Elevated levels of antibodies (IgG4) to *Ascaris lumbricoides* have also been reported (37). However, it is not clear whether these antibodies have any protective role or indicate prior or current infection. It has been suggested that anti-*Ascaris* IgG4 antibody can be used as a marker for the diagnosis of ascariasis (38). Serology is useful in epidemiological studies and its role in diagnosis of ascariasis is debated (39,40). It has been reported that antibody response to infection reflects the intensity of infection and has no protective role (40). High pretreatment specific IgE levels are found to be associated with lower reinfection rates, whereas high pretreatment total IgE levels are associated with higher infection rates (41). It has, therefore, been suggested that specific IgE antibodies may participate in the protection against *A. lumbricoides* and polyclonal IgE may reduce effectiveness of such protective responses (41). An imbalance in T-cell subpopulation that leads to a defective T-cell maturation and a decreased specific anti-*Ascaris* IgE response in malnourished children has been reported (42). This decreased anti-*Ascaris* IgE response can increase susceptibility to infection (42). A highly polarized Th-2 response in *A. lumbricoides* infection in endemic regions has been observed (43). Chronically infected *Ascaris* patients with high parasitic load had reduced cellular activity and lower TNF-α, IFN-γ, and IL-12 responses compared to endemic controls. However, IL-10 and IL-13 responses were similar in all groups. It has, therefore, been suggested that the former type of cytokine profile supports parasitic persistence and the latter type of responses promotes protective immunity (44). Genetic studies have shown that genes on chromosomes 1 and 13 have significant effects on susceptibility to *Ascaris* infection (45).

C. Clinical Features

Symptoms in ascariasis may be due to the migrating larvae or due to the adult worms. Pulmonary migration of larvae is usually asymptomatic. Respiratory symptoms are due to larval pulmonary migration, airway hyper-reactivity, and bronchospasm. Symptomatic pulmonary disease may range from mild cough to Loffler's syndrome (1,46). Loffler's syndrome is a self-limiting inflammation of the lungs and is associated with blood and lung eosinophilia. This syndrome can occur as a result of parasitic infestations (especially ascariasis in children) and exposure to various drugs. Patients may present with general symptoms of malaise, loss of appetite, fever lasting 2–3 days, headache, and myalgia. The respiratory symptoms include chest pain, cough with mucoid sputum, hemoptysis, shortness of breath, and wheezing (47). There may be a rapid respiratory rate and rales can be heard on auscultation. Leucocytosis particularly eosinophilia is an important laboratory finding. Chest radiographs demonstrate unilateral or bilateral, transient, migratory, nonsegmental opacities of various sizes. These opacities are often peripherally situated and appear to be pleural based (48). The severity of symptoms will depend upon the larval burden. Rarely, chronic eosinophilic pneumonia or symptoms of upper airway obstruction can occur (49,50). There were conflicting data about the role of *Ascaris* infection in predisposing children to asthma (51,52). However, a recent study has found no apparent relation between asthma and ascariasis (53).

D. Diagnosis

A diagnosis of pulmonary disease due to Ascariasis can be made in an endemic region in a patient who presents with dyspnea, dry cough, fever, and eosinophilia. Sputum may show Charcot–Leyden crystals and the chest radiograph may reveal fleeting pulmonary infiltrates. Because of the occurrence of respiratory symptoms during larval pulmonary migration, stool examination usually does not show *Ascaris* eggs and stool samples may be negative until 2–3 months after respiratory symptoms occur, unless the patient was previously infected. However, larvae can sometimes be demonstrated in respiratory or gastric secretions (50). It has been suggested that measurement of *Ascaris*-specific IgG4 by ELISA may be useful in the serodiagnosis of ascariasis (39).

E. Treatment

Pulmonary disease due to ascariasis usually does not require any treatment, as it is a self-limiting disease. However, the persistence of gastrointestinal ascariasis may result in repeated episodes of respiratory symptoms due to larval migration. In order to eradicate *A. lumbricoides* from the intestine, specific antihelminthic treatment is given. Mebendazole and albendazole have been found to be equally effective in the treatment of ascariasis (35). Mebendazole is given in a dose of 100 mg twice a day for 3 days. It can be also given as a single dose of 500 mg. Albendazole is given as a single dose of 400 mg. The safety of mebendazole and albendazole during pregnancy has not been established. A single dose of pyrantel pamoate (11 mg/kg, maximum dose 1 g) or piperazine citrate (50–75 mg/kg/day for 2 days) is also useful in the treatment. Pediatric dose is the same as an adult dose. Ivermectin has also been found to be useful (54).

F. Prevention and Control

Health education, good environmental sanitation, appropriate toilet facilities, and clean water supply can have an impact on control of the disease (55). However, it has been observed that these measures may aid in reducing severity of disease, but have no effect on the incidence and prevalence of the disease. Mass treatment of ascariasis with a single dose of 400 mg albendazole given at intervals of 3 months for 2 years has been found to be very effective in the control of ascariasis (56).

III. Pulmonary Ancylostomiasis

Hookworm disease in humans results from infections with two species, *Ancylostoma duodenale* and *Necator americanus*. It has been estimated that more than 1 billion people worldwide are infected with both species of hookworm and the infection is particularly prevalent in tropical and subtropical countries (33). Infection with *N. americanus* is predominantly seen in Central and South America, sub-Saharan Africa, southern China, southern India, and South East Asia. *A. duodenale* infection is predominant in northern India, northern China, and north Africa. However, infection with one parasite can overlap with another in many parts of the world. The adult worm has a buccal capsule armed with teeth (*A. duodenale*) or cutting plates (*N. americanus*) and resides in the upper small intestine attached by buccal capsules to the intestinal mucosa. *N. americanus* is comparatively smaller. The male *N. americanus* is usually between 7 and 9 mm and the females between 9 and 11 mm in length. The male *A. duodenale* measures 8 to 11 mm and females 10–13 mm in length. Hookworm is a habitual blood sucker. *N. americanus* causes a daily per worm blood loss of 0.01–0.04 mL and *A. duodenale* of 0.05–0.30 mL (57,58). Adult *N. americanus* can live for 3–5 years and *A. duodenale* for 1 year (58,59).

A. Life Cycle

Adult female *N. americanus* produces 5000–10,000 eggs per day and female *A. duodenale* produces 10,000–30,000 eggs per day (58,59). Man is the only definitive host. The eggs containing segmented ova with four blastomers are passed out in the feces. A rhabditiform larva develops from each egg in the soil and this larva molts twice and develops into a filariform larva, which is infective to man. The filariform larva penetrates through the intact skin. *N. americanus* larvae can infect man only through the skin, whereas *A. duodenale* larvae can enter the human host via the oral route in addition to the entry through the skin (58). These larvae reach pulmonary circulation through the lymphatics and venules. The larvae then pierce the alveolar walls and ascend the bronchi, trachea, larynx, and pharynx and are ultimately swallowed to reach the upper part of the small intestine. The interval between the time of skin penetration and laying of eggs by adult worms is about 6 weeks. *A. duodenale* larvae can developmentally get arrested in the gut or muscle and restart development when environmental conditions become favorable (60). The arrested larvae can enter the mammary glands from maternal somatic tissue and this is responsible for vertical transmission of ancylostomiasis to infants (61).

B. Immunopathogenesis

Bronchitis and bronchopneumonia can occur when the larvae break through the pulmonary capillaries to enter the alveolar spaces. Chronic blood loss can result in iron deficiency anemia. Pulmonary larval migration can elicit peripheral blood eosinophilia. Hookworm larvae release a family of proteins known as ancylostoma-secreted proteins (ASP). The exact role of ASP in the pathogenesis of the disease is currently not known, though it is highly antigenic (62). Experimental hookworm infection studies have shown humoral antibodies and cellular responses to hookworm antigens, but the exact role of these responses in protective immunity is not known (63). Hookworms can secrete low-molecular weight polypeptides that inhibit clotting factor Xa and tissue factor VIIa (64). These hookworm anticoagulants can facilitate blood loss that results from destruction of capillaries of the intestinal mucosa. Adult hookworms also release a neutrophil inhibitory factor (NIF), which may downregulate invading leucocytes (65).

C. Clinical Features

Ancylostoma dermatitis, which manifests as intense pruritis, erythema, and rash (ground itch) occurs at the site of skin penetration. During pulmonary larval migration, patients may present with fever, cough, wheezing, and transient pulmonary infiltrates in chest radiographs. This is associated with blood and pulmonary eosinophilia. The other characteristic feature is iron deficiency anemia due to chronic blood loss. In severe hookworm anemia, patients may present with fatigue, exertional dyspnea, poor concentration, and cardiac murmurs. During massive infection from oral ingestion of hookworm larvae, patients can present with nausea, vomiting, cough, dyspnea, and eosinophilia and this condition is termed as Wakana disease. Prominent gastrointestinal symptoms in hookworm disease are abdominal pain, nausea, anorexia, and diarrhea.

D. Diagnosis

A direct microscopical examination of stool demonstrates the presence of characteristic hookworm eggs. Concentration method may be used when the infection is light. Eosinophilia in the peripheral blood is a prominent finding. A peripheral blood smear examination will reveal microcytic hypochromic anemia. A polymerase chain reaction (PCR) to differentiate between *A. duodenale* and *N. americanus* has been developed (66).

E. Treatment

Both mebendazole and albendazole are useful in the treatment of hookworm. Mebendazole is given as 100 mg twice daily for 3 days and albendazole is given as a single dose of 400 mg. Pyrantel pamoate at a dose of 11 mg/kg orally (maximum 1 g) as a single dose has also been found to be useful. Recent studies have demonstrated that ivermectin can also be used in the treatment of hookworm infections. Anemia can be treated with oral ferrous sulfate tablets.

IV. Pulmonary Strongyloidiasis

Strongyloides stercoralis is seen worldwide, but common in South America, South East Asia, sub-Saharan Africa, and the Appalachian region of the United States of America (67). In Europe, it has been reported from several countries including the United Kingdom, France, Italy, and Spain (68). It has been estimated that approximately 70 million people are infected with *S. stercoralis* worldwide (33,67). Even if the *S. stercoralis* infections may not be endemic in the general population, it can occur in institutionalized patients such as homes for mentally retarded people (69). The parasitic females live in the wall (mucous membrane) of the small intestine of man, especially in the lamina propria of the duodenum and proximal jejunum. The parasitic males remain in the lumen of the gut and they have no capacity to penetrate the mucus membrane.

A. Life Cycle

Eggs are laid by female parasites and contain larvae ready to hatch. The rhabditiform larvae emanating from the eggs pierce the mucous membrane and reach the lumen of the intestine. These larvae are then passed with the feces and eggs are, therefore, not found in the feces.

The rhabditiform larvae can metamorphose into filariform larvae in the lumen of the bowel. These filariform larvae can penetrate the intestinal epithelium or perianal skin without leaving the host. This is responsible for autoinfection and for persistence of infection 20 to 30 years in persons who have left the endemic areas (70). The unique feature of the life cycle of *S. stercoralis* is that it can complete its life cycle either in the human host or in the soil. The rhabditiform larvae that are voided with the feces can undergo two distinct cycles in the soil: direct (host–soil–host) and indirect cycle. In direct cycle, the rhabditiform larvae directly metamorphose into filariform larvae and can infect man through skin. In indirect cycle, the rhabditiform larvae mature into free-living sexual forms (males and females). A second generation of rhabditiform larvae is then produced and these are then transformed into filariform larvae. The filariform larvae can penetrate directly through the skin, invade the tissues, penetrate into the venous or lymphatic channels, and are carried by the blood stream to the heart and then to the lungs. They pierce the pulmonary capillaries and enter the alveoli. These larvae, then, migrate to the bronchi, trachea, larynx, and epiglottis and are swallowed back into the intestine. In the duodenum and jejunum, they develop into sexual forms to continue the life cycle.

B. Immunopathogenesis

The cutaneous reaction, as a result of the penetration of the skin by the filariform larvae, may be due to immediate hypersensitivity reaction. The cell-mediated immunity that develops following primary infection prevents reinfection (71). As a result, the larvae and adult worms remain confined to the intestine and the tissue invasion is prevented in immunocompetent individuals. When there is immunosuppression, autoinfection is exaggerated and leads to hyperinfection. In this situation, the number of migrating larvae increases tremendously and disseminate to many organs including lungs, meninges, brain, lymph nodes, and kidneys. The parasite can produce hyperinfection syndrome in individuals with deficient cell-mediated immunity as seen in patients with immunosuppressive therapy (especially corticosteroids) and other immune-deficient states (malnutrition, lymphoma, leukemia, etc.) (72,73). Human immunodeficiency virus (HIV)-infected patients are at a higher risk of dissemination and this may occur without elevations of IgE or eosinophils (74).

Newly hatched larvae are found in the Lieberkuhn Crypts within the tunnels formed by the migration of parthenogenic females. A tegument derived from the parasite and host surrounds the larvae and protects the parasite and reduces any disadvantage caused by immaturity. These larvae are capable of active movement through the epithelium and cause mechanical damage to the host (75). The mechanical damage caused by the worms and the host inflammatory response can result in abdominal pain, diarrhea, and malabsorption. These can be aggravated by the associated secondary bacterial infections. During migration of filariform larvae through the lungs, bronchopneumonia and hemorrhages in the alveoli can occur. These areas are infiltrated with eosinophils. This is associated with elevated IgE and eosinophilia in the blood. As the larvae penetrate the intestinal mucosa, gram-negative bacteria from the gut are carried by the larvae on their cuticle. In addition, small breaks in the mucous membrane as the larvae penetrate the intestine also facilitate the entry of enteric bacteria into the blood stream. The inflammation that follows such invasion of larvae leads to disseminated strongyloidiasis and this is usually fatal. It has been suggested that hyperinfection syndrome and disseminated strongyloidiasis can be distinguished from each other (68). In hyperinfection syndrome, severe symptoms are referable to the organs usually involved in parasitic life cycle, the lung, and the intestine. In this situation, the larval load is very high in feces and sputum. In disseminated strongyloidiasis, there is widespread involvement of organs that are not ordinarily part of the life cycle (68). In the lung, massive pulmonary bleeding can occur due to alveolar microhemorrhages. As a result of invasion of bacteria along with larvae, diffuse and patchy bronchopneumonia and pulmonary abscess can occur.

C. Clinical Features

It has been observed that 15–30% of chronically infected people may be asymptomatic (76). Although symptoms in individuals with chronic *S. stercoralis* infection are usually mild, it can persist for many years due to autoinfection. This may occasionally progress to the hyperinfection syndrome with high mortality especially in immunosuppresed individuals. The relative risk of *S. stercoralis* infection is increased in elderly men and patients who had recently used corticosteroids, had a hematologic malignancy, and had prior gastric surgery (77,78). Other risk factors include chronic lung disease, use of histamine blockers, or chronic debilitating illness (79). Strongylodiasis is a chronic relapsing illness of mild to moderate severity characterized by gastrointestinal complaints (diarrhea, pain, tenderness, nausea, vomiting), peripheral blood eosinophilia and hypoalbuminemia (76,80).

Pulmonary signs and symptoms include cough, shortness of breath, wheezing, and hemoptysis (81). In patients at high risk for strongyloidiasis, adult respiratory distress syndrome and septicemia due to intestinal transmural migration of bacteria can occur as a result of pulmonary hyperinfection or disseminated strongyloidiasis (72,76,82,83). In addition, acute anemia, acute renal failure, and systemic inflammatory response syndrome are also reported in hyperinfection (72). Strongyloidiasis can manifest as eosinophilic pleural effusion in both immunocompetent and immunocompromised individuals (84,85). Rare pulmonary manifestations include acute respiratory failure due to respiratory muscle paralysis (86), granulomatous reaction in the lung with interlobular septal fibrosis (87), syndrome of inappropriate secretion of antidiuretic hormone (88), and pulmonary microcalcifications (89). A paradoxic therapeutic response of asthma to glucocorticosteroids, in which bronchial asthma symptoms worsened after treatment with parenteral corticosteroids, has been described in patients with strongyloides superinfections (90). Exacerbations of chronic obstructive pulmonary disease (91) and worsening of symptoms in idiopathic pulmonary fibrosis (92) have also been reported in *S. stercoralis* infection.

D. Diagnosis

In immunocompetent patients with strongyloidiasis, the parasite load is usually low and the larval output is irregular. As a result, the diagnosis of strongyloidiasis by examination of a single stool specimen using conventional techniques usually fails to detect larvae in up to 70% of cases (93). The diagnostic yield can be increased by examination of several stool specimens on consecutive days. Examination of stool by agar plate culture method was found to be superior to direct smear and modified Baermann technique (94–96). *S. stercoralis* larvae can be demonstrated in duodenal aspirate (47). In disseminated disease, larvae and adult parasites can be seen in sputum, urine, bronchoalveolar lavage fluid, and other body fluids (97,98). A serological test using Centers for Disease Control (CDC) enzyme immunoassay (EIA) for detection of antibodies to strongyloidiasis was found to have a sensitivity of 94.6% in patients with proven infection (99).

E. Treatment

Ivermectin, thiabendazole, or albendazole can be used for treatment of strongyloidiasis in immunocompetent individuals without complications (100,101). Ivermectin is given as 200 µg/kg orally for 1 or 2 days. Thiabendazole is given orally as 25 mg/kg twice a day for 2 days. Albendazole 400 mg twice a day for 5 days has been found to be useful in the treatment of strongyloidiasis. As treatment with thiabendazole is effective only in about 70% of patients, it has to be repeated. In immunocompromised individuals with disseminated strongyloidiasis, the dose of thiabendazole has to be doubled and the duration of treatment may be several weeks. In addition, appropriate treatment of bacterial infection as a result of intestinal transmural migration of bacteria has to be instituted. Corticosteroids, if given have to be discontinued or tapered off.

V. Tropical Pulmonary Eosinophilia

Tropical pulmonary eosinophilia (TPE) is characterized by cough, dyspnea, and nocturnal wheezing, diffuse reticulo-nodular infiltrates in chest X rays and marked peripheral blood eosinophilia (102–105). The syndrome results from immunologic hyper-responsiveness to human filarial parasites, *Wuchereria bancrofti* and *Brugia malayi* (104). Tropical pulmonary eosinophilia, one of the main causes of pulmonary eosinophilia in the tropical countries, is prevalent in filarial endemic regions of the world, especially South East Asia (104,106). Most of the patients with acute TPE show remarkable response to a standard 3-week course of diethylcarbamazine citrate (DEC), an antifilarial drug (102,103). However, some individuals develop a chronic form of pulmonary disease that results in interstitial fibrosis and loss of pulmonary function (103,105,107).

Even though TPE as a clinical entity was described only in the 1940s, the earliest report that conformed to the clinical picture of this disease, was in 1916 in a 38-year-old English soldier who had fever, high peripheral blood eosinophilia (>5000 cells/mm^3) and symptoms similar to asthma (108). Subsequently, Roy and Bose (109) and Ghosh (110) reported a group of patients who had asthma, marked leucocytosis with eosinophilia and responded to subcutaneous or intramuscular soamin, suggesting that patients presenting with asthma and marked peripheral blood eosinophilia were a distinct clinical entity. Frimodt-Moller and Barton (111) in 1940 described a group of patients from a sanatorium in south India who had fever, cough, and chest pain, and weight loss in association with massive blood eosinophilia. These patients had extensive bilateral miliary mottling in chest X rays and were wrongly diagnosed as miliary tuberculosis. However, they were in good physical condition and did not have a high mortality as observed in miliary tuberculosis. They described this entity as "a pseudotuberculosis condition associated with eosinophilia."

The name "tropical eosinophilia" to this syndrome was coined by Weingarten in 1943 (112) who described 81 patients with severe spasmodic bronchitis, leucocytosis, and very high eosinophilia and disseminated mottlings of both the lungs. These patients were successfully treated with neoarsphenamine, following the accidental observation that one of his patients with concurrent syphilis was cured of his TPE on being given neoarsphenamine for syphilis. Following the publication of the syndrome by Weingarten, a large number of workers from India and other parts of the World reported the entity under various names (113–117). The disease was also noticed in individuals residing in countries where filariasis was not endemic, but had visited endemic countries earlier (118,119).

A. Epidemiology

Tropical pulmonary eosinophilia, an occult form of filariasis, is endemic in the Indian subcontinent, South East Asia, and South Pacific islands (120). It has been estimated that at least 120 million persons are infected with mosquito-borne lymphatic filariasis worldwide (121). However, TPE is seen in only less than 1% of filarial infections (122). A few studies have been reported from India to know the prevalence of TPE in the community (123–125). In a study of a jail population that included 1183 prisoners, members of staff and their relatives in Patna, it had been observed that the prevalence of pulmonary eosinophilia was 9.9% (123). In another survey of 4282 children in North Arcot Ambedkar district of Tamil Nadu, tropical eosinophilia was found in 23 cases (0.5%) (124). A study of 1754 villagers aged more than 5 years in Puri District of Orissa state had revealed that 69 patients (3.9%) had typical clinical features of TPE and six of them had an eosinophil count above 3000 cells/mm^3 (125). As the number of individuals traveling from filarial endemic areas to other parts of the world has increased tremendously, TPE is being increasingly reported from countries, which are not endemic to filarial infection (118,119). Therefore, TPE should be considered in the differential diagnosis, if a patient traveling from a filarial endemic region presents with "asthma-like" symptoms (126). Conversely, individuals from nonendemic areas visiting filarial endemic regions are more prone to develop TPE, as they do not have natural immunity against filarial infection compared to endemic normal subjects.

B. Etiology

Various studies have shown that filarial infection is the cause of TPE (104,105). Clinically, filarial infections are described in six types: asymptomatic amicrofilaremia, asymptomatic microfilaremia, acute adenolymphangitis, chronic filariasis (hydrocoele, lymphoedema, elephantiasis, and chyluria), renal disease (glomerulonephritis), and occult filariasis (tropical pulmonary eosinophilia) (127). A close epidemiological relationship between filarial infection and TPE was observed, as it had been reported that TPE was most frequently encountered in those regions where filariasis was endemic (103). A positive filarial complement fixation test (FCFT) in TPE using 1% alcoholic extract of dried powder of *Dirofilaria immitis* was described (128), demonstrating high levels of antifilarial antibody in the sera of patients. Intradermal skin tests with *D. immitis* antigens gave immediate positive reactions in patients with TPE (129). Subsequently, many workers used the positive FCFT and intradermal skin tests using *D. immitis* or *D. catis* antigens as a diagnostic test for TPE (130,131). Meyers and Kunwennar (132) and Van der Sar and Hartz (133) found microfilariae in patients with lymphadenopathy and massive peripheral blood eosinophilia. Some of these patients had respiratory manifestations and radiological abnormalities similar to TPE. Histopathological examinations had demonstrated microfilariae in the lungs, liver, and lymph nodes of patients with TPE (134–136). The microfilariae were sheathed and had the anatomical features of *W. bancrofti* (134). Even though microfilariae in the blood are seen very rarely in TPE, Jaggi and Sadana (137) reported microfilaremia in one patient. Experimental studies carried out in a human volunteer by injection of infective larvae of zoonotic filariasis had resulted in a syndrome similar to that of TPE and suggested that the disease was due to filariasis (138).

The usefulness of diethylcarbamazine citrate (DEC), an antifilarial drug, in the treatment of TPE further focuses attention on its filarial etiology (139,140). Elevated concentrations of filarial-specific IgG and IgE have also been reported in TPE (141). Further evidence of human filarial infection is provided by the fact that maximal positive results of leukocyte adhesion phenomenon have been observed in sera from patients with TPE using *W. bancrofti* compared with *D. repens* and *D. immitis* (142). Biopsy of a lump in the spermatic cord in a patient with TPE showed degenerating adult female filarial worm with uteri full of microfilariae (143). Ultrasound examination of the scrotal area of a patient with TPE had demonstrated living adult *W. bancrofti* in the lymphatic vessels of the spermatic cord (144). The demonstration that basophils from patients with TPE released greater amounts of histamine when cells were challenged with *Brugia* or *Wuchereria* antigens than with *Dirofilaria* antigen suggested that TPE resulted from immunologic hyper-responsiveness to human filarial parasites (141).

C. Pathology

The histopathological study in TPE had shown widely scattered nodules of varying size (1–5 mm) over lung surface (136,145). Open lung biopsy studies have demonstrated that three types of histopathological reactions can be seen in TPE (135,146,147): (i) interstitial, peribronchial, and perivascular exudates consisting of histiocytes in patients with a short duration of symptoms (less than 3 weeks), (ii) acute eosinophilic infiltrations of interstitial, peribronchial, and perivascular tissues leading to the formation of eosinophilic abscesses and eosinophilic bronchopneumonia, and granuloma with foreign-body-type giant cells in those with 1–3 months of disease, and (iii) a mixed cell type of infiltration consisting of histiocytes, eosinophils, and lymphocytes with well-marked interstitial fibrosis after 6 months. A predominant histiocytic response developed 2 years after the onset of the disease and ultimately progressed to fibrosis with marked scarring (103). Fine ultrastructural changes include the presence of alveolar macrophages with abundant cytoplasm and increased phagolysosomes, eosinophils with old and young granules, and collagenosis around alveolar cells (148). In the end stage, a picture resembling fibrosing alveolitis with honeycombing might develop in some cases, if untreated (103). Lung biopsies after 1 month's treatment with diethylcarbamazine demonstrate incomplete histological regression, although symptoms subside within 7 days of therapy and peripheral eosinophilia return to normal (146).

D. Pathogenesis

The current concept of the pathogenesis of TPE suggests that it begins with a lung parenchymal inflammation in individuals highly sensitized immunologically to filarial parasites. The microfilariae released from adult worms living in lymphatics are cleared in the pulmonary circulation, degenerate and release their antigenic constituents, which trigger a local inflammatory process (103,136). Though the lung bears the major brunt of the disease as a result of trapping of microfilariae in the pulmonary circulation, the antigenic material released from the microfilariae can reach the systemic circulation and cause extrapulmonary manifestations. Bronchoalveolar lavage (BAL) studies

210   *Vijayan*

have demonstrated that TPE is characterized by intense eosinophilic inflammatory processes in the lower respiratory tract (149). The concentration of eosinophils in the lower respiratory tract is many folds greater than that in the blood, suggesting that eosinophils accumulate selectively in the lung parenchyma (149). Even though the mechanisms responsible for eosinophil accumulation in the lung are unknown, it is likely that the degenerating microfilariae in the lungs are the inciting agent. Electron microscopic examination of lung eosinophils had shown marked alterations consisting of severe degranulation with loss of both the cores and the peripheral portions of the granules, suggesting that eosinophils were in an activated state (149). The activated eosinophils capable of releasing toxic mediators such as major basic protein, eosinophilic cationic protein, eosinophil-derived neurotoxin, peroxidase, and collagenase might be responsible for the pathophysiologic abnormalities in TPE (150–153). The bronchospasm in TPE may result from leukotrienes released by the eosinophils (150). The mediators that orchestrate eosinophilic chemotaxis and activation in TPE are not well characterized. In order to explore the mechanisms underlying the eosinophil-mediated inflammation of TPE, many of the cytokines, chemokines, eosinophilic granular proteins, and leukotrienes were studied in BAL fluid, serum, and supernatants from pulmonary and blood leucocytes (154). Of the many mediators studied, eosinophil-derived neurotoxin (EDN) and macrophage inflammatory protein-1α (MIP-1α) levels were higher for TPE patients than for the non-TPE control groups. EDN levels were also higher in the BAL fluid than in the serum, suggesting compartmentalization of the response. These findings suggest that EDN, an RNAse capable of damaging the lung epithelium, plays an important role in the pathogenesis of TPE (154).

Patients with TPE show striking elevations of total IgE, IgG (hypergamma-globulinemia) and filarial-specific IgG, IgM, and IgE antibodies in peripheral blood and lung epithelial lining fluid (ELF) (149,155). An increase in the number of CD4+ T-helper cells in patients with TPE has been described (156) and it has also been demonstrated that there is an approximately 50-fold increase in the number of B cells capable of producing polyclonal IgE (157). A major IgE-inducing antigen (Bm23–25) of the filarial parasite, *Brugia malayi*, has been identified from patients with tropical pulmonary eosinophilia (158). This Bm23–25 antigen has been found to be the homolog of the enzyme, gamma-glutaryl transpeptidase light chain subunit (159) and expresses mainly in the infective L3 larvae that have been shown to induce specific IgE antibodies in infection-free endemic normal subjects (160,161). In addition, *B. malayi* gamma-glutaryl transpeptidase can induce IgG1 and IgE antibody production in patients with TPE (160). BAL fluid of patients with TPE contains IgE antibodies that recognize *B. malayi* antigen, Bm23–25 (158). The CD4+ T-helper cells from patients with TPE are capable of secreting a mixed phenotypic pattern of cytokines, gamma-interferon, interleukin-2 (IL-2), IL-4, and IL-5 (156).

This observation of mixed phenotypic pattern is in conformity with the findings of elevated IgG1 (controlled by Th-1 cytokines) and IgE (controlled by Th-2 cytokines) induced by *B. malayi* gamma-glutaryl transpeptidase in patients with TPE (160). Experimentally, it has been demonstrated that IL-12 can modulate the T-helper (Th) response in the lungs from Th-2 to Th-1 response. IL-12 decreases IL-4 and IL-5 production and increases gamma-interferon production, thereby downregulating filarial-induced lung immunopathology (162). There is a molecular mimicry between the parasite gamma-glutaryl transpeptidase and the human gamma-glutaryl transpeptidase present on the surface of pulmonary epithelium (158,163). A marked reduction in lung ELF filarial-specific IgG and IgE levels within 6–14 days of therapy with diethylcarbamazine has been observed (155). Immunoblot comparison of the antigen recognition patterns of lung ELF and serum antigens have recognized a distinct subset of filarial-specific antigens recognized by the antibodies in the peripheral blood (155). Thus, the profound antibody response to filarial infection, especially to filarial gamma-glutaryl transpeptidase, observed in the lungs of patients with TPE, plays an important role in the pathogenesis of tropical eosinophilia (161).

E. Clinical Features

Tropical pulmonary eosinophilia is a systemic disease involving mainly the lungs, but other organs such as liver, spleen, lymph nodes, brain, gastrointestinal tract, etc., may also be involved (103,164). The disease occurs predominantly in males, with a male to female ratio of 4:1, and is mainly seen in older children and young adults between the ages 15 and 40 years (103,105). The systemic symptoms include fever, weight loss, and fatigue.

Pulmonary Manifestations

Patients with TPE usually present with respiratory symptoms that include paroxysmal cough, breathlessness, and wheeze and chest pain. The symptoms occur predominantly at night, but can persist during the day. Severe cough can lead to fractured ribs. Sputum is usually scanty, viscous, and mucoid. The sputum often shows clumps of eosinophils (103) and rarely Charcot–Leyden crystals are observed (112). On examination, patients are often breathless. Bilateral scattered rhonchi and rales may be heard on auscultation.

Laboratory Investigations

Leucocytosis with an absolute increase in eosinophils (103,112) in the peripheral blood is the hallmark of TPE. Spontaneous fluctuations in the eosinophil count can occur. Absolute eosinophil counts are usually more than 3000 cells/mm^3 and may range from 5000 to 80,000 (165). Eosinophil count may show diurnal variation with the lowest count at night. The appearance of cytoplasmic vacuoles and degranulations are striking features of blood eosinophils (166–168). These findings together with the observation of increased levels of eosinophilic cations in serum of patients with TPE suggest that blood eosinophils are activated (120,169). During the very early evolution of the disease, there may be only an increase in total leukocyte count without any eosinophilia. In patients with a long-standing history and with recurrences or relapses, and in patients with TPE under the stress of a coincident acute pyogenic infection, the absolute eosinophil count may be below 2000 cells/mm^3(103).

Erythrocyte sedimentation rate is elevated in 90% of cases and returns to normal following specific treatment (103). Microfilariae are rarely seen in the peripheral blood (133). As patients with TPE especially from endemic areas can be simultaneously infected with other helminthic parasites, stool examination may reveal ova or larvae of other helminths (*Ascaris, Ancylostoma,* whipworm, and *strongyloides*) in 20% of patients with TPE. This observation does not deter the physician from making a diagnosis of TPE, if other conditions for diagnosis are fulfilled.

Radiology

The chest radiological features of TPE include reticulo-nodular shadows predominantly seen in mid and lower zones and miliary mottling of 1–3 mm in diameter (Fig. 1) often indistinguishable from miliary tuberculosis. In addition, there may be prominent hila with heavy vascular markings (170–173). Twenty percent of patients have a normal chest radiograph (103). In patients with a long-standing history, a few patients have honeycomb lungs (103). Radiological improvement occurs on specific therapy with DEC, but some degree of radiological abnormality persists in some patients (174,175). CT scan studies have shown bronchiectasis, air trapping, calcification, and mediastinal lymphadenopathy in patients with TPE (176). Rare chest radiological features include pulmonary cavitation (177,178), pneumothorax (177), consolidation (179), pleural effusion (180–182), and cardiomegaly (183).

Lung Function

Lung function tests reveal mainly a restrictive ventilation defect with superimposed airways obstruction (103,107,147,184–188). Single breath carbon monoxide transfer factor (TLCO) is reduced in 88% of untreated patients with TPE (189). The reduction in TLCO is due to reduced pulmonary membrane diffusing capacity (D_m) which itself is due to a reduction in single breath alveolar volume (V_A) (189,190). Pulmonary capillary blood volume (V_c) is normal (190). Following 3 weeks treatment with DEC, although there were significant rise in various pulmonary function parameters, forced expiratory volume in one second (FEV_1), forced vital capacity (FVC), TLCO, D_m, and expiratory flow rates continued to be significantly lower than the control subjects (175,190–192). Single breath

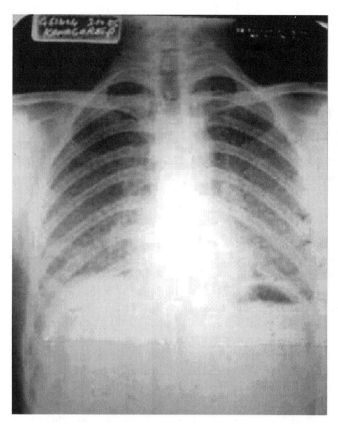

Figure 1 Chest radiograph that shows bilateral diffuse mottling in a patient with tropical pulmonary eosinophilia.

carbon monoxide transfer factor (TLCO) and total lung capacity (TLC) were negatively correlated with total number of inflammatory cells (alveolar macrophages, lymphocytes, eosinophils, and neutrophils) in BAL fluid (193). The lung eosinophils were negatively correlated with TLCO and KCO (diffusion per liter of alveolar volume), but not with FVC, FEV_1, or TLC, whereas alveolar macrophages and lymphocytes were associated with a reduction in lung volumes but not with TLCO, suggesting that different cell types might be responsible for different aspects of lung damage (193).

Arterial hypoxemia ($PaO_2 < 80$ mmHg) was observed in 41% of untreated TPE patients (172,190). Most of them had only mild arterial hypoxemia (174,194–197). Hypocapnia ($PaCO_2 < 35$ mm) was present in 16% of patients (194). Arterial PO_2 and PCO_2 improve following treatment at 1 month and normal PaO_2 and $PaCO_2$ are maintained in most patients 1 year after treatment (174,175). Ventilation–perfusion scintiscanning has demonstrated that hypoxemia in some patients with TPE is due to disturbed ventilation–perfusion relationship (198).

Extrapulmonary Manifestations

Lymphadenopathy may occur in TPE especially in children (103). Rarely, there may be hepatosplenomegaly and may be associated with severe splenic pain (177). Cardiovascular changes, especially electrocardiographic abnormalities (199,200), pericarditis (201), pericardial effusion (202), and cor-pulmonale (203), have also been reported. TPE may also present with gastrointestinal (103), skeletal muscle (204), and central nervous system manifestations (164).

F. Differential Diagnosis

Infestations with helminths (cestodes, nematodes, and trematodes) are the commonest causes of pulmonary eosinophilia in tropical countries (205). Helminths that cause pulmonary eosinophilia frequently are *Ascaris, Ancylostoma, Strongyloides, Toxocara, Schistosoma, Paragonimus, Trichinella*, and *Echinococcus*, besides occult filariasis (120). TPE of filarial etiology may sometimes be clinically indistinguishable from TPE-like syndrome caused by other helminths, except that some of these patients do not respond to DEC. In addition, elevated levels of antifilarial antibodies (IgG, IgG4, and IgE) are also observed in patients with TPE-like syndrome (206). It has also been demonstrated that sera from people of an area, not endemic for filariasis, but harboring intestinal helminths, have antifilarial antibodies that recognize antigens of microfilariae of *W. bancrofti* (207). These observations underscore the need for developing a new diagnostic test to differentiate filarial TPE from TPE-like syndromes caused by other helminths. Other infectious causes of pulmonary eosinophilia include infections with *Brucella, Coccidioides, Corynebacterium pseudotuberculosis*, and *Mycobacterium tuberculosis* (208,209).

Noninfectious causes of pulmonary eosinophilia include allergic bronchopulmonary aspergillosis (ABPA), bronchial asthma, acute eosinophilic pneumonia, chronic eosinophilic pneumonia, idiopathic hypereosinophilic syndrome, cryptogenic pulmonary fibrosis, Wegner's granulomatosis, lymphomatoid granulomatosis, eosinophilic granuloma of the lung, Churg–Strauss syndrome and drug hypersensitivity reactions (6,120). Till a diagnostic test that can differentiate filarial TPE from other TPE-like syndrome is available, the following diagnostic criteria can be used for the diagnosis of TPE: (i) appropriate exposure history (mosquito bite) in an endemic area of filariasis, (ii) a history of paroxysmal nocturnal cough and breathlessness, (iii) chest radiographic evidence of pulmonary infiltrations, (iv) leucocytosis in blood, (v) peripheral blood eosinophils more than 3000 cells/mm^3, (vi) elevated serum IgE levels, (vii) elevated serum antifilarial antibodies (IgG and/or IgE), and (viii) a clinical response to diethylcarbamazine.

G. Treatment

The efficacy of organic arsenicals in the treatment of TPE was reported by Weingarten (112). However, the serious toxicity of arsenicals made it unacceptable for the treatment of TPE. The efficacy of diethylcarbamazine in TPE was proved by Ganatra and Lewis (139) and Danaraj (210). Baker et al. (140) had shown in a controlled trial that DEC in a dose of 5 mg/kg/day for 7 days was sufficient in the treatment of TPE. Danaraj (210) treated patients from Singapore with a higher dose of 18 and 30 mg/kg. The standard treatment recommended by the World Health Organization for treatment of TPE is oral DEC (6 mg/kg/day) for 3 weeks (211). One month after the start of treatment, most patients show marked symptomatic and radiographic improvement, and significant improvement in almost all aspects of lung function (174,175,190–192). However, there is an incomplete reversal of clinical, hematological, radiological, and physiological changes in TPE 1 month after a 3-week course of DEC (174,175,190).

In addition, a mild alveolitis characterized by hypercellular lavage fluid due to a significant increase in alveolar macrophages and eosinophils persists at 1 month (212). Patients evaluated 12 ± 2 months following a standard 3-week course of DEC were found to have mild, persistent symptoms referable to the lung. Chest X-ray abnormalities, blood eosinophilia, elevated serum IgE and filarial-specific IgG, and lung function changes consistent with chronic mild interstitial lung disease (213) persist. These patients have persistent eosinophilic alveolitis and the lower respiratory tract inflammatory cells release spontaneously exaggerated amounts of superoxide (O_2^-) and hydrogen peroxide (H_2O_2) (213). Treatment with prednisolone significantly reduced the lower respiratory tract inflammation and the release of oxidants (214). Patients with chronic eosinophilic alveolitis at 12th month had a significantly lower TLCO compared to patients with normal eosinophils in lower respiratory tract (215). Thus, following a standard 3-week course of DEC therapy, most patients show improvement, but not complete resolution of TPE and many are left with chronic respiratory tract inflammation and a mild form of interstitial lung disease (103,174,213). Relapses following treatment occur in 20% of patients followed for up to 5 years (103). Because of persistent mild interstitial lung disease and high relapse rates in TPE, it has been recommended that repeated monthly courses of DEC at 2–3 monthly intervals for a period of 1–2 years may be useful (103).

Earlier workers had shown that steroids were effective in the treatment of TPE (183,216). Since interstitial lung disease is found to occur in a proportion of patients with TPE despite standard therapy with DEC, a controlled clinical trial is needed to know the optimum dose and duration of DEC therapy with or without steroids. Ivermectin, an antifilarial drug (217), has not been found to be useful in the treatment of tropical pulmonary eosinophilia (218).

H. Prevention and Control

The control of TPE is possible if the mosquito-borne lymphatic filariasis is eliminated. The World Health Organization Assembly in 1997 has passed a resolution proposing elimination of lymphatic filariasis. The strategy proposed is to prevent transmission of parasites through mosquitoes from the blood of infected individuals. The aim is to treat the entire population at risk for lymphatic filariasis with once a year, single-dose treatment with a combination of two drugs (diethylcarbamazine and ivermectin) and to continue to cover the reproductive life span of adult-stage parasites (4–6 years) (219). The combination regimen can be given in the dosage of 6 mg/kg DEC and 400 µg/kg ivermectin. A community-based study from Papua New Guinea has reported the success of such a program (220).

VI. Visceral Larva Migrans

Toxocara larva migrans syndromes are important zoonotic infections (221,222). Certain nematode parasites when entering into an unnatural host (e.g., man) may not be able to complete their life cycle and their progress is arrested in the "unnatural host." If the entry of such parasitic larvae is through skin penetration, it causes cutaneous larva migrans (creeping eruption). If the entry is via oral route, visceral larva migrans results. Cutaneous larva migrans is caused by the parasite, *Ancylostoma brazeliense*, which is a parasite of dogs and cats. The common parasites that cause visceral larva migrans (VLM) and esonophilic lung disease in man are a dog ascarid *(Toxocara canis)* and less commonly a cat ascarid (*Toxocara catis*). Human toxocariasis occurs in all parts of the world wherever there is a large pool of infected dogs (223,224).

A. Life Cycle

Adult *T. canis* and *T. catis* live in the intestines of dogs and cats, respectively. In dogs, there is vertical transmission of larvae from infected pregnant bitches to their puppies. In cats, lactogenic transmission occurs to kittens. Older animals acquire infection by ingestion of eggs of the parasites from contaminated soil. The life cycle is then completed in definitive hosts, dogs, and cats. Eggs, passed by the animals in the feces, embryonate in the soil. These embryonated toxocara eggs, when ingested by an intermediate host (e.g., man), hatch into infective larvae in the intestine. The infective larvae penetrate the intestinal wall and are carried by the circulation to many organs including liver, lungs, muscles, central nervous system, and eye. The progress of the larvae is arrested in these sites of the intermediate host by the formation of a granulomatous lesion. In man, the larvae never develop into adult worms. Therefore, infected man never excretes toxocara eggs in the feces.

B. Immunopathogenesis

Visceral larva migrans (VLM) is characterized by leucocytosis and eosinophilia. The larva induces a granulomatous reaction in the tissues containing eosinophils and multinucleated giant cells. Larvae can get encapsulated within the granuloma where they are either destroyed or persist for many years in a viable state. Granulomata are found in the liver, lungs, central nervous system, and eyes. Later fibrosis and calcification occur. *T. canis* larvae produces excretory-secretary proteins, which may be responsible for inducing a Th-2-type CD4 cellular immune response (225) and this is characterized by eosinophilia and IgE production. *T. canis* larva has a labile mucinous surface coat (226), and eosinophils have been shown to bind on this surface (227). Larval antigens induce the release of histamine (228) and also can cross-react with human A and B blood group antigens (229).

C. Clinical Features

Human toxocariasis can manifest in different forms: visceral larva migrans, ocular larva migrans (OLM), neurological toxocariasis, common toxocariasis, and "covert" toxocariasis (222). Visceral larva migrans is commonly seen in children. However, most children infected with *Toxocara* sp. are asymptomatic.

The main symptoms in patients with visceral larva migrans are fever, cough, wheezing, seizures, anemia, and fatigue. Pulmonary manifestations are reported in 80% of cases and patients may present with severe asthma. Scattered rales and rhonchi are heard on auscultation. There will be intense blood eosinophilia. Skiagram chest may reveal focal patchy infiltrates. In some cases, severe eosinophilic pneumonia may lead to respiratory distress (230–232). Other clinical features include generalized lymph node enlargement, hepatomegaly, and splenomegaly. Ocular larva migrans due to *T. canis* may present with pain in the eyes, white pupil, strabismus or unilateral loss of vision. Neurological manifestations of VLM include eosinophilic meningitis, encephalitis, seizures, arachnoiditis, and myelopathy. Common toxocariasis is described mainly in adults and manifests as weakness, pruritis, rash, difficult breathing, and abdominal pain. This syndrome is associated with eosinophilia, increased total serum IgE level, and elevated antibody titers to *T. canis* (222,233). In "covert" toxocariasis, children present with fever, anemia, headache, abdominal pain, sleep disturbances, nausea, vomiting, pharyngitis, pneumonia, cough, wheeze, cervical lymphadenitis, hepatomegaly, and limb pains (234). A quarter of patients with "covert" toxocariasis have no eosinophilia.

D. Diagnosis

Visceral larva migrans is usually reported in young children with a history of pica. A history of exposure to puppies or dogs supports the diagnosis of

VLM. These children usually present with fever, cough, wheezing, eosinophilia, and hepatomegaly. A skiagram of the chest may show patchy infiltrates. Nonspecific changes include hypergamma-globulinemia and elevated isohemagglutinin titers to A and B blood group antigens. Serological tests by ELISA method using excretory-secretary proteins obtained from cultured *T. canis* may be useful in the diagnosis (235). Cross-reactivity with other helminths limits the usefulness of this test in endemic areas. Detection of IgE antibodies by ELISA (236) and toxocara excretory-secretary antigens by Western blotting procedure (237) has also been reported for diagnosis. However, serodiagnostic procedures cannot distinguish between past and present infections. Histopathological examination of lung or liver biopsy specimens may demonstrate granulomas with eosinophils, multinucleated giant cells, and fibrosis. Since man is not the definitive host of *Toxocara* sp., eggs or larvae cannot be demonstrated in the feces.

E. Treatment

Visceral larva migrans is a self-limiting disease and there may be spontaneous resolution. Therefore, mild to moderately symptomatic patients need not require any drug therapy. Patients with severe VLM can be treated with thiabendazole, mebendazole, or diethylcarbamazine (DEC). Treatment with antihelminthic treatment may exacerbate the inflammatory reactions in the tissues due to the killing of larvae. It is, therefore, advised to combine antihelminthic treatment with corticosteroids. DEC can be given in a dose of 6 mg/kg/day for 21 days (238). Mebendazole is prescribed in a dose of 20–25 mg/kg/day for 21 days (239). Albendazole 10 mg/kg/day for 5 days has been shown to have a moderate effect compared to thiabendazole (240).

F. Prevention

Prevention of contamination of the environment with dog feces containing *T. canis* eggs and exclusion of pet animals from toddler playgrounds may aid in minimizing human toxocariasis.

VII. Pulmonary Trichinellosis

Human trichinellosis is an important food-borne zoonosis. Five species of *Trichinella* (*T. spiralis*, *T. nativa*, *T. nelsoni*, *T. britovi*, and *T. pseudospiralis*) can infect man (241). The most important species that infect man is *T. spiralis*. The parasite has a direct life cycle with complete development in one host (pig, rat, or man). However, two hosts are required to complete the life cycle and for the preservation of the species from extinction. Man gets the infection from raw and partially cooked pork, when infected pig's muscle containing larval trichinellae is eaten by man. The infective larvae in the muscle are surrounded by a host capsule, which is a modified striated muscle known as "nurse" cell. In the stomach, the "nurse" cell is digested and the free larva is liberated. The larvae develop into adults (males and females) in the duodenum and jejunum. The new-born larvae produced by female parasites pass through the lymphatics or blood vessels to reach the striated muscles (242). The larvae undergo encystment in the muscle and a host capsule develops around the larvae. Later on, it may get calcified. The life cycle is completed when infected muscle is ingested by a suitable host.

Th-2 cells play an important role in the pathogenesis of the disease. These cells release IL-5 and IL-4 and these cytokines are responsible for eosinophilia and increased IgE production (243). The common symptoms of trichinellosis are muscle pain, periorbital edema, fever, and diarrhea (244,245). Pulmonary symptoms include dyspnea, cough, and pulmonary infiltrates. Dyspnea may be due to the involvement of the diaphragm (246). Leucocytosis, eosinophilia, and elevated levels of serum muscle enzymes (creatine phosphokinase, lactate dehydrogenase, aldolase, and amino transferase) are important laboratory findings. An enzyme-linked immunosorbant assay (ELISA) for detection of anti-*Trichinella* antibodies using excretory-secretary antigens may be useful in the diagnosis (247). A definitive diagnosis can be made by muscle biopsy (usually deltoid muscle) that may demonstrate larvae of *T. spiralis* (246). Symptomatic treatment of trichinellosis includes analgesics and corticosteroids. Specific treatments with mebendazole 200–400 mg three times a day for 3 days followed by 400–500 mg three times a day for 10 days. Albendazole can be given in a dosage of 400 mg/day for 3 days followed by 800 mg/day for 15 days. Trichinellosis can be prevented by consuming properly cooked pork.

VIII. Pulmonary Schistosomiasis

The schistosomes that cause human disease are *Schistosoma haematobium*, *Schistosoma mansoni*, and *Schistosoma japonicum*. Rarely infections with *Schistosoma intercalatum* and *Schistosoma mekongi* are reported from Africa and the Far East, respectively (248). The schistosome eggs are passed in urine (*S. haematobium*) or in feces (*S. mansoni* and *S. japonicum*) by the infected humans. The eggs released in fresh water are then ingested by snails (intermediate host) in which the eggs hatch and develop into cercariae. The infective cercariae are excreted into the water and these cercariae penetrate human skin or are ingested to penetrate the gut. The final habitat of *S. haematobium* is urinary bladder vesicle beds and of *S. mansoni* and *S. japonicum* in the mesenteric beds. The parasites can cause *Schistosoma* dermatitis at the site of skin penetration. Acute symptoms can develop 3 to 8 weeks after skin penetration (249,250) and manifest as shortness of breath, wheezing, and dry cough. The acute form, also known as Katayama syndrome, may present with fever, chills, weight loss, diarrhea,

abdominal pain, myalgia, and urticaria (250,251). Peripheral blood eosinophilia with mild leucocytosis, abnormal liver function test results and
elevated IgE levels are reported during this phase. Patients with chronic
schistosomiasis present with features of pulmonary hypertension and cor-
pulmonale in patients with *S. haematobium* (252). Hepatosplenomegaly
due to portal hypertension has been reported in patients infected with
S. mansoni or *S. japonicum* (248). Acute schistosomiasis at presentation
can be treated with corticosteroids alone followed by praziquantel (20–30
mg/kg orally in two doses within 12 hours). Chronic schistosomiasis can
also be treated with praziquantel with the same dosage (248) (this volume,
chapter on "Lung Involvement in Schistosomiasis").

IX. Pulmonary Paragonimiasis

Paragonimiasis is caused by infection with *Paragonimus* species and manifest
as subacute or chronic inflammation of the lung. The species that are known to
cause paragonimiasis in man are *P. westermani*, *P. miyazakii*, *P. mexicanus*,
P. skrjabini, *P. africanus*, *P. uterobilateralis*, *P. kellicotti*, *P. phillipinensis*,
and *P. heterotremus* (253–255). Adult worms live in the lungs and the eggs
are voided in the sputum or feces. The eggs hatch in the fresh water to release
miracidiae, which are ingested by the first intermediate host, freshwater snails.
The micracidiae develop into cercariae in the snail and are released into the
water. The cercariae then invade the second intermediate host, crustaceans
(crabs or crayfish) and develop into infective metacercariae. Man gets the
infection, when raw or undercooked crabs or crayfishes infected with infective
metacercariae are ingested (253). The parasite from the human gut passes
through several organs and tissues to reach the lung (253). Pulmonary paragonimiasis manifests as fever, chest pain, chronic cough and hemoptysis (256).
Chest radiographs may show infiltrative, nodular, and cavitating shadows
(257). Pleural effusion or pneumothorax is an important finding in paragonimiasis (258). Peripheral blood eosinophilia and elevated serum IgE levels are
seen in >80% of patients with paragonimiasis (253,258). Paragonimiasis can
be treated with praziquantel (75 mg/kg/day for 3 days), bithionol (30–40
mg/kg in 10 days on alternate days), niclofolan (2 mg/kg as a single dose), or
triclabendazole (20 mg/kg in two equal doses) (253,259) (this volume, chapter
on "Paragonimiasis").

X. Pulmonary Hydatid Disease

The parasite species that are responsible for hydatid disease in man
are *Echinococcus granulosus* and *Echinococcus multilocularis*. The adult
E. granulosus resides in the small intestine of the definitive hosts, mainly
dogs. The intermediate hosts including man are infected by ingestion of

eggs excreted in the feces of the dogs. Hydatid cysts are formed mainly in the liver and lungs. Pulmonary symptoms include cough, fever, and chest pain (260,261). Chest radiographs show solitary or multiple round opacities. Eosinophilia and elevated IgE levels are seen when the hydatid cyst ruptures (7). Treatment of hydatid cysts is essentially surgical. However, pharmacotherapy with albendazole or mebendazole has also been found to be useful (260) (this volume, chapter on "Hydatid Lung Disease").

XI. Pulmonary Eosinophilia in Pulmonary Tuberculosis

Pulmonary eosinophilia in pulmonary tuberculosis is rare. The predominant cells that contribute to granuloma formation in pulmonary tuberculosis are macrophages and lymphocytes (262). In a community-based study, it had been shown that 11% of patients with pulmonary tuberculosis had an associated peripheral blood eosinophilia (263). Muller reported that peripheral blood eosinophilia was twice as frequent in men as in women and the incidence in women was about 6% (264). Blood eosinophilia in tuberculosis was also found to correlate with disease activity (265). Chronic eosinophilic pneumonia in a patient who went on to develop cavitary atypical mycobacterial infection has been reported (266). Pulmonary eosinophilia due to *M. tuberculosis* in two of three patients at the site of the lesion has been reported and the third patient had both peripheral blood and lung eosinophilia (209). There was complete elimination of eosinophilic inflammatory response following successful completion of antituberculosis treatment (209). It had been observed that mice deficient in gamma-interferon (IFN-$\gamma^{-/-}$) or the IFN-γ receptor (IFN-γR$^{-/-}$) are extremely susceptible to infection with mycobacteria (267,268) and there was a striking increase in the number of eosinophils at the site of infection in these mice (267,269). It has been suggested that the accumulation of eosinophils at the site of mycobacterial infection in IFN-$\gamma^{-/-}$ and IFN-γR$^{-/-}$ mice may be due to the elevated levels of Th-2 -cytokines (especially IL-5) produced by lymphocytes of these mice (269,270).

In conformity with these observations, it has been reported that a blockade of eosinophil proliferation and recruitment into the lung by treatment with anti-interleukin-5 monoclonal antibody marginally reduces mycobacterial growth within the lung (271). Further studies are required to know the role of eosinophils in the pathogenesis of tuberculosis (this volume, chapter on "Treatment of Tuberculosis in the Tropics").

XII. Pulmonary Brucellosis

Brucellosis is an important zoonotic disease that is prevalent in many parts of the world (272), including the Mediterranean basin, the Arabian Peninsula, the Indian subcontinent, Mexico, and Central and South America. It causes chronic infection and spontaneous abortions in many animals including cattle, sheep, goats, pigs, and dogs. The disease is caused by a gram-negative coccobacillus of the genus *Brucella*. The species of *Brucella* that infect man are *Brucella abortus*, *Brucella melitensis*, *Brucella suis*, and *Brucella canis*. Transmission of infection to man occurs through direct contact with contaminated animals, ingestion of infected dairy products, and inhalation of infectious aerosol particles (273). The respiratory system is involved when organisms are inhaled. Brucellosis usually presents with undulant fever, night sweats, malaise, weakness, back pain, arthralgia, headache, cough, and peripheral eosinophilia (7). Pulmonary manifestations are rare complications of brucellosis, occurring in only 1–7% of cases (273). The respiratory symptoms include cough, both productive and dry, and dyspnea. Chest radiographs may reveal features of lobar pneumonia, interstitial pneumonitis, and in late stages honeycomb pattern (273).

Other radiographic findings include hilar adenopathy (unilateral or bilateral), granulomas and solitary modules, miliary mottling, cavitation, and penumothorax (7,273). Chronic brucellosis can also manifest as pulmonary infiltrates and eosinophilia (274). Respiratory brucellosis has to be differentiated from pulmonary tuberculosis. Diagnosis of brucellosis can be confirmed by isolation of the organisms from blood, bone marrow, or other tissue culture (273). Serum agglutination test that shows a four-fold or more increase in antibody titer is also diagnostic. Treatment of brucellosis is with a regimen of doxycyclin (100 mg twice daily) plus rifampin (600–900 mg daily) for 6 weeks. A combination of tetracycline for 6 weeks and streptomycin for 2 weeks is an alternate treatment (273).

XIII. Fungus-Induced Eosinophilic Lung Diseases

Eosinophilia due to fungal diseases is rare. However, pulmonary eosinophilia can occur in certain fungal infections especially in coccidiodomycosis, aspergillosis, cryptococcosis, and histoplasmosis. Peripheral blood eosinophilia is seen in most cases (up to 88%) of primary coccidiodomycosis (275,276). Eosinophilia in coccidiodomycosis is usually associated with other hypersensitivity manifestations such as urticaria, erythema multiforme, erythema nodosum, or arthritis. Eosinophilia has also been reported in acute coccidiodal pleural effusion (277). Chronic eosinophilic pneumonia has been observed in cryptococcosis (278) and a transient pneumonitis with eosinophilia has been noted in histoplasmosis (7). Allergic bronchopulmonary mycoses (ABPM) due to hypersensitivity reactions to fungal species are important group of disorders with pulmonary eosinophilia and the most common ABPM is allergic bronchopulmonary aspergillosis (ABPA) (279,280). ABPA is a hypersensitivity reaction to *Aspergillus* species especially to *Aspergillus fumigatus*, *A. flavus* and

A. niger (280). Other fungal species that have been reported to cause ABPM are *Candida albicans* (281), *Curvularia lunata* (282). *Stemphylium lanuginosum* (283), *Pseudallescheria boydii* (284), *Fusarium vasinfectum* (285), and *Helminthosporium* sp.(286). ABPM occurs in patients with asthma who present with unexplained and often fleeting pulmonary infiltrates due to bronchial plugging. The important findings in ABPM include peripheral blood and pulmonary eosinophilia, positive immediate skin reaction to fungal antigens, elevated precipitant antibodies to the fungus, and elevated IgE levels. Chest X rays and CT scan may reveal proximal bronchiectasis. Treatment is with corticosteroids (this volume, chapter on "Fungal Infections in Tropical Countries").

References

1. Loffler W. Zur differential-diagnose der lungeninfiltrieurgen: 11. Uber fluchtige succedan—infiltrate (mit eosinophile). Bietr Klin Tuberk 1932; 79: 368–392.
2. Zumla A, James DG. Immunologic aspects of tropical lung disease. Clin Chest Med 2002; 23:283–308.
3. Reeder WH, Goodrich BE. Pulmonary infiltrate with eosinophilia (PIE syndrome). Ann Intern Med 1952; 36:1217–1240.
4. Crofton JW, Livingston JL, Oswald NC, Roberts ATU. Pulmonary eosinophilia. Thorax 1952; 7:1–35.
5. Leibow AA, Carrington CB. The eosinophilic pneumonias. Medicine 1969; 48:251–285.
6. Allen JN, Davis WB. Eosinophilic lung diseases. Am J Respir Crit Care Med 1994; 150:1423–1438.
7. Savani DM, Sharma OP. Eosinophilic lung disease in the tropics. Clin Chest Med 2002; 23:377–396.
8. Rothenberg ME. Eosinophilia. N Engl J Med 1998; 338:1592–1600.
9. Sanderson CJ. Interleukin-5, eosinophils and disease. Blood 1992; 79: 3107–3109.
10. Collins PD, Marlean S, Griffiths-Johnson DA, Jose PJ, Williams TJ. Co-operation between interleukin-5 and the chemokine eotaxin to induce eosinophil accumulation in vivo. J Exp Med 1995; 182:1169–1174.
11. Wein M, Sterbinsky SA, Bickel CA, Schleismer RP, Bochner BS. Comparison of human eosinophil ligands for P-selectin: ligands for P-selectin differ from those for E-selectin. Am J Respir Cell Mol Biol 1995; 12:315–319.
12. Resnick MB, Weller PF. Mechanism of eosinophil recruitment. Am J Respir Cell Mol Biol 1993; 8:349–355.
13. Kita H, Gleich GJ. Chemokines active on eosinophils—potential roles in allergic inflammation. J Exp Med 1996; 183:2421–2426.
14. Forssmann U, Uguccioni M, Loetscher P, Dahinden CA, Langen H, Thelen M, Baggiolini M. Eotaxin-2, a novel CC chemokine that is selective for the chemokine receptor CCR 3 and acts like eotaxin on human eosinophil and basophil leukocytes. J Exp Med 1997; 185:2171–2176.

15. Simon HU, Yousefi S, Schranz C, Schapowal A, Bachert C, Blaser K. Direct demonstration of delayed eosinophil apoptosis as a mechanism causing tissue eosinophilia. J Immunol 1997; 158:3902–3908.
16. Capron M. Eosinophils and parasites. Ann Parasitol Hum Comp 1991; 66 (suppl 1):41–45.
17. Butterworth A, Wassom D, Gleich GJ, Loegering DA, David JR. Damage to schistosomula of *Schistosoma mansoni* induced directly by eosinophil major basic protein. J Immunol 1979; 122:221–229.
18. Hamann KJ, Gleich GJ, Checkel JL, Loegering DA, McCall JW, Barker RL. In vitro killing of microfilariae of *Brugia pahangi* and *Brugia malayi* by eosinophil granular proteins. J Immunol 1990; 144:3166–3173.
19. Lewis RA, Austen KF, Soberman PJ. Leukotrienes and other products of 5-lipoxygenase pathway: biochemistry and relation to pathobiology in human diseases. N Engl J Med 1990; 323:645–655.
20. Del Prete G. Human Th-1 and Th-2 lymphocytes: their role in the pathophysiology of atopy. Allergy 1992; 47:450–455.
21. Mahanty S, King CL, Kumaraswami V, Regunathan J, Maya A, Jayaraman K, Abrams JS, Ottesen EA, Nutman TB. IL-4 and IL-5 secreting lymphocyte populations are preferentially stimulated by parasite-derived antigens in human tissue invasive nematode infections. J Immunol 1993; 151:3704–3711.
22. Elson LH, Shaw S, Van LRA, Nutman TB. T cell subpopulation phenotypes in filarial infections: CD27 negativity defines a population greatly enriched for Th_2cells. Int Immunol 1994; 6:1003–1009.
23. Elson H, Nutman TB, Metcalfe DD, Prussin C. Flow cytometric analysis for cytokine production identifies T helper 1, T helper 2 and T helper 0 cells within the human CD4 + CD27-lymphocyte subpopulation. J Immunol 1995; 154:4294–4301.
24. Limaye A, Abrams JS, Silver JE, Ottesen EA, Nutman TB. Regulation of parasite-induced eosinophilia: selectively increased interleukin-5 production in helminth-infected patients. J Exp Med 1990; 172:399–402.
25. Hall LR, Mehlotra RK, Higgins AW, Haxhiu MA, Pearlman E. An essential role for interleukin-5 and eosinophils in helminth-induced airway hyper responsiveness. Infect Immun 1998; 66:4425–4430.
26. Dunne DW, Butterworth AE, Fulford AJC, Kariuki HC, Langley JG, Ouma JH, Capron A, Pierce R, Sturrock RF. Immunity after treatment of human schistosomiasis: association between IgE antibodies to adult worm antigens and resistance to reinfection. Eur J Immunol 1992; 22:1483–1494.
27. Hagan P, Wilkins HA, Blumenthal UJ, Hayes RJ, Greenwood BM. Eosinophilia and resistance to *Schistosoma haematobium* in man. Parasite Immunol 1985; 7:625–632.
28. Roberts M, Butterworth AE, Kimau G, Kaman T, Fulford AJ, Dunne DW, Ouma JH, Sturrock RF. Immunity after treatment of human schistosomiasis: association between cellular responses and resistance to reinfections. Infect Immunol 1993; 61:4984–4993.
29. Nutman TB, Kumaraswami V, Ottesen EA. Parasite-specific allergy in human filariasis: insights after analysis of parasite antigen-driven lymphokine production. J Clin Invest 1987; 79:1516–1523.

30. Sartono E, Kruize YCM, Kurniawan A, Meide PH Vander, Partono F, Maizels RM, Yazdanbakhsh M. Elevated cellular immune responses and interferon-gamma release after long-term diethylcarbamazine treatment of patients with human lymphatic filariasis. J Infect Dis 1995; 171:1683–1687.
31. Stoll NR. This wormy world. J Parasitol 1947; 33:1–18.
32. Pawlowski ZS, Davis A. Morbidity and mortality in ascariasis. In: Crompton DWT, Nesheim MC, Pawlowski ZS, eds. Ascariasis and Its Prevention and Control. London: Taylor & Francis, 1989:71–86.
33. Crompton DWT. How much human helminthiasis is there in the world? J Parasitol 1999; 85:379–403.
34. Peng W, Zhou X, Gasser RB. *Ascaris* egg profiles in human faeces: biological and epidemiological implications. Parasitology 2003; 127:283–290.
35. St Georgiev V. Pharmacotherapy of ascariasis. Expert Opin Pharmacother 2001; 2:223–239.
36. Yazicioglu M, Ones U, Yalcin I. Peripheral and nasal eosinophilia and serum total immunoglobulin E levels in children with ascariasis. Turk J Pediatr 1996; 38:477–484.
37. Santra A, Bhattacharya T, Chowdhury A, Ghosh A, Ghosh N, Chatterjee BP, Mazumdar DN. Serodiagnosis of ascariasis with specific IgG4 antibody and its use in epidemiological study. Trans R Soc Trop Med Hyg 2001; 95:289–292.
38. Chatterjee BP, Santra A, Karmarkar PR, Mazumdar DN. Evaluation of IgG4 response in ascariasis by ELISA for serodiagnosis. Trop Med Int Health 1996; 1:633–639.
39. Bhattacharya T, Santra A, Mazumdar DN, Chatterjee BP. Possible approach for serodiagnosis of ascariasis by evaluation of immunoglobulin G4 response using *Ascaris lumbricoides* somatic antigen. J Clin Microbiol 2001; 39: 2991–2994.
40. Palmer DR, Hall A, Haque R, Anwar KS. Antibody isotype responses to antigens of *Ascaris lumbricoides* in a case-control study of persistently infected Bangladeshi children. Parasitology 1995; 111:385–393.
41. Hagel I, Lynch NR, Di Prisco MC, Rojas E, Perez M, Alvarez N. *Ascaris* reinfection of slum children: relation with the IgE response. Clin Exp Immunol 1993; 94:80–83.
42. Hagel I, Lynch NR, Puccio F, Rodriguez O, Luzondo R, Rodriguez P, Sanchez P, Ca CM, Di Prisco MC. Defective regulation of the intestinal helminth *Ascaris lumbricoides* in malnourished children. J Trop Pediatr 2003; 49:136–142.
43. Cooper PJ, Chico ME, Sandoval C, Espinel I, Guevara A, Kennedy MW, Urban JF Jr, Griffin GE, Nutman TB. Human infection with *Ascaris lumbricoides* is associated with a polarized cytokine response. J Infect Dis 2000; 182:1207–1213.
44. Geiger SM, Massara CL, Bethony J, Soboslay PT, Carvalho OS, Correa-Oliveira R. Cellular responses and cytokine profiles in *Ascaris lumbricoides* and *Trichuris trichiura* infected patients. Parasite Immunol 2002; 24:499–509.
45. Williams–Blangero S, VandeBerg JL, Subedi J, Aivaliotis MJ, Rai DR, Upadhayay P, Jha B, Blangero J. Genes on chromosome 1 and 13 have significant effects on *Ascaris* infection. Proc Natl Acad Sci USA 2002; 99:5533–5538.

46. Ford RM. Transient pulmonary eosinophilia and asthma: a review of 20 cases occurring in 5702 asthma sufferers. Am Rev Respir Dis 1996; 93:797–803.
47. Liu LX, Weller PF. Strongyloidiasis and other intestinal nematode infections. Infect Dis Clin North Am 1993; 7:655–682.
48. Citro LA, Gordon ME, Miller WT. Eosinophilic lung disease (or how to slice PIE). Am J Roentgenol Rad Ther Nuc Med 1973; 117:787–797.
49. Rexroth G, Keller C. Chronic course of eosinophilic pneumonia in infection with *Ascaris lumbricoides*. Pneumologie 1995; 49:77–83.
50. Sarinas PS, Chitkara RK. Ascariasis and hookworm. Semin Respir Infect 1997; 12:130–137.
51. Lynch NR, Goldblatt J, Le Souef PN. Parasite infection and the risk of asthma and atopy. Thorax 1999; 54:659–660.
52. Palmer LJ, Celedon JC, Weiss ST, Wang B, Fang Z, Xu X. *Ascaris lumbricoides* infection is associated with increased risk of childhood asthma and atopy in rural China. Am J Respir Crit Care Med 2002; 165:1489–1493.
53. Silva NMT, Andrade J, Tavares-Neto J. Asthma and ascariasis in children aged two to ten living in a low income suburb. J Pediatr (Rio J) 2003; 79:27–32.
54. Belizaro VY, Amarillo ME, de Leon WU, de los Reyes AE, Bugayong MG, Macatangay BJ. A comparison of the efficacy of single dose of albendazole, ivermectin and diethylcarbamazine alone or in combination against *Ascaris* and *Trichuris* spp. Bull World Health Org 2003; 81:35–42.
55. Hosain GM, Saha S, Begum A. Impact of sanitation and health education on intestinal parasite infection among primary school aged children of Sherpur, Bangladesh. Trop Doct 2003; 33:139–143.
56. Fallah M, Mirarab A, Jamalian F, Ghaderi A. Evaluation of two years of mass chemotherapy against ascariasis in Hamadan, Islamic Republic of Iran. Bull World Health Org 2002; 80:399–402.
57. Roche M, Layrise M. Nature and causes of hookworm anemia. Am J Trop Med Hyg 1996; 15:1031–1102.
58. Hoagland KE, Schad GA. *Necator americanus* and *Ancylostoma duodenale*. Life history parameters and epidemiological implications of two sympatric hookworms on humans. Exp Parasitol 1978; 44:36–49.
59. Hotez P. Human hookworm infection. In: Farthing MJG, Keusch GT, Wakelin D, eds. Intestinal Helminths. London: Chapman & Hall, 1995:129–150.
60. Nawalinski TA, Schad GA. Arrested development in *Ancylostoma duodenale*: cause of self-induced infections in man. Am J Trop Med Hyg 1974; 23: 895–898.
61. Yu Sen-Hai, Jiang Ze-xiao, Xu Long-Qi. Infantile hookworm disease in China. A review. Acta Trop 1995; 59:265–270.
62. Hawdon JM, Jones BF, Hoffman D, Hotez PJ. Cloning and expression of *Ancylostoma* secreted proteins. A polypeptide associated with the transition to parasitism by infective hookworm larvae. J Biol Chem 1996; 271: 6672–6678.
63. Ottesen EA. Immune responses in human hookworm infections. In: Schad GA, Warren KS, eds. Hookworm Disease, Current Status and Future Directions. London: Taylor & Francis, 1990:404–416.

64. Cappello M, Clyne LP, MacPhedram P, Hotez PJ. *Ancylostoma* factor Xa inhibitor: partial purification and its identification as a major hookworm-derived anticoagulant in vitro. J Infect Dis 1993; 167:1474–1477.

65. Rien P, Ueda T, Haruta T, Sharma CP, Arnaout MA. The A-domain of B2 integrin CR3 (CD11b/CD18) is a receptor for the hookworm-derived neutrophil adhesion inhibitor (NIF). J Cell Biol 1994; 127:2081–2091.

66. Howdon JM. Differentiation between the human hookworm *Ancylostoma duodenale* and *Necator Americanus* using PCR-RFLP. J Parasitol 1996; 82:642–647.

67. Genta RM. Global prevalence of strongyloidiasis: critical review with epidemiologic insights into the prevention of disseminated disease. Rev Infect Dis 1989; 5:755–767.

68. Sanchez P, Guzman AP, Guillen SM, Adell RI, Estruch AM, Gonzalo IN, Olmos CR. Endemic strongyloidiasis on the Spanish Mediterranean coast. Q J Med 2001; 94:357–368.

69. Braun TI, Fekete T, Lynch A. Strongyloidiasis in an institution for mentally retarded adults. Arch Intern Med 1988; 148:634–636.

70. Scowden EB, Schaffner W, Stone WJ. Overwhelming strongyloidiasis: an unappreciated opportunistic infection. Medicine (Baltimore) 1978; 57:527–544.

71. Neva FA. Biology and immunology of human strongyloidiasis. J Infect Dis 1986; 153:397–406.

72. Casati A, Cornero G, Muttini S, Tresoldi M, Gallioli G, Torri G. Hyperacute pneumonitis in a patient with overwhelming *Strongyloides stercoralis* infection. Eur J Anesthesiol 1996; 13:498–501.

73. Genta RM, Miles P, Fields K. Opportunistic *Strongyloides stercoralis* infection in lymphoma patients. Report of a case and review of the literature. Cancer 1989; 63:1407–1411.

74. Lessman KD, Can S, Talavera W. Disseminated *Strongyloides stercoralis* in human immunodeficiency virus-infected patients: treatment failure and review of literature. Chest 1993; 104:119–122.

75. Dionisio D, Manneschi LI, di Lollo S, Orsi A, Tani A, Papucci A, Esperti F, Leoncini F. *Strongyloides stercoralis*: ultra structural study of newly hatched larvae within human duodenal mucosa. J Clin Pathol 2000; 53:110–116.

76. Wehner JH, Kirsch CM. Pulmonary manifestations of strongyloidiasis. Semin Respir Infect 1997; 12:122–129.

77. Alzer PD, Milder JE, Banwell JG, Kilgore G, Klein M, Parker R. Epidemiologic features of *Strongyloides stercoralis* infection in an endemic area of United States. Am J Trop Med Hyg 1982; 31:313–319.

78. Davidson RA, Fletcher RH, Chapman LE. Risk factors for strongyloidiasis. A case-control study. Arch Intern Med 1984; 144:321–324.

79. Woodring JH, Halfhill H II, Berger R, Reed JC, Moser N. Clinical and imaging features of pulmonary strongyloidiasis. South Med J 1996; 89:10–19.

80. Milder JE, Walzer PD, Kilgore G, Rutherford I, Klein M. Clinical features of *Strongyloides stercoralis* infection in an endemic area of the United States. Gastroenterology 1981; 80:1481–1488.

81. Nwokolo C, Imohiosen E. Strongyloidiasis of respiratory tract presenting as "asthma". Br Med J 1973; 2:153–154.

82. Woodring JH, Halfhill H II, Reed JC. Pulmonary strongyloidiasis: clinical and imaging features. Am J Roentgenol 1994; 162:537–542.
83. Ghoshal UC, Ghoshal U, Jain M, Kumar A, Aggarwal R, Misra A, Ayyagiri A, Naik SR. *Strongyloides stercoralis* infestation associated with septicemia due to intestinal transmural migration of bacteria. J Gastroenterol Hepatol 2002; 17:1331–1333.
84. Goyal SB. Intestinal strongyloidiasis manifesting as eosinophilic pleural effusion. South Med J 1998; 91:768–769.
85. Premanand R, Prasad GV, Mohan A, Gururajkumar A, Reddy MK. Eosinophilic pleural effusion and presence of filariform larva of *Strongyloides stercoralis* in a patient with metastatic squamous cell carcinoma deposits in the pleura. Indian J Chest Dis Allied Sci 2003; 45:121–124.
86. da Silva OA, Amarol CF, da Silveira JC, Lopez M, Pittella JE. Hypokalemic respiratory muscle paralysis following *Strongyloides stercoralis* hyperinfection: a case report. Am J Trop Med Hyg 1981; 30:69–73.
87. Lin AL, Kessimian N, Benditt JO. Restrictive pulmonary disease due to interlobar septal fibrosis associated with disseminated infection by *Strongyloides stercoralis*. Am J Respir Crit Care Med 1995; 151:205–209.
88. Reddy TS. Syndrome of inappropriate secretion of antidiuretic hormone and nonpalpable purpura in a woman with *Strongyloides stercoralis*. Am J Med Sci 2003; 325:288–291.
89. Caceres MA, Genta RM. Pulmonary microcalcification associated with *Strongyloides stercoralis*. Chest 1988; 94:862–865.
90. Sen P, Gil C, Estrellas B, Middleton JR. Corticosteroid-induced asthma: a manifestation of limited hyperinfection syndrome due to *Strongyloides stercoralis*. South Med J 1995; 88:923–927.
91. Ossorio MA, Brovon PE, Fields CL, Roy TM. Exacerbation of chronic obstructive pulmonary disease due to hyperinfection with *Strongyloides stercoralis*. J Ky Med Assoc 1990; 88:233–237.
92. Marriota S, Pallone G, Li Bianchi E, Gilardi G, Bisetti A. *Strongyloides stercoralis* hyperinfection in a case of idiopathic pulmonary fibrosis. Panminerva Med 1996; 38:45–47.
93. Siddiqui AA, Berk SL. Diagnosis of *Strongyloides stercoralis* infection. Clin Infect Dis 2001; 33:1040–1047.
94. Koga K, Kasuya S, Khamboonruang C, Sukavat K, Nakamura Y, Tani S, Ieda M, Tomita K, Hattan N, Mori M, Makino S. An evaluation of the agar plate method for the detection of *Strogyloides stercoralis* in northern Thailand. J Trop Med Hyg 1990; 93:183–188.
95. Hernadez-Chavarria F, Avendano L. A simple modification of the Baermann method for diagnosis of strongyloidiasis. Mem Inst Oswaldo Cruz (Rio de Janeiro) 2001; 96:805–807.
96. De Kaminsky RG. Evaluation of three methods for laboratory diagnosis of *Strogyloides stercoralis* infection. J Parasitol 1993; 79:277–280.
97. Chu E, Whitlock WL, Dietrich RA. Pulmonary hyperinfection syndrome with *Strogyloides stercoralis*. Chest 1990; 97:1475–1477.
98. Williams J, Ninley D, Dralle W, Berk SL, Verghese A. Diagnosis of pulmonary strongyloidiasis by bronchoalveolar lavage. Chest 1988; 94:643–644.

99. Loutfy MR, Wilson M, Keystone JS, Kain KC. Serology and eosinophil count in the diagnosis and management of strongyloidiasis in a non-endemic area. Am J Trop Med Hyg 2002; 66:749–752.
100. Datry A, Hilmarsdoltir I, Mayorga-Sagastume R, Lyaguobi M, Gaxotte P, Biligui S, Chodakewitz J, Neu D, Danis M, Gentilini M. Treatment of *Strongyloides stercoralis* infection with ivermectin compared with albendazole: results of an open study of 60 cases. Trans R Soc Trop Med Hyg 1994; 88:344–345.
101. Pitisuttihum P, Supanaranoud W, Chindanoud A. A randomized comparative study of albendazole in chronic strongyloidiasis. South East Asian J Trop Med Public Health 1995; 26:735–738.
102. Vijayan VK. Tropical pulmonary eosinophilia. Indian J Chest Dis Allied Sci 1996; 38:169–180.
103. Udwadia FE. Tropical eosinophilia. In: Herzog H, ed. Pulmonary Eosinophilia: Progress in Respiration Research. Basel: S. Karger, 1975:35–155.
104. Neva FA, Ottesen EA. Tropical (Filarial) eosinophilia. N Engl J Med 1978; 298:1129–1131.
105. Ottesen EA, Nutman TB. Tropical pulmonary eosinophilia. Ann Rev Med 1992; 43:417–424.
106. Ottesen EA. Immunological aspects of lymphatic filariasis and onchocerciasis. Trans R Soc Trop Med Hyg 1984; 73(suppl):9–18.
107. Poh SC. The course of lung function in treated tropical eosinophilia. Thorax 1974; 29:710–712.
108. Low GC. An interesting case of eosinophilia. Trans R Soc Trop Med Hyg 1916; 9:77–81.
109. Roy NC, Bose CC. Effectiveness of soamin in cases of asthma associated with eosinophilia. Calcutta Med J 1918; 12:268–277.
110. Ghosh BN. Soamin in the treatment of asthma. Glasgow Med J 1918; 39:343–348.
111. Frimodt-Moller C, Barton RM. A pseudo-tuberculosis condition associated with eosinophilia. Indian Med Gaz 1940; 75:607–613.
112. Weingarten RJ. Tropical eosinophilia. Lancet 1943; 1:103–105.
113. Chaudhari RN. Eosinophil lung. Indian Med Gaz 1943; 78:575–577.
114. Danaraj TJ. Eosinophilic lung. Med J Malaysia 1947; 1:278–280.
115. Sussman HL. Tropical eosinophilia. S Afr Med J 1947; 21:863–866.
116. Viswanathan R. Pulmonary eosinophiliosis. Quart J Med 1948; 17:257–270.
117. Hodes PJ, Wood FC. Eosinophilic lung (Tropical eosinophilia). Am J Med Sci 1945; 210:288–295.
118. Stuiver PC, Wismans PJ, Schornagel R. Tropical eosinophilia is an important disease in the Netherlands. Ned Tijdschr Geneeskd 1991; 135:283–286.
119. Hayashi K, Horiba M, Shindou J, Sumida T, Takekoshi A. Tropical eosinophilia in a man from Sri Lanka. Nihon Kyobu Shikkan Gakkai Zasshi 1996; 34:1411–1415.
120. Spry CJF, Kumaraswami V. Tropical eosinophilia. Semin Hematol 1982; 19:107–115.
121. World Health Organization, Division of Control of Tropical Diseases. Lymphatic filariasis infection and disease: control strategies. Report of a

WHO/CTD/TDR consultative meeting held at the Universiti Sains Malaysia, Penang, Malaysia, 22–24 Aug 1994 (TDR/CTD/FIL/PENANG/94.1). 1994: 1–30.

122. Johnson S, Wilkinson R, Davidson RN. Tropical respiratory medicine. IV: acute tropical infection and the lung. Thorax 1994; 49:714–718.

123. Viswanathan R, Prasad M, Prasad S, Saran R, Sinha TRBPN, Sinha SP. Morbidity survey of jail population. Part I. Incidence of certain chronic respiratory diseases with special reference to pulmonary eosinophiliosis. Indian J Chest Dis 1965; 7:142–145.

124. Ray D, Abel R, Selvaraj KG. Epidemiology of pulmonary eosinophilia in rural South India: a perspective study, 1981–86. J Epidemiol Community Health 1993; 7:469–474.

125. Kar SK, Mania J. Tropical pulmonary eosinophilia in an Orissa village. Natl Med J India 1993; 6:64–67.

126. Jiva TM, Israel RH, Poe RH. Tropical pulmonary eosinophilia masquerading as acute bronchial asthma. Respiration 1996; 63:55–58.

127. WHO Expert Committee on Filariasis. Fifth Report, Lymphatic Filariasis: the Disease and Its Control. WHO Technical Report Series 821. Geneva: World Health Organization, 1992:1–71.

128. Danaraj TJ, de Silva LS, Schacher JF. The serological diagnosis of eosinophilic lung (Tropical eosinophilia). Am J Trop Med Hyg 1959; 8:151–159.

129. Danaraj TJ, Schacher JF. I/D test with *Dirofilaria immitis* extract in eosinophilic lung (Tropical eosinophilia). Am J Trop Med Hyg 1959; 8:640–643.

130. Donohugh DC. Tropical eosinophilia: an etiology enquiry. N Engl J Med 1963; 269:1357–1364.

131. Saran R. Intradermal and gel diffusion tests with *Dirofilarial* antigens in tropical pulmonary eosinophilia. Indian J Chest Dis Allied Sci 1976; 18:90–94.

132. Meyers FM, Kunwennar W. Over hypereosinophilic en over een merkwaardiegen Vorm Van filariasis. Geneesk Tiddsdr Ned Ind 1939; 79:853–873.

133. Van Der Sar A, Hartz P. The syndrome tropical eosinophilia and microfilaria. Am J Trop Med Hyg 1945; 25:83–96.

134. Webb JKB, Job CK, Gault EW. Tropical eosinophilia. Demonstration of microfilariae in lung, liver and lymph nodes. Lancet 1960; 1:835–842.

135. Joshi VV, Udwadia FE, Gadgil RK. Etiology of tropical eosinophilia: a study of lung biopsies and review of published reports. Am J Trop Med Hyg 1969; 18:231–240.

136. Danaraj TJ, Pachecco G, Shanmugaratnam K, Beaver PC. The etiology and pathology of eosinophilic lung (Tropical eosinophilia). Am J Trop Med Hyg 1966; 15:183–189.

137. Jaggi OP, Sadana GS. Microfilariae detected in peripheral blood in tropical eosinophilia: a preliminary report. Indian J Chest Dis 1972; 14:197–201.

138. Buckley JJC. Tropical pulmonary eosinophilia in relation to filarial infections (*Wuchereria* sp.) of animals. Trans R Soc Trop Med Hyg 1958; 52:335–336.

139. Ganatra RD, Lewis RA. Diethylcarbamazine (Hetrazan) in tropical eosinophilia. India J Med Sci 1955; 9:672–681.

140. Baker SJ, Rajan KJ, Davadutta S. Treatment of tropical eosinophilia: a controlled trial. Lancet 1959; 2:144–147.

141. Ottesen EA, Neva FA, Paranjape RS, Tripathy SP, Thiruvengadam KV, Beaver MA. Specific allergic sensitization to filarial antigens in tropical pulmonary eosinophilia. Lancet 1979; 1:1158–1161.
142. Viswanathan R, Bagai RC, Saran R. Leukocyte adhesion phenomenon in pulmonary eosinophilia (Tropical eosinophilia). Am Rev Respir Dis 1973; 107:298–300.
143. Perera CS, Perera LM, de Silva C, Abeywickreme W, Dissanaike AS, Ismail MM. An eosinophilic granuloma containing an adult female *Wuchereria* in a patient with tropical pulmonary eosinophilia. Trans R Soc Trop Med Hyg 1992; 86:542.
144. Dreyer G, Noroes J, Rocha A, Addiss D. Detection of living adult *Wuchereria bancrofti* in a patient with tropical pulmonary eosinophilia. Braz J Med Biol Res 1996; 29:1005–1008.
145. Viswanathan R. Post mortem appearances in tropical eosinophilia. Indian Med Gaz 1947; 82:49–50.
146. Udwadia FE, Joshi VV. A study of tropical eosinophilia. Thorax 1964; 19: 548–554.
147. Udwadia FE. Tropical eosinophilia: a correlation of clinical, histopathologic and lung function studies. Dis Chest 1967; 52:531–538.
148. Manghani DK, Dastur DK, Udwadia FE. The lung in tropical eosinophilia compared to that in pulmonary hypertension. Fine structural basis in respiratory disability. Zentralbl Pathol 1992; 138:108–118.
149. Pinkston P, Vijayan VK, Nutman TB, Rom WN, O'Donnell KM, Cornelius MJ, Kumaraswami V, Ferrans VJ, Takemura T, Yenokida G, Thiruvengadam KV, Tripathy SP, Ottesen EA, Crystal RG. Acute tropical pulmonary eosinophilia: characterization of the lower respiratory tract inflammation and its response to therapy. J Clin Invest 1987; 80:216–225.
150. Gliech GJ, Loegering DA. Immunobiology of eosinophils. Ann Rev Immunol 1984; 2:429–459.
151. Ayers GH, Altman LC, Gleich G, Loegering DA, Baker CB. Eosinophil and eosinophil granule mediated pneumocyte injury. J Allergy Clin Immunol 1985; 76:595–604.
152. Weller PF. Immunobiology of eosinophils. N Engl J Med 1991; 324: 1110–1118.
153. Davis WB, Fells GA, Sun S, Gadek JE, Venet A, Crystal RG. Eosinophil-mediated lung injury of lung parenchymal cells and interstitial matrix. J Clin Invest 1984; 74:269–278.
154. O'Bryan L, Pinkston P, Kumaraswami V, Vijayan VK, Yenokida G, Rosenberg HF, Crystal RG, Ottesen EA, Nutman TB. Localized eosinophil degranulation mediates disease in tropical pulmonary eosinophilia. Infect Immun 2003; 71:1337–1342.
155. Nutman TB, Vijayan VK, Pinkston P, Steel R, Crystal RG, Ottesen EA. Tropical pulmonary eosinophilia: analysis of antifilarial antibody localized to the lung. J Infect Dis 1989; 160:1042–1050.
156. Nutman TB, Kumaraswami V. Regulation of the immune response in lymphatic filariasis: perspectives on acute and chronic infection with *Wuchereria bancrofti* in South India. Parasite Immunol 2001; 23:389–399.

157. King CL, Poindexter RW, Ragunathan J, Fleisher TA, Ottesen EA, Nutman TB. Frequency analysis of IgE secreting B-lymphocytes in individuals with normal or elevated serum IgE levels. J Immunol 1991; 146:1478–1483.

158. Lobos E, Ondo A, Ottesen EA, Nutman TB. Biochemical and immunologic characterization of a major IgE-inducing filarial antigen of *Brugia malayi* and implications for the pathogenesis of tropical pulmonary eosinophilia. J Immunol 1992; 149:3029–3034.

159. Lobos E, Zahn R, Weiss N, Nutman TB. A major allergen of lymphatic filarial nematodes is a parasite homolog of the gamma-glutaryl transpeptidase. Mol Med 1996; 2:712–724.

160. Lobos E, Nutman TB, Hothersall JS, Moncada S. Elevated immunoglobulin E against recombinant *Brugia malayi* gamma-glutaryl transpeptidase in patients with bancroftian filariasis: association with tropical pulmonary eosinophilia or putative immunity. Infect Immun 2003; 71:747–753.

161. Freedman DO, Nutman TB, Ottesen EA. Protective immunity in bancroftian filariasis: selective recognition of a 43-KD larval stage antigen by infection-free individuals in an endemic area. J Clin Invest 1989; 83:14–22.

162. Mehlotra RK, Hall L, Higgins AW, Dreshaj IA, Haxhiu MA, Kazura JW, Pearlman E. Interleukin-12 suppresses filarial-induced pulmonary eosinophilia deposition of major basic protein and airway hyperresponsiveness. Parasite Immunol 1998; 20:455–462.

163. Gounni AS, Spanel-Borowski K, Palacios M, Heusser C, Moncada S, Lobos E. Pulmonary inflammation induced by a recombinant *Brugia malayi* gamma-glutaryl transpeptidase homolog: involvement of human autoimmune process. Mol Med 2001; 7:344–354.

164. Ravindran M. Tropical eosinophilia presenting with neurological features. Br Med J 1979; 2:1262.

165. Cooray JH, Ismail MM. Re-examination of the diagnostic criteria of tropical pulmonary eosinophilia. Respir Med 1999; 93:655–659.

166. Saran R, Sanyal RK. Diurnal variations in eosinophil count and vacuolization of eosinophil cells in tropical eosinophilia. Indian J Chest Dis 1973; 15:209–213.

167. Bhaskaran CS, Reddy MK. Cytoplasmic vacuoles of eosinophils in tropical eosinophilia. Indian J Chest Dis Allied Sci 1979; 21:31–34.

168. Saran R. Cytoplasmic vacuoles of eosinophils in tropical pulmonary eosinophilia. Am Rev Respir Dis 1973; 108:1283–1285.

169. Spry CJF. Alterations in blood eosinophil morphology, binding capacity for complexed IgG and kinetics in patients with tropical (filarial) eosinophilia. Parasite Immunol 1980; 3:1–11.

170. Kamat SR, Pimparkar SD, Store SD, Warrier NVU, Fakey YC. Study of clinical, radiological and pulmonary function patterns and response to treatment in pulmonary eosinophilia. Indian J Chest Dis 1970; 12:91–100.

171. Basu SP. X-ray appearance in lung fields in tropical eosinophilia. Indian Med Gaz 1954; 89:212–217.

172. Islam N. Radiological features of tropical eosinophilia. J Trop Med Hyg 1965; 68:117–180.

173. Khoo FY, Danaraj TJ. The roentgenographic appearances of eosinophilic lung. Am J Roentgenol 1960; 86:251–259.
174. Vijayan VK. Tropical Eosinophilia: Bronchoalveolar Lavage and Pulmonary Pathophysiology in Relation to Treatment. Ph.D. dissertation, University of Madras, Madras, India, 1988.
175. Vijayan VK, Kuppurao KV, Sankaran K, Venkatesan P, Prabhakar R. Tropical eosinophilia: clinical and physiological response to diethylcarbamazine. Respir Med 1991; 85:17–20.
176. Sandhu M, Mukhopadhyay S, Sharma SK. Tropical pulmonary eosinophilia: a comparative evaluation of plain chest radiography and computed tomography. Austral Radiol 1996; 40:32–37.
177. Menon NK. Tropical eosinophilia: atypical manifestations. Indian J Chest Dis 1963; 5:231–236.
178. Islam N, Haq N. Eosinophilic lung abscess. Br Med J 1962; 1:1810–1811.
179. Raj B, Gupta KB, Chawla RK, Janmeja AJ. Tropical pulmonary eosinophilia presenting as pneumonic consolidation. Indian J Chest Dis Allied Sci 1987; 29:175–177.
180. Purohit SD, Jain SK, Sharma TN, Agnihotri S, Talwar KL. Pulmonary eosinophilia presenting with bilateral pleural effusion and consolidation. Indian J Chest Dis Allied Sci 1984; 26:126–129.
181. Boornazian JS, Fagan MJ. Tropical pulmonary eosinophilia associated with pleural effusion. Am J Trop Med Hyg 1985; 34:473–475.
182. Oyamada Y, Funae O, Kamegaya Y, Soejima K, Nakamura M, Mori S, Yamaguchi K, Kanazawa M, Okusawa E, Yamasawa F. A case of tropical eosinophilia with pleural effusion. Nihon Kyobu Shikkan Gakkai Zasshi 1995; 33:451–455.
183. Kamat SR, Warrier NVU, Store SD, Karandikar KN, D'sa E, Hoskote VR. Clinical studies in pulmonary eosinophilia. I. Comparative study of response to diethylcarbamazine and corticosteroid drugs. Indian J Chest Dis Allied Sci 1976; 18:221–232.
184. Azad Khan AK, Patra RWJ, Banu SA, Rabee ME. Spirometry in tropical pulmonary eosinophilia. Br J Dis Chest 1970; 64:107–109.
185. Nesarajah MS. Pulmonary function in tropical eosinophilia. Thorax 1972; 27:185–187.
186. Ray D. Lung function in tropical eosinophilia. Indian J Chest Dis 1974; 16: 368–373.
187. Abdulla AK, Siddique MA, Qureshi MA, Khan A. Ventilatory impairment in tropical eosinophilia and its comparison with asthma. Indian J Chest Dis Allied Sci 1977; 19:82–87.
188. Sharma SK, Pande JN, Khilnani GC, Verma K, Khanna M. Immunologic and pulmonary function abnormalities in tropical pulmonary eosinophilia. Indian J Med Res 1995; 101:98–102.
189. Vijayan VK, Kuppurao KV, Sankaran K, Venkatesan P, Prabhakar R. Diffusing capacity in acute untreated tropical eosinophilia. Indian J Chest Dis Allied Sci 1988; 30:71–77.
190. Vijayan VK, Kuppurao KV, Sankaran K, Venkatesan P, Prabhakar R. Pulmonary membrane diffusing capacity and capillary blood volume in tropical eosinophilia. Chest 1990; 97:1386–1389.

191. Kuppurao KV, Vijayan VK, Venkatesan P, Sankaran K. Maximal expiratory flow rates in tropical eosinophilia. Biomedicine 1992; 12:59–62.
192. Kuppurao KV, Vijayan VK, Venkatesan P, Sankaran K. Effect of treatment on maximal expiratory flow rates in tropical eosinophilia. Ceylon Med J 1993; 38:78–80.
193. Vijayan VK, Sankaran K, Venkatesan P, Kuppurao KV. Correlation of lower respiratory tract inflammation with changes in lung function and chest roentgenograms in patients with untreated tropical pulmonary eosinophilia. Singapore Med J 1991; 32:122–125.
194. Vijayan VK, Kuppurao KV, Venkatesan P, Prabhakar R. Arterial hypoxemia in acute tropical pulmonary eosinophilia. Lung India 1988; 6:183–185.
195. Mathur KS, Nagarath SP, Kishore B, Rastogi SP. A study of ventilatory function and arterial blood gases in tropical eosinophilia. Indian J Chest Dis 1969; 11:1–4.
196. Ray D. Relapsing tropical eosinophilia. Indian J Chest Dis Allied Sci 1977; 19:65–71.
197. Ray D. Arterial desaturation in tropical eosinophilia. Indian J Chest Dis Allied Sci 1984; 26:34–37.
198. Ray D, Jayachandran CA. Ventilation-perfusion scintiscanning in tropical pulmonary eosinophilia. Chest 1993; 104:497–500.
199. Vakil RJ. Cardiovascular involvement in tropical eosinophilia. Br Heart J 1961; 23:578–586.
200. Johny KV, Ananthachari MD. Cardiovascular changes in tropical eosinophilia. Am Heart J 1965; 69:591–598.
201. Singh M, Sharma SK, Patney RM. Tropical eosinophilic pericarditis. Indian Heart J 1974; 26:261–263.
202. D'Arbera VSE. Tropical eosinophilia: some atypical cases of clinical interest. Med J Malaya 1958; 12:559–562.
203. Quah BS, Anuar AK, Rowani MR, Pennie RA. Cor pulmonale: an unusual presentation of tropical eosinophilia. Ann Trop Pediatr 1997; 17:17–18.
204. Kedarnath, Agarwal SN. An unusual case of tropical eosinophilia. J Trop Med Hyg 1963; 66:175–177.
205. Spry CJF. Lung diseases associated with eosinophils. In: Kay AB, Goetzl EJ, eds. Current Perspective in Allergy. Edinburgh: Churchill Livingstone, 1982: 67–77.
206. Rocha A, Dreyer G, Poindexter RW, Ottesen EA. Syndrome resembling tropical eosinophilia but of non-filarial etiology: serological findings with filarial antigens. Trans R Soc Trop Med Hyg 1995; 89:573–575.
207. Alves LC, Brayner FA, Silva LF, Pimentel RC, Rocha A, Peixoto CA. Immunocytochemical localization of antigens recognized by tropical pulmonary eosinophilia and individuals with intestinal helminth antisera in microfilaria of *Wuchereria bancrofti*. J Submicrose Cytol Pathol 2002; 34:211–216.
208. Vijayan VK. Allergic bronchopulmonary helminthiasis (ABPH). Lung India 1991; 9:145–148.
209. Vijayan VK, Reetha AM, Jawahar MS, Sankaran K, Prabhakar R. Pulmonary eosinophilia in pulmonary tuberculosis. Chest 1992; 101:1708–1709.

210. Danaraj TJ. The treatment of eosinophilic lung (tropical eosinophilia) with diethylcarbamazine. Q J Med 1958; 27:243–263.
211. Joint WPRO/SEARO Working Group on Brugian Filariasis. Final Report. Manila: WHO, 1979:1–47.
212. Vijayan VK, Sankaran K, Venkatesan P, Prabhakar R. Effect of diethylcarbamazine on the alveolitis of tropical eosinophilia. Respiration 1991; 58: 255–259.
213. Rom WN, Vijayan VK, Cornelius MJ, Kumaraswami V, Prabhakar R, Ottesen EA, Crystal RG. Persistent lower respiratory tract inflammation associated with interstitial lung disease in patients with tropical pulmonary eosinophilia following treatment with diethylcarbamazine. Am Rev Respir Dis 1990; 142:1088–1092.
214. Vijayan VK. Role of steroids in chronic tropical eosinophilia: a bronchoalveolar lavage study [abstr]. Indian J Chest Dis Allied Sci 1987; 29:vii.
215. Vijayan VK. Changes in respiratory function and lung inflammation in patients with tropical eosinophilia one year after treatment with diethylcarbamazine. Indian J Clin Pharmacol Therap 1997; 15:5–7.
216. Sanjivi KS, Thiruvengadam KV, Friedman HC. Tropical eosinophilia treated with cortisone. Dis Chest 1955; 28:88–90.
217. Ottesen EA, Vijayasekaran V, Kumaraswami V, Perumal Pillai SV, Sadanandam A, Frederik S, Prabhakar R, Tripathy SP. A controlled trial of ivermectin and diethylcarbamazine in lymphatic filariasis. N Engl J Med 1990; 322: 1113–1117.
218. Vijayan VK. Ivermectin in the treatment of tropical eosinophilia [abstr]. Chest 2000; 118(suppl 4):247s.
219. Ottesen EA. Major progress toward eliminating lymphatic filariasis. N Engl J Med 2002; 347:1885–1886.
220. Bockarie MJ, Tisch DJ, Kasteus W, Alexander ND, Dimber Z, Bockarie F, Ibam E, Alpres MP, Kazura JW. Mass treatment to eliminate filariasis in Papua New Guinea. N Engl J Med 2002; 347:1841–1848.
221. Beaver PC, Syncler CH, Carrera GM. Chronic eosinophilia due to visceral larva migrans. Pediatrics 1952; 9:7–19.
222. Magnaval JF, Glickman LT, Dorchies P, Morassin B. Highlights of human toxocariasis. Korean J Parasitol 2001; 39:1–11.
223. Glickman LT, Schantz PM. Epidemiology and pathogenesis of zoonotic toxocariasis. Epidemiol Rev 1981; 3:230–250.
224. Thompson DE, Bundy DAP, Cooper ES, Schantz PM. Epidemiological characteristics of *Toxocara canis* infection of children in a Caribbean community. Bull World Health Org 1986; 64:283–290.
225. Del Prete GF, De Carli M, Mastromauro C, Biagiotti R, Macchia D, Falagiani P, Ricci M, Romagnani S. Purified protein derivative of *Mycobacterium tuberculosis* and excretory-secretary antigen(s) of *Toxocara canis* expand in vitro human T cells with stable and opposite (type 1 T helper or type 2 T helper) profile of cytokine production. J Clin Invest 1991; 88: 346–350.
226. Blaxter ML, Page AP, Rudin W, Maizels RM. Nematode surface coats: actively evading immunity. Parasitol Today 1992; 8:243–247.

227. Badley JE, Grieve RB, Rockey JH, Glickman LT. Immuno-mediated adherence of eosinophils to *Toxocara canis* infective larvae. The role of excretory-secretary antigens. Parasite Immunol 1987; 9:133–143.
228. Windelborg NB, Lind P, Hansen B, Nansen P, Schiotz PO. Larval exoantigens from ascarid nematodes are potent inducers of histamine release from human blood basophils. Clin Exp Allergy 1991; 21:725–732.
229. Smith HV, Kusel JR, Girdwood RW. The productions by human A and B blood group like substances by in vitro maintained second stage *Toxocara canis* larvae. Their presence on the outer larval surfaces and in their excretions/secretions. Clin Exp Immunol 1983; 54:625–633.
230. Feldman GJ, Parker HW. Visceral larva migrans associated with the hypereosinophilic syndrome and the onset of severe asthma. Ann Intern Med 1992; 116:838–840.
231. Roig J, Romeu J, Riera C, Texido A, Domingo C, Morera J. Acute eosinophilic pneumonia due to toxocariasis with broncho alveolar lavage findings. Chest 1992; 102:294–296.
232. Bartelink AK, Kortbeek LM, Huidekoper HJ, Meulenubelt J, Van Knapen F. Acute respiratory failure due to toxocara infections. Lancet 1993; 342:1234.
233. Glickman LT, Magnaval JF, Domanski LM, Shofer FS, Lauria SS, Gottstein B, Brochier B. Visceral larva migrans in French adults: a new disease syndrome? Am J Epidemiol 1987; 125:1019–1034.
234. Nathwani D, Laing RB, Currie PF. "Covert" toxocariasis-a cause of recurrent abdominal pain in childhood. Br J Clin Pract 1992; 46:271.
235. Spieser F, Gottstein B. A collaborative study on larval excretory/secretary antigens of *Toxocara canis* for immunodiagnosis of human toxocariasis with ELISA. Acta Trop 1984; 41:361–372.
236. Magnaval JF, Fabre R, Maurieres P, Charlet JP, De Larrard B. Evaluation of an immunenzymatic assay detecting specific anti-*Toxocara* immunoglobulin E for diagnosis and post treatment follow up of human toxocariasis. J Clin Microbiol 1992; 30:2269–2274.
237. Magnaval JF, Fabre R, Maurieres P, Charlet JP, De Larrard B. Application of the Western-blotting procedure for the immunodiagnosis of human toxocariasis. Parasitol Res 1991; 77:697–702.
238. Rasmussen LN, Dirdal M, Birkeback NH. "Covert toxocariasis" in a child treated with low-dose diethylcarbamazine. Acta Paediatr 1993; 82:116–118.
239. Magnaval JF. Comparative efficacy of diethylcarbamazine and mebendazole for the treatment of human toxocariasis. Parasitology 1995; 110:529–533.
240. Sturchler D, Schubarth P, Gualzata M, Gottstein B, Orettli A. Thiabendazole vs. albendazole in treatment of toxocariasis: a clinical trial. Ann Trop Med Parasitol 1989; 83:473–478.
241. Pozio E, La Rosa G, Murrell KD, Lichtenfels JR. Taxonomic revision of the genus *Trichinella*. J Parasitol 1992; 78:654–659.
242. Despommier DD. How does *Trichinella spiralis* make itself at home? Parasitol Today 1998; 14:318–323.
243. Dessein AJ, Parker WL, James SL, David JR. IgE antibody and resistance to infection. I. Selective suppression of the IgE antibody response in rats diminishes

the resistance and the eosinophil response in Trichinella spiralis infections. J Exp Med 1981; 153:423–436.

244. Capo V, Despommier DD. Clinical aspects of infections with *Trichinella* spp. Clin Microbiol Rev 1996; 9:47–54.

245. Sheldon JH. An outbreak of trichinosis near Wolverhampton. Lancet 1941; 1:203–205.

246. Bruschi F, Murrell K. Trichinellosis, Guerrant RL, Walker DH, Weller PF, eds. Tropical Infectious Diseases: Principles, Pathogens and Practice. Vol. 2, Elsevier Science Health Science Div. Philadelphia: Churchill Livingstone, 1999:917–925.

247. Engvall E, Ljungstrom I. Detection of human antibodies to *Trichinella spiralis* by enzyme-linked immunosorbent assay (ELISA). Acta Pathol Microbiol Scand 1975; 83:231–237.

248. Schwartz E. Pulmonary schistosomiasis. Clin Chest Med 2002; 23:433–443.

249. Schwartz E, Rozenman J, Perelman N. Pulmonary manifestations of early *Schistosoma* infection in nonimmune travelers. Am J Med 2000; 109:718–722.

250. Walt F. The Katayama syndrome. S Afr Med J 1954; 28:89–93.

251. Doherty JF, Moody AH, Wright SG. Katayama fever; an acute manifestation of schistosomiasis. Br Med J 1996; 313:1071–1072.

252. Morris W, Knauer M. Cardiopulmonary manifestations of schistosomiasis. Semin Respir Infect 1997; 12:159–170.

253. Nakamura-Uchiyama F, Mukae H, Nawa Y. Paragonimiasis: a Japanese perspective. Clin Chest Med 2002; 23:409–420.

254. Blair D, Xu ZB, Agatsuma T. Paragonimiasis and the genus paragonimus. Adv Parasitol 1999; 42:113–222.

255. King CH. Pulmonary flukes. In: Mahamoud AAF, ed. Lung Biology in Health and Disease: Parasitic Lung Disease. New York: Marcel Dekker, 1997: 157–169.

256. Xu ZB. Studies on clinical manifestations, diagnosis and control of paragonimiasis in China. Southeast Asian J Trop Med Public Health 1991; 22(suppl 1): 345–348.

257. Suwanik R, Harinasuta C. Pulmonary paragonimiasis: an evaluation of roentgen findings in 38 positive sputum patients in an endemic area in Thailand. Am J Roentgenol 1959; 81:236–244.

258. Mukae H, Taniguchi H, Matsumoto N, Liboshi H, Ashitani J, Matsukura S, Nawa Y. Clinicoradiologic features of pleuropulmonary *Paragonimus westermani* on Kyushu Island, Japan. Chest 2001; 120:514–520.

259. Velez ID, Ortega JE, Velasquez LE. Paragonimiasis: a review from Columbia. Clin Chest Med 2002; 23:421–431.

260. Gottstein B, Reichen J. Hydatid lung disease (echinococcosis/hydatidosis). Clin Chest Med 2002; 23:397–408.

261. Blanton R. Pulmonary echinococcosis. In: Mahmoud AAF, ed. Lung Biology in Health and Disease: Parasitic Lung Diseases. New York: Marcel Dekker, 1997:171–189.

262. Dannenbergh AM Jr. Pathogenesis of tuberculosis. In: Fishman AP, ed. Pulmonary Diseases and Disorders. New York: McGraw-Hill Book Co., 1980:1264–1281.

263. Ray D, Abel R. Hypereosinophilia in association with pulmonary tuberculosis in a rural population in South India. Indian J Med Res 1994; 100:219–222.

264. Muller GL. Clinical Significance of the Blood in Tuberculosis. New York: Commonwealth Fund, 1943:95–121.

265. Schwarz E. Die Lehre von der allgemeinen und ortlichen eosinophilie. Ergeb Allg Pathol Anat 1914; 7:137–187.

266. Wright JL, Pare PD, Hammond M, Donevan RE. Eosinophilic pneumonia and atypical mycobacterial infections. Am Rev Respir Dis 1983; 127:497–499.

267. Cooper AM, Dalton DK, Stewart TA, Griffin JP, Russel DG, Orme IM. Disseminated tuberculosis in interferon γ gene-disrupted mice. J Exp Med 1993; 178:2243–2247.

268. Flynn JL, Chan JC, Triebold KJ, Dalton DK, Sterwart TA, Bloom BR. An essential role for interferon γ in resistance to *Mycobacterium tuberculosis* infection. J Exp Med 1993; 178:2249–2254.

269. Erb K, Kirman J, Delahunt B, LeGros G. Infection of mice with *M. bovis* BCG induces both Th$_1$ and Th$_2$ immune responses in the absence of interferon-γ signaling. Eur Cytokine Netwroks 1999; 10:147–153.

270. Murray PJ, Young RA, Daley GQ. Hematopoietic remodeling in interferon-γ-deficient mice infected with mycobacteria. Blood 1998; 91:2914–2924.

271. Kirman J, Zakaria Z, McCoy K, Delahunt B, LeGros G. Role of eosinophils in the pathogenesis of *Mycobacterium bovis* BCG infection in gamma interferon receptor-deficient mice. Infect Immun 2000; 68:2976–2978.

272. Corbel M. Brucellosis: an overview. Emerg Inf Dis 1997; 3:213–221.

273. Pappas G, Bosilkovski M, Akritidis N, Mastora M, Krteva L, Tsianos E. Brucellosis and the respiratory system. Clin Inf Dis 2003; 37:e95–e99.

274. Elsom KA, Ingelfinger FJ. Eosinophilia and pneumonitis in chronic brucellosis: a report of two cases. Ann Intern Med 1942; 16:995–1002.

275. Drutz DR, Catanzaro A. Coccidiodomycosis: part 2. Am Rev Respir Dis 1978; 118:727–771.

276. Lombard CM, Tazelaar HD, Krasne DL. Pulmonary eosinophilia in coccidiodal infections. Chest 1987; 91:734–736.

277. Lonky SA, Catanzaro A, Moser KM, Einstein A. Acute coccidiodal pleural effusions. Am Rev Respir Dis 1976; 114:681–688.

278. Starr JC, Che H, Montgomery J. Cryptococcal pneumonia simulating chronic eosinophilic pneumonia. South Med J 1995; 68:345–346.

279. Greenberger PA. Allergic bronchopulmonary aspergillosis and fungoses. Clin Chest Med 1988; 9:599–608.

280. Honson KFW, Moon AJ, Plummer NS. Bronchopulmonary aspergillosis: a review and report of eight cases. Thorax 1952; 7:317–333.

281. Lee TM, Greenberger PA, Oh S, Patterson R, Roberts M, Liotta JL. Allergic bronchopulmonary asperginosis: case report and suggested diagnostic criteria. J Allergy Clin Immunol 1987; 80:816–820.

282. McAleer R, Kroenert DB, Elder JL, Froudist JH. Allergic bronchopulmonary disease caused by *Curvularia lunata* and *Dreschslera hawaiiensis*. Thorax 1981; 36:338–344.

283. Benatar SR, Allan B, Hewitson RP, Don RA. Allergic bronchopulmonary stemphyliosis. Thorax 1980; 35:515–518.

284. Miller MA, Greenberger PA, Amerian R, Toogood JH, Noskin GA, Roberts M, Patterson R. Allergic bronchopulmonary mycosis caused by *Pseudallescheria boydii*. Am Rev Respir Dis 1993; 148:810–812.
285. Backman KS, Roberts M, Patterson R. Allergic bronchopulmonary mycosis caused by *Fusarium vasinfectum*. Am J Respir Crit Care Med 1995; 152: 1379–1381.
286. Hendrick DJ, Ellithorpe DB, Lyon F, Hattier P, Salvaggio JE. Allergic bronchopulmonary helminthosporiasis. Am Rev Respir Dis 1982; 126: 935–938.

10

Immunopathogenesis of Malaria

S. K. JINDAL

Department of Pulmonary Medicine, Postgraduate Institute of Medical
   Education and Research,
Chandigarh, India

Malaria continues to pose a threat to human life. It is an important cause of morbidity and mortality. Malaria accounts for over 1 million deaths. Since only seriously affected individuals are likely to die, the total magnitude of those infected runs into several millions. Different estimates of the number of infected individuals vary from 150 to about 300–500 million. The more severe infections, especially with *Plasmodium falciparum*, may involve multiple organs besides the liver and the hematopoietic system. The occurrence of the lung complications and the frequent requirement for assisted ventilation for the critically sick patients has aroused great interest in the disease in pulmonary literature.

There is a wide clinical and pathological spectrum of malaria varying from that of mild disease to fatal illness. These differences are at least partly attributable to the immune status of an individual. Specific immunity may develop in some individuals suffering from repeated parasitic exposures; others without any history of previous exposure may demonstrate nonspecific immunity. Development of resistance of the parasite to antimalarial drugs and comorbidities associated with infection are other important issues, which determine the disease outcome. It is therefore, important to understand the basic immunology and pathogenesis of malaria.

There is an enormous body of data which have appeared in the published literature on the immunopathology of malaria. Some of these data have been analyzed in several elegant reviews in the last few years (1–5). This information has greatly helped to define the disease mechanisms, and plan its management with the development of newer antimalarial drugs. It is even more crucial for the advent of an effective antimalarial vaccine, which remains the obvious goal of all immunological research in malaria.

I. The Malaria Parasite

There are four species of the malaria parasite (i.e. the *Plasmodium*), which can cause infection in humans. Although *P. vivax* is the most common form, it is the *P. falciparum*, which is the most important in view of its life-threatening complications and involvement of other organs including the brain and the lungs.

The malarial parasite cycles through the hepatocytes and the erythrocytes of the human host and, thereafter, the gastrointestinal system of the carrier mosquito. It has got a sexual and an asexual phase, which occur in the mosquito and two asexual phases, which occur in human liver cells and red blood cells, respectively. Each phase ends with the production of an invasive form, which enters the host cells to establish the next phase. Through the entire journey, it faces several physical, biochemical, immunological, and nonimmunological barriers. It is the fight between the parasite's selective effects and the host's defenses, which determine the outcome.

Ultrastructurally, the plasmodium contains various organelles, which perform one or more specialized metabolic functions. *P. falciparum* is genetically more closely related to malaria parasites from rats and birds than to other human *Plasmodium* species (6). It has a nucleus, which contains about 0.02 pg of DNA corresponding to a total of approximately 10 million base pairs, which is about 10 times more than the genome of a typical bacterium. More than 80% of the bases in *P. falciparum* DNA are constituted by the adenine–thymine base pair (A+T), which is the highest recorded for a living organism. This is responsible for a more restricted genetic code of the organism.

A large number of antigen proteins are synthesized and released during the life cycle of the parasite. Many of these antigens have polymorphic structure, therefore causing a rapid variation between different strains and isolates of *P. falciparum*. It is because of this great clonal antigenic variation that a diverse repertoire of antibodies are required to achieve an effective immunity against the parasite (7).

II. Pathogenesis of Malaria

P. falciparum possesses the ability to invade red blood cells of all ages and capacity to adhere to vascular endothelium. These two features of invasion and adherence in disease pathogenesis are primarily responsible for most of the serious problems attributed to falciparum malaria (2).

A. Erythrocyte Invasion

It is the invasive merozoite form of the parasite, which enters the erythrocytes. There is an initial invagination of the red cell membrane caused by the pushing of the parasite adhered to the surface receptors, eventually forming a vacuole and resulting in invasion after multiple receptor ligand interactions (8). A number of surface proteins on the merozoite are involved in this process. *P. falciparum* erythrocyte membrane protein 1 (PfEMP1) is an important antigen involved in parasitic binding (9). Surface proteins 2, 3, and 4 are also involved (10).

Erythrocytic invasion results in parasitemia, which induces severe inflammatory response. Hyperparasitemia is generally responsible for the severity of symptoms although there is no direct correlation. Both the presence of a severe disease with low parasite counts as well as asymptomatic children with hyperparasitemia are known to occur.

B. Adhesion Mechanisms

Adhesive mechanisms between the infected erythrocytes and the cells play an important role in disease virulence. The various adhesive interactions include cyto adhesion, rosetting, autoagglutination, clumping, etc.

Cyto Adhesion

The infected erythrocytes (IE) have a great propensity to adhere to the vascular endothelium of various organs. This is attributed to the development of electron dense exuberances (knobs) on the surfaces of IEs containing histidine-rich proteins such as thrombospondin, intracellular adhesion molecule 1 (ICAM1), and CD36. The sequestrated IEs cause mechanical blockade and ischemic injury to the organ. The local release of inflammatory mediators is responsible for several metabolic derangements (11).

Sequestration may occur in brain, kidneys, lungs, heart, skeletal muscles, and other organs. Although sequestration generally involves the asexual forms, the gametocytes are also reported to show cytoadherence (12). This is an important factor for maturation of gametocytes in the human host before they are transmitted to the mosquito vector. Both the sequestration and the subsequent tissue injury would finally result in clinical manifestations of organ dysfunction. The various mediators that are liberated include both proinflammatory and anti-inflammatory cytokines (13). The inflammatory cytokines such as tumor necrosis factor-α (TNF-α), interleukin-1 (IL-1), interleukin-6 (IL-6), and interferon-γ (IFN-γ) play an important role in causing disease severity (14,15). High levels of circulating cytokines have been shown in severe cases of malaria in several reports. TNF-α has been linked to the occurrence of cerebral malaria. But there is recent evidence, which supports the overproduction of lymphotoxin-α (LT-α) rather than TNF-α, which causes this problem (16). IFN-γ is also linked to the onset of cerebral malaria. IFN-γ is also able to upregulate TNF-α production and promote the quinolinic acid pathway of tryptophan metabolism. Quinolinic acid is neurotoxic and contributes to the development of cerebral malaria.

The inflammatory cytokines, especially TNF, induce nitric oxide (NO) generation from vascular endothelium (17). NO crosses the blood brain barrier to produce neurotoxicity, and also exerts direct toxic effects on the parasite through oxidative stress (18).

Rosetting

The infected erythrocytes bind two or more uninfected erythrocytes resulting in rosette formation. This phenomenon is seen mostly with the sequestered parasites in the interal organs. Rosetting is most common with *P. falciparum* but can occur with *P. vivax*, *P. malariae*, and *P. ovale* (19).

The correlation of rosette formation with disease severity is controversial. It is supported in a few while disputed in other studies. It is possible that rosetting promotes progressive erythrocyte invasion and a higher degree of parasitemia. On the other hand, rosetting may help the IEs, who use the uninfected erythrocytes as "shields" to avoid recognition by the immune system (20).

Agglutination and Other Adhesions

IEs have a tendency to form large agglutinates by adhering to other IEs (autoagglutination) or to noninfected erythrocytes (giant rosetting) (21). Similarly, the IEs can adhere together with the help of thrombocytes, which act as "bridges" (clumping) (22). All three adhesive phenomena have potential to cause ischemic and chemical insults.

IEs may also adhere to the cells of immune system such as the monocytes, macrophages, and myeloid dendritic cells (23). This may impair the function of these cells and cause a relative immune deficiency state.

III. Immunopathogenesis of Malarial Acute Lung Injury: Increased Vascular Permeability

While vascular adhesion and sequestration are important in cerebral malaria, it is the increased permeability that plays a major role in the development of pulmonary edema (24–27). This complication is at considerable variance from several other manifestations of severe malaria.

Some of the important mediators, which have been believed to be involved in causing increased permeability, are the histamine, kinins, complement activation, TNF, and the oxygen free radicals (26,27). Elevated levels of histamine, kallikrein, and bradykinin were found in animal and human subjects with malaria. Their exact role in contributing to pulmonary edema is not clear.

Endothelial damage caused by the oxygen free radicals and other mediators such as TNF increases permeability. They may also cause neutrophil activation, hemolysis, and dyserythropoiesis.

Complement activation and immune complex formation have been shown to occur in human disease but no vasculitis is seen. Immune complexes of IgM, C3, C4, and malarial antigen have been shown in the kidneys and the lungs in a mouse model (28). Similar phenomena could occur in human pulmonary edema and disseminated intravascular coagulation (DIC).

Elevated levels of endotoxin seen in human malaria are possibly ascribable to coexistent bacterial infection since the parasite itself does not contain it (26,28). Endotoxin may cause hemolysis-related endothelial injury, release of TNF, and occurrence of DIC (29).

The microvascular damage in the lungs is responsible for acute lung injury (ALI) or acute respiratory distress syndrome (ARDS). The changes include a severe congestion of pulmonary capillaries, thickened alveolar septae, diffuse pulmonary edema, focal hyaline membrane formation, and scattered intra-alveolar hemorrhages (30). The illness is caused exclusively by the intraerythrocyte asexual forms of the parasite. Besides the sequestered IEs and release of inflammatory mediators, ALI is also contributed by other phenomena happening simultaneously, i.e. DIC, endotoxins from bacterial sepsis, cardiac dysfunction and reduced oxygen uptake. Presence of other risk factors such as an immunocompromised state, pregnancy, extremes of age, acidosis, and thrombocytopenia may also promote the occurrence of pulmonary edema.

IV. Immunity to Malaria

Not all individuals infected with the parasite develop severe malaria. This is attributed to the presence of immunity, which may be either specific, i.e., developed after repeated exposures to the parasite or nonspecific immunity due to the presence of innate or acquired factors.

A. Specific Immunity

Exposures to the parasitic infection in endemic areas are likely to occur right from infancy. In fact, there is evidence to suggest the presence of immunity in children born to immune mothers. The child is relatively protected for about 3 months after birth (31). Both the immunological and epidemiological data suggest that the primary malarial infection in an infant induces low levels of IFN-γ and TNF-α in an innate way and also primes the antigen-specific T cells. The primary infection may cause a mild disease with minimal clinical symptoms, but the parasites are cleared very soon through opsonization by maternal antibodies and cytokine-mediated parasite killing. The normal physiological barriers including the fetal hemoglobin and the dietary deficiencies also act against the parasite (32). The child may become parasitemic and develop more symptoms if the infection is heavy. But the disease is never as severe as in adults. It is commonly believed that a very young infant behaves like an immune adult.

On reinfection after the first few months, the children may also develop a more severe infection but remain relatively healthy. There is an increased production of IFN by the malaria-primed T cells, and upregulation of TNF-α and/or LT leading to cerebral malaria. The severity of attacks decline in spite of the high parasite counts after the fourth year (33).

Repeated infections induce effective antiparasitic immunity. The fall in antigen concentrations as well as the dampening of proinflammatory cytokine cascade causes switching of the Th1 (IFN-γ producing) to a regular T-cell phenotype producing IL-10 and TGF-β cytokines. This enables the clinically immune individuals to clear infection without the risk of overproduction of harmful inflammatory mediators. But complete immunity to parasitization is probably never achieved.

There is no protective immunity in adults of a malaria-free region who travel to an endemic area. They are likely to suffer from severe disease from the presence of cross-reactively primed T cells due to their exposures to cross-reacting microbes such as *Toxoplasma gondii*, tetanus toxoid, adenovirus, mycobacteria, streptococcal, and fungal antigens (34,35). The cross-reactively primed $\alpha\beta$T cells make significant amounts of IFN-γ but do not offer any protection. In fact, they further promote the disease pathology. Such exposures are fewer in children who have lower levels of cross-reactively primed cells. The disease therefore is less severe in nonimmune children exposed to the parasite in endemic areas. It is the downregulation of nonprotective cross-reactive T-cell response, which is important in clinical immunity.

B. Nonspecific Immunity

Nonspecific immunity is the resistance to *Plasmodium* infection in previously nonexposed individuals. There are several factors, which contribute to the presence of this nonspecific immunity. This could be either due to innate, i.e., genetic or acquired, factors.

Innate Immunity

Gene polymorphism and immune responses are known to determine the occurrence, severity, and outcome of malaria. There is evidence to say that the cytokine profile in the first few hours of malaria infection predicts the course and final outcome (36,37). There is therefore, a likelihood of a pre-existing, cross-reactively primed effector memory T cell or an innate immune system.

The rapid response in IFN-γ and TNF-α, which occurs following *P. falciparum* infection, is derived principally from NK cells (38). Subsequently, $\gamma\delta$T cells and eventually $\alpha\beta$T cells also begin to secrete IFN-γ. But there is considerable variation in NK-mediated IFN-γ production. It is not clear whether a strong and early IFN-γ response may correlate with avoidance of hyperparasitemia or conversely with an excessive inflammatory reaction contributing to disease pathology. But the existing data suggest that NK cells are necessary to "kick start" the inflammatory response (39). This activation of NK cells by *P. falciparum* is dependent upon IL-12 and IL-18 derived from monocyte macrophages or dendritic cells (38).

Innate resistance to malaria also depends upon the "internal environment" faced by the parasite in the red blood cell. Some of the genetic differences, which determine this resistance, are relatively well characterized. Only those genetic variants of red cells, which have achieved a polymorphic status, are important in malaria.

Polymorphic status can be described when the alternative versions of the same gene coexist in a population at high frequencies, not attributable to the repeated occurrence of the mutation producing the variant gene. It is believed that the carriers of the genes (heterozygotes) have an advantage against malaria that balances the disadvantage of the homozygote state—"the malaria hypothesis" (40). There are several red cells polymorphisms, which support a malaria hypothesis (40). Most of the geographic differences in malarial epidemiology have been explained on the basis of these polymorphisms.

Hemoglobin Variants

Red cell polymorphic conditions, which affect the structure of betaglobin chain of hemoglobin include HbS, HbC, and HbE. The frequency of HbS is high in areas with high malarial endemicity. Individuals who are heterozygotes for HbS (AS) have a strong protection against the clinical effects of malaria (41). There is no protection, however, against the susceptibility to infection.

Similarly HbC and HbE have protective effects. Possibly, both the heterozygotes and the homozygotes show the reduced parasitic growth although the mechanisms are not clear.

Miscellaneous Red Cell Polymorphisms

Thalassemias are characterized by a reduced rate of production of one or more of the globin chains of Hb. There is good evidence in favor of a reduced parasite growth in both α and β thalassemia. The mechanisms of protection are not known.

Several other red cell polymorphic states, which resist malaria, include the deficiency of glucose-6 phosphate dehydrogenase (G6PD) enzyme, Duffy-negative blood group system, and red cell cytoskeletal abnormalities. G6PD is a χ-chromosome-linked enzyme. Protection against malaria is present in heterozygote, both male and female, individuals. Similarly, red cells from Duffy-negative individuals are resistant to infection with *P. vivax*, possibly preventing their entry into the red cells. Hereditary ovalocytosis, an autosomal dominant condition, is also highly resistant to invasion by both *P. vivax* and *P. falciparum*.

Other Host Cell Polymorphisms

Human leukocyte antigens (HLA) constitute a highly polymorphic group of proteins involved in immune response. Reduced susceptibility to malaria is shown in the presence of both HLA class 1 antigen (HLA BW53) and HLA class II haplotypes (DRBI 1302-DQBI 0501) (42).

A few other polymorphisms, which are shown to affect malaria, include those affecting the gene coding for TNF-α and intracellular adhesion molecule 1 (ICAM-1). ICAM-1 polymorphism is associated with an increased risk of cerebral malaria. On the other hand, different polymorphisms affecting TNF-α are associated with protection as well as increased susceptibility (43).

Acquired Nonspecific Immunity

The acquired factors important in causing resistance to malaria are somewhat puzzling. Severe malaria is extremely uncommon in the presence of severe under-nutrition, e.g., marasmus or Kwashiorkar, and in the presence of deficiencies of nutrients such as iron, riboflavin, and para-aminobenzoic acid. Possibly, the parasite growth gets inhibited due to nutritional deficiencies in extremely starved individuals (44). Interestingly, exacerbations occur when these deficiencies are supplemented. On the other hand, poor nutritional status is also known to increase susceptibility to malaria. Similarly, the presence of acquired immunosuppression, e.g., due to human immunodeficiency virus (HIV) infection is known to cause clinical malaria (45). Acute malaria is also reported to upregulate HIV replication leading to higher plasma viral loads (45). Malaria along with tuberculosis and bacterial infection is identified as the leading cause of HIV-related morbidity across sub-Saharan Africa (46).

The extensive community use of antimalarial drugs such as chloroquin is also included among acquired causes of resistance to malaria (44).

V. Antimalarial Vaccination

Development of an effective vaccine is in the center stage of all immunological research on malaria. There are at least three observations, which have raised high hopes of antimalarial vaccination:

    i.   demonstration of specific immunity against malaria in people living in endemic areas;

    ii.   successful use of specific immunoglobulins for cure of malaria; and

    iii.   protection shown by vaccination with attenuated sporozoites.

There are enormous problems with vaccine development. One major difficulty is the production of thousands of antigens by the parasite throughout its life cycle. It is difficult to identify the antigens, which can be targeted by the vaccine. It is also important to develop a multistage vaccine, which can block different stages of the parasite life cycle. A vaccine against the pre-erythrocytic stages of the parasite will find its use for short-term visitors to endemic areas but without any sterilizing immunity in the long term.

It is important to combine several antigens of different stages of the parasite in a multicomponent, multistage vaccine, which can be used for both the travelers and the people living in the endemic areas (47,48). It should also prevent serious morbidity and mortality. Such a vaccine is probably required to target the parasites in the red blood cells. But clinical assessment of potential vaccines to be used in the blood stages has somewhat lagged behind.

Vaccines against the mosquito stage of malaria life cycle is an attractive group of vaccines, which are likely to be developed relatively more rapidly. These vaccines generate antibodies against the male and female gametocytes in the human host. These antibodies ingested by the mosquito together with the parasite, block the parasitic growth in the mosquito. This type of transmission blocking vaccines would confer immunity in the community rather than in an individual (44,49). They will possibly find use along with other multistage vaccines.

There are several vaccines against malaria in different phases of trials (50). While the results of the early trials were generally disappointing in nature, good humoral and cell-mediated responses have been shown more recently. Most of the currently used vaccines utilize multiepitope approaches. In addition to the use of multiple potential antigen combinations, an increasing range of alternative modes of delivery have been used. These have included the insertion of genes for vaccine antigens into a plasmid, modified bacteria or live vector viruses (such as vaccinia). Use of recombinant proteins, synthetic peptides, and direct DNA vaccines are other potential alternatives.

A meta-analysis of randomized controlled trials in endemic areas of four types of malaria vaccines has been recently made available (51). The vaccines included SPf 66 and MSP/RESA against the asexual stages of the plasmodium and CS-NANP and RTS, S against the sporozoite stages. No protection was reported by SPf 66 against *P. falciparum* in Africa, while modest reduction in attacks was seen in other regions. No protection was seen with the use of CS-NANP vaccines while RTS, S and MSP/RESA showed promising results.

There is no final word on an effective and ideal antimalaria vaccine. The trials are time consuming, technically difficult and costly to conduct. In spite of all these problems, it continues to remain an essential goal to achieve for both the scientists and the health administrators.

References

1. Artavanis-Tsakonas K, Tongren JE, Riley EM. The war between the malaria parasite and the immune system: immunity, immunoregulation and immuno-pathology. Clin Exp Immunol 2003; 133:145–152.
2. Heddini A. Malaria pathogenesis: a jigsaw with an increasing number of pieces. Inter J Parasitol 2002; 32:1587–1598.
3. deSouza JB, Riley EM. Cerebral malaria: the contribution of studies in animal models to our understanding of immunopathogenesis. Microbes Infect 2002; 4:291–300.
4. Dimopoulos G. Insect immunity and its implications in mosquito–malaria interactions. Cell Microbiol 2003; 5:3–14.
5. Greenwood B. The molecular epidemiology of malaria. Trop Med Int Health 2002; 7:1012–1021.
6. Knell AJ. Malaria. Oxford: Oxford University Press, 1991:35–60.
7. Molineaux L. *Plasmodium falciparum* malaria: some epidemiological implications of parasite and host diversity. Ann Trop Med Parasitol 1996; 90:379–393.
8. Ward GE, Chitnis CE, Miller LH. The invasion of erythrocytes by malaria merozoites. In: Russel D, ed. Strategies for Intracellular Survival of Microbes. London: WB Saunders, 1994:155–190.
9. Yipp BG, Baruch DI, Brady C, Murray AG, Looareesuwan S, Kubes P, Ho M. Recombinant PfEMP1 peptide inhibits and reverses cytoadherence of clinical *Plasmodium falciparum* isolates in vivo. Blood 2003; 101:331–337.
10. Marshall VM, Coppel RL, Anders RF, Kemp DJ. Two novel alleles within subfamilies of the merozoite surface antigen 2 (MSP-2) of *Plasmodium falciparum*. Mol Biochem Parasitol 1992; 50:181–184.
11. MacPherson GG, Warrell ML, White NJ, Looareesuwan S, Warrell DA. Human cerebral malaria. A quantitative ultrastructural analysis of parasitized erythrocyte sequestration. Am J Pathol 1985; 119:385–401.
12. Hayward RE, Tiwari B, Piper KP, Baruch DI, Day KP. Virulence and transmission success of the malaria parasite *Plasmodium falciparum*. Proc Natl Acad Sci USA 1999; 96:4563–4568.
13. Torre D, Spermanza F, Martegani R. Role of proinflammatory and anti-inflammatory cytokines in the immune response to *Plasmodium falciparum* malaria. Lancet Infect Dis 2002; 2:719–720.

14. Grau GE, Taylor TE, Molyneux ME, Wirima JJ, Vassalli P, Hommel M, Lambert PH. Tumor necrosis factor and disease severity in children with falciparum malaria. N Engl J Med 1989; 320:1586–1591.
15. Molyneux M, Taylor T, Wirima J, Grau G. Tumor necrosis factor, interleukin-6 and malaria. Lancet 1991; 337:1098.
16. Engwerda CR, Mynott TL, Sawhney S, DeSouza JB, Bickle QD, Kaye PM. Locally upregulated lymphotoxin alpha, not systemic tumor necrosis factor alpha, is the principle mediator of murine cerebral malaria. J Exp Med 2002; 195:1371–1377.
17. Anstey NM, Weinberg JB, Hassanali MY, Mwaikambo ED, Manyenga D, Misukonis MA, Arnelle DR, Hollis D, McDonald MI, Granger DL. Nitric oxide in Tanzanian children with malaria: inverse relationship between severity and nitric oxide production/nitric oxide synthase type 2 expression. J Exp Med 1996; 184:557–567.
18. Clark IA, Rockett KA, Cowden WB. Possible role of nitric oxide in conditions clinically similar to cerebral malaria. Lancet 1992; 340:894–896.
19. Lowe B, Msobo M, Bull P. All four species of human malaria form rosettes. Trans R Soc Trop Med Hyg 1998; 92:526.
20. Kaul DK, Roth EF Jr, Nagel RL, Howard RJ, Handunnetti SM. Rosetting of *Plasmodium falciparum*-infected red cells with uninfected cells enhance vasooclusion in an ex vivo microvascular system. Blood 1991; 78:812–819.
21. Roberts DJ, Pain A, Kai O, Kortok M, Marsh K. Autoagglutination of malaria-infected red blood cells and malaria severity. Lancet 2000; 355: 1427–1428.
22. Pain A, Ferguson D, Kai O, Urban B, Lowe B, Marsh K, Roberts D. Platelet-mediated clumping of *Plasmodium falciparum*-infected erythrocytes is a common adhesive phenotype and is associated with severe malaria. Proc Natl Acad Sci USA 2001; 98:1805–1810.
23. Urban BC, Roberts DJ. Malaria, monocytes, macrophages and myeloid dendritic cells: sticking of infected erythrocytes switches off host cells. Curr Opin Immunol 2002; 14:458–465.
24. Warrell DA. Pathophysiology of severe falciparum malaria in man. Parasitology 1987; 94(suppl):S53–S76.
25. Jindal SK, Aggarwal AN, Gupta D. Adult respiratory distress syndrome in the tropics. Clin Chest Med 2002; 23:445–455.
26. WHO Malaria Action Programme. Severe and complicated malaria. Trans R Soc Trop Med Hyg 1986; 80(suppl):3–50.
27. Bambery P, Jindal SK, Kaur U. Pulmonary complications of malaria. In: Sharma OP, ed. Lung Disease in the Tropics. New York: Marcel Dekker Inc., 1991:101–133.
28. Weiss ML, Kubat K. *Plasmodium berghei*: a mouse model for the "sudden death" and "malaria lung" syndromes. Exp Parasitol 1983; 56:143–151.
29. Warrell DA. Pathophysiology of severe falciparum malaria in man. Parasitology 1987; 94(suppl):S29–S51.
30. Brooks MH, Kiel FW, Sheehy TW, Barry KG. Acute pulmonary edema in falciparum malaria. N Engl J Med 1968; 279:732–737.

31. Fried M, Nosten F, Brockman A, Brabin BJ, Duffy PE. Maternal antibodies block malaria. Nature 1998; 395:851–852.
32. Riley EM, Wagner GE, Akanmori BD, Koram KA. Do maternally acquired antibodies protect infants from malaria infection? Parasite Immunol 2001; 23:51–59.
33. Gupta S, Snow RW, Donnelly CA, Marsh K, Newbold C. Immunity to non-cerebral severe malaria is acquired after one or two infections. Nat Med 1999; 5:340–343.
34. Riley EM. Is T-cell priming required for initiation of pathology in malaria infections? Immunol Today 1999; 20:228–233.
35. Currier J, Sattabongkot J, Good MF. "Natural" T cells responsive to malaria, evidence implicating immunological cross-reactivity in the maintenance of TCR alpha beta+ malaria-specific responses from non-exposed donors. Int Immunol 1992; 4:985–994.
36. Choudhury HR, Sheikh NA, Bancroft GJ, Katz DR, De Souza JB. Early non-specific immune responses and immunity to blood stage non-lethal *Plasmodium yoelii* malaria. Infect Immun 2000; 68:6127–6132.
37. De Souza JB, Williamson KH, Otani T, Playfair JH. Early gamma interferon responses in lethal and nonlethal murine blood-stage malaria. Infect Immun 1997; 65:1593–1598.
38. Artavanis-Tsakonas K, Riley KM. Innate immune response to malaria, rapid induction of IFN-gamma from human NK cells by live *Plasmodium falciparum* infected erythrocytes. J Immunol 2002; 169:2956–2963.
39. Carnaud C, Lee D, Donnars O, Park SH, Beavis A, Koezuka Y, Bendelac A. Cutting edge. Cross talk between cells of the innate immune system: NKT cells rapidly activate NK cells. J Immunol 1999; 163:4647–4650.
40. Weatherall DJ. Common genetic disorders of the red cell and the 'malaria hypothesis'. Ann Trop Med Parasitol 1987; 81:539–548.
41. Bayoumi RA. The sickle-cell trait modifies the intensity and specificity of the immune response against *P. falciparum* malaria and leads to acquired protective immunity. Med Hypoth 1987; 22:287–298.
42. Hill AV, Allsopp CE, Kwiatkowski D, Austey NM, Twumasi P, Rowe PA, Bennet S, Brewster D, McMichael AJ, Greenwood BM. Common West African HLA antigens are associated with protection from severe malaria. Nature 1991; 352:595–600.
43. Knight JC, Udalova I, Hill AL, Greenwood BM, Peshu N, Marsh K, Kwiatkowski D. A polymorphism that affects OCT-1 binding to the TNF promoter region is associated with severe malaria. Nat Genet 1999; 22:145–150.
44. March K. Immunology of malaria. In: David W, ed. Malariology. London: Arnold, 2002:252–267.
45. Rowland Jones SL, Lohman B. Interaction between malaria and HIV infection—an emerging public health problem. Microbes Infect 2002; 4:1265–1270.
46. Holmes CB, Losina E, Walensky RP, Yazdanpanah Y, Freedberg KA. Review of human immuno-deficiency virus type 1 related opportunistic infections in sub-Saharan Africa. Clin Infect Dis 2003; 36:652–662.
47. Genton B, Corradin G. Malaria vaccines from the laboratory to the field. Curr Drug Targets Immune Endocr Metab Disord 2002; 2:255–267.

48. Moore SA, Surgey EG, Cadwgan AM. Malaria vaccines: where are we and where are we going? Lancet Infect Dis 2002; 2:737–743.
49. Whitty CJM, Rowland M, Sanderson F, Mutabingwa TK. Malaria. BMJ 2002; 325:1221–1224.
50. Chauhan VS, Bhardwaj D. Current status of malaria vaccine development. Adv Biochem Eng Biotechnol 2003; 84:143–182.
51. Graves P, Gelband H. Vaccine for preventing malaria. Cochrane Database Syst Rev 2003; CD 000129.

11

Pulmonary and Critical Care Aspects of Severe Malaria

ARUNABH TALWAR and
ALAN M. FEIN

Division of Pulmonary and Critical Care
Medicine, Department of Internal
Medicine, North Shore University
Hospital,
Manhasset, New York, U.S.A.

GAUTAM AHLUWALIA

Department of Medicine, Dayanand
Medical College and Hospital,
Ludhiana, India

I. Introduction

Malaria is an enormous global public health problem resulting in nearly 500 million febrile episodes per year and approximately 1 million deaths annually worldwide (1–3). There have been increasing number of cases of complicated and fatal malaria around the world, especially in developing nations. Poor primary health care, failure of mosquito eradication programs, and emerging drug resistance in endemic areas has all contributed to its morbidity and mortality. Increased global travel, migration, and poor compliance of prescribed chemoprophylaxis have also contributed to the magnitude of the disease in nonendemic areas (4–6). Nearly 1500 cases of malaria are reported each year in the United States; approximately 60% are among U.S. travelers. It is estimated that one of every 100 U.S. travelers with malaria diagnosed and reported to National Malaria Surveillance System dies and *P. falciparum* is responsible for nearly all deaths (7).

Human malaria is caused by four species of *Plasmodia*: *P. falciparum*, *P. vivax*, *P. ovale*, and *P. malariae*. Human infection by all four *Plasmodia* sp. occurs by transmission of sporozoites via a bite from an infected anopheline mosquito. Worldwide, the majority of malaria infection is caused by either *P. falciparum* or *P. vivax*, and most malaria-associated deaths are due to *P. falciparum* (5,6). Mixed infection due to more than one malarial species occurs in 5–7% of infections. The severity and manifestations of malarial infestation are usually governed by the infecting species, magnitude of parasitemia, and the cytokines released as a result of the infection (8). Delay in diagnosis and timely initiation of appropriate treatment may also increase morbidity and mortality.

II. Pathophysiology

The virulence of *P. falciparum* is attributed to its propensity to produce heavy parasitemia and its ability to cytoadhere to the vascular endothelium, which leads to the sequestration of parasitized red blood cells in the microvasculature of the vital organs (8). The organ-specific sequestration of mature, late-stage *P. falciparum* parasites in deep vascular endothelium has been considered a central process in the pathophysiology of severe malaria, a concept supported by a number of autopsy studies (Fig. 1) (9).

The parasitized red cells develop the property of cytoadherence, which is enhanced by tumor necrosis factor (TNF) and other cytokines (10). Therefore, the noninfected red cells may stick around parasitized red cells forming rosettes and aggravating the mechanical obstruction (11). As in sepsis, malaria is associated with release of a variety of toxins that can trigger the activation of host immune factors including proinflammatory cytokines, oxygen free radicals, and nitric oxide; all of which can result in damage to host tissues. Similar to many serious infections, the raised levels of proinflammatory cytokines correlate with disease severity and outcome (12,13).

The parasites release various proteins such as *P. falciparum* erythrocyte membrane protein 1 (PfEMP-1) on the surface of the parasitized red cells, which bind to the receptors like intercellular adhesion molecule (ICAM-1) and CD36 on the endothelium of the cerebral venules causing cytoadherence of parasitized cells (11,14).

The peripheral sequestration of parasitized red blood cells in the capillary bed of the end organs along with production of cytokines from host are responsible for specific complications encountered with *P. falciparum* infection. In African children with cerebral malaria, the plasma concentrations of tumor necrosis factor-alpha, interleukin (IL)-1 alpha, and other proinflammatory cytokines IL-1 [beta], IL-6, and IL-10 have been observed to closely correlate with the severity of the disease as reflected by parasitemia, hypoglycemia, case fatality, and neurological sequel (10). They may also be responsible for fever, hypoglycemia, coagulopathy, and leucocytosis (10,15,16). Interestingly, the development of cytoadherence property is specific to a particular strain. Therefore, cerebral malaria is caused only by *P. falciparum* infection (17,18).

The microvascular dysfunction partly explains the multiple organ dysfunction syndrome (MODS) associated with severe falciparum malaria. The clinical manifestations of MODS include acute respiratory distress syndrome (ARDS), altered sensorium, and/or acute hepatorenal failure (19,20).

Data from case series of adults admitted with severe falciparum malaria to intensive care units in India (21), Malaysia (22), South Africa (16), and France (23), all provide evidence of multiorgan failure as major risk factor for death. In severe malaria, mortality rate is 6.4% when one or fewer organs fail but increases to 48.8% with presence of two or more organ dysfunction (21). The similarity between severe malaria to the pathogenesis of bacterial sepsis is clearly evident. Severe malaria due to *P. falciparum* like bacterial sepsis results hyperdynamic circulatory state, characterized by tachycardia, high cardiac output, hypotension and a reduced systemic vascular resistance (10,19). In fulminant cases, the hemodynamic status is characterized by a low cardiac output, high systemic vascular resistance and refractory hypotension—similar to a terminal bacterial sepsis.

III. Clinical Features

Clinically *P. falciparum* malaria is classified either as acute and uncomplicated or severe and complicated. The other three species though cause an acute febrile episode but hardly ever lead to complications and multiorgan dysfunction. The severity of clinical manifestations in malaria is also dependent upon degree of parasitemia as well as the immune status of the host. The incubation period (the interval between infection and the first symptom) usually ranges from 7 to 14 days (mean 12 days) and correlates with the primary hepatic (exo-erythrocytic) phase of infection.

During the asexual erythrocytic phase, patients may develop paroxysms of pyrexia. The typical tertian or subtertian periodicity (48 hours or 36 hours between fever spikes) is seen infrequently with falciparum malaria. A high irregularly spiking, continuous or remittent fever, or daily (quotidian) paroxysm is more usual as the asynchronous cycle of multiplication of *P. falciparum* results in less marked periodicity. Classically, the paroxysmal episodes are described as cold, hot, and sweating stages. The patient feels inexplicably cold even in a hot environment. The spectrum of rigor varies from shivering to violent shaking with teeth chattering associated with intense peripheral vasoconstriction. The rapid increase in core temperature may trigger febrile convulsions in young children. The rigor lasts up to 1 hour and is followed by hot flushes and signs of peripheral cardiovascular collapse (palpitations, tachypnea, prostration, postural syncope). At this time, the temperature reaches its peak. The last stage is characterized by drenching sweat and the fever defervesces over the next few hours. The paroxysm lasts 8 to 12 hours, after which the patient may be remarkably well. The other common prodromal symptoms are headache, backache, dizziness, postural hypotension, nausea, vomiting, abdominal discomfort, and diarrhea. These nonspecific symptoms often result in a diagnostic dilemma. On physical examination, anemia and minimal icterus may be present. The abdomen examination may reveal hepatosplenomegaly.

Nonimmune patients tend to present with fulminant manifestations of the illness at a lesser degree of parasitemia. A primary attack in a nonimmune individual may be brief, severe, and occasionally fatal, and the patient may present to the emergency room in a state of hemodynamic instability. Therefore, malaria is an important differential diagnosis in patients with acute febrile illness in developing countries. In the nonendemic countries, most patients with falciparum malaria present within 3 months of arrival from the endemic zones.

In the nonendemic countries, a high index of suspicion of the disease is essential, especially in recently traveled individuals presenting with fever of unknown origin (19). In an appropriate clinical setting, it is better to empirically institute antimalarial therapy in an appropriate critically ill patient when other diagnosis have been considered and excluded.

A.   Major Manifestations of Severe Falciparum Malaria and Critical Care Medicine

The common complications of severe malaria include acute renal failure, disseminated intravascular coagulation, acute respiratary distress syndrome (ARDS), hypoglycemia, anemia, and cerebral malaria (Tables 1 and 4) (24). *P. falciparum* is responsible for the most severe forms of malaria and accounts for approximately 80% of deaths due to this disease. The mortality rate of uncomplicated falciparum malaria is approximately 0.1%. The mortality in *P. falciparum* malaria parallels the degree of parasitemia (14,15).

Bruneel et al. (23) studied 188 adults (93 with severe malaria) admitted to a 1200-bed teaching hospital in Paris between 1988 and 1999. All had *P. falciparum* parasites in blood smears and were admitted to intensive care (ICU). All cases were treated with intravenous quinine and intensive monitoring, with titration of PaCO2 to 35–40 mmHg, elevated head of bed, normalization of glucose, sedation, and mannitol as appropriate. Of those 93 patients with severe malaria, there were 10 fatalities (11%), all of which took no malaria prophylaxis. Average falciparum parasitemia was 18.2% among fatalities. Mean time to malaria diagnosis was 4 days. The mean ICU stay was 7.5 days (4–13 days). Forty patients needed mechanical ventilation and 12 developed ARDS. Shock occurred in 24 patients. Pneumonia and bacteremia were documented in 14% of cases. Four criteria were associated with mortality: unarousable coma,

ARDS, shock, and acidosis ($p < 0.001$ for all four). Similar results have been reported from endemic areas. Tran et al. (25) in a study of 560 Vietnamese with severe malaria reported an overall mortality rate of 15% (83 of 560 patients).

B. Cerebral Malaria

Although the clinical presentation of cerebral malaria may be quite similar to other encephalopathies, clinical case definition of cerebral malaria includes unarousable coma and/or evidence of *P. falciparum* infection (5,6). However, the other encephalopathies should be excluded by appropriate investigations. The onset of cerebral malaria may be quite abrupt. The patient develops an acute febrile illness associated with acute or subacute onset of altered sensorium and/or a generalized tonic-clonic seizure. Convulsions, usually generalized and often repeated, occur in approximately 50% pediatric patients with cerebral malaria. Occasionally, delirium and confusion may precede the coma. Focal seizures and localizing neurological signs are very uncommon. Signs of mild meningism may be present but neck rigidity and photophobia are rare manifestations, unlike meningoencephalitis. The patient may also complain of localized or diffuse headache and/or vomiting. Papilledema is rare and retinal hemorrhages are seen in only 10–15% of cases. Although brain swelling is common in cerebral malaria, it results from intravascular space occupation provided by the large biomass of parasitized erythrocytes and not from cerebral edema (26).

The mortality ranges from 10% to 50% with treatment. Postcerebral malaria sequel is more frequent in the pediatric population (27) and include delirium, agitation, transient paranoid psychosis, ataxia, and epilepsy. The neurological sequel in adults include cranial nerve lesions and extrapyramidal features.

C. Hypoglycemia

The characteristic metabolic dysfunction of severe malaria is hypoglycemia and is a poor prognostic sign (28). The potential mechanisms for hypoglycemia include impaired hepatic gluconeogenesis and metabolic demands of the parasite. Iatrogenic factors like quinine also contribute to the occurrence of hypoglycemic episodes as these are potent stimulant of pancreatic insulin secretion (29,30). In malaria, glucose consumption is also increased by fever, infection, anaerobic glycolysis, and the metabolic demands of the malaria parasites. Moreover, glycogen reserves are depleted in children and pregnant women predisposing these individuals on quinine therapy to severe hypoglycemia.

D. Acute Renal Failure

Acute renal failure commonly occurs in *P. falciparum* malaria although its rare occurrence has been reported in *P. vivax* malaria. Acute renal failure in falciparum malaria is mostly due to acute tubular necrosis (ATN) though acute glomerulonephritis (AGN) has also been reported. The incidence of ATN is estimated at between 1% and 4% of all cases of falciparum malaria (31). It lasts from few days to several weeks, and is occasionally nonoliguric type. The pathogenesis of renal injury is hypothesized due to erythrocyte sequestration interfering with renal microcirculatory flow and metabolism. Several other factors including catecholamine release, cytoadherence of parasitized erythrocytes and associated hemorrhagic changes, intravascular coagulation, intravascular hemolysis, rhabdomyolysis, hyperbilirubinemia, and severe hyperpyrexia have been implicated in the pathogenesis of ARF in malaria (31). Hyperparasitemia, jaundice, and hemoglobinuria are also associated with a high risk of acute tubular necrosis. The presence of renal failure is a poor prognostic parameter, but is completely reversible with early aggressive fluid management and/or renal replacement therapy (32,33).

E. Metabolic/Lactic Acidosis

Although a number of factors may contribute to the acidosis of severe malaria including anemia, impairment of tissue perfusion by sequestration of parasitized red blood cells, poorly deformable nonparasitized red blood cells, impaired hepatic and renal function, and derangements in glucose and organic acid metabolism (28); the most common cause of acidosis in critically ill children worldwide is shock caused by hypovolemia (34). Furthermore, volume expansion with either saline or albumin was associated with correction of both hypovolemia and metabolic acidosis (35), supporting the conclusion that such children are hypovolemic and might benefit from resuscitation with fluids. The presence of acidosis is a poor prognostic sign in patients of severe malaria (36). The main pathophysiological mechanism responsible for acidosis is lactic acidosis. Lactic acidosis is caused by the combination of anaerobic glycolysis in tissues where sequestered parasites interfere with microcirculatory flow, lactate production by the parasites, and a failure of hepatic and renal lactate clearance (28). The plasma concentrations of bicarbonate or lactate are one of the best biochemical prognosticators in severe malaria (34). Dondrop et al. (28,37) have suggested that unidentified acids other than lactate also contribute to anion gap metabolic acidosis seen in severe malaria.

F. Pulmonary Manifestations in Malaria

There is a wide variety of pulmonary disease in malaria from asymptomatic respiratory alkalosis with tachypnea to ADRS (38). Common presenting symptoms include cough (77%), dyspnea (32%), expectoration (29%), and chest pain (15%) (39). In one study, 17% of children with severe malaria admitted to the hospital had respiratory distress with a mortality of 13.9%, as compared to 3.5% in the total population with malaria (36).

Pulmonary edema due to fluid overload and heart failure secondary to anemia may occur. However, this is true only in minority of patients. In one study, only one in ten in one series had an elevated capillary pulmonary wedge pressure; the remainder had a physiologic picture consistent with noncardiogenic pulmonary edema (38). In addition, secondary bacterial pneumonia also contributes to the morbidity and mortality. Depressed mental status, vomiting, seizures, renal failure, and aspiration in patients with severe malaria may predispose to bacterial infection. Pleural effusions in malaria are rather uncommon (40,41). These effusions are usually not large enough to effect respiratory function.

ARDS is a devastating constellation of clinical, radiological and pathological signs characterized by failure of gas exchange and refractory hypoxia and occurs in 3–30% of patients with severe malaria (42,43). ARDS is defined as acute lung injury with an arterial oxygen tension/fractional inspired oxygen ratio of 200 mmHg or less (Table 3) (44). Acute lung injury (ALI) is defined as the acute onset of bilateral pulmonary infiltrates with an arterial oxygen tension/fractional inspired oxygen ratio of 300 mmHg or less, with a pulmonary arterial wedge pressure of 18 mmHg or less, and no evidence of left arterial hypertension. Charoenpan et al. (45) found that patients with ARDS have a high cardiac index and considerable reduction in systemic and peripheral vascular resistance. ARDS/ALI usually occurs due to *P. falciparum* but can occur occasionally due to *P. vivax* (46) and *P. ovale* (47). However, the prognosis in the two clinical situations is vastly different. In patients with vivax or ovale malaria, the patients usually recover, whereas in *P. falciparum* malaria, mortality rate is >80% (20,23,43,48).

The acute lung injury (ALI) usually occurs a few days into the disease course. It may develop rapidly, even after initial response to antimalarials treatment and clearance of parasitemia. The first indications of impending pulmonary edema include tachypnea and dyspnea, followed by hypoxemia accompanied by the development of bilateral infiltrates and ultimately resulting in respiratory failure requiring intubation (43). Patients often have coexisting complications of severe malaria (6).

The hallmark of ARDS is inflammation in the lung. Inflammatory response involves both humoral and cellular elements. In the early stages of ARDS, sequestration of activated neutrophils and parasites in pulmonary microvasculature is associated with intraluminal fibrin and platelet aggregation. Subsequently, injury to alveolar capillary membrane leads to increased pulmonary vascular permeability resulting in further pulmonary inflammation and noncardiogenic pulmonary edema (45). The other postulated mechanisms include volume overload from renal failure (48) and a neurogenic component in patients with cerebral involvement leading to ARDS (42).

G. Hematological Abnormalities

The pathophysiology of the anemia of falciparum malaria is both complex and multifactorial, and results in a condition, which is a major cause of mortality and morbidity in patients, especially children and pregnant women, living in malarial endemic areas. Two clinical presentations predominate: severe acute malaria in which anemia supervenes, and severe anemia in patients in whom there have been repeated attacks of malaria. The major mechanisms are those of red cell destruction and decreased red cell production.

Potential causes of hemolysis (49) include loss of infected cells by rupture or phagocytosis, removal of uninfected cells due to antibody sensitization or other physicochemical membrane changes, and increased reticuloendothelial activity, particularly in organs such as the spleen. In addition, disseminated intravascular coagulation (DIC) (50) may be present contributing to further hematological derangements. In less than 5% of patients with severe malaria, significant bleeding with evidence of disseminated intravascular coagulation may be the presenting feature. Hematemesis, presumably from stress ulceration or acute gastric erosions, may also occur. The pathophysiology of DIC includes impaired synthesis of clotting factors and thrombocytopenia. These manifestations are correlated with the degree of parasitemia (6).

"Blackwater fever" is a rare but acute complication due to a rapid and massive intravascular hemolysis of parasitized and nonparasitized red blood cells resulting in hemoglobinuria and acute onset anemia. It is accompanied with high fever, hepatic involvement, and is often fatal due to renal failure. In fact, after the hemolysis, the parasites are difficult to detect in blood.

The other hematological abnormality in severe malaria is characterized by subacute presentation of anemia resulting from hemolysis as well as reduced synthesis of red blood cells due to bone marrow involvement. Decreased production results from marrow hypoplasia seen in acute infections, and dyserythropoiesis, a morphological appearance, which in functional terms results in ineffective erythropoiesis. The erythrocyte survival is reduced even after the disappearance of parasitemia due to increased splenic clearance of nonparasitized as well as parasitized red cells. In severe malaria, both infected and uninfected red cells show reduced deformability, which correlates with prognosis and development of anemia. In some patients, anemia can develop rapidly and transfusion is often required. Anemia may also be a consequence of antimalarial drug resistance, which results in repeated or continued infection (6). Slight coagulation abnormalities are common in falciparum malaria. In fact, mild thrombocytopenia is usual and is attributable to sequestration in the spleen, rather than to a production defect in the marrow or immune-mediated lysis (6,51,52).

H. Liver Dysfunction

Hyperbilirubinemia is almost invariably associated with malarial acute renal failure and this pattern usually results from the complication of hemolysis and intrahepatic cholestasis (51) rather than hepatocellular necrosis. It is more common among adults than children and results from hemolysis, hepatocyte injury, and cholestasis. When accompanied by other vital organ dysfunction (especially renal impairment), liver dysfunction carries a poor prognosis (52). Hepatic dysfunction contributes to hypoglycemia, lactic acidosis, and impaired drug metabolism (15,51).

I. Splenic Rupture

Spontaneous rupture of the spleen is an uncommon but often fatal complication of malaria. Interestingly, *P. vivax* is more closely associated with splenic rupture than *P. falciparum*. The exact pathogenesis of spleen rupture is not known. However, three potential hypotheses have been suggested. The first mechanism is increase in intrasplenic tension due to cellular hyperplasia and engorgement. Secondly, the spleen may be compressed by the abdominal musculature during physiological activities such as sneezing, coughing, and defecation. Finally, vascular occlusion due to reticular endothelial hyperplasia results in thrombosis and infarction. This leads to interstitial and subcapsular hemorrhage and stripping of the capsule, which lead to further subcapsular hemorrhage. Subsequently, the distended capsule ruptures. Most patients present with an acute abdomen. The treatment of choice in patients of splenic rupture is splenectomy (6).

J. "Algid Malaria" and/or Nosocomial Infections

The most common infections in patients with severe malaria are aspiration pneumonia and primary gram-negative bacteremia possibly due to impaired splanchnic vasoconstriction (19,43). The term "algid malaria" is used for severe malaria complicated with hypovolemic shock and septicemia. In endemic area, *Salmonella* bacteremia has been associated specifically with *P. falciparum* infections.

Aspiration pneumonia following seizures is an important cause of death in cerebral malaria. In few patients, it may be difficult to differentiate aspiration pneumonia from ARDS. The other complications of a comatose patient viz. catheter-induced urinary tract infection and nosocomial respiratory infection may aggravate the clinical condition. In fact, transient malaria-induced immunosuppresion may contribute to the occurrence and severity of bacterial infections. In most severely ill patients, bacteremia and/or pneumonia should be treated aggressively (5,53,54).

IV. Diagnosis

Microscopy still remains the investigation of choice for diagnosing malaria. The thick smear is more sensitive in diagnosing malaria, and the thin smear allows species differentiation and staging of parasite differentiation. The thin smear also allows quantification of the percentage of parasitized red cells. Mixed plasmodial infection (*P. vivax* and *P. falciparum*) must be excluded by repeated and meticulous examination of blood smears (55). However, microscopy is operator dependent, requires expertise, and is also time consuming. Therefore, rapid assays are being developed to hasten the diagnostic work-up, especially in critically ill patients.

Polymerase chain reaction (PCR)-based techniques, based upon the detection of nucleic acid sequences (DNA or mRNA) specific to *Plasmodium* species have the ability to detect parasitemia levels as low as 5 parasites/μL (56). The technique has high sensitivity and specificity (57). The disadvantages of these techniques are that they are expensive, labor intensive, take hours to complete, and requires significant technical expertise. PCR may ultimately have a role in monitoring the efficacy of antimalarial therapy and diagnosing therapeutic failure early stage (58).

Fluorescent microscopy viz. QBC Malaria Test System (Becton Dickinson, Sparks, Maryland, U.S.A.) is also being used to identify malaria parasites (57). In this assay, a sample of blood is mixed in a capillary tube with acridine orange, microcentrifuged and analyzed under fluorescent microscopy. Although it gives results more quickly than traditional microscopy, species identification can be more problematic with this assay (59). This technique is useful in the critically ill patient as preparing, spinning, and reading the sample requires 10 minutes. However, in comparison to thin- and thick-smear analysis, the sensitivity of QBC system is 70–100% and specificity is 85–95% (57,60). The limitations of QBC system are the cost of the fluorescent microscope and tabletop centrifuge, especially in the developing world.

More recently, a number of rapid diagnostic tests have been developed that detect parasite antigens in peripheral blood. The first of these tests detect malaria histidine-rich protein II antigen (61,62). The initial prototype versions of these assays detected only HRPII of *P. falciparum*, but newer-generation assays detect antigens of both *P. falciparum* and *P. vivax* (63). The other group of assays detect plasmodial lactate dehydrogenase (pLDH) via immunochromatographic detection or via enzymatic reaction (36,64–66). The diagnostic potential of the various HRP and pLDH rapid assays are comparable. As compared to thin- and thick-blood-smear analysis, these assays have a sensitivity of approximately 90–95% and specificity of 85–95% (57,67).

Although the rapid diagnostic assays offer a number of attributes that make them suitable for use in the developing world (minimally trained personnel, not much requirement of equipment and easy visual reading of the samples), they also have a number of disadvantages that limit their utility: (i) They are unreliable in the presence of low-level parasitemia. The sensitivity of these tests is much lower in the presence of low-level parasitemia (less than 100 parasites per microliter of blood). (ii) They may give false-positive reactions in individuals with positive rheumatoid factor (especially HRP-detecting assays) (68). At the present time, none of the above-mentioned rapid tests are approved for use in United States. An approved rapid test nonetheless will be useful for a positive test might speed initiation of antimicrobial therapy (69). In addition, in the setting of severe malaria, blood and urine cultures should be sent to rule out any bacterial coinfection.

V. Management

The effective care of severe malaria includes early administration of antimalarial therapy, supportive therapy, and management of complications that are present at admission or develop during treatment. Hospitalization and parenteral administration of antimalarial agents is necessary for patients with severe malaria.

A. Antimalarial Therapy

Quinidine Gluconate and Quinine Dihydrochloride

All patients with severe malaria are assumed to be chloroquine resistant irrespective of the clinical presentation. In most developing countries, quinine dihydrochloride is the parenteral agent of choice for treating individuals with severe malaria. The only drug currently approved and available in the United States for severe malaria is quinidine gluconate (Table 2). It is important to appreciate that quinidine is more potent than quinine against malaria, but it is more cardiotoxic (70).

Quinine dihydrochloride may be administered intravenously or intramuscularly. Quinidine gluconate, a class IA antiarrhythmic agent, should be administered intravenously. Both intravenous quinidine and quinine should be delivered by continuous infusion; when they are administered by rapid or bolus injection, they can induce fatal hypotension (30). Quinine is given as an intravenous infusion over 4 hours. If the patient remains seriously ill or in acute renal failure for more than 48 hours, the maintenance doses of quinine or quinidine should be reduced by 30–50% to prevent toxicity of the drugs.

Treatment should be started with a loading dose infusion of 20 mg/kg quinine salt in 5% dextrose. The maximum loading dose of 1.4 g quinine can be given over 4 hours. After 8–12 hours, maintenance dosage at 10 mg/kg quinine salt should be administered up to a maximum of 700 mg. The dose should be repeated at intervals of 8–12 hours until the patient can take drugs orally.

The loading dose of quinidine gluconate is 10 mg/kg loading dose (maximum 600 mg) IV in normal saline slowly over 1–2 hours, followed by continuous infusion of 0.02 mg/kg/min until oral therapy can be started. The loading dose should not be given if the patient has received quinine, quinidine, or mefloquine during the previous 24 hours. Mefloquine should not be used for severe malaria, since no parenteral form is available. Intravenous therapy with quinine or quinidine should be administered only till the patient is not able to take oral medications (30). In Asia, a 7-day course of tetracycline or doxycyclin is administered to adults and clindamycin to children or pregnant women. In African countries, sulfadoxin-pyrethamine is used but its efficacy is decreasing. However, it is prudent to administer at least 5–7 days of quinine.

Quinine can also be administered intramuscularly but results in muscle necrosis; the hydrochloride form is less irritant than the dihydrochloride form. The patients with cardiac disease should be monitored by an electrocardiogram (ECG) with special emphasis on QRS duration and QTc. Individuals receiving parenteral quinidine should also be monitored electrocardiographically. If the QTc interval increases more than 25% above the baseline reading, then the infusion rate should be reduced. The intravenous administration of quinine or quinidine can induce hypoglycemia, which usually occurs 24 hours after treatment is initiated and most frequently affects pregnant women and children (30,71).

Artemisinin Derivatives

Artemisinin or Qinghaosu ("ching-how-soo") is the active principal of the Chinese medicinal herb *Artemisia annua.* The artemisinin derivatives are efficacious and widely used overseas for treating severe malaria. A water-soluble ester called artesunate and two oil-soluble preparations called artemether and arteether are being used. Artemisinin derivatives can also be given via rectal suppository if parenteral therapy is unavailable (72). The artemisinins have a number of unique properties including their extremely rapid mode of action, their broad range of activity on all asexual and sexual forms of the parasite, and their low tendency to induce parasite resistance (73), relative ease of administration and potentially lesser side effects, especially hypoglycemia (25). However, its potential benefit over quinine is blunted by its slow and erratic absorption, especially in patients who are in shock, as artemether and arteether have to be administered intramuscularly.

There is increasing evidence that, artemisinin derivatives are better than quinine (74,75). In the recent individual patient data, meta-analysis of 1919 adults and children entered into randomized comparisons of artemether and quinine, mortality was significantly lower in artemether-treated adults (76).

Artesunate is relatively preferable over artemether, as it can be administered both by the intravenous as well as intramuscular route. It should be given as a loading dose 2.4 mg/kg, then 1.2 mg/kg intravenously 12-hourly to a total dose of 600 mg. It can be given intramuscularly in children. Artemether is given as a loading dose 3.2 mg/kg intramuscularly, then 1.6 mg/kg intramuscularly daily to a total of 640 mg. As with quinine, the oral formulation should be instituted as soon as possible. The dose of arteether is 2.4 mg/kg/day administered intramuscularly once daily for three consecutive days. But these drugs are not available in most temperate countries.

B. Supportive Management

Besides antimalarial therapy, ancillary supportive management is also important in improving the outcome of patients with severe malaria. If possible, the patients must be managed in a critical care unit for intensive monitoring of cardiorespiratory and neurological status. Antipyretics and cold sponging do adequate control of temperature. Hyperpyrexia itself may lead to coma and convulsions. Convulsions, vomiting, and aspiration pneumonia further complicate the clinical condition if adequate care and precautions are not undertaken.

The control of seizures should be achieved by using intravenous diazepam, phenytoin sodium or phenobarbital. Though phenobarbitone is an effective method for controlling convulsions, the risk of respiratory arrest increases with phenobarbitone and the patients should be closely monitored for this complication (77).

Hypoglycemia is very common in malaria, especially in pregnancy, which if not treated promptly can be fatal (28). Intravenous 10% or 25% dextrose followed by continuous dextrose infusion is given till the blood sugar returns to normal. Hypokalemia is a common complication of severe malaria; however, it is often not apparent on admission. On correction of acidosis, plasma potassium decreases precipitously, and thus careful, serial monitoring of serum potassium with adequate supplementation is suggested in patients with severe malaria complicated by acidosis (78).

Malaria has many features in common with the sepsis syndrome with high levels of proinflammatory cytokines, which may be associated with increased vascular permeability, pathologic vasodilatation, and increased loss of intravascular fluids favoring the development of intravascular volume depletion (34,79). Particularly, in children, volume depletion is present at admission in the majority of children with severe malaria complicated with acidosis. Volume expansion corrects the hemodynamic abnormalities and is associated with improved organ function (35). The group of children with highest mortality are those who have severe anemia (hemoglobin <5 g/dL), impaired consciousness, and acidosis, which have a case fatality rate of 35% (36). The widely perceived fear of aggravating increased intracranial pressure in cerebral malaria and of precipitating pulmonary edema has resulted in the use of maintenance requirement fluid regimens, with volume expansion only being considered in children who have hypotension or signs of dehydration (6). Over hydration can be prevented by judicious monitoring of central venous pressure and/or pulmonary artery wedge pressure. To avoid pulmonary edema, the pulmonary capillary wedge pressure should be maintained between 12 and 16 mmHg or the central venous pressure between 10 and 12 cmH$_2$O. The urine output rate should be kept above 30 mL/hr by continuing fluid administration. A reasonable goal is to maintain a mean arterial blood pressure of >60 mmHg.

Deteriorating respiratory status requires mechanical ventilation for adequate management of the airway. Hopefully, early positive pressure ventilation will help prevent the high mortality associated with ARDS in severe malaria (74). The Acute Respiratory Distress network (ARDS net) trial showed that implementation of a lung protective strategy by lowering of tidal volumes and application of appropriate positive end expiratory pressure (PEEP) in the volume assist control mode in mechanically ventilated ALI/ARDS patients could decrease mortality from 40% to 31% (80,81). The role of prone position and use of inhaled nitric oxide still remains to be studied further (81). Injudicious volume overload and hypoalbuminemia may aggravate pulmonary capillary wedge leakage and aggravate ARDS in comatose patients. It seems most reasonable to maintain the lowest pulmonary artery occlusive pressure in ARDS patients that still maintains adequate circulating blood volume, mean arterial perfusion pressures, and cardiac output to provide sufficient oxygen delivery. Other clinical variables such as central venous pressure, urinary output, acid–base status, and lactate, serum urea nitrogen, and serum creatinine levels may help in judging the adequacy of a patient's intravascular volume, especially if central vascular pressure measurements are not available. Vasopressor use is especially important when systemic perfusion pressures are inadequate to maintain organ blood flow (82). Use of pulmonary toilet, aspiration precautions, patient positioning including intermittent prone positioning, and recruitment maneuvers are useful therapeutic complements for maintaining functional residual capacity and decreasing shunt. During ventilation care must be taken to maintain a PaCO$_2$ below 30 mmHg since a rise in PaCO$_2$ may increase intracranial pressure and precipitate death (26).

Associated bacterial sepsis is reported in 10–30% of ARDS patients who have malaria (43,83,84). It has been suggested that the infections early in the course of disease are due to splanchnic ischemia and transmigration of enteric organisms and later may occur as nosocomial infections (85). Furthermore, a pronounced general immunosuppression has been reported in malaria patients, which may predispose them to opportunistic infections (86). Bacterial coinfection occur more commonly in children and should always be suspected and treated empirically with broad-spectrum antibiotics, until the results of cultures are available.

Patients showing early signs of renal failure should be treated conservatively. A meticulous record of fluid requirement is necessary. However, the patients should be subjected to early dialysis if the urine output does not increase and there is further deterioration of renal function tests. In a study performed in Vietnam, mortality in patients with malaria and renal failure was 75% without dialysis and 26% when dialysis was available (32). Recent studies have demonstrated a significantly lower mortality with hemofiltration compared with peritoneal dialysis (30,33). Although low-dose dopamine augments renal blood flow in healthy volunteers (87) and patients with life-threatening infections like severe malaria (88), a recent, large, multicenter, randomized trial demonstrated that low-dose dopamine administered to critically ill patients who are at risk of renal failure does not confer clinical significant protection from renal dysfunction (89). There is no justification in using low-dose dopamine in treating critically ill patients with severe malaria as renal protection strategy. In renal failure, the dose of the intravenous quinine in renal failure should not be decreased in the first 48 hours; however, if it needs to be given beyond that the dose should be reduced to half or one-third of the initial dose (6). Artemisinin drugs do not require any dose modification in the presence of acute renal failure.

Despite appropriate medical treatment, the mortality in patients with a greater than 10% parasitemia ranges from 20% to 40% when cerebral or renal function is impaired and up to 80% in the presence of ARDS (90). It has been argued that in these cases, the use of exchange transfusion (ET) can achieve a prompt reduction in parasitemia, and may improve prognosis. The main advantages of ET are rapid correction of the anemia, decrease in the level of parasites, elimination of several cytokines and parasite toxins. Other advantages associated with the ET are that it ensures an adequate fluid balance and homodynamic status and absence of interference with drug therapy (90). However, ET treatment is still considered a matter of debate because some authors consider that similar results to that achieved with ET could be obtained with chemotherapy alone (91). A single inadequately powered study in eight subjects reported no benefit with ET (92). A recent meta-analysis, which reviewed eight quasirandomized studies, concluded that adjunct exchange transfusion did not improve survival

Table 1 Clinical and Laboratory Features of Severe and Complicated Falciparum Malaria in Adults

Criterion
Coma[a]
Impaired consciousness
Prostration/extreme weakness
Multiple convulsions
Hyperbilirubinemia[b]
Pulmonary edema
Acute renal failure
Severe anemia[c]
Acute intravascular hemolysis with hemoglobinuria
Spontaneous bleeding
Hypoglycemia[d]
Shock
Acidemia/acidosis[e]
Hyperlactemia[f]
Parasitemia $\geq$4% to $\geq$20%[g]

[a]Unarousable coma defines cerebral malaria.
[b]Total bilirubin $\geq$3 mg/dL.
[c]In adults: Hb <7 g/dL, Hct <20% (children: Hb <5 g/dL,/Hct < 15%).
[d]Whole blood glucose <2.2 mmol/L.
[e]pH <7.35/plasma bicarbonate <15 mmol/L.
[f]Plasma lactate >5 mmol/L.
[g]Depends on malaria-acquired immunity (i.e., $\geq$4% in nonimmune persons).
Source: From Ref. 6.

as compared to antimalarial chemotherapy alone, but patients receiving exchange transfusion were sicker and had higher level of parasitemia (93). The WHO-endorsed guidelines for management of severe falciprum malaria recommend that exchange transfusion be considered in nonimmune individuals only if pathogen-free compatible blood and facilities for safe exchange and adequate clinical monitoring are available (6). However, we agree with Ridle et al. (93) that whether exchange transfusion is really beneficial in severe malaria still needs to be proven in a randomized controlled trial.

With a mortality of 15–20% despite parenteral antimalarial treatment, cerebral malaria is a considerable therapeutic challenge. Raised intracranial pressure (ICP) is frequently detected in African children with cerebral malaria (94). Treatment of raised ICP remains controversial.

Mannitol reduces the ICP, but no randomized controlled trial has been conducted to show that it reduces sequelae and mortality. Corticosteroids have not been shown to be of any benefit in cerebral malaria and their use is associated with significant side effects (83).

Table 2 Recommended Regimens for Initial Parentral Treatment for Severe Falciparum Malaria

Drug	Loading dose	Maintenance dose	Comments
Quinine dihydrochloride salt (available outside United States) reconstituted in 5% dextrose	20 mg/kg over 4 hr followed 8 hr later by maintenance dose[a]	10 mg/kg diluted in 10 ml/kg 5% dextrose saline IV over 4 hr repeated every 8 hr[a]	If hemodialysis is performed, then quinine is administered after dialysis. Monitor blood glucose because of hypoglycemia
Quinindine gluconate (available in United States), reconstituted in normal saline	10 mg/kg IV infused over 1–2 hr followed immediately by maintenance dose[a]	0.02 mg/kg/min continuous infusion[a]	Electrocardiographic monitoring is mandatory; slow or stop infusion if QRS >25% baseline value or QTc interval >500 msec
Artesunate	2.4 mg/kg IV bolus[b]	1.2 mg/kg IV daily[b]	Artesunic acid 60 mg is dissolved in 0.6 mL 5% NaHCO₃, diluted to 3–5 mL 5% glucose, and given immediately by IV bolus injection for atleast 3 days followed by oral antimalarial drugs
Artemether	3.2 mg/kg IM[b]	1.6 mg/kg IM daily[b]	
Arteether	2.4 mg/kg IM[b]	2.4 mg/kg IM daily[b]	

[a]Intravenous (IV) medication given for at least 24 hours but oral antimalarial treatment should be substituted as soon as the patient is stable and can take oral therapy to complete the course. In renal failure, the dose of the intravenous quinine in renal failure should not be decreased in the first 48 hours; however, if it needs to be given beyond that, the dose should be reduced to half or one-third of the initial dose.
[b]Parentral therapy should be given for at least 3 days, but oral antimalarial treatment should be substituted as soon as the patient is stable and can take oral therapy to complete the course.

Table 3 Defining Criterion for Acute Lung Injury and Acute Respiratory Distress Syndrome

	Timing	Oxygenation	PA chest radiograph	Pulmonary artery wedge pressure
Acute lung injury	Acute onset	PaO_2/FiO_2 $\leq 300\,mmHg^a$	Bilateral infiltrates[b]	<18 mmHg or no clinical evidence of left atrial hypertension
ARDS	Acute onset	PaO_2/FiO_2 $\leq 200\,mmHg^a$	Bilateral infiltrates[b]	<18 mmHg or no clinical evidence of left atrial hypertension

[a]Irrespective of the level of positive end-expiratory pressure.
[b]Abnormal chest radiographic findings may lag behind functional disturbances.
Abbreviations: FiO_2, concentration of inspired oxygen; PA, posteroanterior; PaO_2, partial pressure of oxygen in arterial blood.

Table 4 Differences Between Severe Malaria in Adults and Children

Symptoms and signs	Adults	Children
Cough	Uncommon	Common in early stage
Convulsion	Indicates cerebral malaria or hypoglycemia	Indicates cerebral malaria, hypoglycemia but may be nonspecific consequence of fever
Duration of symptoms	Several days	Usually 1–2 days
Jaundice	Common	Uncommon
Anemia	Not so common	Common
Pulmonary edema/ARDS	Common	Rare
Acute renal failure	Common	Rare
Hypoglycemia	Common in pregnant women, or with quinine therapy, sometimes may be present without quinine therapy	Common before treatment
Seizure	Less common	Frequent
Development of unconsciousness	Insidious	Rapid
Coma recovery time	Slow, usually 2–4 days	Rapid (usually 1–2 days)
CSF pressure	Usually normal	Variable, raised
Neurological sequelae	Uncommon	Occurs in about 10% cases

Source: From Ref. 6.

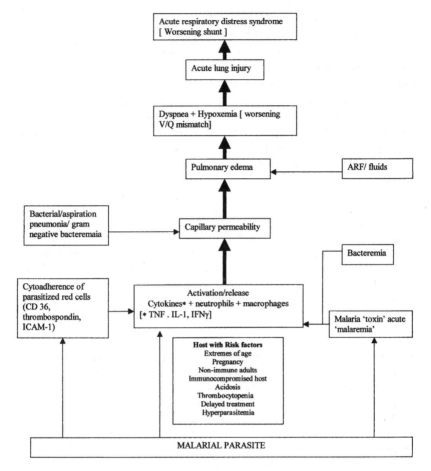

Figure 1 Schematic summary of the possible pathophysiologic steps of malaria-related ALI and ARDS.

In pregnancy, both symptomatic and asymptomatic malaria can cause morbidity and mortality to both mother and the unborn fetus. Primigravida women in endemic areas and nonimmune pregnant women (particularly during second and third trimester) are at greatest risk. Pregnant women with malaria are particularly prone to hypoglycemia, pulmonary edema, and anemia.

VI. Conclusion

Severe malaria is associated with significant morbidity and mortality. The management includes prompt administration of appropriate parenteral antimalarial agents and early recognition and treatment of the complications. In children, the complications include metabolic acidosis (often caused by hypovolemia), hypoglycemia, hyperlactiacidemia, severe anemia, seizures, and raised intracranial pressure. In adults, renal failure and acute respiratory failure are more common causes of death. Admission to critical or intensive care units may help reduce the mortality, and the frequency and severity of sequelae related to severe malaria. Providers must educate travelers about the need for appropriate chemoprophylaxis and personal protection measures if they travel to malarious areas. Clinicians should have a high index of suspicion, especially with travelers to areas where malaria is rampant.

References

1. Breman JG. The ears of the hippopotamus: manifestations, determinants, and estimates of the malaria burden. Am J Trop Med Hyg 2001; 64(1–2 suppl): 1–11.
2. Olliaro P, Cattani J, Wirth D. Malaria, the submerged disease. JAMA 1996; 275(3):230–233.
3. Filler S, et al. Malaria surveillance—United States, 2001. MMWR Surveill Summ 2003; 52(5):1–14.
4. Kain KC, Keystone JS. Malaria in travelers. Epidemiology, disease, and prevention. Infect Dis Clin North Am 1998; 12(2):267–284.
5. World Health Organization, Division of Control of Tropical Diseases. Severe and complicated malaria. Trans R Soc Trop Med Hyg 1990; 84(suppl 2): 1–65.
6. World Health Organization, Communicable Diseases Cluster. Severe falciparum malaria. Trans R Soc Trop Med Hyg 2000; 94(suppl 1):S1–S90.
7. Newman RD, et al. Malaria-related deaths among US travelers, 1963–2001. Ann Intern Med 2004; 141(7):547–555.
8. White NJ, Ho M. The pathophysiology of malaria. Adv Parasitol 1992; 31: 83–173.
9. Pongponratn E, et al. An ultrastructural study of the brain in fatal *Plasmodium falciparum* malaria. Am J Trop Med Hyg 2003; 69(4):345–359.
10. Kwiatkowski D, et al. TNF concentration in fatal cerebral, non-fatal cerebral, and uncomplicated *Plasmodium falciparum* malaria. Lancet 1990; 336(8725): 1201–1204.
11. Baruch DI, et al. Identification of a region of PfEMP1 that mediates adherence of *Plasmodium falciparum* infected erythrocytes to CD36: conserved function with variant sequence. Blood 1997; 90(9):3766–3775.
12. Moormann AM, et al. Malaria and pregnancy: placental cytokine expression and its relationship to intrauterine growth retardation. J Infect Dis 1999; 180(6):1987–1993.
13. Clark IA, Cowden WB. The pathophysiology of falciparum malaria. Pharmacol Ther 2003; 99(2):221–260.

14. Reeder JC, et al. The adhesion of *Plasmodium falciparum*-infected erythrocytes to chondroitin sulfate A is mediated by *P. falciparum* erythrocyte membrane protein 1. Proc Natl Acad Sci USA 1999; 96(9):5198–5202.
15. Lichtman AR, et al. Pathophysiology of severe forms of falciparum malaria. Crit Care Med 1990; 18(6):666–668.
16. Vogetseder A, et al. Time course of coagulation parameters, cytokines and adhesion molecules in *Plasmodium falciparum* malaria. Trop Med Int Health 2004; 9(7):767–773.
17. Clark IA, Cowden WB. Why is the pathology of falciparum worse than that of vivax malaria? Parasitol Today 1999; 15(11):458–461.
18. Pouvelle B, et al. Cytoadhesion of *Plasmodium falciparum* ring-stage-infected erythrocytes. Nat Med 2000; 6(11):1264–1268.
19. Bruneel F, et al. Shock complicating severe falciparum malaria in European adults. Intensive Care Med 1997; 23(6):698–701.
20. Blumberg L, et al. Predictors of mortality in severe malaria: a two year experience in a non-endemic area. Anaesth Intensive Care 1996; 24(2):217–223.
21. Krishnan A, Karnad DR. Severe falciparum malaria: an important cause of multiple organ failure in Indian intensive care unit patients. Crit Care Med 2003; 31(9):2278–2284.
22. Koh KH, Chew PH, Kiyu A. A retrospective study of malaria infections in an intensive care unit of a general hospital in Malaysia. Singapore Med J 2004; 45(1):28–36.
23. Bruneel F, et al. The clinical spectrum of severe imported falciparum malaria in the intensive care unit: report of 188 cases in adults. Am J Respir Crit Care Med 2003; 167(5):684–689.
24. Mohanty S, et al. Complications and mortality patterns due to *Plasmodium falciparum* malaria in hospitalized adults and children, Rourkela, Orissa, India. Trans R Soc Trop Med Hyg 2003; 97(1):69–70.
25. Tran TH, et al. A controlled trial of artemether or quinine in Vietnamese adults with severe falciparum malaria. N Engl J Med 1996; 335(2):76–83.
26. Looareesuwan S, et al. Magnetic resonance imaging of the brain in patients with cerebral malaria. Clin Infect Dis 1995; 21(2):300–309.
27. Brewster DR, Kwiatkowski D, White NJ. Neurological sequelae of cerebral malaria in children. Lancet 1990; 336(8722):1039–1043.
28. Krishna S, et al. Lactic acidosis and hypoglycaemia in children with severe malaria: pathophysiological and prognostic significance. Trans R Soc Trop Med Hyg 1994; 88(1):67–73.
29. Molyneux ME, et al. Effect of rate of infusion of quinine on insulin and glucose responses in Malawian children with falciparum malaria. BMJ 1989; 299(6699):602–603.
30. White NJ. The treatment of malaria. N Engl J Med 1996; 335(11):800–806.
31. Sitprija V. Nephropathy in falciparum malaria. Kidney Int 1988; 34(6): 867–877.
32. Trang TT, et al. Acute renal failure in patients with severe falciparum malaria. Clin Infect Dis 1992; 15(5):874–880.
33. Phu NH, et al. Hemofiltration and peritoneal dialysis in infection-associated acute renal failure in Vietnam. N Engl J Med 2002; 347(12):895–902.

34. Day NP, et al. The pathophysiologic and prognostic significance of acidosis in severe adult malaria. Crit Care Med 2000; 28(6):1833–1840.
35. Maitland K, et al. Response to volume resuscitation in children with severe malaria. Pediatr Crit Care Med 2003; 4(4):426–431.
36. Marsh K, et al. Indicators of life-threatening malaria in African children. N Engl J Med 1995; 332(21):1399–1404.
37. Dondorp AM, et al. Unidentified acids of strong prognostic significance in severe malaria. Crit Care Med 2004; 32(8):1683–1688.
38. James MF. Pulmonary damage associated with falciparum malaria: a report of ten cases. Ann Trop Med Parasitol 1985; 79(2):123–138.
39. Rajput R, et al. Pulmonary manifestations in malaria. J Indian Med Assoc 2000; 98(10):612–614.
40. Al-Ibrahim MS, Holzman RS. Bilateral pleural effusions with *Plasmodium falciparum* infection. Am J Trop Med Hyg 1975; 24(6 Pt 1):910–912.
41. Sirivichayakul C, et al. Pleural effusion in childhood falciparum malaria. Southeast Asian J Trop Med Public Health 2000; 31(1):187–189.
42. Baud M, et al. Acute respiratory distress syndrome due to falciparum malaria in a pregnant woman. Intensive Care Med 1997; 23(7):787–789.
43. Gachot B, et al. Acute lung injury complicating imported *Plasmodium falciparum* malaria. Chest 1995; 108(3):746–749.
44. Bernard GR, et al. Report of the American-European consensus conference on ARDS: definitions, mechanisms, relevant outcomes and clinical trial coordination. The Consensus Committee. Intensive Care Med 1994; 20(3):225–232.
45. Charoenpan P, et al. Pulmonary edema in severe falciparum malaria. Hemodynamic study and clinicophysiologic correlation. Chest 1990; 97(5):1190–1197.
46. Curlin ME, et al. Noncardiogenic pulmonary edema during vivax malaria. Clin Infect Dis 1999; 28(5):1166–1167.
47. Lee EY, Maguire JH. Acute pulmonary edema complicating ovale malaria. Clin Infect Dis 1999; 29(3):697–698.
48. Losert H, et al. Experiences with severe *P. falciparum* malaria in the intensive care unit. Intensive Care Med 2000; 26(2):195–201.
49. Phillips RE, Pasvol G. Anaemia of *Plasmodium falciparum* malaria. Baillieres Clin Haematol 1992; 5(2):315–330.
50. Sharma SK, et al. Haematological and coagulation profile in acute falciparum malaria. J Assoc Phys India 1992; 40(9):581–583.
51. Dash SC, et al. Falciparum malaria complicating cholestatic jaundice and acute renal failure. J Assoc Phys India 1994; 42(2):101–102.
52. Wilairatana P, Looareesuwan S, Charoenlarp P. Liver profile changes and complications in jaundiced patients with falciparum malaria. Trop Med Parasitol 1994; 45(4):298–302.
53. Matteelli A, et al. Epidemiological features and case management practices of imported malaria in northern Italy 1991–1995. Trop Med Int Health 1999; 4(10):653–657.
54. Hocqueloux L, et al. Fatal invasive aspergillosis complicating severe *Plasmodium falciparum* malaria. Clin Infect Dis 2000; 30(6):940–942.
55. Perren A, Beretta F, Schubarth P. ARDS in *Plasmodium vivax* malaria. Schweiz Med Wochenschr 1998; 128(25):1020–1023.

56. Postigo M, Mendoza-Leon A, Perez HA. Malaria diagnosis by the polymerase chain reaction: a field study in south-eastern Venezuela. Trans R Soc Trop Med Hyg 1998; 92(5):509–511.

57. Hanscheid T. Diagnosis of malaria: a review of alternatives to conventional microscopy. Clin Lab Haematol 1999; 21(4):235–245.

58. Ciceron L, et al. Development of a *Plasmodium* PCR for monitoring efficacy of antimalarial treatment. J Clin Microbiol 1999; 37(1):35–38.

59. Tanpradist S, et al. Comparison between microscopic examination, ELISA and quantitative buffy coat analysis in the diagnosis of falciparum malaria in an endemic population. Southeast Asian J Trop Med Public Health 1995; 26(1): 38–45.

60. Wang X, et al. Field evaluation of the QBC technique for rapid diagnosis of vivax malaria. Bull World Health Organ 1996; 74(6):599–603.

61. Funk M, et al. MalaQuick versus ParaSight F as a diagnostic aid in travellers' malaria. Trans R Soc Trop Med Hyg 1999; 93(3):268–272.

62. Gaye O, Diouf M, Diallo S. A comparison of thick smears, QBC malaria, PCR and PATH falciparum malaria test trip in *Plasmodium falciparum* diagnosis. Parasite 1999; 6(3):273–275.

63. Tjitra E, et al. Field evaluation of the ICT malaria P.f/P.v immunochromato-graphic test for detection of *Plasmodium falciparum* and *Plasmodium vivax* in patients with a presumptive clinical diagnosis of malaria in eastern Indonesia. J Clin Microbiol 1999; 37(8):2412–2417.

64. Rock EP, et al. Comparative analysis of the *Plasmodium falciparum* histidine-rich proteins HRP-I, HRP-II and HRP-III in malaria parasites of diverse origin. Parasitology 1987; 95(Pt 2):209–227.

65. Piper R, et al. Immunocapture diagnostic assays for malaria using Plasmodium lactate dehydrogenase (pLDH). Am J Trop Med Hyg 1999; 60(1):109–118.

66. Palmer CJ, et al. Evaluation of the Optimal test for rapid diagnosis of *Plasmodium vivax* and *Plasmodium falciparum* malaria. J Clin Microbiol 1998; 36(1):203–206.

67. Jelinek T, et al. Sensitivity and specificity of dipstick tests for rapid diagnosis of malaria in nonimmune travelers. J Clin Microbiol 1999; 37(3):721–723.

68. Iqbal J, Sher A, Rab A. *Plasmodium falciparum* histidine-rich protein 2-based immunocapture diagnostic assay for malaria: cross-reactivity with rheumatoid factors. J Clin Microbiol 2000; 38(3):1184–1186.

69. Moody A. Rapid diagnostic tests for malaria parasites. Clin Microbiol Rev 2002; 15(1):66–78.

70. Sabchareon A, et al. In vivo and in vitro responses to quinine and quinidine of *Plasmodium falciparum*. Bull World Health Org 1988; 66(3):347–352.

71. Phillips RE, et al. Hypoglycaemia and antimalarial drugs: quinidine and release of insulin. Br Med J (Clin Res Ed) 1986; 292(6531):1319–1321.

72. Birku Y, Makonnen E, Bjorkman A. Comparison of rectal artemisinin with intravenous quinine in the treatment of severe malaria in Ethiopia. East Afr Med J 1999; 76(3):154–159.

73. Maitland K, Makanga M, Williams TN. Falciparum malaria: current therapeutic challenges. Curr Opin Infect Dis 2004; 17(5):405–412.

74. White NJ. The management of severe falciparum malaria. Am J Respir Crit Care Med 2003; 167(5):673–674.
75. Pittler MH, Ernst E. Artemether for severe malaria: a meta-analysis of randomized clinical trials. Clin Infect Dis 1999; 28(3):597–601.
76. The Artemether-quinine meta analysis study group. A meta-analysis using individual patient data of trials comparing artemether with quinine in the treatment of severe falciparum malaria. Trans R Soc Trop Med Hyg 2001; 95:1–14.
77. Crawley J, et al. Effect of phenobarbital on seizure frequency and mortality in childhood cerebral malaria: a randomised, controlled intervention study. Lancet 2000; 355(9205):701–706.
78. Maitland K, et al. Hypokalemia in children with severe falciparum malaria. Pediatr Crit Care Med 2004; 5(1):81–85.
79. Day NP, et al. The prognostic and pathophysiologic role of pro- and antiinflammatory cytokines in severe malaria. J Infect Dis 1999; 180(4):1288–1297.
80. The Acute Respiratory Distress Syndrome Network. Ventilation with lower tidal volumes as compared with traditional tidal volumes for acute lung injury and the acute respiratory distress syndrome. N Engl J Med 2000; 342(18):1301–1308.
81. Flores JC, et al. Severe acute respiratory distress syndrome in a child with malaria: favorable response to prone positioning. Respir Care 2004; 49(3): 282–285.
82. Rosenberg AL. Fluid management in patients with acute respiratory distress syndrome. Respir Care Clin N Am 2003; 9(4):481–493.
83. Hoffman SL, et al. High-dose dexamethasone in quinine-treated patients with cerebral malaria: a double-blind, placebo-controlled trial. J Infect Dis 1988; 158(2):325–331.
84. Warrell DA, White NJ, Warrell MJ. Dexamethasone deleterious in cerebral malaria. Br Med J(Clin Res Ed) 1982; 285(6355):1652.
85. Molyneux ME, et al. Reduced hepatic blood flow and intestinal malabsorption in severe falciparum malaria. Am J Trop Med Hyg 1989; 40(5):470–476.
86. Harbarth S, et al. Septic shock due to cytomegalovirus infection in acute respiratory distress syndrome after falciparum malaria. J Travel Med 1997; 4(3):148–149.
87. Holmes CL, Walley KR. Bad medicine: low-dose dopamine in the ICU. Chest 2003; 123(4):1266–1275.
88. Day NP, et al. Effects of dopamine and epinephrine infusions on renal hemodynamics in severe malaria and severe sepsis. Crit Care Med 2000; 28(5): 1353–1362.
89. Bellomo R, et al. Low-dose dopamine in patients with early renal dysfunction: a placebo-controlled randomised trial. Australian and New Zealand Intensive Care Society (ANZICS) Clinical Trials Group. Lancet 2000; 356(9248): 2139–2143.
90. Miller KD, Greenberg AE, Campbell CC. Treatment of severe malaria in the United States with a continuous infusion of quinidine gluconate and exchange transfusion. N Engl J Med 1989; 321(2):65–70.
91. Hoontrakoon S, Suputtamongkol Y. Exchange transfusion as an adjunct to the treatment of severe falciparum malaria. Trop Med Int Health 1998; 3(2): 156–161.

92. Vanchon F, Walff M, Clair B, Regnier B. Treatment of severe malaria by exchange transfusion. N Engl J Med 1990; 322:58.
93. Riddle MS, et al. Exchange transfusion as an adjunct therapy in severe *Plasmodium falciparum* malaria: a meta-analysis. Clin Infect Dis 2002; 34(9): 1192–1198.
94. Newton CR, et al. Intracranial hypertension in Africans with cerebral malaria. Arch Dis Child 1997; 76(3):219–226.

12

Pleuropulmonary Amebiasis

ALEJANDRO SANCHEZ and
A. WILCOX

Los Angeles County-University of Southern
California Medical Center,
Los Angeles, California, U.S.A.

OM P. SHARMA

Keck School of Medicine, University of
Southern California,
Los Angeles, California, U.S.A.

Amebiasis, an infection caused by the protozoan *Entamoeba histolytica,* is the third leading parasitic cause of death in developing countries (second to malaria and schistosomiasis) (1). The disease has a variable picture and may cause acute or chronic symptoms. At one extreme it may remain asymptomatic, on the other it can blossom into a devastating multisystem disorder involving the liver, chest, brain, and almost any other tissue system. Because the major presenting symptoms in pleuropulmonary amebiasis are pulmonary in nature, the illness is easily confused with other lung ailments including pulmonary tuberculosis, bacterial lung abscess, and pulmonary carcinoma. Delay in diagnosis remains a major factor in the severity of the illness, so familiarity with the pleuropulmonary complications of amebiasis is important.

I. History

Entamoeba was first described in 1875 by Losch (2) of St. Petersburg, Russia. He named the organism *Amoeba coli.* Kartulis (in Egypt, 1886), Koch and Gaffky (Egypt, 1887), and Halva (Prague, 1887) associated amoebae with intestinal and hepatic lesions in patients with diarrhea. In the United States, Osler was the first to report in 1890 the association of amebic dysentery and liver abscess. Simon (3) in 1890 described a patient in whom the liver abscess had ruptured into the lung; *A. coli* were observed in the sputum. Schaudinn in 1903 named the species *Entamoeba histolytica* (tissue-destroying) and differentiated it from *Entamoeba coli*. Brumpt (4) in 1925 was the first to recognize that *E. histolytica* was comprised of two species; the pathogenic *E. histolytica* and the non-pathogenic *E. dispar*. In 1976, Sargeaunt et al. (5) demonstrated distinct isoenzyme patterns of *Entamoeba* that supported Brumpt's assumption.

Losch treated patients with amebiasis with quinine enemas. In the early 19th century, Indian physicians used ipecacuanha for the treatment of dysentery. Later, the active ingredient of ipecacuanha was found to be emetine. In 1912, Rogers (6) in Calcutta first treated amebic dysentery and liver abscess with emetine injections. Emetine is no longer used because it has been associated with significant toxicity. Subsequently, chloroquine (associated with a higher relapse rate than metronidazole) (7), dihydroemetine (8), and metronidazole (9) were introduced.

II. The Parasite

E. histolytica is a pseudopod-forming nonflagellate protozoan parasite. The organism has a life cycle with three distinct stages: trophozite, precyst, and cyst. The cyst is the infective stage, which remains viable in water up to 4 weeks. In contrast, trophozoites are degenerated within minutes outside the body and rapidly destroyed by the low gastric pH. If the cyst is ingested, usually from fecally contaminated food, water, and fingers, it passes through the stomach. Excystation occurs in the lower small bowel. Four trophozoites are formed from a cyst. Trophozoites multiply and move along the intestinal canal until conditions favorable for colonization are found, commonly in the large bowel. Colonization is facilitated by the galactose N-acetyl-D-galactosamine (Gal/GalNAc)-specific lectin that allows trophozites to adhere to colonic mucins (10). Once in the colon, *E. histolytica* can remain either a commensal or become a pathogen. In the presence of diarrhea, the parasite does not become encysted. However, with slow gut motility, the trophozoites that travel toward the rectum discharge food vacuoles and other cytoplasmic inclusions and become precysts. The precyst then acquires a wall and develops into a mature quandrinucleate cyst. Both precyst and cyst are infectious.

E. histolytica has a worldwide distribution. It is estimated that 10% of the world's population is infected with *E. histolytica*. Annually, 35–50 million cases of symptomatic amebiasis are reported. It is second only to malaria in mortality due to parasitic infection (11). The disease is endemic in Mexico, the western portion of South America, South Africa, Egypt, India, and Southeast Asia. It is prevalent in tropical regions, where invasive disease is more frequent and severe. Contributing factors for this geographic distribution include malnutrition, crowding, poor sanitation, and lower socioeconomic status.

In the United States, the prevalence of amebiasis is less than 5%. In 1993, a total of 2970 cases of amebiasis were reported to the Center for Diseases Control; one-third were Hispanic immigrants (12). Antiamebic antibodies were found in 4% of healthy U.S. military recruits (13). The incidence is higher in institutionalized individuals for *Entamoeba* infection (up to 73%) (14). Prevalence rates in homosexuals have ranged from 20% to 50%, although invasive disease was uncommon, probably because the nonpathogenic *E. dispar* was the predominant species encountered (15,16). A minor epidemic of amebiasis in Colorado was related to the use of enema in a chiropractic clinic (17). The majority of cases in the south and southwestern United States occur in immigrants from Mexico and Latin American countries (18,19) In general, severe disease is likely to attack the very young and old.

Immunity to *E. histolytica* is associated with an intestinal IgA response against the Gal/GalNAc lectin. This effective immunological attack reduces the new infection rate by 86% over 1 year (20).

As mentioned above, HIV is an associated risk factor for amebiasis. In Japan, the homosexual population was found to have high levels of antibodies to *E. histolytica* (21). Recently, Lowther et al. (15) reported a 3.3% prevalence of Entameba infection among HIV-infected persons. HIV infection, however, does not lead to increases in invasive amebiasis. A murine model of amebic colitis has shown that the depletion of CD4 T cells decreases the severity of the disease.

III. Pleuropulmonary Complications

The incidence of pleuropulmonary complications of amebiasis varies considerably (Table 1). In 1935, Oschner and DeBakey (16) reported an incidence of 13.5% in their 59 cases of amebic liver abscess. An incidence of 15.7% was found in another series of 95 patients with amebic liver abscess (22). Radke (23) found only one patient with pulmonary disease in 101 cases of amebiasis. Webster (24,25) observed an incidence of 6.3% among 95 patients with intestinal amebiasis in 1956 and 4.0% among 249 patients in 1959. Shaw (26) estimated that 15% of his patients with amebic liver abscess had thoracic involvement. Twenty percent of DeBakey and Ochsner (27) patients with amebic liver abscess had intrathoracic extension. In an analysis of 2074 cases of amebic liver abscess, Adams and MacLeod (28) was able to separate out 146 cases with rupture into the

Table 1 Incidence of Pleuropulmonary Complications

Author	Number of patients with			Incidence of complications
	Amebiasis	ALA	PPA	
Oschner, 1935	388	59	7	11.9% of ALA, 1.8% of amebiasis
Oschner and Debakey, 1936		95	15	15.7% of ALA
Debakey and Oschner, 1951		176	35	19.9% of ALA
Radke, 1951	101		1	0.99% of amebiasis
Kean et al., 1956		90	22	24.4% of ALA
Webster, 1956	95	24	6	20.8% of ALA, 6.3% of amebiasis
Webster, 1960	249	48	10	18.8% of ALA, 4% of amebiasis
Adams and MacLeod, 1977		2074	146	7% of ALA
Vergese et al., 1979	1534	686	23	3.35% of ALA
Nwafo and Egbue, 1981		44	38	86% of ALA
Adeyemo and Aderounmu, 1984		33	22	66.7% of ALA

Abbreviations: ALA, amebic liver abscess; PPA, pleuropulmonary amebiasis.

chest. In one study of fatal amebiasis, 41 of 90 cases with amebic liver abscess had rupture; in 22 patients, the disease extended into the chest (29).

Pleuropulmonary amebiasis, like amebic liver disease, occurs predominantly in men; male:female ratio varies from 9:1 to 15:1 (16,30). It predominantly affects people between the ages of 20 and 50 years (31,32).

IV. Pathogenesis

Pulmonary involvement is almost always secondary to intestinal infection, although a few isolated case reports suggest that the organism might have been inhaled before producing bronchial and pulmonary changes (33,34). From the small bowel, amebae may reach the lung by direct extension or hematogenous spread.

Trophozoites invade the portal circulation and travel to the liver via the portal vein. Hepatic abscesses may form by lytic activity of the parasites. Progression of the abscess may incorporate the diaphragm and pleuropulmonary complications may then occur by direct extension. As the hepatic abscess enlarges upwards, adhesions are formed between the surface of liver and the diaphragm and, later, the diaphragm and the base of the lung. Thus, the involvement of the pleura or the lung depends upon the extent to which the subdiaphragmatic and pleural spaces lead to an amebic empyema, in which a rupture into the lung may produce an abscess, consolidation, or a hepatobronchial fistula. Most pleuropulmonary complications are due to direct extension of amebic liver abscess. Hepatic abscesses may also induce inflammatory changes in the adjacent areas without causing definite parasitic invasion or perforation (35).

Hematogenous dissemination occasionally occurs either through the portal system and hepatic veins or through the inferior hemorrhoidal veins and inferior vena cava. In rare cases, the route is via the lymphatic ducts into the thoracic duct and the lung lesions.

Ochsner and DeBakey (22) first classified pleuropulmonary amebiasis into hematogenous pulmonary abscess without liver involvement (14.3%), hematogenous pulmonary abscess and an independent liver abscess (10.4%), pulmonary abscess extending directly from a liver abscess (37.2%), hepato-bronchial fistula with little pulmonary involvement (19.6%), and empyema extending from a liver abscess (17.6%). There are four main types of pleur-opulmonary involvement: (1) serous effusion with or without atelectasis, (2) consolidation or lung abscess, (3) empyema, and (4) hepatobronchial fistula.

V. Clinical Features

Because pleuropulmonary amebiasis is commonly secondary to amebic liver abscess, it is important to know the clinical presentations of amebic liver abscess. The liver abscess may appear suddenly or, more commonly, follow an insidious course. Patients complain of malaise, fever, night sweats, abdominal discomfort, anorexia, and/or abdominal pain to the right upper quadrant. Infrequently, an abrupt onset may produce a clinical picture of an acute abdomen. Some patients may experience ill health and weight loss for many months and in a small number of patients, fever may be the only man-ifestation (36). Chest symptoms are present in approximately 25% of the patients with amebic liver abscess. Pulmonary symptoms occasionally dom-inate the clinical presentation and these symptoms depend upon the type and extent of pleuropulmonary involvement. Inflammation of the pleura may cause pleuritic chest pain, right shoulder pain, hiccups, or a nonpro-ductive cough. Sudden rupture of a liver abscess into the chest may produce tearing sensation in the chest, dyspnea, or cough. Patients with a hepato-bronchial fistula may cough up "anchovy paste," chocolate-colored, or creamy contents of amebic liver abscess.

The liver is tender and enlarged in nine of every ten patients. The point of maximum tenderness can often be detected either in the intercostal space or over the enlarged liver. The dullness to percussion with diminished air entry at the right base is usually due to a raised diaphragm or accumula-tion of pleural fluid. Percussion may demonstrate a fixed raised diaphragm.

A large abscess may produce visible bulging in the right intercostal space. Diarrhea occurs in less than 20% of the patients.

VI. Laboratory Abnormalities

In general, the laboratory studies in patients with pleuropulmonary amebiasis are abnormal but nonspecific. Normochromic anemia is common. Leukocytosis occurs in three-quarters of patients; eosinophilia is rare. Although the alkaline phosphatase and liver transaminases are often elevated, however, the normal liver function tests do not exclude the diagnosis of liver or pulmonary amebiasis. Hypoalbuminemia is present in more than half of the patients. Serum bilirubin levels are usually normal.

More than 90% of patients with pleuropulmonary amebiasis or amebic liver abscess have positive antiamebic antibody titers. Occasionally, the antibody test is negative in the very early course of the disease, but it almost always becomes positive if repeated after 1–2 weeks. A positive serological result, however, does not differentiate between active tissue invasion and previous infection. Serological tests may be positive for 2 years or more after effective treatment. Specific and sensitive stool assays to detect *E. histolytica* are now available.

VII. Radiographic Findings

The radiographic features of pleuropulmonary amebiasis are not specific for the disease. However, the combination of radiographic features, history, and physical examination may suggest the diagnosis.

Elevation of the right hemi-diaphragm is among the common findings. This abnormality occurs in about 50% of patients with amebic liver abscess, but the reported incidence varies between 30% and 86% (37,38). The lateral chest radiograph may show a diaphragmatic hump situated in the front, back, or in the middle of the diaphragm. The anterior locations are common.

A triangular area of consolidation with its base against the diaphragm and the apex pointing upwards toward the hilum may be present. Cavitation may occur in a consolidated area. A hazy crescentic shadow, less dense than the liver, may be seen above the right dome of the diaphragm.

Pleural effusion can be small, moderate, or massive. Small effusions might be seen only on lateral or lateral decubitus films. Occasionally, they produce only a minor blunting of the right costophrenic angle. If a hepatobronchial fistula is formed, an air-containing cavity may be present under the diaphragm.

Occasionally, a pulmonary abscess may be seen distant from the liver. This may occur in any lobe and usually indicates hemotogenous dissemination. Fluoroscopy or the diaphragm may reveal decreased or absent diaphragmatic motility. The Diagnostic pneumoperitoneum, which differentiates the elevated diaphragm due to liver abscess from the pleural effusion caused by primary pulmonary disease, is rarely used nowadays.

Noninvasiveness, diagnostic accuracy, and cost effectiveness have made ultrasound a test of choice. About one-third of patients with amebic liver abscesses have the ultrasound pattern that is highly suggestive, although not pathognomonic, of hepatic amebic abscess (39). The following are the characteristic features of an amebic liver abscess:

1. It is round or oval.
2. It has no significant wall echoes (abrupt transition from normal hepatic parenchyma to the amebic lesion).
3. It is less echogenic than normal hepatic parenchyma. Fine homogenouslow level echoes are seen throughout the lesion at high gain.
4. It is located peripherally.
5. Distal sonic enhancement of echoes is observed behind the lesions.

Ralls et al. tell us that when all of the above features are present, sonographers should consider amebic liver abscess, even when the diagnosis is not suspected clinically. Although the complete pattern is seen in only one-third of patients with amebic liver abscesses, 90% of the lesions fulfill at least three of the five criteria given above.

Pleural disease was present in 18.9% of patients with amebic liver abscess who underwent ultrasound examination (40).

Amebic liver abscess typically appears as a well-defined, rounded, low-density lesion on a computed tomographic (CT) scan. The margin of the abscess may be smooth or nodular and one or more internal septa may be present. Occasionally, a dense rim around the periphery of the amebic liver abscess may be seen after enhancement (41). A feature of amebic liver abscess that helps differentiate it from other focal hepatic lesions is its tendency to extend beyond the surface of the liver. Radin and co-workers (42) found that only five of their 23 patients (21%) did not have any extrahepatic extension; pleural effusion was present in nine (39%) patients. Although CT is superior to ultrasound in determining the extent of disease, it is less specific and more expensive.

Magnetic resonance imaging (MRI) can be used for imaging amebic liver abscess but more costly when compared to CT scan. Ralls and colleagues studied 12 patients with amebic liver abscess. They were not able to identify any specific patterns to differentiate an amebic liver abscess from other hepatic lesions (43). One patient with amebic empyema showed increased pleural intensity on both T1- and T2-weighted images, compared to low signal intensity with T1-weighted sequence and a high signal intensity with T2-weighted sequence in patients with sympathetic effusions.

VIII. Diagnosis

Pleuropulmonary amebiasis should be included in the differential diagnosis of patients with unexplained right pleural effusion or consolidation, particularly in individuals who either live in or have come from an endemic area.

Demonstration of *E. histolytica* from sputum, bronchoalveolar lavage fluid, or pleural fluid establishes the diagnosis of pleuropulmonary amebiasis. Unfortunately, *E. histolytica* is present in less than 10% of patients. *E. gingivalis*, on oral commensal, should be differentiated from *E. histolytica*. An ultrasound scan, liver scan, or CT scan is helpful in confirming the presence of a liver abscess. The US and CT studies may also demonstrate small pleural effusions. Serological tests should be always performed in patients with suspected pleuropulmonary amebiasis, which are present in 70–90% of patients. The gel diffusion test has a sensitivity of >95% for infection (44). The serum indirect hemagglutination antibody (IHA) is nearly 100% sensitive for infection (45). An enzyme-linked immunosorbent assay (ELISA) has been developed that is as sensitive as the IHA test (46). One major limitation to this approach is that patients remain positive for years after infection, making it difficult to distinguish new from old infection. Once the diagnosis is established, the patients are treated with antiamebic drugs. If the patient responds to the treatment, the diagnosis of amebiasis is established. Occasionally, a pyogenic infection also responds to metronidazole.

IX. Treatment

Therapy for amebiasis is based on whether the disease is invasive or noninvasive. Noninvasive disease may be treated with luminal agents paromomycin or diloxanide furoate (Table 2). Nitroimidazoles, particularly metronidazole, are the mainstay of therapy for invasive infection. This agent has good penetration into the liver and pleural space. In mild to moderate intestinal disease the response rate is up to 90% (47). In severe amebic colitis, it may be necessary to add broad-spectrum antibiotics to treat intestinal bacteria that may have gained access into the peritoneum. After the treatment of intestinal disease, parasites may persist in the intestinal lumen in as many as 40–60% (48). Therefore, nitroimidazole treatment should be followed with one of the luminal agents.

The treatment of amebic empyema is controversial. Surgical management has played a major role in patients with advanced disease. Ibarra-Perez and Selma-Lema cautioned that even though both emetine and

Table 2 Drug Therapy for the Treatment of Amebiasis

Drug	Adult dosage	Pediatric dosage	Side effects
Amebic liver abscess (followed by a luminal agent)			
Metronidazole	750 mg PO 3 times a day for 7–10 days	35–50 mg/kg/day in 3 divided doses for 7–10 days	Anorexia, nausea, vomiting, diarrhea, abdominal distress, disulfuram-like intolerance reaction with alcohol
Tinidazole (not available in US)	800 mg PO 3 times a day for 5 days	60 mg/kg/day for 5 days (max dose 2 g)	Similar as metronidazole
Amebic colitis (followed by luminal agent)			
Metronidazole	750 mg PO 3 times a day for 7–10 days	35–50 mg/kg/day in 3 divided doses for 7–10 days	Same as amebic liver abscess
Asymptomatic intestinal colonization (luminal agents)			
Paromomycin	25–35 mg/kg/ day in 3 divided doses for 7 days	25–35 mg/kg/day in 3 divided doses for 7 days	Diarrhea, GI distress
Or second-line agent			
Diloxanide furoate (not available in US)	500 mg PO 3 times a day for 10 days	20 mg/kg/day in 3 divided doses for 10 days	Flatulence, nausea, vomiting, pruritus, urticaria

metronidazole were effective, patients remained toxic and dyspneic as long as the chest remained undrained. He recommended drainage with a large-bore chest tube connected to strong suction (49).

Verghese et al. commented that thickening occurred that was out of proportion to the duration of the disease and required closed thoracotomy with insertion of a large tube. Continuous suction was required. He found repeated chest taps inadequate (50). Ragaheb and colleagues (51) described five patients with empyema who, despite repeated chest tube thoracentesis and drainage, required decortication. Rasaretnam et al. reported that even though the response to closed thoracotomy was dramatic, complete lung expansion was achieved in only 37% of patients. They reported that if complete expansion did not occur by the ninth day, it would probably not occur and decortication would be necessary (52).

Stephen and Uragoda (53), on the other hand, contend that amebic infection differs from pyogenic infection in that tissue reaction is minimal, unless secondary bacterial infection is present. They recommend repeated needle aspirations. Chest tube insertion is indicated if pus is thick and persistent. In their series of 22 patients with empyema, only one required decortication. The patient also had a secondary infection. Imari treated five patients with empyema with repeated aspiration and emetine therapy (54). Similarly, Adams and MacLeod treated all their patients with pleural effusion by aspiration and amebicidal drugs. Surgical intervention was rarely required (28).

X. Conclusion

Invasive amebiasis is the third leading cause of death due to parasitic disease in the world secondary to parasitic disease. Although, predominantly occurring in tropical and developing countries, it can be expected to be seen more frequently in developed countries. The increase in immigrant populations, increase in global travel, and the ever-increasing crowding conditions (which may lead to the breakdown of the public sanitation network) (56) may contribute to the presentation of cases to unfamiliar physicians. Pleuropulmonary
complications are second to extraintestinal complications (second to hepatic involvement), one must consider the diagnosis in high-risk patients presenting with pulmonary disease and initiate amebicidal therapy. Delay in diagnosis may lead to higher mortality rates.

References

1. Walsh JA. Prevalence of *Entamoeba histolytica* infection. In: Ravdin JI, ed. Amebiasis: Human Infection by *Entamoeba histolytica.* New York: Churchill Livingstone, 1988:93–105.
2. Losch FA. Massive development of amebas in the large intestine. Am J Trop Med Hyg 1875; 24:383–392.
3. Simon CE. Abscess of the liver: perforation into the lung; *Amoeba coli* in sputum. Bull J Hopkins Hosp 1890; 1:97.

4. Brumpt E. Etude sommaire de l' "Entamoeba sidpar" n. sp. Amibe akystes quadrninucleees, parasite de l'homme. Bull Acad Med 1925; 94:943–952.

5. Sargeaunt P, et al. The differentiation of invasive and non-invasive *Entamoeba histolytica* by isoenzyme electrophoresis. Trans R Soc Trop Med Hyg 1978; 72:519–521.

6. Rogers L. The rapid cure of amoebic dysentery and hepatitis by hypodermic injections of soluble salts of emetine. Br Med J 1912; 1:14–24.

7. Conan NJ. Chloroquine in amebiasis. Am J Trop Med 1979; 28:107–110.

8. Brossi A, Braumann N, Choparddit J. Syntheseversuche in der Emetine-Reihe: 4. mitteilung Racmisches 2-Dehydroemetine. Helv Chim Acta 1959; 42:772.

9. Powell SJ, et al. Metroniadazole in amoebic dysentery and amoebic liver abscess. Lancet 1966; 2:1329–1331.

10. Petri WA, Mann BJ, Haque R. The bittersweet interface of parasite and host:lectin-carbohydrate interactions during human invasion by the parasite *Entamoeba histolytica*. Ann Rev Microbiol 2002; 56:39–64.

11. WHO/PAHO/UNESCO. Report of a consultation of experts on amoebiasis. Wkly Epidemiol Rec 1997; 14:97–99.

12. Center for Disease Control. Summary of notifiable diseases, United States. MMWR Morb Mortal Wkly Rep 1994; 42:1–73.

13. Cuyadero R, Kagan IG. The prevalence of antibodies to parasitic diseases in sera of young Army recruits from the United States and Brazil. Am J Epidemiol 1967; 86:330–340.

14. Petri WA, Ravddin JI. Amebiasis in institutionalized populations. In: Ravdin JI, ed. Amebiasis: Human Infection of *Entamoeba histolytica*. New York: Churchill Livingstone, 1988:576–581.

15. Lowther SA, Dworkin MS, Hanson DL. The Adult and Adolescent Spectrum of HIV Disease Project. *Entamoeba histolytica/ Entamoeba dispar* infections in human immunodefiency virus-infected patients in the United States. Clin Infect Dis 2000; 30:955–959.

16. Oschner A, Debakey M. Diagnosis and treatment of amebic abscess of liver: study based on 4484 collected and personal cases. Am J Digest Dis Nutr 1935; 2:47–51.

17. Istre GR, et al. An outbreak of amebiasis spread by colonic irrigation at a chiropractic clinic. N Engl J Med 1982; 309:339–342.

18. White AC, Atmar RL. Infections in Hispanic immigrants. Clin Infect Dis 2002; 34:1627–1632.

19. Shandera WX, et al. Hepatic amebiasis among patients in a public teaching hospital. South Med J 1998; 91:829–837.

20. Haque R, et al. Innate and acquired resistance to amebiasis in Bangladeshi children. J Infect Dis 2002; 186:547–552.

21. Takeuchi T, Okuzawa E, Nozake T. High seropositivity of Japanese homosexual mens for amebic infection. J Infect Dis 1989; 159:808.

22. Oschner A, Debakey M. Pleuropulmonary complications of amebiasis. J Thoracic Surg 1936; 5:225–258.

23. Radke RA. Amebiasis with hepatic abscess and pleuropulmonary involvement. US Armed Forces Med J 1951; 22:437–444.

24. Webster BH. Pulmonary complications of amebiasis. Dis Chest 1956; 30: 315–325.
25. Webster BH. Pleuropulmonary amebiasis. A review with an analysis of ten cases. Am Rev Respir Dis 1960; 81:683–688.
26. Shaw RR. Thoracic complications of amebiasis. Surg Gynecol Obstet 1949; 88:753–762.
27. DeBakey ME, Ochsner A. Hepatic amebiasis: a 20 year experience and analysis of 263 cases. Int Abstr Surg 1951; 92:209–231.
28. Adams EB, MacLeod N. Invasive amebiasis 11. Medicine 1977; 56:325–334.
29. Kean BH, et al. Fatal amebiasis: report of 148 fatal cases from Armed Forces Institute of Pathology. Ann Intern Med 1956; 44:831–843.
30. Bookless AS. Thoracic amoebiasis. J R Army Med Corps 1950; 94:52–60.
31. Daniels AC, Childress ME. Pleuropulmonary amebiasis. Calif Med 1956; 85:369–375.
32. Kubitschek KR, et al. Amebiasis presenting as pleuropulmonary disease. West J Med 1985; 142:203–207.
33. Matthew NT, Ananthachari MC. Pleuropulmonary amoebiasis. J Assoc Physicians India 1964; 12:839–844.
34. Minetto E, Prinotti C. Etat de mal asthmatique dasns un cas d'amebiase bronchique. Ann Otolaryngol 1965; 82:223–225.
35. Rhode FC, Riveros O. Thoracic complications of amoebic liver abscess. Br J Dis Chest 1979; 73:302–304.
36. DeCock CK, Reynolds TB. Amebic and pyogenic liver abscess. In: Schiff L, Schiff E, eds. Diseases of the Liver. Philadelphia: JB Lippincott, 1987: 1235–1253.
37. Nanda RB, Hoon RS. Amoebic liver abscess. Med J Armed Forces India 1976; 32:404–412.
38. Nwafo DC, Egbue MO. Intrathoracic manifestations of amoebiasis. Ann R Coll Surg Engl 1981; 63:126–128.
39. Ralls PW, et al. Sonographic findings in hepatic amebic abscess. Radiology 1982; 145:123–126.
40. Ralls PW, Colleti PM, Benson R, Raval JK, Radin DR, Boswell WD, Halls JM. Imaging in hepatic amebic abscess. In: Ravdin JI, ed. Amebiasis. Human Infection by *Entamoeba histolytica*. New York: Churchill Livingstone, 1988.
41. Baert AL, Wackenheim A, Jeanmart L. Atlas of Pathological Computer Tomography. Abdominal Computer Tomography. Vol. 2. New York, Springer-Verlag, 1980:116.
42. Radin DR, et al. CT of amebic liver abscess. AJR 1988; 150:1297–1301.
43. Ralls, et al. Medical treatment of hepatic amebic abscess: rare need of percutaneous drainage. Radiology 1987; 165:805–807.
44. Proctor EM. Laboratory diagnosis of amebiasis. Clin Lab Med 2001; 11: 829–859.
45. Milgram EA, Healy GR, Kagan IG. Studies on the use of the indirect hemagglutination test in the diagnosis of amebiasis. Gastroenterology 1966; 50: 645–649.
46. Sathar MA, et al. Evaluation of an enzyme-linked immunosorbent assay in the serodiagnosis of amoebic liver abscess. S Afr Med J 1988; 74:625–628.

47. Petri WA. Therapy of intestinal protozoa. Trends Parasitol 2003; 11:523–526.
48. Haque H, et al. Amebiasis. N Engl J Med 2003; 348:1565–1573.
49. Ibarra-Perez C, Selma-Lema M. Diagnosis and treatment of amebic "empyema." Am J Surg 1977; 134:283–287.
50. Verghese M, et al. Management of thoracic amebiasis. J Thorac Cardio Surg 1979; 78:757–760.
51. Ragaheb MI, et al. Intrathoracic presentation of amebic liver abscess. Ann Thorac Surg 1976; 22:483–489.
52. Rasaretnam R, et al. Pleural empyema due to ruptured amoebic liver abscess. Br J Surg 1974; 61:713–715.
53. Stephen SJ, Uragoda CG. Pleuropulmonary amoebiasis. Br J Dis Chest 1970; 64:96–106.
54. Imari AJ. Pleuropulmonary amebiasis in Iraq. Dis Chest 1965; 47:17–19.
55. Barwick RS, Uzicanin A, Lareau S, et al. Outbreak of amebiasis in Tbilisi Republic of Georgia, 1988. In: Program and Abstracts of the Annual Meeting of the American Society of Tropical Medicine and Hygiene, Washington, DC, 29 Nov.–2 Dec. 1999. Northbrook, IL: 1999.

13

Paragonimiasis

FUKUMI NAKAMURA-UCHIYAMA and YUKIFUMI NAWA

Parasitic Diseases Unit, Department of Infectious Diseases, Faculty of Medicine,
Miyazaki University,
Kiyotake, Miyazaki, Japan

I. Introduction

Paragonimiasis is a subacute to chronic inflammatory lung disease caused by infection with lung flukes, *Paragonimus* species. Human infection occurs mainly by ingesting freshwater crabs/crayfishes contaminated with metacercariae (infective larvae) of *Paragonimus* spp. so that the disease is a typical food-borne parasitic zoonosis. Baelz found the first human case of paragonimiasis in Japan by detecting *Paragonimus westermani* eggs in sputum of a patient with hemoptysis. Subsequently, other species has been reported to cause human infection. Till now, at least the following nine species are known to cause human paragonimiasis: *P. westermani*, *P. skrjabini*, *P. heterotremus*, *P. miyazakii*, *P. caliensis*, *P. mexicanus*, *P. africanus*, *P. uterobilateralis*, and *P. kellicotti* (1–3). Clinical findings of paragonimiasis is often confused with pulmonary tuberculosis, lung malignancy, or other infectious diseases. The key to the diagnosis is just an awareness of this disease not only in endemic but also in nonendemic areas. Because of the increase in number of overseas travelers, popularization of ethnic dishes, and the expansion of worldwide trading of food materials, sporadic cases have been found in nonendemic areas

(4). In this review, we will elucidate the current status of paragonimiasis from the data of our laboratory and literal survey.

II. Geographical Distribution and Genetics

Among the nine species causing human paragonimiasis, *P. westermani* distributes in Asia; west to Pakistan and east to Japan and the Philippines, north up to south-east Russia and south down to Indonesia and possibly Papua New Guinea, and has probably the widest distribution of any member of the genus. *P. heterotremus* is endemic in China, Thailand, Laos, and Vietnam. Distribution of *P. miyazakii* and *P. skrjabini* is limited, the former in Japan and the latter in northern China. Distribution of *P. mexicanus*, which is the most common species of human infection in America, is also limited to Mexico and Central and South America (5). Several reports described that *P. caliensis* distributed also in Central and South America to cause human paragonimiasis. However, we could not find out subsequent reports since the first record appeared in 1968 (6). Although *P. kellicotti* is commonly found in wild mammals in North America, autochthonous human cases were rare because of the lacking of food habits of ingesting freshwater crabs or crayfishes in this area. Recently, however, American patients infected with *P. kellicotti* have been reported (7–9). *P. uterobilateralis* is the dominant species in Nigeria and is also found in Cameroon, Liberia, and southern Africa. *P. africanus* is endemic in Cameroon, Equatorial Guinea, and Ivory Coast (5).

Chromosome analysis revealed that there are two types of *P. westermani*, the diploid and the triploid types. There are some morphological differences between them (5). More importantly, they have biological differences such as the migration route and the development in the final hosts. Thus, though it has not been proven yet, human cases infected with either diploid or triploid type may present with different clinical manifestations (10). In addition, the infectivity of *Paragonimus* spp. seems to be affected by geographical isolation of the worm and their intermediate hosts. When rats were infected with *P. heterotremus* of the Chinese, Indian, or the Thai strain, the Chinese and Indian strain migrate into the lung parenchyma to form worm cyst, whereas the Thai strain was unable to develop into mature adults (11). For the taxonomic interest, various isozymes or regions of genomic DNA have been analyzed (12–24).

III. Incidence and Epidemiology

A. Life Cycle of *Paragonimus*

Paragonimus spp. widely distribute in tropical to temperate climate zones of the world and their life cycle is maintained well in wild animals. As shown

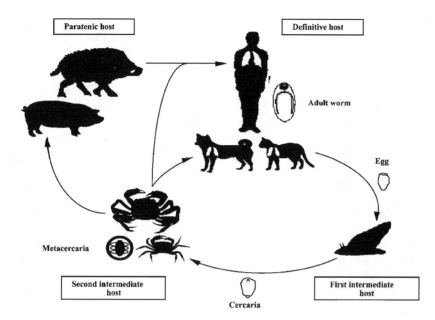

Figure 1 Life cycle of *Paragonimus* spp. *Source*: From Ref. 4.

in Figure 1, adult worms in the lungs of definitive hosts lay eggs, which are voided from the host either in sputum or in stool. Eggs develop in freshwater and release miracidiae that invade the freshwater snail, the first intermediate host. In the snail host, the parasite progress their stage to sporocysts, rediae, and cercariae. Then cercariae emerged from the snail invade crustaceans (crabs or crayfishes; the second intermediate host) where they become metacercariae. Infection occurs most commonly by the ingestion of raw or partially cooked freshwater crabs or crayfishes that contain the infective larvae, metacercariae (4). As an unusual route of human infection, consumption of raw meat of wild boars, which serve as a paratenic host, has been reported from Japan (25,26).

B. Endemic Countries

Since paragonimiasis is a typical food-borne zoonosis, endemic areas are focally distributed in Asia, some parts of Latin America and Africa closely related to the cultural food habits and traditional medicines. It has been estimated that 195 million people are at risk, of which 20.7 million people are infected in worldwide (2).

In Africa, paragonimiasis is endemic in Cameroon and Nigeria. In west Cameroon in 1965, paragonimiasis was present in 10.6% of 256 people examined (27). Recent survey in the southwest province of Cameroon revealed that 1.1% of the people examined were *P. africanus* egg-positive in sputum and stool (28). Age distribution of the patients was ranged from 2 to 19 years without sex difference (29). The decline in the prevalence from 5.6% in 1977 to 2.56% in 2001 was observed in neighborhood area (29,30). Most of the patients were under 20 years and males were more affected than females. In the previous report, the highest prevalence of paragonimiasis in Cameroon was among 10- to 29-year-old females. This was because of the people's belief that the crabs are a valuable aid to fertility (29). Sometimes political and economical status affects the disease epidemiology. Until 1970, only five cases of paragonimiasis had been reported from Nigeria. As a result of the lack of food, crab consumption increased during the Nigerian Civil War (1967–1970) and subsequent economic austerity, paragonimiasis emerged in this country (31,32). The prevalence was 16.8% in Igwan Basin in the mid 1980s, 12.27% and 8.7% in two areas of Cross River Basin in the late 1990 by sputum examination (32–34). Although male to female ratio was different depending on their role and activity in a society, most of patients were under 30 years of age.

Peru and Ecuador are the two well-known endemic areas of paragonimiasis mexicanus in Latin America. A total of 310 cases were reported in Peru from 1910 to 1980. Among those 135 cases were from the department of Cajamarca where residents ingest raw crabs mixed with lemon juice, locally called "ceviche" (35). In the late 1960s, 54/159 (33.9%) of the people examined showed positive reaction for paragonimiasis by skin test. *Paragonimus* eggs were detected in the sputum of 3/29 (10.3%) persons examined (36). Recently, the prevalence of paragonimiasis in this area is declining: only 2/77 (2.6%) and 0.5% of school children were positive with skin test and stool/sputum examination, respectively. However, the prevalence of infection in freshwater crabs was still high (17.5%). Thus, the risk of *Paragonimus* infection has still been persisting in this area (36). In Ecuador, the first case of paragonimiasis was recorded in 1921, since then over 800 cases were reported until 1976 (3). In routine sputum screening for tuberculosis conducted by the Ministry of Public Health, 252 cases were diagnosed as having paragonimiasis during 1988 and 1992 in the province of Esmeraldas where 42.6% of freshwater crabs were contaminated with *P. mexicanus* metacercariae (37). Infected freshwater crabs distributed in 15 of the 22 provinces of Ecuador and one-fifth of the total population is at risk of infection (2).

Among Asian countries, China, Korea, the Philippines, Thailand, and Laos are the major endemic areas of paragonimiasis. However, precise epidemiological data are limited from those countries. In China, *Paragonimus* infection distributed in 433 counties of 22 province in a nationwide survey with a coverage of 30 provinces/autonomous regions/municipalities (38) and it was estimated that 20 million people were infected (2). In Sorsogon, the Philippines, 26 (16.3%) out of 160 people were positive for *Paragonimus* eggs in sputum. More importantly 12 of 26 paragonimiasis patients were registered as tuberculosis

(39). Misdiagnosis between paragonimiasis and tuberculosis is a serious problem not only in the Philippines but also in other countries because of their mimicking clinical findings and overlapping of endemic areas (3). In northern Thailand, nowadays only 0.51% (2/391) of the examined residents were positive for *P. heterotremus* eggs in sputum (40). In Korea at least 2 million people had contracted paragonimiasis as determined by skin test in 1959 (12.9% of 9711 examined). Recently, nationwide survey for paragonimiasis has not been performed in Korea. Based on those figures, the prevalence is presumed to be less than 2% (41). In the late 1980s, the referral system by enzyme-linked immunosorbent assay (ELISA) has been run efficiently in Korea and since 1989, 70–120 paragonimiasis cases have been diagnosed annually (41).

In Japan, overall prevalence of skin-test positive was 3.5% of 146,698 people from seven prefectures during 1954 and 1968. The majority of patients were children without sex difference and the major source of infection was freshwater crabs. As a result of nationwide survey, treatment and prevention campaigns, the prevalence of paragonimiasis drastically decreased to the extent that *Paragonimus* eggs were not detected in stool samples submitted for regular health checking in the early 1980s. However, new cases have been re-emerging from the late 1980s. Since 1986 till now, we have experienced over 200 cases of paragonimiasis, most of which were infected with *P. westermani* and very few with *P. miyazakii*. Particularly, in the recent 3 years, >30 cases have been found every year. The major source of *Paragonimus* infection replaced from freshwater crabs to wild boar meat. The recent patients in Japan are mostly middle-aged men because of their conservative affinity to eat raw wild boar meat (4).

C. Other Countries

Paragonimus spp. widely distribute in tropical to temperate climate zones of the world where the people are at risk of infection. For instance, autochthonous cases have been reported from many countries: Liberia (42,43), Guinea (42–44), and Gabon (45,46) in Africa; Mexico (47), Costa Rica (48,49), Venezuela (50), and Honduras (51) in Latin America. Recently, Benin (52) in Africa, Colombia (53) in Latin America, and India (54,55) and Vietnam (56,57) in Asia were added as new endemic areas.

In America and Australia, most of paragonimiasis patients were the emigrants/refugees from endemic areas or those who have eaten contaminated food materials in the endemic areas or imported from endemic areas. Thus, exotic species such as *P. westermani* or *P. heterotremus*, which are not distributed there, are the most likely cause of the disease (58–64). In addition, American patients infected with *P. kellicotti* have been reported from North America where this species distributes in (7–9).

Even in endemic countries imported paragonimiasis cases or patients infected from imported crabs has been reported (65,66). From France, a nonendemic area, one patient recently reported seemed to be infected while visiting to Japan (67). Along with the globalization of traveling and food trading together with the popularization of ethnic dishes, paragonimiasis can be seen all over the world.

IV. Clinical Manifestations

A. Migration Route of *Paragonimus*

To obtain better understanding on clinical manifestations of paragonimiasis, it is important to know the biological nature of this parasite. In the definitive host, *Paragonimus* worms move dynamically from the small intestine to the lungs via several organs (Fig. 2). Metacercariae ingested by definitive hosts excyst in the small intestine and penetrate into the abdominal cavity across

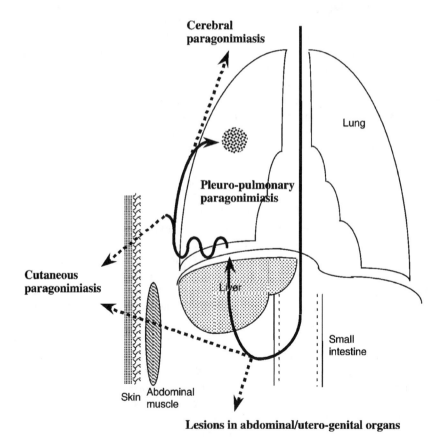

Figure 2   Migration route of *Paragonimus* in humans. *Source*: Adapted from Ref. 4.

the intestinal wall. Since juvenile worms lodged in paratenic hosts have the same ability, when they are ingested, they penetrate into abdominal cavity. From the abdominal cavity, juvenile worms penetrate through diaphragm into the pleural cavity. This migration process takes few weeks. When worms migrate finally in the lungs, solid worm cysts are formed gradually as a result of the host immune responses against the worm components/metabolites. Within the worm cyst, they become mature adults at around 6 weeks and start laying eggs.

Some species pass through additional organs during their way of migration. For example, *P. westermani*, *P. heterotremus*, and *P. kellicotti* migrate once into abdominal muscles. They stay there for a week or more, then they re-enter into the abdominal cavity and go toward the diaphragm (5). In experimental infection in the definitive host animals, *P. skrjabini*, *P. westermani*, and *P. miyazakii* migrate into liver; this phase might be essential for the development of *P. miyazakii* (5,68,69). Human cases of liver involvement infected with the former two species have been reported (68,70,71).

Paragonimus worms may accidentally migrate into unexpected sites. For example, they may migrate across abdominal muscles or pleural wall into the covering skin or through mediastinal soft tissues to the brain. On rare occasions, the worms migrate into urogenital organs or remain in the abdominal cavity to form granulomatous lesions.

B. Clinical Findings

Paragonimiasis is divided into two clinical types, pleuropulmonary and extra-pulmonary paragonimiasis, depending on the sites affected (Fig. 2). Because of the complex migration route, patients express various symptoms depending on the location of worms. Other factors affecting clinical findings are the density of infection and the duration of disease.

Pleuropulmonary Paragonimiasis

Symptoms

Regardless of *Paragonimus* species, main complaints of pleuropulmonary paragonimiasis are respiratory symptoms such as cough, hemosputum, chest pain and dyspnea. Some patients present nonspecific symptoms such as fever, abdominal pain, diarrhea, etc. Clinical manifestations appeared in several reports from various countries are summarized in Table 1 (28,34,53,55,59,72,73). Though over 80% of patients in all the listed countries showed respiratory symptoms, the incidence of each symptom varied ranging from 6.7% to 100%. Asymptomatic cases were noted in American and Japanese reports. Those variances in clinical findings may reflect the worm burden and the timing of diagnosis.

Table 1 Clinical Manifestations of Paragonimiasis Patients from Several Reports

Causative species	Cameroon 2003	Nigeria 2001	Colombia 2000	America 1983	India 1986	Korea 1992	Japan 2001
	P. africanus	*P. uterobilateralis*	*Paragonimus* spp.		*P. westermani*		
Respiratory symptoms (+)	100	ND	100	92.0	ND	ND	79.3
• Cough	100	79.7	100	92.0	61.5	63.3	33.3
• Hemosputum	43.3	77.1	88	64.0	94.9	60.0	20.0
• Chest pain	60.0	48.4	22	ND	61.5	38.0	23.3
• Dyspnea	ND	51.6	22	24.0	ND	38.0	6.7
Non-respiratory symptoms	Yes	ND	ND	ND	Yes	ND	Yes
Asymptomatic	0	ND	0	8.0	ND	ND	17.2
Radiographic abnormalities (+)	73.3	Not included in this study	95.8	92.0	87.2	ND	93.3
• Infiltration	40.0		ND	44	61.5	45	10.0
• Nodular lesions	10.0		ND	20	7.7	25	16.7

• Cavitation	10.0	8.3	20	12.8	ND	6.7
• Other parenchymal lesions	16.7	Cotton-like appearance (most frequent)	24	7.7	ND	0
• Pleural effusion	0	0	48	10.3	28	63.3
• Pneumothorax	0	0	ND	0	8	6.7
• Other pleural lesions	0	0	ND	0	ND	0
No radiographic abnormalities	26.7	4.2	8.0 / 52.0	12.8	ND	6.7
Egg (+) ratio	100 (S/F)	100 (S)	(S)	84.6 (S), 25.6 (F)	38.0 (S)	10 (S/BF)
Diagnosis detection / IDT	Egg detection; Serological test/egg detection	Egg detection; Serological test	Egg detection	detection/CF	Egg	BF

Number shows positive rates (%) of the subjects examined.

Abbreviations: ND, not determined or data not mentioned; S, sputum; F, feces; BF, samples obtained by bronchoscopy; CF, complement fixation test; IDT, intradermal test. *Source:* From Refs. 28, 34, 53, 55, 59, 72, 73.

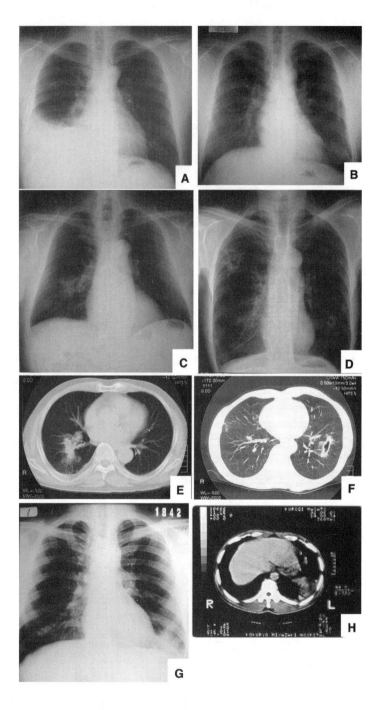

Figure 3   (*Caption on facing page*)

Radioimaging Findings

By chest radiograph, paragonimiasis patients have various abnormalities. In case of Nigeria, the most common shadows are well-defined patches of cavitation, ill-defined cotton wool lesions, streaky shadows, or bubble cavitations in lung parenchyma (74). Predominance of parenchymal lesions in chest radiograph was also recently reported from Cameroon and Colombia (Table 1). Different from those countries, relatively higher proportion of patients with pleural effusion were reported from America, India, and Korea. In Japan, pleurisy in chest radiography was the most frequent finding (Table 1). One possible reason for this difference in the incidence of pleural lesions is that only egg-positive patients were subjected to the study in African and Latin American countries, whereas patients in other countries were diagnosed by a combination of egg detection and immunological tests.

Chest radiographic appearances reflect the localization of worms along their way of migration: pleural lesions such as pleural effusion and pneumothorax are expected to appear at the early stage of the disease, whereas parenchymal lesions such as infiltration, nodular and cavitating lesions develop at the later stage (Fig. 3) (4,72,75). Pleurisy is also common in low-density infection because a single worm in the pleural cavity fails to migrate into lung parenchyma (76). Paragonimiasis patients recently found in Japan and Korea had low-density grade infection and were diagnosed at relatively early stage. Taken all these together, none of the symptoms and chest radiography findings are specific for paragonimiasis. Complication of tuberculosis and paragonimiasis was also reported (77). It is difficult to differentiate paragonimiasis from lung cancer, tuberculosis, or other infectious lung diseases by merely symptoms and chest radiography (4). Recently, a case of pulmonary paragonimiasis mimicking lung cancer on positron emission tomography with fluorodeoxyglucose (FDG-PET) imaging was reported (78).

Paragonimiasis patients do not present any specific findings on computed tomography (CT) and bronchoscopic examination. In rare occasion,

---

Figure 3 (*Facing page*) Various findings of chest radiography and CT of paragonimiasis patients. (**A**) Pleural effusion and (**B**) pneumothorax found in the chest radiography of paragonimiasis westermani patients. (**C, E**) Infiltrations or nodular lesions in the chest radiography and CT from a patient infected with *P. westermani*. (**D**) Mixed parenchymal lesions including cotton-wool lesions in right upper lung field and cavitating lesions in left lower lung field seen in the chest radiography of a patient infected with *P. westermani*. (**F**) A cavitating lesion in the chest CT from the same patient shown in (**D**). (**F, H**) Lung lesions of paragonimiasis miyazakii patients. Note that there are no differences in chest radiographic appearances regardless of the causative species.

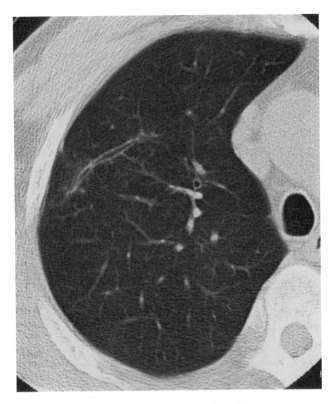

Figure 4   A worm migration truck detected on chest CT.

worm migration truck is detected not only on CT (Fig. 4) but also on chest radiograph as linear opacities, extending from pleura to the lung, running differently from the linear shadow of the bronchovascular bundle. According to Im et al., CT may reveal the presence of an intracystic worm (73). By bronchoscopic examination, stenosis of congested and edematous bronchi are seen in the majority of patients who have parenchymatous lesions (79). In their study, four (30.8%) of 13 patients were egg-positive in usual sputum examination. Eggs were found in six bronchoalveolar lavage (BAL) fluid and/or brushing samples (66.7%) from nine patients who received broncho-scopic examination. Among them, two patients were egg-positive only in BAL fluid or brushing samples.

Laboratory Examinations

Peripheral blood eosinophilia and elevated total IgE level in serum are the important parameters for paragonimiasis and also for other helminthic diseases. Over 80% of paragonimiasis patients showed eosinophilia and/or hyper-IgE (79,80). Despite remarkable eosinophilia, total white blood cell count remains in the normal range or slightly elevated. The degree of eosino-philia is correlated with the stage of the disease. Patients who have pleurisy show significantly higher eosinophilia than those who have parenchymal lesions on chest radiography (4,72). However, the lack of eosinophilia should not be used to rule out the possibility of paragonimiasis or any other hel-minthic diseases. Some patients having parenchymal lesions show normal eosinophil count in their peripheral blood. Those patients would refer to lung surgeons under the suspicion of having lung cancer. When a pulmonary mass lesion is detected in patients who live in paragonimiasis endemic areas, para-gonimiasis should always be considered for differential diagnosis (81). Total IgE level in serum has no correlation with the stage of paragonimiasis (72).

Extrapulmonary Paragonimiasis

Extrapulmonary involvement can be seen along with the normal or aberrant migration of the worms (Fig. 2). Though cutaneous and cerebral paragoni-miasis are the classically known types of extrapulmonary paragonimiasis, every other organs/tissues are possibly involved. A combined pleuropul-monary and extrapulmonary involvement can occur in heavy infection (64,82–84).

Cutaneous Paragonimiasis

A slow-moving induration/swelling is a characteristic lesion in cutaneous paragonimiasis. Such a lesion is preferentially seen on the abdominal or ante-rior chest wall and often precedes the development of lung lesions (84,85). Not only *Paragonimus* spp. but also other parasites such as *Gnathostoma* spp. and *Spirometra* spp. cause similar mobile skin lesions. Since the geogra-phical distributions of these parasites overlap each other, combinations of immunoserological tests and/or skin biopsy together with the history of patient's eating habits should always be considered for differential diagnosis. A juvenile worm is sometimes found in the biopsied specimen of the skin (51,86).

Cerebral Paragonimiasis

Symptom of cerebral paragonimiasis varies depending on the clinical stages. In the acute phase, hemiplegia, and convulsive seizures may appear in asso-ciation with nonspecific symptom including fever, headache, nausea, and vomiting. In the chronic phase, the Jacksonian-type convulsion and/or visual disturbance are found as a result of space occupying lesions (87). It is difficult to distinguish this disease from other central nervous system (CNS) diseases, especially from brain tumors or from other parasitic infec-tions in CNS such as cysticercosis or echinococcosis (88). The early diagno-sis of cerebral paragonimiasis is extremely important because the disease can be curative with appropriate chemotherapy. The most common and characteristic CT or MR imaging findings in the active stage of cerebral paragonimiasis are conglomerated, multiple ring-shaped enhancements with surrounding edema of variable degree, resembling "grape clusters." Sometimes, cerebral hemorrhage is an initial finding (48,89). Together with radio-imaging findings immunoserological tests are useful for the diagnosis. Chronic cerebral paragonimiasis may be suspected by the presence of a "soap-bubble" or "egg-shell" appearance with scattered calcifications on the plain radiographs, CT, or MR of the skull (88). Parasite-specific antibodies are usually not detected in chronic cerebral paragonimiasis.

Other Extrapulmonary Paragonimiasis

Other extrapulmonary sites affected by *Paragonimus* infection are the liver (70,71), peritoneal cavity (90–93), urogenital organs (94–96), pericardial cavity (49,97), breast (98,99), lymph nodes (100), and eye (101). Although most of these cases are found by chance in a postoperative histopathological examination under the diagnosis of nonparasitic diseases, some cases developed acute symptoms depending on the sites affected. In case of *P. skrjabini* infection, which is endemic only in north China, pulmonary symptoms are relatively infrequent (68). Most outstanding clinical manifestations are the migrating subcutaneous nodules, and lesions in the liver, pleura, orbit, brain, and pericardium. In acute ectopic infection, immunoserological tests must be performed for differential diagnosis. Ectopic lesions in urogenital organs are occasionally found by ultrasonographic observations (91,94). Two cases of paragonimiasis of the breast were confirmed by demonstrating many parasite eggs through fine needle aspiration (98,99).

V. Diagnosis

Definitive diagnosis for paragonimiasis can be achieved by detecting characteristic *Paragonimus* eggs in sputum or stool. However, sputum or stool examination is not useful in the early stage of disease, low-density infection, or extrapulmonary infections. Various immunoserological methods have been developed for the diagnosis of paragonimiasis. Skin test as well as stool/sputum examination had been widely used for epidemiological survey in the 1960s because these methods are simple, cheap, and still highly specific. However, since positive skin reaction remains for many years even after successful treatment of the disease, this test is inadequate to discriminate whether an individual case must be treated or not (102). Other immunological methods such as precipitation reaction in gels (Ouchterlony's method and immunoelectrophoresis) (103,104), a complement fixation test (105,106), and an indirect hemagglutination test (107) have gradually been replaced by more sensitive and specific methods like ELISA (108) or enzyme-linked immunoelectrotransfer blotting method (EITB) (109). Attempts were made successfully to detect circulating antigen in serum (110,111) or parasite-specific antigen and DNA in feces of experimentally infected cats (112).

ELISA and EITB have been applied most commonly for the immuno-diagnosis of paragonimiasis. These systems are aimed primarily to detect parasite-specific IgG or sometimes IgE antibodies using somatic or excre-tory-secretory (ES) antigens. To monitor the clinical course of an individual patient or to evaluate the efficacy of treatment, quantitative measurement of parasite-specific IgG or IgE antibody by microplate ELISA or EITB is quite useful. Recently, we have found that the detection of parasite-specific IgM antibody is useful for the diagnosis of paragonimiasis at the early stage (72). Along with the progress of analytical methods and molecular biology, purified or recombinant proteins have been applied for immunoserological tests to obtain high sensitivity and specificity. For example, when antigens purified from *P. heterotremus* somatic extract by affinity chromatography using specific monoclonal antibody (MoAb) were used for antibody detec-tion, the sensitivity and the specificity was 73.7% and 99.2%, respectively. When affinity purified ES antigen was used in the same assay system, sensiti-vity and specificity were both 100% (110). Cysteine proteases purified from *P. westermani* ES products also increased the sensitivity to paragonimiasis sera and reduced the cross-reactivity to fascioliasis sera (113). Cystatin cap-ture ELISA or protein A immunocapture assay can reduce laborious and time-consuming antigen purification processes and applicable for immuno-diagnosis of paragonimiasis and fascioliasis (114,115). The ELISA/EITB using a recombinant protein of yolk ferritin or 28-kDa cruzipain-like cysteine protease of *P. westermani* revealed that the specificity and the sensitivity were 100% and 88.2%, and 98% and 86.2%, respectively (116,117). Purified or recombinant antigens having a specific epitope can contribute to high speci-ficity but not to high sensitivity in ELISA/EITB because patient's serum con-tains polyclonal antibodies against parasite components with various affinity and avidity. Although recombinant protein may overcome the difficulties of collecting parasites and of purification, its production system is expensive and unaffordable in developing countries.

Sputum or stool examination for detecting *Paragonimus* eggs and skin test are still being used in epidemiological survey in developing countries (Table 1). If seroepidemiological survey were conducted in these countries, a bulk of hidden cases will be disclosed. The dot-ELISA/EITB methods are suitable for this purpose because these methods do not need special tools like ELISA plate reader. Multiple-dot ELISA system was developed for the first step of parasite antibody screening because a panel of various para-site antigens can be spotted onto a small piece of nitrocellulose membrane (Fig. 5). This method is useful for the diagnosis not only for parago-nimiasis but also for other parasitic diseases. For example, pulmonary spar-ganosis (118,119) and gnathostomiasis (120) were diagnosed successfully by this method.

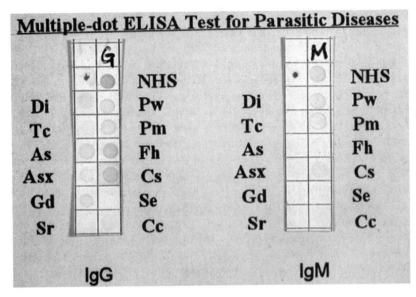

Figure 5 Multiple-dot ELISA test for parasitic diseases. Not only IgG but also IgM antibodies were detected via this method. Patients' body fluids such as serum, pleural effusion, cerebrospinal fluid and cyst fluid could be examined by this method.

VI. Treatment

In the 1960s to 1970s, bithionol has been used extensively for the treatment of paragonimiasis. Due to the requirement of long-term administration and its relatively severe side effects bithionol has gradually been replaced by a new trematodicidal drug, praziquantel (121). Praziquantel is currently the first choice of drug for pulmonary and extrapulmonary paragonimiasis regardless of the causative *Paragonimus* species (4). A dose of 75 mg/kg/day for 3 days is recommended to obtain nearly 100% cure rate. At this dose, it has only mild and transient side effects, if any. When patients are treated with insufficient doses, the cure rate reduced significantly (122). In patients having pleural effusion, pleural fluid must be extensively drained off before starting chemotherapy. Insufficient drainage or delayed diagnosis of paragonimiasis often cause complication such as chronic empyema or insufficient inflation of lungs (123) and sometimes patients should receive for surgical treatment (124).

Triclabendazole is a highly efficient agent for human fascioliasis and listed in WHO essential drugs. According to the drug information, the exact mechanisms of the action of triclabendazole against trematodes have not been fully elucidated. The only information available at the present is that triclabendazole and its active sulfoxide metabolite readily penetrate the tegument of flukes and rapidly inhibit its motility and interfere with its microtubular structure and function. This drug has recently been found to have a parasiti-cidal effect on experimental infection with *P. uterobilateralis* and *P. skrjabini* in rats (125,126) and *P. westermani* in dogs (127). Not only in experimental infection but also in clinical trials, the efficacy of triclabendazole for human paragonimiasis was evaluated. Patients infected with *P. africanus* in Camer-oon were effectively treated with 10 mg/kg at a single dose of triclabendazole (128). However, in the study in Ecuador, where the patients were infected with *P. mexicanus*, the overall cure rates of the different triclabendazole dose were 87.5% by a single dose of 10 mg/kg and 100% by 5 mg/kg/day for 3 days and also by 10 mg/kg twice on 1 day (129). In consistence with the results of Ecua-dor, the cure rate of a single dose of 10 mg/kg for paragonimiasis westermani patients in Japan was 63.6% (130). All patients infected with *P. skrjabini* were cured by a dose of 10 mg/kg for 3 days in China (126). Among those studies, the dosage of the drug and the parameters of evaluation, i.e., egg examination or immunoserological methods, were different from each other. Further eva-luation of triclabendazole against paragonimiasis under the same regimen must be performed.

VII. Clinical Presentation

A. Pulmonary Paragonimiasis

Thirty years old previously healthy female admitted to a regional hospital complaining abdominal pain and fever on January 30, 2003. The patient ate raw wild boar meat at the end of November 2002. Laboratory data on admission revealed that the white blood cell count was 7400/mm^3 with 8.9% eosinophils and CRP was 1.19 mg/dL. A small amount of abdominal fluid was detected on abdominal CT. No other abnormalities were found out. The patient's symptoms resolved spontaneously without any treatment. However, the degree of eosinophilia increased to 19.4% (WBC count was 9200/mm^3) on February 18, 2003. Although the patient was discharged on February 19, 2003, readmission was required to the same hospital for com-plaint of right chest pain on March 10, 2003. At that time, laboratory data were as follows: total WBC, 14000/mm^3 (39.0% neutrophils, 2.9% mono-cytes, 13.0% lymphocytes, 45% eosinophils, 0.1% basophils); total serum IgE, 387 IU/mL; CRP, 3.44 mg/dL. On chest radiography, right cost-phrenic angle was slightly dull. An infiltration shadow in right lower lung field was seen on both chest radiography and CT (Fig. 6A, B). Cytological examination of the BALF sample showed 0.2% neutrophils, 4.2% lymphocytes, 87.8% eosinophils, 5.0% histiocytes, and 2.8% macrophages. Parasite eggs were not detected in stool, sputum, or BALF samples. Since paragonimiasis was strongly suspected, the patient's serum was examined by a multiple-dot ELISA test. It showed strong positive reaction against *P. westermani* antigen with slight cross-reaction to other trematodes, *P. miyazakii*,

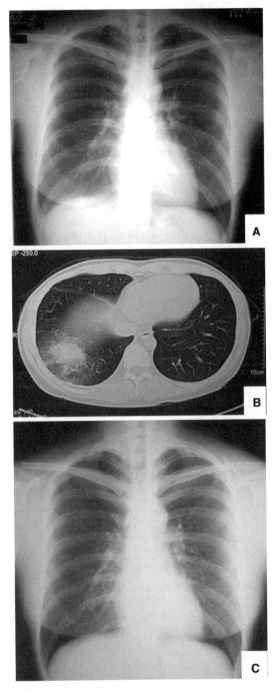

Figure 6   A case of typical pleuropulmonary paragonimiasis westermani. Chest radiography and CT on March 10, 2003 (**A, B**). Chest radiography 4 months after the chemotherapy (**C**).

Clonorchis sinensis, and *Fasciola hepatica*. The patient was successfully treated with praziquantel at a dose of 75 mg/kg/day for 3 days. The number of eosinophil turned normal range within 6 weeks after the treatment. The lung lesion almost disappeared (Fig. 6C) and the serum antibody titer decreased significantly within 4 months after the treatment; IgG-ELISA values (O.D. at 405 nm) of 900-fold diluted patient's sera against *P. westermani* antigen was 1.32 before treatment and 0.53 after treatment.

B. Extrapulmonary Paragonimiasis

A thirty-two-year-old female was admitted to a regional hospital complaining of a right breast tumor in November 2002. The patient was born in Thailand and immigrated to Japan 4 years ago. Since then the patient never goes back to her home country but often eats freshwater crabs and freshwater fishes cooked in Thai-style. Aspiration biopsy from the nodule was performed at the end of December 2002. Aspiration fluid appeared bloody in color. By microscopic observation, the aspirated fluid contained numerous eosinophils, Charcot–Leyden crystals, and parasite eggs of which unidentified species (Fig. 7). Since the nodule gradually enlarged, aspiration biopsy was reperformed on February 5, 2003. Laboratory examination of the aspiration fluid gave the same findings as before. No abnormalities were found out in chest radiography. Serum and the aspiration biopsy fluid of the patient were sent to our laboratory for diagnosis on March 18, 2003. Most of eggs were distorted during processing. Relatively intact eggs were thin-shelled having flattened operculum at one end (Fig. 7A). Not only the egg shape but also its size helps us to identify the parasite species. When 10 eggs were measured microscopically, the average size of eggs and their range were 74.9 (70.0–77.5) × 46.9(41.7–53.0) mm. From these results, they were identified as *P. miyazakii* eggs. By a multiple dot-ELISA test, the patient's serum gave positive reaction against *P. westermani* and *P. miyazakii*. Binding inhibition

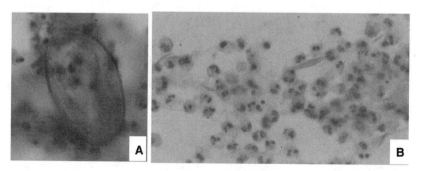

Figure 7 A case of extrapulmonary paragonimiasis miyazakii. Eggs (**A**) and Charcot–Leyden crystals (**B**) found in the aspiration biopsy specimen from the left breast mass.

test in ELISA revealed that her serum had specific antibody against *P. miya-zakii*. Laboratory data at the start of PZQ treatment were as follows: total WBC, 7700/mm^3 (44.0% neutrophils, 3.0% monocytes, 33.0% lymphocytes, 19.0% eosinophils, 1.0% basophils); CRP, 0.1 mg/dL. Three weeks after the praziquantel treatment (75 mg/kg/day for 3 days) the breast lesion disappeared and white blood cell and eosinophil count turned normal.

VIII. Immunology

Immune responses against *Paragonimus* or other helminth infections are characterized as the Th2-type response seen as the elevation of total IgE level in serum and peripheral blood eosinophilia in both experimental models and clinical cases (4,131). Th2-related cytokines and molecules such as IL-5 and soluble CD23/FcεRII, low-affinity receptor for IgE, in serum and culture supernatants of the peripheral blood mononuclear cells were elevated in cutaneous paragonimiasis patients. In their peripheral mononuclear cells, mRNA expression of IL-4, IL-5, IL-10, and IL-13 were also elevated before treatment and decreased after the chemotherapy (132,133). In pleural effusion of patients with paragonimiasis, IL-5 and thymus and activation-regulated chemokine (TARC) were elevated and were assumed to play important roles in mediating eosinophilic inflammation (134,135).

Antibody-dependent cell-mediated cytotoxicity (ADCC) is one of the important host defense mechanisms against helminth parasites (136). Parasite-specific IgE antibody mediates schistosomula killing by macrophages and eosinophils in vitro (137,138). Contribution of parasite-specific IgE in the protective immunity against *Schistosoma* was also reported from the epidemiological study (139). In *S. hematobium* infection, specific IgE production was blocked by early production of IgG4 against the worm and egg antigens, so that protective immunity was established only during reinfection (139). Antibodies including IgE directly act as effectors on functional and morphological impediment of tegument of *P. westermani* metacercariae (140). In contrast, anti-IgE monoclonal antibody treatment, which completely blocked IgE antibody production, did not affect the worm burden in mice infected with *P. westermani* (141). According to Pritchard (142), excessive amount of nonspecific IgE induced by parasite infection would be beneficial to parasite because these molecule occupy FcεRII on macrophage or eosinophils and disarm the effector cells. In fact, the amount of parasite-specific IgE was only 10% of the total IgE in helminth infection (143,144). Thus, further study is necessary to clarify the role of specific and nonspecific IgE antibody in *Paragonimus* infection.

Parasite-specific IgG and eosinophils are also involved in ADCC mechanism against helminth parasites (136). However, cystain proteases secreted by newly excysted *P. westermani* metacercariae (PwNEM) are capable of degrading IgG to attenuate the effector function of human eosinophils activated by immobilized IgG in vitro (145,146). The high concentration of cysteine proteases of PwNEM directly induced eosinophil apoptosis (147). These immune evasion mechanisms may contribute to successful parasitism in the host. On the other hand, when human eosinophils were treated with lower dose of cysteine proteases from PwNEM, significant level of IL-8 production was observed in vitro. IL-8 can prolongate eosinophil survival and may contribute to eosinophil accumulation to parasite-infected lesions, though such effects were not observed by the treatment of cells with higher concentration (148). Thus, cysteine proteases secreted by PwNEM have biphasic effects against eosinophils; higher dose of proteases is beneficial for parasites to accelerate eosinophil apoptosis, whereas low dose of protease regulate eosinophil survival through the autocrine production of GM-CSF resulting in the elicitation of eosinophilic inflammatory responses at the worm-infected lesion in human paragonimiasis (149). Similarly, intraperitoneal injection with the low dose of neutral thiol proteases from *P. westermani* metacercariae induce accumulation of eosinophils and high dose treatment induce immunosuppressive effects in mice (150,151). These biphasic effects of *Paragonimus*-derived proteases may not simply be explained by the dose of antigen because the subtype of proteases secreted by *Paragonimus* are variable and stage specifically expressed along with the development during the migration in the host. More complexly, the susceptibility of mammalian host is determined by not only *Paragonimus* species but also geographical heterogeneity in the genotype (5,10,11).

Experimentally, the number of *P. westermani* worms recovered from immunized dogs was significantly lower than that from unimmunized dogs (152). Interestingly, protective immunity against *P. westermani* was acquired by intraperitoneal injection of the metacercariae but failed by oral administration of the larvae (K. H. Park, J. W. Shin, personal communication). Since there are many cases of repeated *Paragonimus* infection in humans, the protective immunity against *Paragonimus* in humans may not work strongly or parasite has some ability to evade the host immune responses.

IX. The Future

Because of its complex life cycle and wide distribution in the world, it is particularly impossible and difficult to completely eradicate *Paragonimus*. Also it is extremely difficult to change the traditional food habits of the people living in the endemic areas; paragonimiasis will remain forever. A major clinical problem is that paragonimiasis is often ignored not only by physicians but also by diagnosticians. As mentioned above, paragonimiasis can be seen all over the world and often confused with tuberculosis, lung malignancy, and other infectious diseases. To avoid high-cost diagnostic examinations and unnecessary treatment, correct and straightforward diagnosis is necessary. Clinicians should always be aware of the possibility of paragonimiasis when patients have pulmonary lesions.

Acknowledgments

This work is supported in part by a Grant-in-Aid for Scientific Research KH42074 and KH42075 from the Ministry of Health, Welfare and Labor. Our special thanks go to Drs. K. Hiromatsu (Parasitic Diseases Unit, Department of Infectious Diseases, Faculty of Medicine, University of Miyazaki), M. Yoshikawa (Department of Parasitology, Nara Medical University) and H. Mukae (Second Department of Internal Medicine, Nagasaki University School of Medicine) for their valuable advice on this study. We thank also Drs. J. Ashitani (Third Department of Internal Medicine, School of Medicine, University of Miyazaki), T. Hiratsuka (Department of Respiratory Medicine, National Miyazaki-Higashi Hospital), K. Fukutani (Department of Internal Medicine, San-in Rosai Hospital), and N. Ariga (Department of Surgery, National Mito Hospital) for providing us the clinical cases and diagnostic imaging. Excellent technical assistance of Ms A. Tanaka for immunodiagnosis is gratefully acknowledged.

References

1. Marty AM, Neafie RC. Paragonimiasis. In: Mayers WM, ed. Pathology of Infectious Diseases. Vol.1. Helminthiasis. Washington, D.C.: American Forces Institute of Pathology, 2000:49–67.
2. WHO. Control of foodborne trematode infections. Report of a WHO Study Group. World Health Org Tech Rep Ser 1995; 849:1–157.
3. Toscano C, Hai YS, Mott KE. Paragonimiasis and tuberculosis, diagnostic confusion: a review of literature. Trop Dis Bull 1995; 92:R1–R26.
4. Nakamura-Uchiyama F, Mukae H, Nawa Y. Paragonimiasis: a Japanese perspective. Clin Chest Med 2002; 23:409–420.
5. Blair D, XuZB, Agatsuma T. Paragonimiasis and the genus *Paragonimus*. Adv Parasitol 1999; 42:113–222.
6. Little MD. *Paragonimus caliensis* sp. n. and paragonimiasis in Colombia. J Parasitol 1968; 54:738–746.
7. Castilla EA, Jessen R, Sheck DN, Procop GW. Cavitary mass lesion and recurrent pneumothoraces due to *Paragonimus kellicotti* infection: North American paragonimiasis. Am J Surg Pathol 2003; 27:1157–1160.
8. DeFrain M, Hooker R. North American paragonimiasis: case report of a severe clinical infection. Chest 2002; 121:1368–1372.
9. Procop GW, Marty AM, Scheck DN, Mease DR, Maw GM. North American paragonimiasis. A case report. Acta Cytol 2000; 44:75–80.

10. Kanazawa T, Hata H, Kojima S, Yokogawa M. *Paragonimus westermani*: a comparative study on the migration route of the diploid triploid types in the final hosts. Parasitol Res 1987; 73:140–145.

11. Narain K, Rekha Devi K, Mahanta J. A rodent model for pulmonary paragonimiasis. Parasitol Res 2003; 91:517–519.

12. Agatsuma T, Habe S. Electrophoretic studies on enzymes of diploid and triploid *Paragonimus westermani*. Parasitology 1985; 91(Pt 3):489–497.

13. Agatsuma T, Ketudat P, Thaithong S, Shibahara T, Sugiyama H, Habe S, Terasaki K, Kawashima K. Electrophoretic analysis of a natural population of the Thai *Paragonimus heterotremus* and its genetic relationship to the three Japanese species *P. miyazaki*, *P. ohirai* and *P. westermani*. Parasitol Res 1992; 78:463–468.

14. Zillmann U, Sachs R, Ebert F. Isoenzymes of the lung fluke *Paragonimus uterobilateralis* from Liberia. Trop Med Parasitol 1987; 38:320–322.

15. Agatsuma T. Electrophoretic demonstration of polymorphism of glucosephosphate isomerase in natural populations of *Paragonimus miyazakii*. J Parasitol 1981; 67:452–454.

16. Agatsuma T, Iwagami M, Sato Y, Iwashita J, Hong SJ, Kang SY, Ho LY, Su KE, Kawashima K, Abe T. The origin of the triploid in *Paragonimus westermani* on the basis of variable regions in the mitochondrial DNA. J Helminthol 2003; 77:279–285.

17. Iwagami M, Rajapakse RP, Paranagama W, Agatsuma T. Identities of two *Paragonimus* species from Sri Lanka inferred from molecular sequences. J Helminthol 2003; 77:239–245.

18. Park GM, Im KI, Yong TS. Phylogenetic relationship of ribosomal ITS2 and mitochondrial COI among diploid and triploid *Paragonimus westermani* isolates. Korean J Parasitol 2003; 41:47–55.

19. Iwagami M, Monroy C, Rosas MA, Pinto MR, Guevara AG, Vieira JC, Agatsuma Y, Agatsuma T. A molecular phylogeographic study based on DNA sequences from individual metacercariae of *Paragonimus mexicanus* from Guatemala and Ecuador. J Helminthol 2003; 77:33–38.

20. Sugiyama H, Morishima Y, Kameoka Y, Kawanaka M. Polymerase chain reaction (PCR)-based molecular discrimination between *Paragonimus westermani* and *P. miyazakii* at the metacercarial stage. Mol Cell Probes 2002; 16:231–236.

21. Iwagami M, Ho LY, Su K, Lai PF, Fukushima M, Nakano M, Blair D, Kawashima K, Agatsuma T. Molecular phylogeographic studies on *Paragonimus westermani* in Asia. J Helminthol 2000; 74:315–322.

22. van Herwerden L, Blair D, Agatsuma T. Multiple lineages of the mitochondrial gene NADH dehydrogenase subunit 1 (ND1) in parasitic helminths: implications for molecular evolutionary studies of facultatively anaerobic eukaryotes. J Mol Evol 2000; 51:339–352.

23. van Herwerden L, Blair D, Agatsuma T. Intra- and interindividual variation in ITS1 of *Paragonimus westermani* (trematoda: digenea) and related species: implications for phylogenetic studies. Mol Phylogenet Evol 1999; 12:67–73.

24. Blair D, Agatsuma T, Watanobe T, Okamoto M, Ito A. Geographical genetic structure within the human lung fluke, *Paragonimus westermani*, detected from DNA sequences. Parasitology 1997; 115(Pt 4):411–417.

25. Miyazaki I, Habe S. A newly recognized mode of human infection with the lung fluke, *Paragonimus westermani* (Kerbert 1878). J Parasitol 1976; 62:646–648.

26. Miyazaki I, Hirose H. Immature lung flukes first found in the muscle of the wild boar in Japan. J Parasitol 1976; 62:836–837.

27. Vogel H, Crewe W. Observation of the lung fluke infection in Cameroon (West Africa). Z Tropenmed Parasitol 1965; 16:109–125.

28. Moyou-Somo R, Tagni-Zukam D. Paragonimiasis in Cameroon: clinicoradiologic features and treatment outcome. Med Trop (Mars) 2003; 63:163–167.

29. Kum PN, Nchinda TC. Pulmonary paragonimiasis in Cameroon. Trans R Soc Trop Med Hyg 1982; 76:768–772.

30. Moyou-Somo R, Kefie CA, Dreyfuss G, Dumas M. An epidemiological study of pleuropulmonary paragonimiasis among pupils in the peri-urban zone of Kumba town, Meme Division, Cameroon. BMC Public Health 2003; 3:40.

31. Nwokolo C. Outbreak of paragonimiasis in Eastern Nigeria. Lancet 1972; 1:32–33.

32. Udonsi JK. Endemic *Paragonimus* infection in upper Igwun Basin, Nigeria: a preliminary report on a renewed outbreak. Ann Trop Med Parasitol 1987; 81:57–62.

33. Arene FO, Ibanga E, Asor JE. Epidemiology of paragonimiasis in Cross River basin, Nigeria: prevalence and intensity of infection due to *Paragonimus uterobilateralis* in Yakurr local government area. Public Health 1998; 112: 119–122.

34. Ibanga ES, Eyo VM. Pulmonary paragonimiasis in Oban community in Akamkpa Local Government Area, Cross River State, Nigeria: prevalence and intensity of infection. Trans R Soc Trop Med Hyg 2001; 95:159–160.

35. Ibanez N, Fernandez E. Actual state of the paragonimiasis in Peru. Bol Peruano Parasitol 1980; 2:12–18.

36. Cornejo W, Huiza A, Espinoza Y, Alva P, Sevilla C, Centurion W. Paragonimosis in the Cajabamba and Condebamba districts, Cajamarca, Peru. Rev Inst Med Trop Sao Paulo 2000; 42:245–247.

37. Vieira JC, Blankespoor HD, Cooper PJ, Guderian RH. Paragonimiasis in Ecuador: prevalence and geographical distribution of parasitisation of second intermediate hosts with *Paragonimus mexicanus* in Esmeraldas province. Trop Med Parasitol 1992; 43:249–252.

38. Yu SH, Xu LQ, Jiang ZX, Xu SH, Han JJ, Zhu YG, Chang J, Lin JX, Xu FN. Nationwide survey of human parasite in China. Southeast Asian J Trop Med Public Health 1994; 25:4–10.

39. Belizario V, Guan M, Borja L, Ortega A, Leonardia W. Pulmonary paragonimiasis and tuberculosis in Sorsogon, Philippines. Southeast Asian J Trop Med Public Health 1997; 28(suppl 1):37–45.

40. Waree P, Polseela P, Pannarunothai S, Pipitgool V. The present situation of paragonimiasis in endemic area in Phitsanulok Province. Southeast Asian J Trop Med Public Health 2001; 32(suppl 2):51–54.

41. Cho SY, Kong Y, Kang SY. Epidemiology of paragonimiasis in Korea. Southeast Asian J Trop Med Public Health 1997; 28(suppl 1):32–36.

42. Sachs R, Voelker J. Human paragonimiasis caused by *Paragonimus uterobilateralis* in Liberia and Guinea, West Africa. Tropenmed Parasitol 1982; 33:15–16.
43. Monson MH, Koenig JW, Sachs R. Successful treatment with praziquantel of six patients infected with the African lung fluke, *Paragonimus uterobilateralis.* Am J Trop Med Hyg 1983; 32:371–375.
44. Simarro PP, Alamo A, Sima FO, Roche J, Mir M, Ndong P. Endemic human paragonimiasis in Equatorial Guinea. Detection of the existence of endemic human paragonimiasis in Equatorial Guinea as a result of an integrated sanitary programme. Trop Geogr Med 1991; 43:326–328.
45. Petavy AF, Cambon M, Demeocq F, Dechelotte P. A Gabonese case of paragonimiasis in a child. Bull Soc Pathol Exot Filiales 1981; 74:193–197.
46. Sachs R, Kern P, Voelker J. *Paragonimus uterobilateralis* as the cause of 3 cases of human paragonimiasis in Gabon. Tropenmed Parasitol 1983; 34:105–108.
47. Lamothe Argumedo R. Human pulmonary paragonimiasis in Mexico. Salud Publica Mex 1986; 28:37–40.
48. Brenes Madrigal R, Rodriguez-Ortiz B, Vargas Solano G, Ocamp Obando EM, Ruiz Sotela PJ. Cerebral hemorrhagic lesions produced by *Paragonimus mexicanus.* Report of three cases in Costa Rica. Am J Trop Med Hyg 1982; 31:522–526.
49. Saborio P, Lanzas R, Arrieta G, Arguedas A. *Paragonimus mexicanus* pericarditis: report of two cases review of the literature. J Trop Med Hyg 1995; 98:316–318.
50. Alarcon de Noya B, Abreu G, Noya O. Pathological and parasitological aspects of the first autochthonous case of human paragonimiasis in Venezuela. Am J Trop Med Hyg 1985; 34:761–765.
51. Brenes RR, Little MD, Raudales O, Munoz G, Ponce C. Cutaneous paragonimiasis in man in Honduras. Am J Trop Med Hyg 1983; 32:376–378.
52. Aka NA, Allabi AC, Dreyfuss G, Kinde-Gazard D, Tawo L, Rondelaud D, Bouteille B, Avode G, Anagonou SY, Gninafon M, Massougbodji A, Dumas M. Epidemiological observations on the first case of human paragonimiasis and potential intermediate hosts of *Paragonimus* sp. in Benin. Bull Soc Pathol Exot 1999; 92:191–194.
53. Velez ID, Ortega J, Hurtado MI, Salazar AL, Robledo SM, Jimenez JN, Velasquez LE. Epidemiology of paragonimiasis in Colombia. Trans R Soc Trop Med Hyg 2000; 94:661–663.
54. Singh TS, Mutum S, Razaque MA, Singh YI, Singh EY. Paragonimiasis in Manipur. Indian J Med Res 1993; 97:247–252.
55. Singh TS, Mutum SS, Razaque MA. Pulmonary paragonimiasis: clinical features, diagnosis and treatment of 39 cases in Manipur. Trans R Soc Trop Med Hyg 1986; 80:967–971.
56. De NV, Cong LD, Kino H, Son DT, Vien HV. Epidemiology, symptoms and treatment of paragonimiasis in Sin Ho district, Lai Chau province, Vietnam. Southeast Asian J Trop Med Public Health 2000; 31(suppl 1):26–30.
57. De NV, Murrell KD, Cong le D, Cam PD, Chau le V, Toan ND, Dalsgaard A. The food-borne trematode zoonoses of Vietnam. Southeast Asian J Trop Med Public Health 2003; 34(suppl 1):12–34.

58. Johnson JR, Falk A, Iber C, Davies S. Paragonimiasis in the United States. A report of nine cases in Hmong immigrants. Chest 1982; 82:168–171.
59. Johnson RJ, Johnson JR. Paragonimiasis in Indochinese refugees. Roentgenographic findings with clinical correlations. Am Rev Respir Dis 1983; 128:534–538.
60. Yee B, Hsu JI, Favour CB, Lohne E. Pulmonary paragonimiasis in Southeast Asians living in the central San Joaquin Valley. West J Med 1992; 156: 423–425.
61. Rangdaeng S, Alpert LC, Khiyami A, Cottingham K, Ramzy I. Pulmonary paragonimiasis. Report of a case with diagnosis by fine needle aspiration cytology. Acta Cytol 1992; 36:31–36.
62. Burton K, Yogev R, London N, Boyer K, Shulman ST. Pulmonary paragonimiasis in Laotian refugee children. Pediatrics 1982; 70:246–248.
63. Sharma OP. The man who loved drunken crabs. A case of pulmonary paragonimiasis. Chest 1989; 95:670–672.
64. Meehan AM, Virk A, Swanson K, Poeschla EM. Severe pleuropulmonary paragonimiasis 8 years after emigration from a region of endemicity. Clin Infect Dis 2002; 35:87–90.
65. Obara A, Nakamura-Uchiyama F, Hiromatsu K, Nawa Y. Paragonimiasis cases recently found among immigrants in Japan. Intern Med 2004; 43: 388–392.
66. Vuong PN, Bayssade-Dufour C, Mabika B, Ogoula-Gerbeix S, Kombila M. *Paragonimus westermani* pulmonary distomatosis in Gabon. First case. Presse Med 1996; 25:1084–1085.
67. Guiard-Schmid JB, Lacombe K, Osman D, Meynard JL, Febvre M, Meyohas MC, Frottier J. Paragonimiasis: a rare little known disease. Presse Med 1998; 27: 1835–1837.
68. Hu X, Feng R, Zheng Z, Liang J, Wang H, Lu J. Hepatic damage in experimental and clinical paragonimiasis. Am J Trop Med Hyg 1982; 31:1148–1155.
69. Yokogawa M. *Paragonimus* and paragonimiasis. Adv Parasitol 1969; 7:375–387.
70. Sasaki M, Kamiyama T, Yano T, Nakamura-Uchiyama F, Nawa Y. Active hepatic capsulitis caused by *Paragonimus westermani* infection. Intern Med 2002; 41:661–663.
71. Nabeshima K, Inoue T, Sekiya R, Tanigawa M, Koga Y, Imai J, Nawa Y. Intrahepatic paragonimiasis—a case report. Jpn J Parasitol 1991; 40:296–300.
72. Nakamura-Uchiyama F, Onah DN, Nawa Y. Clinical features of paragonimiasis cases recently found in Japan: parasite-specific immunoglobulin M and G antibody classes. Clin Infect Dis 2001; 32:e151–e153.
73. Im JG, Whang HY, Kim WS, Han MC, Shim YS, Cho SY. Pleuropulmonary paragonimiasis: radiologic findings in 71 patients. AJR Am J Roentgenol 1992; 159:39–43.
74. Ogakwu M, Nwokolo C. Radiological findings in pulmonary paragonimiasis as seen in Nigeria: a review based on one hundred cases. Br J Radiol 1973; 46:699–705.
75. Im JG, Kong Y, Shin YM, Yang SO, Song JG, Han MC, Kim CW, Cho SY, Ham EK. Pulmonary paragonimiasis: clinical and experimental studies. Radiographics 1993; 13:575–586.

76. Yokogawa M. *Paragonimus* and paragonimiasis. In: Morishita KK, Matsubayashi HY, eds. Progress of Medical Parasitology in Japan. Vol. 1. English ed. Tokyo: Meguro Parasitological Museum, 1964:63–156.
77. Ishikawa R, Higa T, Yoshida A, Kumamoto K, Ishikawa N, Tomita M, Maruyama H, Nawa Y. A case report of pulmonary paragonimiasis with pulmonary tuberculosis. Jpn J Parasitol 1995; 44:254–257.
78. Watanabe S, Nakamura Y, Kariatsumari K, Nagata T, Sakata R, Zinnouchi S, Date K. Pulmonary paragonimiasis mimicking lung cancer on FDG-PET imaging. Anticancer Res 2003; 23:3437–3440.
79. Mukae H, Taniguchi H, Matsumoto N, Iiboshi H, Ashitani J, Matsukura S, Nawa Y. Clinicoradiologic features of pleuropulmonary *Paragonimus westermani* on Kyusyu Island, Japan. Chest 2001; 120:514–520.
80. Nakamura-Uchiyama F, Onah DN, Nawa Y. Clinical features and parasite-specific IgM/IgG antibodies of paragonimiasis patients recently found in Japan. Southeast Asian J Trop Med Public Health 2001; 32(suppl 2):55–58.
81. Tomita M, Matsuzaki Y, Nawa Y, Onitsuka T. Pulmonary paragonimiasis referred to the Department of Surgery. Ann Thorac Cardiovasc Surg 2000; 6:295–298.
82. Ashitani J, Kumamoto K, Matsukura S. *Paragonimiasis westermani* with multifocal lesions in lungs and skin. Intern Med 2000; 39:433–436.
83. Okamoto M, Miyake Y, Shouji S, Fujikawa T, Tamaki A, Takeda Z, Nawa Y. A case of severe *Paragonimiasis miyazakii* with lung and skin lesions showing massive egg production in sputum and faeces. Jpn J Parasitol 1993; 42: 429–433.
84. Dainichi T, Nakahara T, Moroi Y, Urabe K, Koga T, Tanaka M, Nawa Y, Furue M. A case of cutaneous paragonimiasis with pleural effusion. Int J Dermatol 2003; 42:699–702.
85. Mizuki M, Mitoh K, Miyazaki E, Tsuda T. A case of *paragonimiasis westermani* with pleural effusion eight months after migrating subcutaneous induration of the abdominal wall. Nihon Kyobu Shikkan Gakkai Zasshi 1992; 30:1125–1130.
86. Ogata K, Miyagi T, Inoue S, Imai J, Nawa Y. Cutaneous paragonimiasis—a case report. Jpn J Parasitol 1990; 39:63–66.
87. Toyonaga S, Kurisaka M, Mori K, Suzuki N. Cerebral paragonimiasis—report of five cases. Neurol Med Chir (Tokyo) 1992; 32:157–162.
88. Im JG, Chang KH, Reeder MM. Current diagnostic imaging of pulmonary and cerebral paragonimiasis, with pathological correlation. Semin Roentgenol 1997; 32:301–324.
89. Cha SH, Chang KH, Cho SY, Han MH, Kong Y, Suh DC, Choi CG, Kang HK, Kim MS. Cerebral paragonimiasis in early active stage: CT and MR features. AJR Am J Roentgenol 1994; 162:141–145.
90. Shimao Y, Koono M, Ochiai A, Fujito A, Ide H, Kobayashi T, Maruyama H, Itoh H, Nawa Y. A case report of intraperitoneal granuloma due to occult infection with *Paragonimus* sp. Jpn J Parasitol 1994; 43:315–317.
91. Jeong YY, Kang HK, Oh BR, Ryu SB. Paragonimiasis mimicking urachal cyst. J Comput Assist Tomogr 1998; 22:91–92.

92. Jeong WK, Kim Y, Kim YS, Park DW, Park CK, Baek HK, Park YW. Hetero-topic paragonimiasis in the omentum. J Comput Assist Tomogr 2002; 26: 1019–1021.

93. Lee SC, Jwo SC, Hwang KP, Lee N, Shieh WB. Discovery of encysted *Paragonimus westermani* eggs in the omentum of an asymptomatic elderly woman. Am J Trop Med Hyg 1997; 57:615–618.

94. Hahn ST, Park SH, Kim CY, Shinn KS. Adrenal paragonimiasis simulating adrenal tumor—a case report. J Korean Med Sci 1996; 11:275–277.

95. Lee YH, Park EH, Kim WC, Choi YD, Park JH. A case of pelvic paragoni-miasis combined with myoma uteri and pelvic inflammatory disease. Korean J Parasitol 1993; 31:295–297.

96. Lin CM, Chen SK. Paragonimus calcified ova mimicking left renal staghorn stone. J Urol 1993; 149:819–820.

97. Iwahashi N, Suzuki F, Tamura S, Kawai Y, Miyake M, Matsuda Y, Maeda J, Nakano T, Hada T, Higashino K. A case of paragonimiasis miyazakii with bilateral pleural and pericardial effusion. Nihon Kyobu Shikkan Gakkai Zasshi 1991; 29:1047–1051.

98. Jun SY, Jang J, Ahn SH, Park JM, Gong G. Paragonimiasis of the breast. Report of a case diagnosed by fine needle aspiration. Acta Cytol 2003; 47:685–687.

99. Fogel SP, Chandrasoma PT. Paragonimiasis in a cystic breast mass: case report and implications for examination of aspirated cyst fluids. Diagn Cytopathol 1994; 10:229–231.

100. Xialong J, Weihua L. Inguinal lymph node infection with paragonimiasis. Hum Pathol 1991; 22:842.

101. Wang WJ, Xin YJ, Robinson NL, Ting HW, Ni C, Kuo PK. Intraocular para-gonimiasis. Br J Ophthalmol 1984; 68:85–88.

102. Choi DW. *Paragonimus* and paragonimiasis in Korea. Kisaengchunghak Chapchi 1990; 28(suppl):79–102.

103. Katamine D, Imai J, Iwamoto I. Immunological study on paragonimiasis. Agar-gel precipitin reactions in paragonimiasis. Trop Med 1968; 10:28–38.

104. Tsuji M. On the immunoelectrophoresis for helminthological researches. Jpn J Parasitol 1974; 23:335–345.

105. Chung HL, Weng HC, Hou TC, Ho LY. The value of complement fixation test and intradermal test in the diagnosis of paragonimiasis. Chin Med J 1955; 73:47–54.

106. Sadun EH, Buck AA, Walton BC. The diagnosis of *Paragonimiasis westermani* using purified antigens in intradermal and complement fixation tests. Mil Med 1959; 124:187–195.

107. Pariyanonda S, Maleewong W, Pipitgool V, Wongkham C, Morakote N, Intapan P, Thirakharn B, Boonphadung N. Serodiagnosis of human paragoni-miasis caused by *Paragonimus heterotremus*. Southeast Asian J Trop Med Public Health 1990; 21:103–107.

108. Waikagul J. Serodiagnosis of paragonimiasis by enzyme-linked immunosor-bent assay and immunoelectrophoresis. Southeast Asian J Trop Med Public Health 1989; 20:243–251.

109. Slemenda SB, Maddison SE, Jong EC, Moore DD. Diagnosis of paragonimiasis by immunoblot. Am J Trop Med Hyg 1988; 39:469–471.
110. Maleewong W, Intapan PM, Priammuenwai M, Wongkham C, Tapchaisri P, Morakote N, Chaicumpa W. Monoclonal antibodies to *Paragonimus heterotremus* and their potential for diagnosis of paragonimiasis. Am J Trop Med Hyg 1997; 56:413–417.
111. Zhang Z, Zhang Y, Shi Z, Sheng K, Liu L, Hu Z, Piessens WF. Diagnosis of active *Paragonimus westermani* infections with a monoclonal antibody-based antigen detection assay. Am J Trop Med Hyg 1993; 49:329–334.
112. Maleewong W, Intapan PM, Wongkham C, Wongratanacheewin S, Tapchaisri P, Morakote N, Chaicumpa W. Detection of *Paragonimus heterotremus* in experimentally infected cat feces by antigen capture-ELISA and by DNA hybridization. J Parasitol 1997; 83:1075–1078.
113. Ikeda T, Oikawa Y, Nishiyama T. Enzyme-linked immunosorbent assay using cysteine proteinase antigens for immunodiagnosis of human paragonimiasis. Am J Trop Med Hyg 1996; 55:435–437.
114. Ikeda T. Cystatin capture enzyme-linked immunosorbent assay for immunodiagnosis of human paragonimiasis and fascioliasis. Am J Trop Med Hyg 1998; 59:286–290.
115. Ikeda T. Protein A immunocapture assay detecting antibodies to fluke cysteine proteinases for immunodiagnosis of human paragonimiasis and fascioliasis. J Helminthol 2001; 75:245–249.
116. Kim TY, Joo IJ, Kang SY, Cho SY, Kong Y, Gan XX, Sukomtason K, Hong SJ. Recombinant *Paragonimus westermani* yolk ferritin is a useful serodiagnostic antigen. J Infect Dis 2002; 185:1373–1375.
117. Yun DH, Chung JY, Chung YB, Bahk YY, Kang SY, Kong Y, Cho SY. Structural and immunological characteristics of a 28-kilodalton cruzipain-like cysteine protease of *Paragonimus westermani* expressed in the definitive host stage. Clin Diagn Lab Immunol 2000; 7:932–939.
118. Ishii H, Mukae H, Inoue Y, Kadota JI, Kohno S, Uchiyama F, Nawa Y. A rare case of eosinophilic pleuritis due to sparganosis. Intern Med 2001; 40:783–785.
119. Tanaka S, Maruyama H, Ishiwata K, Nawa Y. A case report of pleural sparganosis. Parasitol Int 1997; 46:73–75.
120. Miyamoto N, Mishima K, Nagatomo K, Ishikawa N, T O, Eto T, Kobayashi T, Maruyama H, Nawa Y. A case report of serologically diagnosed pulmonary gnathostomiasis. Jpn J Parasitol 1994; 43:397–400.
121. Rim HJ. Therapy of fluke infections in the past. A review. Arzneimittelforschung 1984; 34:1127–1129.
122. Rim HJ. Paragonimiasis: experimental and clinical experience with praziquantel in Korea. Arzneimittelforschung 1984; 34:1197–1203.
123. Norimatsu Y. Paragonimiasis. J Ther 1993; 73:2435–2438.
124. Tomita M, Ishinari H, Matsuzaki Y, Shibata K, Koga Y, Yamaguchi R, Mukae H, Masumoto H, Matsukura S, Maruyama H, Nawa Y. A case of chronic pleural empyema by *Paragonimus westermani* infection resistant to chemotherapy and cured by surgical decortication. Jpn J Parasitol 1996; 45: 242–246.

125. Weber P, Buscher G, Buttner DW. The effects of triclabendazole on the lung fluke, *Paragonimus uterobilateralis* in the experimental host *Sigmodon hispidus*. Trop Med Parasitol 1988; 39:322–324.

126. Gao J, Liu Y, Wang X, Hu P. Triclabendazole in the treatment of *Paragonimiasis skrjabini*. Chin Med J (Engl) 2003; 116:1683–1686.

127. Liu Y, Gao J, Wang X, Yu D, Su Q. Experimental observation of effects of triclabendazole on *Paragonimus westermani* infection in dogs. Chin Med J (Engl) 1999; 112:345–348.

128. Ripert C, Couprie B, Moyou R, Gaillard F, Appriou M, Tribouley-Duret J. Therapeutic effect of triclabendazole in patients with paragonimiasis in Cameroon: a pilot study. Trans R Soc Trop Med Hyg 1992; 86:417.

129. Calvopina M, Guderian RH, Paredes W, Chico M, Cooper PJ. Treatment of human pulmonary paragonimiasis with triclabendazole: clinical tolerance and drug efficacy. Trans R Soc Trop Med Hyg 1998; 92:566–569.

130. Nakamura-Uchiyama F, Nawa Y. Efficacy of triclabendazole in patients with fascioliasis and paragonimiasis westermani. Clin Parasitol 2003; 14:107–109.

131. Min DY, Ryu JS, Shin MH. Changes of IgE production, splenic helper and suppressor T lymphocytes in mice infected with *Paragonimus westermani*. Korean J Parasitol 1993; 31:231–238.

132. Matsumoto T, Kimura S, Yamauchi M, Nawa Y, Miike T. Soluble CD23 and IL-5 levels in the serum and culture supernatants of peripheral blood mononuclear cells in a girl with cutaneous paragonimiasis: case report. Ann Trop Paediatr 1998; 18:49–53.

133. Hatano Y, Katagiri K, Ise T, Yamaguchi T, Itami S, Nawa Y, Takayasu S. Expression of Th1 and Th2 cytokine mRNAs in freshly isolated peripheral blood mononuclear cells of a patient with cutaneous paragonimiasis. J Dermatol Sci 1999; 19:144–147.

134. Taniguchi H, Mukae H, Matsumoto N, Tokojima M, Katoh S, Matsukura S, Ogawa K, Kohno S, Nawa Y. Elevated IL-5 levels in pleural fluid of patients with *Paragonimiasis westermani*. Clin Exp Immunol 2001; 123:94–98.

135. Matsumoto N, Mukae H, Nakamura-Uchiyama F, Ashitani JI, Abe K, Katoh S, Kohno S, Nawa Y, Matsukura S. Elevated levels of thymus and activation-regulated chemokine (TARC) in pleural effusion samples from patients infested with *Paragonimus westermani*. Clin Exp Immunol 2002; 130:314–318.

136. Pearce EJ, Scott PA, Sher A. Immune regulation in parasitic infection and disease. In: Paul WE, ed. Fundamental Immunology. Philadelphia: Lippincott-Raven Publishers, 1999:1271–1294.

137. Capron M, Spiegelberg HL, Prin L, Bennich H, Butterworth AE, Pierce RJ, Ouaissi MA, Capron A. Role of IgE receptors in effector function of human eosinophils. J Immunol 1984; 132:462–468.

138. Auriault C, Capron M, Capron A. Activation of rat and human eosinophils by soluble factor(s) released by *Schistosoma mansoni* schistosomula. Cell Immunol 1982; 66:59–69.

139. Hagan P, Blumenthal UJ, Dunn D, Simpson AJ, Wilkins HA. Human IgE, IgG4 and resistance to reinfection with *Schistosoma haematobium*. Nature 1991; 349:243–245.

140. Min DY, Ahn MH, Kim KM, Leem MH, Park SY. The effects of antibodies and complement in macrophage-mediated cytotoxicity on metacercariae of the lung fluke, *Paragonimus westermani*. Kisaengchunghak Chapchi 1990; 28:91–100.

141. Shin MH, Min HK. Effects of anti-IgE mAb on serum IgE, Fc epsilon RII/ CD23 expression on splenic B cells and worm burden in mice infected with *Paragonimus westermani*. Korean J Parasitol 1997; 35:47–54.

142. Pritchard DI. Immunity to helminths: is too much IgE parasite—rather than host-protective? Parasite Immunol 1993; 15:5–9.

143. Rousseaux-Prevost R, Capron M, Bazin H, Capron A. IgE in experimental schistosomiasis. II. Quantitative determination of specific IgE antibodies against *S. mansoni*: a follow-up study of two strains of infected rats. Correlation with protective immunity. Immunology 1978; 35:33–39.

144. Dessaint JP, Bout D, Wattre P, Capron A. Quantitative determination of specific IgE antibodies to *Echinococcus granulosus* and IgE levels in sera from patients with hydatid disease. Immunology 1975; 29:813–823.

145. Chung YB, Yang HJ, Kang SY, Kong Y, Cho SY. Activities of different cysteine proteases of *Paragonimus westermani* in cleaving human IgG. Korean J Parasitol 1997; 35:139–142.

146. Shin MH, Kita H, Park HY, Seoh JY. Cysteine protease secreted by *Paragonimus westermani* attenuates effector functions of human eosinophils stimulated with immunoglobulin G. Infect Immun 2001; 69:1599–1604.

147. Shin MH. Excretory-secretory product of newly excysted metacercariae of *Paragonimus westermani* directly induces eosinophil apoptosis. Korean J Parasitol 2000; 38:17–23.

148. Shin MH, Lee SY. Proteolytic activity of cysteine protease in excretory-secretory product of *Paragonimus westermani* newly excysted metacercariae pivotally regulates IL-8 production of human eosinophils. Parasite Immunol 2000; 22:529–533.

149. Shin MH, Seoh JY, Park HY, Kita H. Excretory-secretory products secreted by *Paragonimus westermani* delay the spontaneous cell death of human eosinophils through autocrine production of GM-CSF. Int Arch Allergy Immunol 2003; 132:48–57.

150. Hamajima F, Yamamoto M, Tsuru S, Yamakami K, Fujino T, Hamajima H, Katsura Y. Immunosuppression by a neutral thiol protease from parasitic helminth larvae in mice. Parasite Immunol 1994; 16:261–273.

151. Hamajima F, Yamakami K, Tsuru S. Experimental eosinophil accumulation in mice by a thiol protease from metacercariae of *Paragonimus westermani*. Jpn J Parasitol 1986; 35:63–65.

152. Chyu I. Studies on the experimental paragonimiasis. II. Immunological study on dog paragonimiasis. Kyoto Daigaku Kekkaku Kenkyusho Kiyo 1962; 5:251–259.

14

Hydatid Lung Disease

BRUNO GOTTSTEIN

Institute of Parasitology, Vetsuisse Faculty
and Faculty of Medicine,
University of Bern,
Bern, Switzerland

JÜRG REICHEN

Department of Clinical Pharmacology,
University Hospital of Bern,
Bern, Switzerland

I. Introduction

Two *Echinococcus* species exhibit medical relevance as causative agent of pulmonary forms of echinococcosis. Most importantly, infections with *Echinococcus granulosus* result in "cystic hydatid disease" or "cystic echinococcosis (CE)," which affects the lungs in a considerable ratio of cases. *Echinococcus multilocularis*, causing "alveolar echinococcosis" (AE), affects the lungs relatively rarely and then usually upon metastasizing from primary hepatic lesions.

E. *granulosus* is a small cestode tapeworm living predominantly in dogs and other canine final hosts (life cycle shown in Fig. 1). Tapeworm eggs shed in their feces are infective for intermediate hosts, including humans beside mainly many domestic animal species (e.g., sheep, goats, cattle horses, pigs, and others). Ingestion of *E. granulosus* eggs by intermediate hosts is followed by the release of an oncosphere; this larva is subsequently transported through blood or lymph to primary target organs. The effect of the hepatic and pulmonary capillary sieves in retaining the parasite is largely responsible for the main distribution of the disease in the liver and

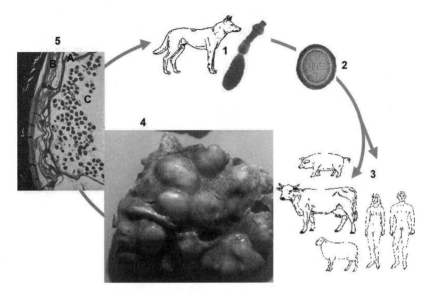

Figure 1   Life cycle of *Echinococcus granulosus*. Adult tapeworms parasitize in the small intestine of definitive hosts, mainly dogs [1]. Parasite eggs [2] are shed with the feces, being infectious for intermediate hosts including many domestic animal species, man can accidentally act as intermediate host as well [3]. Hydatid cysts formation occurs predominantly in the liver and lungs [4]. Histologically, the cyst by itself consists of a very thin inner germinal layer (**A**), externally protected by an acellular laminated layer (**B**) of variable thickness [5]. The endogenous formation of brood capsules and protoscolices (**C**) is a prerequisite for termination of the life cycle, which occurs when definitive hosts ingest protoscolex-containing hydatid cysts.

lungs. Within the affected organ(s), the oncosphere matures into a vesicle, which grows expansively by concentric enlargement. A fully mature hydatid cyst, normally fluid-filled and unilocular, represents the final stage within the intermediate host. The cyst consists of an inner germinal and nucleated syncytial layer supported externally by a carbohydrate-rich acellular laminated layer of variable thickness, surrounded by a host-produced fibrous adventitial layer. Daughter cysts may develop within larger primary cysts, leading to the classical segmentation of a cyst as found upon imaging rocedures. Endogenous formation of brood capsules and protoscolices terminate the maturation of cysts, such protoscolices would grow to the adult stage once ingested by a definitive host.

   The natural life cycle of *E. multilocularis* involves predominantly red and arctic foxes as definitive hosts, domestic dogs and house cats can also become infected and—due to their close contact with human beings—may represent an important infection source in highly endemic areas (life cycle shown in Fig. 2). In the definitive host, egg production starts as early

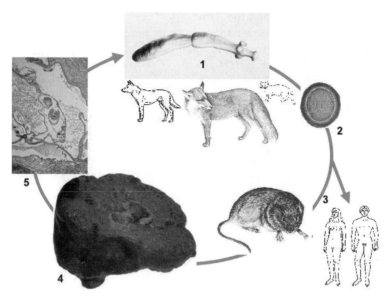

Figure 2 The life cycle of *E. multilocularis* involves predominantly foxes as definitive hosts [1], but other carnivores such as dogs or cats can become infected as well. When parasite eggs [2], shed by the feces of definitive hosts, are ingested by a suitable intermediate host [3] including various rodents and accidentally man, the parasite metacestode will primarily establish in the liver. Metastases may form in adjacent organs such as lungs among other sites. Macroscopically, the typical lesion is characterized by a dispersed mass of fibrous tissue with a multitude of interconnected vesicles ranging from a few millimetres to centimetres in size [4]. The peroral uptake of protoscoleces-containing metacestodes [5] be definitive hosts—e.g., when eating infected mice—terminates the life cycle.

as 28 days after infection. Following egg ingestion by an intermediate host (including normally rodents, but accidentally also humans), an oncosphere is released, which will enter the intestinal venous and lymphatic system. Subsequently, most of the oncospheres will develop in the liver; some may rarely reach lungs or other organs. The parasite then further develops by cellular proliferation, vesicularization, and endogenous and exogenous budding from the primary metacestode tissue, this occurs in a progressive, tumor-like manner. AE will primarily occur within the liver tissue in most cases. Primary lung affection without liver involvement is not described. However, subsequent metastasis formation from the liver may occur into the lungs or other adjacent or distant tissues in approximately 20% of AE cases.

II. Epidemiology and Genetics

E. granulosus has basically a worldwide distribution; however, relevant public health problems focus predominantly on countries of South and Central

America, the European and the African part of the Mediterranean area, the Middle East and some sub-Saharan countries, Russia, China, and some other Asian areas. Most cases observed in Central Europe and the United States are related to immigration of persons from highly endemic areas. Various strains of *E. granulosus* have been described so far, differing especially also in infectivity to humans. The most relevant for human infection are the sheep and the cattle strain (1).

The main areas affected by *E. multilocularis* are all restricted to the northern hemisphere. For America, they include specifically the subarctic regions of Alaska and Canada and some other central states of the United States, for Europe central and eastern France, Switzerland, Austria, and Germany, for Asian the whole zone of tundra, from the White Sea eastwards to the Bering strait, covering large parts of the Soviet Union, and some parts of China and northern Japan (2). The European endemic areas were claimed to have extended north- and eastwards, now also including countries such as Belgium, the Netherlands, Poland, Czechia, and Slovakia (3).

Concerning *E. granulosus*, infection risk was shown to associate to genetically fixed differences in pathogenicity between parasite genotypes from different host species. Thus, identification of strain-specific nucleotide sequences for a number of genes of *E. granulosus* has enabled up to nine genotypes (strains) to be characterized. Although the dog–sheep strain appears responsible for the majority of zoonotic CE infections, recent studies also indicate human infections with camel and pig genotypes (4). Genetic heterogeneity appears much less in *E. multilocularis* (5).

Some evidence has been found in animal intermediate hosts that susceptibility to larval infection with *Echinococcus* spp. is restricted by individual host factors. The search for respective susceptibility markers in human patients, based on MHC class II (DR, DQ, and DP) polymorphism, indicated some association between AE and HLA: In patients with progressive disease, DR3 and DQ2 was more frequent; the HLA DR11 antigen was associated with a reduced risk for disease development in AE; an increase of DR13 was noted in the group of cured AE patients (6,7). For *E. granulosus*, the carriage of HLA-B5 and B18 antigens determined a high risk of infection of the lungs and liver, conversely, HLA-B27 antigen appeared less frequently in such patients than in healthy controls (8).

III. Clinical Presentation

A. CE

The early phase following primary infection is always asymptomatic. Dependent upon the size and the site of the developing hydatid cyst, the infection can remain asymptomatic for months, years, or even longer. After a highly variable incubation period, the infestation may become symptomatic due to a range of different events:

a. The growing cyst exerts pressure on or induces dysformation of adjacent tissues, thus inducing dysfunction of the affected organ or vascular compromise. Thus, infestation of the lungs may then present with chronic cough, hemoptysis, bilioptysis, pneumothorax, pleuritis, lung abscess, and parasitic lung embolism.

b. A cyst may rupture and spill its content into the adjacent site. When a cyst ruptures, there is an abrupt onset of cough, expectoration and fever, sometimes followed by an acute hypersensitivity, thus representing a life-threatening manifestation. After the cyst has ruptured into the bronchial tree its membrane may float on the fluid within the cyst give rise to the classic "water-lily sign." This sign may also be seen in pleural fluid when rupture of the cyst into the pleural space has resulted in hydropneumothorax (9).

c. The cyst can become superinfected, either intracystic or subphrenic, both being an indication for rapid surgical intervention (10).

The majority of patients with CE—independent of the affected organ—have single organ involvement with solitary cysts. Simultaneous involvement of two or more organs is observed in 10–15% of patients, dependent on the geographical origin of the patient and the strain of the parasite, respectively. Approximately 10% of hepatic CE cases occur in children, whereas the rate of lung affection is significantly increased among this group of young patients and may reach 50% (11). Primary symptoms in patients with pulmonary CE include cough, fever, and chest pain (12). Cysts in the lungs are multiple in 20–30% of patients. The size of such cysts ranges from 1 to over 20 cm in diameter (9). The majority of pulmonary cysts are located in the lower lobes, more often posteriorly than anteriorly. Approximately 50% of cysts are localized in the right lung, 40% in the left lung, and 10% bilaterally.

Lung cysts are relatively often bacterially infected and this is best detected by CT scanning (13). Superinfection such as by *Haemophilus influenzae* eventually required lobectomy (12). Bronchial fistulization is an important event in the evolution of the cyst. Intrapleural rupture constitutes a rare eventuality, but it is often as characteristic as it is severe. Secondary, metastatic hydatidosis, due to breaking of a primary visceral cyst in a vein or heart, is rare (14). Rothlin (15) reported about a recurring hydatid cyst of the liver located in segment 8 adjacent to both inferior vena cava and right hepatic vein. During the operation, after application of traction on the liver the patient suddenly went into cardiac arrest. Following a Trendelenburg operation, a massive embolus of echinococcal material was revealed in the paracentral branches of the pulmonary artery. Resuscitation was unsuccessful. The conclusions from this and other similar deaths (Fig. 3) were that an adequate incision is mandatory, no traction on the liver should be necessary, and total vascular exclusion of the liver before cyst drainage and extracorporal bypass appears necessary (15).

B. AE

The initial phase of primary *E. multilocularis* infection is always hepatic and asymptomatic. Dependent upon the size and the site of the developing parasite lesion, the infection may remain asymptomatic for years or even decades (5–15 years). Subsequently, the infection may become symptomatic due to a range of different events: the growing parasite tissue exerts pressure on or induces dysformation of adjacent tissues and induces complication by dysfunction of the affected organ. Growth can also be expansive—thus invading, e.g., the lungs through the diaphragm. With regard to this rare event of secondary pulmonary involvement, symptoms may mimic those of lung cancer (16–19).

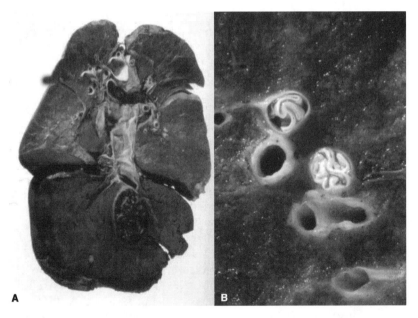

Figure 3 Autopsy findings of an intraoperatively deceased patients with cystic echinococcosis of multiple organ affection. A large hepatic cyst invading the *cava inferior* is shown, resulting also in a massive *E. granulosus* embolism within the central *Arteria pulmonalis* (**A**). Multiple folded *E. granulosus* cyst wall layers lead to embolism within the pulmonary arteria (**B**). *Source*: Courtesy of Prof. R. Ammann, University Hospital of Zürich.

IV. Pathogenesis

A. CE

CE is clinically related to the presence of a well-delineated spherical primary cysts, most frequently formed in the liver and lungs (60% and 20–30% of cases, respectively), and much less frequently in the kidney, bone, heart, spleen, pancreas, and organs of the head and neck including the brain. Pathogenetically, tissue damage and organ dysfunction results mainly from the gradual process of space-occupying repression or displacement of vital host tissue or whole organs. Conversely to the liver and other organs, lung affection remains longly asymptomatic in most cases, unless cyst rupture or leakage occurs (see below). The histology of a typical hydatid cyst demonstrates the germinal layer as primary site of parasite development, surrounded by a parasite-derived thick laminated layer strongly stainable with periodic acid Schiff's solution (Fig. 1). The germinal layer may form protoscolices and brood capsules within the cyst lumen. Granulae, calcareous corpuscles, and occasionally free daughter cysts are often observed. The parasite may evoke an immune response, which will be involved in the formation of a host-derived adventitious capsule. Accidental rupture of cysts can be followed by a massive release of cyst fluid and dissemination of protoscolices, resulting occasionally in anaphylactic reactions and in multiple secondary CE, as protoscolices have the potential to develop into secondary cysts.

B. AE

The *E. multilocularis* metacestode (larva) will develop in infected human patients primarily in the liver. Occasionally, secondary lesions may form metastases in the lungs, brain, and other organs (20). Formation of echinococcal lung metastases may become a problem within recurrence of AE in the liver graft after liver transplantation (21). An exceptional form of hepatic AE with metastasis of the right atrium has been reported by Etievent et al. (18). This cardiac location of the parasitosis was revealed by attacks of pulmonary embolism, which produced secondary pulmonary lesions. This case suggested that pulmonary metastases of AE of the liver might be due to the migration of parasitic clots from the hepatic veins.

Principally, typical AE lesions appears macroscopically as a dispersed mass of fibrous tissue (Fig. 2) with a conglomerate of scattered cavities ranging each from a few millimeters to centimeters in size (22). In advanced chronic cases, a central necrotic cavity can be formed, which contains a viscous fluid with rarely a bacterial superinfection. The lesion often contains focal zones of calcification localized within the metacestode tissue. Parasite proliferation is usually accompanied by a granulomatous host reaction including a vigorous synthesis of fibrous and germinative tissue in the periphery of the metacestode, but also of regressive changes centrally. The host mechanisms modulating the course of infection are most likely of immunological nature and include primarily T-cell interactions and respective (pro) inflammatory cytokine and chemokine activities, e.g., resulting in NO-mediated periparasitic immunosuppression (23) and T-cell independent antibody synthesis (23).

V. Immunology

A. CE

Immunologically, during the early stage of CE the parasite activates complement, and hence complement-dependent inflammatory responses. However, on differentiation into the hydatid cyst, the parasite exposes to the host its laminated layer that does not activate complement strongly (24). Mechanisms inhibiting complement activation on the cyst wall have been elucidated, contributing to the understanding of how the inflammatory response is controlled during CE. Basically, the host–parasite relationship is sustained as a dynamic equilibrium between parasite growth and acquired immunity, the balance being subject to mutual regulation and including the possibility of spontaneous rejection of the parasite (25). Immunoregulatory events have been linked to the generation of T-suppressor populations and to impairing the accessory action of macrophages in lymphoproliferative responses. Local immune modulation by the parasite has been shown to enhance susceptibility to mycobacterial infections close to the site of parasite lesions (26). The coexistence of elevated quantities of IFN-γ, IL-4, IL-5, IL-6, and IL-10 observed in most of hydatid patients supports Th1 and Th2 cell activation in CE. In particular, Th1 cell activation seemed to be more related to protective immunity, whereas Th2 cell activation to susceptibility to disease (27). Thus, Ortona et al. (28) were postulating the following features to be characteristic for the host–parasite relationship in CE: (1) immunoglobulin isotype profiles differ in patients with distinct clinical outcomes of the disease; in particular, antigen B is the antigen of choice to detect specific IgG4, which is the immunoglobulin isotype most clearly associated with the progression of the disease; (2) Th1/Th2 cell activation is involved in the clinical outcome of E. granulosus infection and, in particular Th2 response, is associated with susceptibility to the disease, whereas a Th1 response is associated with protective immunity.

B. AE

In AE, the host mechanisms modulating the course of infection are most likely of immunological nature and include primarily T-cell interactions and respective (pro) inflammatory cytokine and chemokine activities, e.g., resulting in NO-mediated periparasitic immunosuppression (23) or development of protection (29) in mice or modulating the course of disease in human patients (30,31). Cellular immunity in controlling the metacestode growths kinetics is strongly suggested by the intense granulomatous infiltration observed around the hepatic parasite lesions in infected patients and in experimental mouse models (32,33). It has been shown that a regressive versus a progressive course of disease correlated with a respective granuloma cell composition and with the relative ratios of T-lymphocyte subpopulations in the periparasitic areas of hepatic lesions (34). Furthermore, the role of immunity in the control of alveolar echinococcosis has been substantially demonstrated by the rapid fatal outcome of an *E. multilocularis* infection in an HIV-coinfected immunodeficient patient (35). Nevertheless, the biological significance of CD4+ and CD8+ T cells and of B cells in modulating the growth behavior of *E. multilocularis* is still poorly understood.

VI. Clinical and Laboratory Diagnostic Features

In most cases of CE and AE, imaging procedures together with serology will yield the diagnosis. For CE, there are a variety of radiographic images upon chest X ray (Fig. 4). Computed tomography (CT) and magnetic resonance imaging (MRI) can recognize certain details of the lesions and discover others that are not visible by conventional radiography (Fig. 5). CT allows ready distinction of hydatid cysts from soft tissue nodules by demonstrating a thin-walled fluid-filled cyst. CT can also visualize signs of the onset of complications, such as incipient membrane detachment or small bubbles located in the cyst wall (36). MR imaging also allows reliable differentiation, as the cyst has low signal intensity on T1-weighted images and high signal intensity on T2-weighted MR images (9). For pulmonary

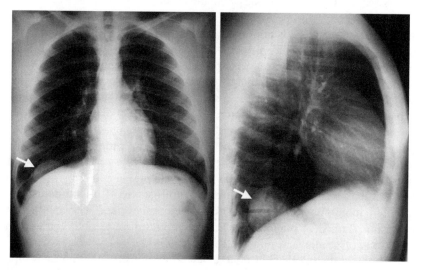

Figure 4 Pulmonary CE in a 14-year-old girl. Chest X ray presents an unruptured solitary cyst (*white arrow*) in the inferior lobe of the right lung. *Source*: Courtesy of P. Vock, University Hospital of Berne.

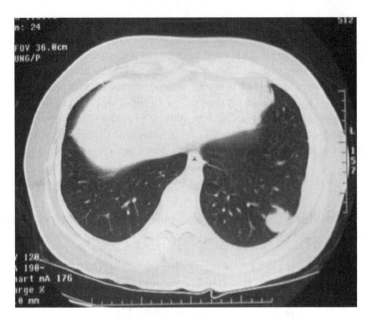

Figure 5 Pulmonary CE in a 37-year-old woman. CT of the chest presents an unruptured cyst in the inferior lobe of the right lung (*white arrow*). Beside this cyst, the patient additionally exhibited multiple hepatic cysts of variable size. One year before being admitted to the clinic in Switzerland, the patient had undergone thoracotomy for a hydatid cyst in the right lung in an Albanian clinic. *Source*: Courtesy of J. Reichen, Department of Clinical Pharmacology, University of Berne.

sites, U.S. examination is unhelpful in most cases, but it can sometime confirm the cystic nature of a parenchymatous mass that is juxtaparietal (36). It will display an anechoic area with posterior strengthening.

Over-all diagnostic imaging features of hydatid cysts include separation of the parasite germinal/laminated layer from the surrounding host capsule and internal daughter cysts. In the differential diagnosis, fiber optic bronchoscopy may help to distinguish from bronchogenic carcinoma and pulmonary tuberculosis mimicking CE (37). If aspiration cytology is performable, trichrome staining of the filtrated aspirate reveals the acid-fast hooklets (38). Cytology appears particularly helpful in detecting pulmonary (39) involvement. Viability of aspirated protoscolices can be determined by microscopic demonstration of flame cell activity and Trypan Blue dye exclusion. Transient pneumonitis and pneumothorax can be seen as complications of needle aspiration (12).

Immunodiagnostic tests for the detection of serum antibodies or circulating antigens are used to support the clinical diagnosis of CE (40). The indirect hemagglutination tests (IHAT) and the enzyme-linked immunosorbent assay (ELISA) using *E. granulosus* hydatid fluid antigen are diagnostically relatively sensitive for hepatic cases (85–98%). For pulmonary cyst localization, the diagnostic sensitivity is markedly lower (50–60%), for multiple organ localization very high (90–100%). These tests are usually used for a primary serological screening. Specificity of such tests increases considerably when using, e.g., the antigen-5-precipitation (arc-5-test) or immunoblotting for a relatively specific 8 kDa/12 kDa hydatid fluid polypeptide antigen (41,42). Beside problems of diagnostic sensitivity and specificity due to cross-reactions, there is accumulating evidence for false-positive antibody reactions not only related to infections with heterologous helminth species, but also to malignancies (42–44), and the presence of anti-P1 antibodies (45).

The demonstration of parasite-specific IgE has attracted particular attention due to its well-known relevance in helminthic diseases (46,47). Hypersensitivity reactions in CE vary widely from benign urticaria and short episodes of shaking chills or fever to potentially fatal bronchial spasms, angioneurotic edema, and anaphylactic shock. The latter occurs most frequently after the spontaneous rupture of the hydatid cyst or incidental to surgery. In a study of Ortona et al. (28), about 20% of patients reported a history of allergic manifestations of unknown origin during infection; however, a higher percentage of patients had IgE specific to hydatid antigens. IgE, which decreases rapidly in serum of patients after surgery or successful chemotherapy, was claimed to be a useful marker of the outcome of CE (48). The same authors suggested also to use cytokine monitoring in the clinical follow-up of patients after therapy (28), while the use of antigen-specific lymphocyte transformation assays appeared less suitable (49).

Monoclonal antibodies (Mabs) generated against different parasite antigens have been used for the diagnosis of CE by detection of circulating antigens in patients' sera or of native proteins in biopsies. Such Mabs have been mainly directed against two major *E. granulosus* antigens, named antigen 5 (Ag5) and antigen B (AgB) (50,51). Principally, detection of circulating antigens—by the use of Mabs—has been proposed as an early marker for hydatid infection, being also relevant as a method for postsurgical follow-up of patients, and to monitor the growth dynamics and/or the activity of cysts (50). Anti-Ag5 Mabs were also used for the detection of the respective antigen in diagnostic fine needle aspiration biopsies (FNAB) from patients with suspected CE (52).

Early diagnosis of persons with asymptomatic echinococcosis is a prerequisite for efficient management of the disease. Consequently, screening may be offered to populations at risk. The currently optimal epidemiological tool to be used includes ultrasonographic examination for abdominal cystic echinococcosis combined with an appropriate immunodiagnosis (40,53,54).

The primary manifestations of *E. multilocularis* are related to the liver, which is affected in 92–100% of all cases. The most frequent presenting symptoms include nonspecific abdominal pain, hepatomegaly and jaundice. In about 15%, the parasite is incidentally discovered in asymptomatic patients, or there are only unspecific symptoms such as fatigue and weight loss (2). Thus, lung manifestation always succeeds an already diagnosed primary hepatic AE and thus does not require primary diagnostic tools, but rather imaging procedures to characterize the localization and extent of the secondary pulmonary lesions (Figs. 6 and 7). For this purpose, among the imaging procedures, CT and MRI are of greatest diagnostic

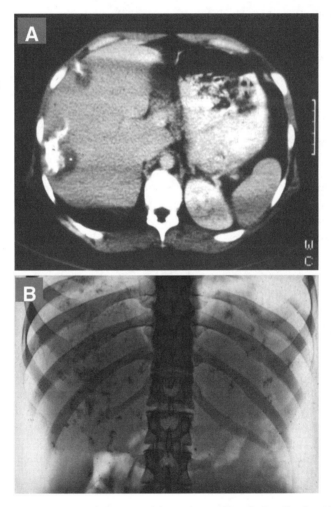

Figure 6 In most cases, AE starts with a primary hepatic localization. At a later stage, dissemination of the parasite may occur, including metastasis formation in the lungs. (**A**) Upper abdominal CT showing the presence of multiple AE lesions affecting various organs/sites, including the lungs. (**B**) Chest X ray presenting multiple pulmonary AE lesions. *Source*: Courtesy of J. Reichen, Department of Clinical Pharmacology, University of Berne.

(A)   **(B)**

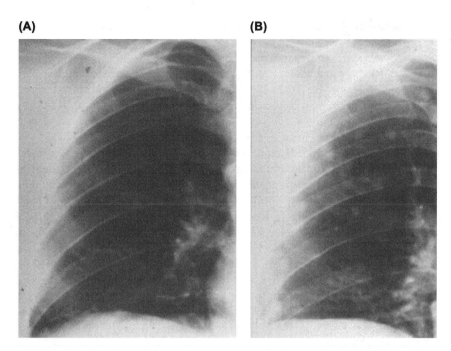

Figure 7 Multiple peripheral *E. multilocularis* lesions within the right lung as shown in 1983 (**B**), which could not be visualized 4 years before in 1979 (**A**). *Source*: Courtesy of Prof. R. Ammann, University Hospital of Zürich.

value, none of those being uniquely superior (54). The percentage of calcifications in AE lesions increases from 33% to 100% as the disease progresses (55–57). Applying to hepatic as well as pulmonary lesions, histopathological and immunohistochemical procedures to analyze surgically resected samples or biopsies obtained by fine-needle aspiration (FNAB) include the use of species-specific Mabs such as MAbG11 or molecular techniques such as PCR (both methods discussed in the section below), beside conventional histology, with PAS being the best staining method to characterize the typical laminated layer of the parasite (58).

Complementary to imaging procedures, immunodiagnosis represents a valuable secondary diagnostic tool to confirm the nature (and species) of the etiologic agent (40,59,60). In general, serological tests are more reliable in the diagnosis of AE than CE. The use of purified *E. multilocularis* antigens (such as the Em2 antigen, or recombinant antigens II/3-10, EM10, or Em18) exhibit diagnostic sensitivities ranging between 91% and 100%, with over-all specificities of 98–100%. These antigens allow to discriminate between AE and CE with a reliability of 95% (59,61,62). Specific serological tests such as discussed below exhibit operating characteristics, which allow performing reliable seroepidemiological studies to detect early, asymptomatic cases of AE (63–66).

Serological methods have been assessed for their value in the surveillance of operated or pharmacologically treated patients. Conventional serological tests (such as in EmII/3-10-ELISA or Em18-ELISA) exhibited some prognostic value, as a decrease of serum antibody concentrations after radical surgery correlated with the clinical course (67,68). Relatively limited clinical use of such tests appeared for patients with partial, palliative, or no surgery (69,70).

Molecular biological techniques such as the polymerase-chain reaction (PCR) have been developed and introduced for the diagnostic identification of *E. multilocularis*-specific nucleic acids in the last few years. The primary diagnostic identification of parasite materials in biological specimens (resections or biopsies) and also the assessment of the viability of parasite samples following chemotherapy or other treatment were both addressed. The *E. multilocularis* nucleic acid sequence pAL1 served to derive oligonucleotide primers suitable for use in PCR amplification (71), allowing the differentiation between *E. multilocularis* and *E. granulosus* and other parasite material of any stage and origin. These primers have been diagnostically used to detect *E. multilocularis*-DNA in lesions occurring especially in complicated cases of extrahepatic AE, e.g., pancreatic AE (58) or AE of other sites (72).

VII. Treatment

For both CE and AE, treatment is essentially surgical. In general, chemotherapy is used as a complement to operative treatment to avoid recurrence.

Surgery of CE has two objectives: to remove the parasite and to treat the bronchipericyst pathology and other associated lesions. The prognosis has changed during the last few years, and results are now commonly satisfactory. The most frequent complications are pleural infection and prolonged air leakage. Operative mortality does not exceed 1–2%. Despite the low mortality and the limited recurrence rate, it is necessary to remember the invading character of pulmonary hydatid disease, which sometimes makes therapy difficult and questionable (14).

A. Surgery of CE

Pulmonary cysts are often the result of infected or ruptured hepatic cysts. About 40% of patients present with complications, mainly infection but also pneumothorax (73). In these cases, surgical treatment is mandatory. Perforated cysts appear radiologically in approximately 10–30% of cases (74), but perforated hydatid cysts may also exit behind various radiological appearances. The radiological appearance of hydatid cysts includes hydroaeric cysts, sign of the camelote, air crescent sign, pneumothorax, solitary opacity, and pleural effusion (75). Overall, the lung conserving surgical approach is the treatment of choice for most patients with pulmonary CE.

Treatment consists of parenchyma-preserved methods such as cystectomy and closure of bronchial openings. Obliteration of the residual cavity by imbricating structures from within (capittonage) is attempted in some of the patients, but capittonage provided no advantage in operations for pulmonary hydatid cysts (76). Pulmonary resections include lobectomy, segmentectomy, polisegmentectomy, and bilobectomy, by decreasing frequency. Sometimes a two-stage procedure is necessary (73). PAIR (puncture, aspiration, injection of an heminthicide and reaspiration) has been propagated for certain hepatic forms of CE. For pulmonary CE, this technique is not indicated, with a few exceptions (77). Recurrence of pulmonary disease after surgery appears to be rare (73,78,79). As a placebo-controlled trial of albendazole in pulmonary hydatid disease showed cure in 45% in the verum group as opposed to zero in the placebo group, a primary pharmacotherapy can be considered in uncomplicated cases (80).

It remains unclear what to do with asymptomatic patients detected at screening or with imaging for unrelated medical problems. In one small series of 28 patients followed for over 10 years, 75% of patients remained free of symptoms (81).

Whatever surgical procedure is chosen, care has to be taken to avoid spillage of cyst content, which is the main predictor of recurrent disease. To achieve this, the perisurgical cavity area should be carefully protected, and the cyst evacuated and sterilized with scolicidal agents. Pretreatment with benzimidazole compounds—optionally complemented with praziquantel—has been proposed to avoid the use of dangerous scolicidal agents and to decrease the rate of recurrence (82–84).

B. Surgery of AE

The following strategies are commonly accepted for treatment of AE: (i) The first choice of treatment is radical surgical resection of the entire parasitic lesion from the liver and other affected organs (e.g., lungs) in all operable cases. Excision of the parasitic lesion has to follow the rules of radical tumor surgery. (ii) Concomitant chemotherapy in all cases after radical surgery or after nonsurgical interventional procedures. (iii) long-term chemotherapy of inoperable or only partially resectable cases and all patients after liver transplantation. Presurgical chemotherapy is not indicated in cases of AE.

Radical resection is possible only in 15–58% of AE cases (2,17). Even in presumed radical surgery, recurrences can occur in 10–20% (16,85).

C. Pharmacotherapy of CE

Two benzimidazole compounds—mebendazole and albendazole—and praziquantel, have activity against *E. granulosus* in vitro and in animal models

(86,87). No controlled studies have ever been performed in man so far. Albendazole appears preferable to mebendazole because of its better bioavailability (88,89). Both drugs penetrate into the cysts (82, 90), but sometimes heroic doses are needed to achieve a therapeutic plasma concentration of mebendazole (91), the generally accepted therapeutic levels are around 250 nmol/L. The former use of albendazole in cycles of 4 weeks, followed by a drug-free interval of 2 weeks, has been more and more replaced by a continuous treatment (2,92). Thus, in a small comparative study, 6/6 patients on continuous therapy showed cyst involution, while relapse occurred in the cycling group (93). Side effects of the two drugs appear to be similar and include mainly leucopoenia, hair loss and hepatotoxicity (94,95). For both benzimidazoles, it appears likely that they act not truly parasiticidal in vivo but rather parasitostatic, although the effect can be visualized much more rapidly in cystic than in alveolar echinococcosis (Fig. 8). Short-term treatment is clearly inadequate since also with albendazole treatment for three weeks 50% viable cysts were found in a prospective study (96). The drug has also been used in children (97) and the response rate of 51% is comparable with that seen in adult series. The summarized success rate, as defined above and referring to albendazole, ranges from 66% to 100%. Complete cyst disappearance was observed in 22% of patients with hepatic cysts (98). In a triple blind parallel-randomized clinical trial, 20 patients with 179 *E. granulosus* pulmonary cysts were entered into comparing the effects of albendazole versus placebo (80). Fifteen patients (150 cysts) completed 6 months of treatment; four patients (26 cysts) were in the placebo group, and 11 patients (124 cysts) in the albendazole treatment group. Ten of 11 patients (91%) in the treatment group showed either cure or improvement. In the placebo group, only one of four (25%) showed spontaneous improvement, but cure did not occur. In the treatment group, 88 of 124 cysts (71%) showed improvement compared to four of 26 (15.4%) in the placebo group. This study suggested that patients suffering from uncomplicated hydatid disease should be given a trial of albendazole before surgery is considered (80).

The beneficial effects of praziquantel medication (additional to benzimidazoles) have been suggested and discussed (82,86,99).

The combination may be of particular interest since it appears more potent than either agent alone in an animal model of peritoneal spillage in vivo (86). However, Piens et al. (100) treated nine patients prior to surgery with two 10-day courses of praziquantel. The drug could not be detected in the cyst fluid and as many cysts remained vital as in an untreated control group, shedding doubt on the efficacy of praziquantel alone as a scolicidal agent. This may be due to the fact that praziquantel acts on protoscolices but not on the germinal layer.

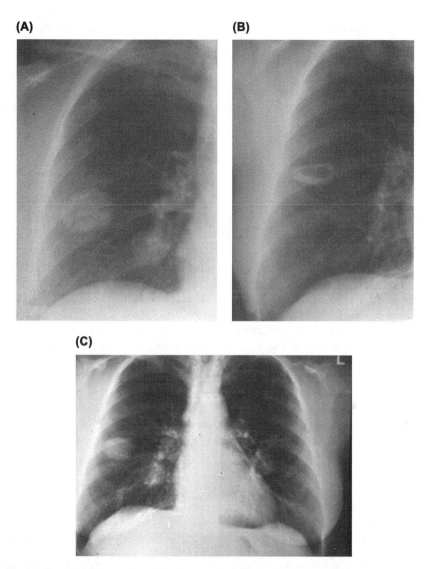

Figure 8 Multiple cystic lesions in the lungs before mebendazole therapy (**A**) and circular shadows (**B**) remaining after 4 months of mebendazole therapy in a patient with hepatic and pulmonary cyst involvement. No significant difference was seen after 1 month of mebendazole medication (**C**). *Source*: Courtesy of Prof. R. Ammann, University Hospital of Zürich.

D. Pharmacotherapy of AE

Only few compounds exhibit a significant activity against *E. multilocularis* (101), they include mebendazole, albendazole, and praziquantel. Although praziquantel was the most effective scolicidal agent, it did not inhibit meta-cestode growth and did not affect germinal layer activity. Albendazole was the most active agent in inhibiting metacestode growth (101). For alben-dazole, recent experience indicated that continuous treatment was well tolerated for about 1 to 6 years, and proved to be superior to discontinuous treatment for AE associated with obstructive jaundice (102). The daily dosage for albendazole and mebendazole treatment is the same as for CE. For mebendazole, plasma drug levels should reach > 250 nmol/L ($=74$ ng/mL). Generally, duration of treatment is at least 2 years in cases after radical surgery or continuously for many years in inoperable cases or in cases with incomplete resection.

Assessing efficacy in treatment of *E. multilocularis* is even more diffi-cult than in *E. granulosus*, since viability of the parasite cannot easily be judged in vivo, spontaneous death of parasite has been described (65), and radiological regression is rare (103). Therefore, radiological progres-sion and/or death are the only hard endpoints as treatment failures (104). With regard to respective assessments, a preliminary but promising ap-proach has been described by Reuter et al. (55) who were measuring peri-cystic metabolic activity by PET to assess and follow-up patients with AE. For albendazole, recent experience indicated that continuous treatment was well tolerated for about 1 to 6 years, and proved to be superior to discontin-uous treatment for AE associated with obstructive jaundice (102).

Acknowledgment

This work was supported by Grant No. 31–63615.00 from the Swiss National Science Foundation.

References

1. Thompson RCA, McManus DP. Towards a taxonomic revision of the genus *Echinococcus*. Trends Parasitol 2002; 18:452–457.
2. Eckert J, Gemmel MA, Meslin FX, Pawlowski ZS. WHO/OIE Manual on Echinococcosis in Humans and Animals: a Public Health Problem of Global Concern. Paris: OIE/WHO, 2001.
3. Deplazes P, Eckert J. Veterinary aspects of alveolar echinococcosis—a zoonosis of public health significance. Vet Parasitol 2001; 98:65–87.
4. Scott JC, Stefaniak J, Pawlowski ZS, McManus DP. Molecular genetic analy-sis of human cystic hydatid cases from Poland. Identification of a new geno-typic group (G9) of *Echinococcus granulosus*. J Parasitol 1997; 114:37–43.
5. Haag KL, Zaha A, Araújo AM, Gottstein B. Reduced genetic variability within coding and non-coding regions of the *Echinococcus multilocularis* genome. Parasitology 1997; 115:521–529.

6. Gottstein B, Bettens F. Association between HLA-DR13 and susceptibility to alveolar echinococcosis. J Infect Dis 1994; 169:1416–1417.
7. Eiermann TH, Bettens F, Tiberghien P, Schmitz K, Beurton I, Bresson-Hadni S, Ammann RW, Goldmann SF, Vuitton DA, Gottstein B, Kern P. HLA and alveolar echinococcosis. Tissue Antigens 1998; 52:124–129.
8. Shcherbakov AM. Human echinococcosis: the role of histocompatibility antigens in realizing infestations and the characteristics of their course. Med Parazitol 1993; 5:13–18.
9. Özhan MH. Pulmonary hydatidosis: state of the art. Int Arch Hydatidosis 2001; 34:11.
10. Salinas JC, Torcal J, Lozano R, et al. Intracystic infection of liver hydatidosis. Hepatogastroenterol 2000; 47:1052–1055.
11. Rebhandl W, Turnbull J, Felberbauer FX, et al. Pulmonary echinococcosis (hydatidosis) in children: results of surgical treatment. Pediatr Pulmonol 1999; 27:336–340.
12. Lamy AL, Cameron BH, Le Blanc JG, et al. Giant hydatid lung cysts in the Canadian northwest: outcome of conservative treatment in three children. J Pediatr Surg 1993; 28:1140–1143.
13. Kervancioglu R, Bayram M, Elbeyli L. CT findings in pulmonary hydatid disease. Acta Radiol 1999; 40:510–514.
14. Ramos G, Orduna A, Garcia-Yuste M. Hydatid cyst of the lung: diagnosis and treatment. World J Surg 2001; 25:46–57.
15. Rothlin MA. Fatal intraoperative pulmonary embolism from a hepatic hydatid cyst. Am J Gastroenterol 1998; 93:2606–2607.
16. Akinoglu A, Demiryurek H, Guzel C. Alveolar hydatid disease of the liver: a report on thirty-nine surgical cases in eastern Anatolia, Turkey. Am J Trop Med Hyg 1991; 45:182–189.
17. Ammann RW, Eckert J. Cestodes: *Echinococcus*. Gastroenterol Clin North Am 1996; 25:655–689.
18. Etievent JP, Vuitton D, Allemand H, et al. Pulmonary embolism from a parasitic cardiac clot secondary to hepatic alveolar echinococcosis. J Cardiovasc Surg 1986; 27:671–674.
19. Wilson JF, Rausch RL. Alveolar hydatid disease: a review of clinical features of 33 indigenous cases of *E. multilocularis* infection in Alaskan Eskimoes. Am J Trop Med Hyg 1980; 29:1340–1355.
20. Lampl L, Hamperl WD. Curative en-bloc resection (lung, diaphragm, liver, adrenal gland and thoracic wall) for *Echinococcus multilocularis*. Report of an unusual disease course. Langenbecks Arch Chir 1992; 377:68–70.
21. Bresson-Hadni S, Miguet JP, Lenys D, et al. Recurrence of alveolar echinococcosis in the liver graft after liver transplantation. Hepatology 1992; 16:279–280.
22. Gottstein B, Felleisen R. Protective immune mechanisms against the metacestode of *Echinococcus multilocularis*. Parasitol Today 1995; 11:320–326.
23. Dai WJ, Gottstein B. Nitric oxide-mediated immunosuppression following murine *Echinococcus multilocularis* infection. Immunology 1999; 97:107–116.
24. Ferreira AM, Irigoin F, Breijo M, et al. How *Echinococcus granulosus* deals with complement. Parasitol Today 2000; 16:168–172.

25. Dixon JB. Echinococcosis. Comp Immunol Microbiol Infect Dis 1997; 20:87–94.

26. Ellis ME, Sinner W, Asraf AM, et al. Echinococcal disease and mycobacterial infection. Ann Trop Med Parasitol 1991; 85:243–251.

27. Rigano R, Profumo E, Siracusano A. New perspectives in the immunology of *Echinococcus granulosus* infection. Parassitologia 1997; 39:275–277.

28. Ortona E, Rigano R, Buttari B, Delunardo F, Ioppolo S, Margutti P, Profumo E, Teggi A, Vaccari S, Siracusano A. An update on immunodiagnosis of cystic echinococcosis. Acta Trop 2003; 85:165–171.

29. Godot V, Harraga S, Podoprigora G, Liance M, Bardonnet K, Vuitton DA. IFN alpha-2a protects mice against a helminth infection of the liver and modulates immune responses. Gastroenterology 2003; 124(5):1441–1450.

30. Eger A, Kirch A, Manfras B, Kern P, Schulz-Key H, Soboslay PT. Pro-inflammatory (IL-1beta, IL-18) cytokines and IL-8 chemokine release by PBMC in response to *Echinococcus multilocularis* metacestode vesicles. Parasite Immunol 2003; 25(2):103–105.

31. Harraga S, Godot V, Bresson-Hadni S, Mantion G, Vuitton DA. Profile of cytokine production within the periparasitic granuloma in human alveolar echinococcosis. Acta Trop 2003; 85(2):231–236.

32. Emery I, Liance M, Deriaud E, Vuitton D, Houin R, Leclerc C. Characterization of T-cell immune responses of *Echinococcus multilocularis* infected C57BL/6 mice. Parasite Immunol 1996; 18:463–472.

33. Gottstein B, Hemphill A. Immunopathology of echinococcosis. Chem Immunol 1997; 66:177–208.

34. Bresson-Hadni S, Liance M, Meyer JP, Houin R, Bresson JL, Vuitton D. Cellular immunity in experimental *Echinococcus multilocularis* infection. II. Sequential and comparative phenotypic study of the periparasitic mononuclear cells in resistant and sensitive mice. Clin Exp Immunol 1990; 82:378–383.

35. Sailer M, Soelder B, Allerberger F, Zaknun D, Feichtinger H, Gottstein B. Alveolar echinococcosis of the liver in a six-year-old girl with acquired immunodeficiency syndrome. J Pediatr 1997; 130:320–323.

36. Pawlowski ZS, Eckert J, Vuitton DA, et al. Echinococcosis in humans: clinical aspects, diagnosis and treatment. In: Eckert J, Gemell MA, Meslin FX, et al., eds. WHO/OIE Manual on Echinococcosis in Humans and Animals: a Public Health Problem of Global Concern. Paris: WHO and OIE, 2001:20–71.

37. Kilinc O, Sakar A, Yorgancioglu A, et al. Interesting pulmonary hydatid cyst cases mimicking other pulmonary diseases. Int Arch Hydatidosis 2001; 34:189.

38. Hira PR, Lindberg LG, Francis I, et al. Diagnosis of cystic hydatid disease: role of aspiration cytology. Lancet 1988; ii:655–657.

39. Frydman CP, Raissi S, Watson CW. An unusual pulmonary and renal presentation of echinococcosis. Report of a case. Acta Cytol 1989; 33:655–658.

40. Siles-Lucas S, Gottstein B. Review: molecular tools for the diagnosis of cystic and alveolar echinococcosis. Trop Med Int Health 2001; 6:463–475.

41. Liance M, Janin V, Bresson-Hadni S, Vuitton DA, Houin R, Piarroux R. Immunodiagnosis of *Echinococcus* infections: confirmatory testing and

species differentiation by a new commercial WesternBlot. J Clin Microbiol 2000; 38:3718–3721.

42. Poretti D, Felleisen E, Grimm F, et al. Differential immunodiagnosis between cystic hydatid disease and other cross-reactive pathologies. Am J Trop Med Hyg 1999; 60:193–198.

43. Pfister M, Gottstein B, Cerny T, et al. Immunodiagnosis of echinococcosis in cancer patients. Clin Microbiol Infect 1999; 5:693–697.

44. Dar FK, Buhidma MA, Kidwai SA. Hydatid false positive serological test results in malignancy. BMJ 1984; 288:1197.

45. Ben-Ismail R, Rouger P, Carme B, et al. Comparative automated assay of anti-P1 antibodies in acute hepatic distomiasis (fasciolasis) and in hydatidosis. Vox Sang 1980; 38:156–168.

46. Pinon JM, Poirriez J, Lepan J, et al. Value of isotypic characterization of antibodies of *Echinococcus granulosus* by enzyme-linked immuno-filtration assay. Eur J Clin Microbiol 1987; 6:291–295.

47. Wattal C, Mohan C, Agarwal SC. Evaluation of specific immunoglogulin E by enzyme-linked immunosorbent assay in hydatid disease. Int Arch Allergy Appl Immunol 1987; 87:98–100.

48. Rigano R, Profumo E, Ioppolo S, Notargiacomo S, Ortona E, Teggi A, Siracusano A. Immunological markers indicating the effectiveness of pharmacological treatment in human hydatid disease. Clin Exp Immunol 1995; 102:281–285.

49. Bonifacino R, Carter SD, Craig PS, Almeida I, Da Rosa D. Assessment of the immunological surveillance value of humoral and lymphocyte assays in severe human cystic echinococcosis. Trans R Soc Trop Med Hyg 2000; 94(1):97–102.

50. Ferragut G, Ljungstrom I, Nieto A. Relevance of circulating antigen detection to follow-up experimental and human cystic hydatid infections. Parasite Immunol 1998; 20:541–549.

51. Lightowlers MW, Liu D, Haralambous A, et al. Subunit composition and specificity of the major cyst fluid antigens of *Echinococcus granulosus*. Mol Biochem Parasitol 1989; 37:171–182.

52. Stefaniak J. Fine needle aspiration biopsy in the differential diagnosis of the liver cystic echinococcosis. Acta Tropica 1997; 67:107–111.

53. MacPherson CNL, Romig T, Zehyle E, et al. Portable ultrasound scanner versus serology in screening for hydatid cysts in a Nomadic population. Lancet 1987; ii:259–261.

54. Shambesh MA, Craig PS, Macpherson CN, et al. An extensive ultrasound and serologic study to investigate the prevalence of human cystic echinococcosis in northern Libya. Am J Trop Med Hyg 1999; 60:462–468.

55. Reuter S, Nüssle K, Kolokythas O, et al. Alveolar liver echinococcosis: a comparative study of three imaging techniques. Infection 2001; 29:119–125.

56. Ammann RW, Hoffmann AF, Eckert J. Swiss study of chemotherapy of alveolar echinococcosis—review of a 20-year clinical research project. Schweiz Med Wochenschr 1999; 129:323–332.

57. Kasai Y, Koshino I, Kawanishi N, et al. Alveolar echinococcosis of the liver. Studies on 60 operated cases. Ann Surg 1980; 192:145–152.

58. Diebold-Berger S, Khan H, Gottstein B et al. Cytologic diagnosis of isolated pancreatic alveolar hydatid disease with immunologic and PCR analyses—a case report. Acta Cytolo 1997; 41:1381–1386.

59. Gottstein B, Jacquier P, Bresson-Hadni S, et al. Improved primary immuno-diagnosis of alveolar echinococcosis in humans by an enzyme-linked immuno-sorbent assay using the Em2plus-antigen. J Clin Microbiol 1993; 31:373–376.

60. Lightowlers M, Gottstein B. Immunodiagnosis of echinococcosis. In: Thompson RCA, Lymbery AJ, eds. Echinococcus and Hydatid Disease. Wallingford: CAB International, 1995.

61. Frosch PM, Frosch M, Pfister T, Schaad V, Bitter-Suermann D. Cloning and characterisation of an immunodominant major surface antigen of Echinococcus multilocularis. Mol Biochem Parasitol 1991; 48:121–130.

62. Xiao N, Mamuti W, Yamasaki H, Sako Y, Nakao M, Nakaya K, Gottstein B, Schantz PM, Lightowlers MW, Craig PS, Ito A. Evaluation of recombinant Em18 and affinity-purified Em18 for serological differentiation alveolar echi-nococcosis from cystic echinococcosis and other parasitic infections. J Clin Microbiol 2003; 41:3351–3353.

63. Bresson-Hadni S, Laplante J, Lenys D, et al. Seroepidemiologic screening of Echinococcus multilocularis infection in a European area endemic for alveolar echinococcosis. Am J Trop Med Hyg 1994; 51:837–846.

64. Gottstein B, Saucy F, Deplazes P, et al. Is a high prevalence of Echinococcus multilocularis in wild and domestic animals associated with increased disease incidence in humans? Emerg Inf Dis 2001; 7:408–412.

65. Rausch RL, Wilson JF, Schantz PM, et al. Spontaneous death of Echinococcus multilocularis: Cases diagnosed serologically by Em2-ELISA and clinical sig-nificance. Am J Trop Med Hyg 1987; 36:576–585.

66. Romig T, Kratzer W, Kimmig P, et al. An epidemiological survey of human alveolar echinococcosis in southwestern Germany. Am J Trop Med Hyg 1999; 6:566–573.

67. Gottstein B, Bettens F, Parkinson AJ, Wilson F. Immunological parameters associated with susceptibility or resistance to alveolar hydatid disease in Yupiks/Inupiats. Arctic Med Res 1996; 55:14–19.

68. Sako Y, Nakao M, Nakaya K, Yamasaki H, Gottstein B, Lightowers MW, Schantz PM, Ito A. Alveolar echinococcosis: characterization of diagnostic antigen Em18 and serological evaluation of recombinant Em18. J Clin Micro-biol 2002; 40:2760–2765.

69. Gottstein B, Tschudi K, Eckert J, et al. Em2-ELISA for the follow-up of alveolar echinococcosis after complete surgical resection of liver lesions. Trans R Soc Trop Med Hyg 1989; 83:389–393.

70. Lanier AP, Trujillo DE, Schantz PM, et al. Comparison of serologic tests for the diagnosis and follow-up of alveolar hydatid disease. Am J Trop Med Hyg 1987; 37:609–615.

71. Gottstein B, Mowatt MR. Sequencing and characterization of an Echinococcus multilocularis DNA probe and its use in the polymerase chain reaction. Mol Biochem Parasitol 1991; 44:183–194.

72. Reuter S, Seitz HM, Kern P, et al. Extrahepatic alveolar echinococcosis with-out liver involvement: a rare manifestation. Infection 2000; 28:187–192.

73. Safioleas M, Misiakos EP, Dosios T, et al. Surgical treatment for lung hydatid disease. World J Surg 1999; 23:1181–1185.

74. Kondov G, Spirovski Z, Joves S, et al. Surgical treatment of hydatid cysts in the pleural space. Int Arch Hydatidosis 2001; 34:186.

75. Altiay G, Tabakoglu E, Köse S, et al. Radiological appearances of our pulmonary hydatid cysts cases. Int Arch Hydatidosis 2001; 34:180.

76. Turna A, Yilmaz MA, Haciibrahimoglu G, Kutlu CA, Bedirhan MA. Surgical treatment of pulmonary hydatid cysts: is capitonnage necessary? Ann Thorac Surg 2002; 74(1):191–195.

77. Mawhorter S, Temeck B, Chang R, et al. Nonsurgical therapy for pulmonary hydatid cyst disease. Chest 1997; 112:1432–1436.

78. Cangiotti L, Giulini S M, Muiesan P, et al. Hydatid disease of the liver: long-term results of surgical treatment. J Chir 1991; 12:501–504.

79. Novick RJ, Tchervenkov CI, Wilson JA, et al. Surgery for thoracic hydatid disease: a North American experience. Ann Thorac Surg 1987; 43:681–686.

80. Keshmiri M, Baharvahdat H, Fattahi SH, et al. A placebo controlled study of albendazole in the treatment of pulmonary echinococcosis. Eur Respir J 1999; 14:503–507.

81. Frider B, Larrieu E, Odriozola M. Long-term outcome of asymptomatic liver hydatidosis. J Hepatol 1999; 30:228–231.

82. Cobo F, Yarnoz C, Sesma B, et al. Albendazole plus praziquantel versus albendazole alone as a pre-operative treatment in intra-abdominal hydatisosis caused by *Echinococcus granulosus*. Trop Med Int Health 1998; 3:462–566.

83. Messaritakis J, Psychou P, Nicolaidou P, Karpathios T, Syriopoulou B, Fretzayas A. High mebendazole doses in pulmonary and hepatic hydatid disease. Arch Dis Child 1991; 66:532–533.

84. Morris DL. Pre-operative albendazole therapy for hydatid cyst. Br J Surg 1987; 74:805–806.

85. Partensky C, Landraud R, Valette P-J, et al. Radical and nonradical hepatic resection for alveolar echinococcosis: report of 18 cases. World J Surg 1990; 14:654–659.

86. Chinnery JB, Morris DL. Effect of albendazole sulphoxide on viability of hydatid protoscolices in vitro. Trans R Soc Trop Med Hyg 1986; 80: 815–817.

87. Taylor DH, Morris DL. Combination chemotherapy is more effective in post-spillage prophylaxis for hydatid disease than either albendazole or praziquantel alone. Br J Surg 1989; 76:954.

88. Braithwaite PA, Roberts MS, Allan RJ, et al. Clinical pharmacokinetics of high dose mebendazole in patients treated for cystic hydatid disease. Eur J Clin Pharmacol 1982; 22:161–169.

89. Marriner SE, Morris DL, Dickson B, et al. Pharmacokinetics of albendazole in man. Eur J Clin Pharmacol 1986; 30:705–708.

90. Luder PJ, Robotti G, Meister FP, et al. High oral doses of mebendazole interfere with growth of larval echinococcus multilocularis lesions. J Hepatol 1985; 1:369–377.

91. Luder PJ, Siffert B, Witassek F, et al. Treatment of hydatid disease with high oral doses of mebendazole. Long-term follow-up of plasma mebendazole levels and drug interactions. Eur J Clin Pharmacol 1986; 31:443–448.

92. Horton RJ. Albendazole in treatment of human cystic echinococcosis: 12 years of experience. Acta Trop 1997; 64:79–93.

93. Luchi S, Vincenti A, Messina F, et al. Albendazole treatment of human hydatid tissue. Scand J Infect Dis 1997; 29:165–167.

94. Cotting J, Zeugin T, Steiger U, et al. Albendazole kinetics in patients with echinococcosis: delayed absorption and impaired elimination in cholestasis. Eur J Clin Pharmacol 1990; 38:605–608.

95. Davis A, Dixon H, Pawlowski ZS. Multicentre clinical trials of benzimidazole carbamates in human cystic echinococcosis (phase 2). Bull World Health Organ 1986; 67:503–508.

96. Aktan AO, Yalin R. Preoperative albendazole treatment for liver hydatid disease decreases the viability of the cyst. Eur J Gastroenterol Hepatol 1996; 8:877–879.

97. French CM. Mebendazole and surgery for human hydatid disease in Turkana. East Afr Med J 1984; 61:113–119.

98. Morris DL, Dykes PW, Marriner S, et al. Albendazole: objective evidence of response in human hydatid disease. JAMA 1985; 253:2053–2057.

99. Henriksen TH, Klungsoyr P, Zerihun D. Treatment of disseminated peritoneal hydatid disease with praziquantel. Lancet 1989; 1:272.

100. Piens MA, Persat F, May, et al. Praziquantel in human hydatidosis. Evaluation by preoperative treatment. Bull Soc Pathol Exot Filiales 1989; 82:503–512.

101. Taylor DH, Morris DL, Reffin D, et al. Comparison of albendazole, mebendazole and praziquantel chemotherapy of *Echinococcus multilocularis* in a gerbil model. Gut 1989; 30:1401–1405.

102. Wang X, Liu Y, Yu D. Continuous therapy with albendazole for hepatic alveolar echinococcosis associated with obstructive jaundice. Chung Hua Nei Ko Tsa Chih 1996; 35:261–264.

103. Luder PJ, Witassek F, Weigand K, et al. Treatment of cystic echinococcosis (*Echinococcus granulosus*) with mebendazole: assessment of bound and free drug levels in cyst fluid and of parasite vitality in operative specimens. Eur J Clin Pharmacol 1985; 28:279–285.

104. Ammann R, Tschudi K, von Ziegler M, et al. Langzeitverlauf bei 60 Patienten mit alveolaerer Echinokokkose unter Dauertherapie mit Mebendazol (1976–1985). Klin Wochenschr 1988; 66:1060–1073.

15

Lung Involvement in Schistosomiasis

ELI SCHWARTZ

Center for Geographic and Tropical Medicine,
   Sheba Medical Center,
Tel-Hashomer, Israel and
Division of Internal Medicine, Sackler Faculty of Medicine,
   Tel Aviv University, Tel Aviv, Israel

I. Introduction

Schistosomiasis, also named bilharziasis, is one of the most prevalent infectious diseases in the world. It is endemic in more than 70 countries, mainly in the less developed countries, and is estimated to place about 20% of the endemic population at risk. Thus, the number of people affected are estimated to be ~200 millions (1).

The schistosomes are a group of trematodes (flukes), some of which are pathogenic to humans. The principal parasites that affect humans are *Schistosoma hematobium*, *S. mansoni*, and *S. japonicum*; less prevalent are *S. intercalatum* in Africa and *S. mekongi* in the Far East. The most prevalent area for schistosomiasis is Africa, where *S. hematobium* and *S. mansoni* dominate.

The clinical aspects of schistosomal infection depend on the species. *S. hematobium* that resides mainly in the vesicle bed and gives rise to genitourinary symptoms, while the other species that reside in the mesentrium vasculature manifest in range of gastrointestinal symptoms and could lead to portal hypertension.

As it is, the lungs seem to be a noninvolved organ. However, from long time it is known that a late consequence of schistosoma infection can be pulmonary hypertension due to ectopic migration of schistosomal eggs to the pulmonary vasculature. A recent phenomenon is the lung involvement in early (several weeks after exposure) infection. This phenomena, which seems to be an immunological reaction, is seen mainly in returning travelers (nonimmune population) who contract the disease while have been exposed in fresh water in endemic areas. Physicians practicing in the developed countries have a higher chance to encounter these patients; thus, vigilance to the disease and its treatment is deserved.

The clinical picture of the disease in "nonimmune" travelers can be considerably different from that in the endogenous populations, thus increasing the challenge of diagnosis and management. The literature on the disease among travelers is scarce, and even less information exists on pulmonary involvement. This review will focus thoroughly on the pulmonary manifestation of schistosomiasis in travelers, but includes also the chronic pulmonary manifestation, which occurs among the people of the endemic areas.

II. Incidence and Epidemiology

As mentioned above, approximately 200 million people are affected by the disease, most of them are in Africa. Some foci exist in Brazil (*S. mansoni*) and in the Far East (*S. mekongi*). Figure 1 presents the global distribution of schistosome species. In the recent decades, schistosomiasis has been gaining attention in the developed countries, after increasing numbers of returning travelers have been presenting at medical facilities with variety of symptoms due to schistosomiasis. In most cases, the disease was acquired in sub-Saharan Africa, and once back in the developed world, it becomes a medical challenge to Western doctors less familiar with the disease.

The incidence of schistosomiasis among travelers can only be guessed at from circumstantial evidence. The Center of Diseases Control and Prevention (CDC, Atlanta) and the International Society of Travel Medicine (ISTM) keep a database—GeoSentinel—that collects data of morbidity among returning travelers from a network of 25 travel and tropical clinics around the world (2). According to GeoSentinel, schistosomiasis is one of the 10 leading causes of morbidity among travelers, accounting for 6% of the cases to sub-Saharan Africa. Other data point to schistosomiasis as being a significant cause for morbidity among travelers to Africa who had contact with fresh water bodies. A study done at Lake Malawi, one of the major infected freshwater lakes, showed that there was a correlation between the rate of infection and the days of exposure, with an estimate

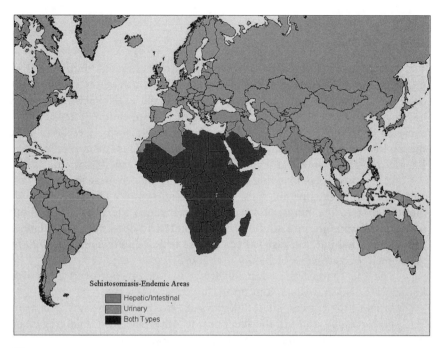

Figure 1 World distribution of *Schistosoma* species according to clinical presentation.

of up to 95% infection of travelers who stayed longer than 7 days (3). It is reported that 55–100% of travelers on rafting tours in African rivers became infected, most of whom were symptomatic (4–7).

A. Incidence of Pulmonary Involvement

The incidence of pulmonary involvement in the early stages of *Schistosoma* infection is unknown. In several series of travelers with Katayama fever, coughing was reported in over 40% of the infected persons (7–9). In these series, radiographic evaluation had not been done. However, in a series we recently published, eight out of 60 patients with schistosomiasis had pulmonary involvement with radiographic findings (10). Since not all patients presented at our clinic at the onset of their early symptoms, this suggests that pulmonary involvement may occur more commonly than previously recognized.

The incidence of lung involvement among patients with chronic schistosomiasis was assessed in several autopsy series. Eggs deposition in lungs of infected people was found in more than 30% of them; however, signs of pulmonary hypertension was found in less than 5% (11).

III. Pathophysiology

A. *Schistosoma* Life Cycle

The life cycle of *Schistosoma* involves two hosts: humans and snails. An infected human sheds the schistosome eggs into fresh water via the urine or feces. Snails, the intermediate hosts, ingest the eggs that subsequently hatch and go through a number of cycles of multiplication. They are then excreted into the water as cercariae, the infective form. Cercariae have the ability to penetrate human skin, or if ingested, to penetrate the gut. People mostly get infected while swimming in contaminated water.

In the process of invading the human skin, the cercariae lose their tails and change into the juvenile form, called schistosomule. The schistosomule migrate first to the lungs, and within 1 week reach the liver. After about 6 weeks, they mature into adult flukes that mate and descend via the venules to their final habitat: the vesicle beds in case of *S. hematobium* infection; the mesenteric beds in case of *S. mansoni* and *S. japonicum*.

The life span of the adult fluke is a matter of controversy, but it is known to be several years, and up to 30 years.

Most of the eggs an adult fluke lays are excreted by the host (via urine in *S. hematobium,* and via the feces in the other species). These eggs are important from the public health point of view, since they are the cause of the spreading of the disease. The minority of the eggs will remain stuck in the host tissue, causing granuloma formation around them. These granulomas are what cause the clinical symptoms of schistosomiasis.

IV. Clinical Manifestations of Schistosomiasis

A. General

The clinical manifestations can be divided into three major stages: The first stage occurs within 24 hours after skin penetration by the cercariae and is manifest as a pruritic papular rash (swimmer's itch; *Schistosoma* dermatitis).

The second stage usually occurs 3–8 weeks after infection during the maturation of the adult fluke. This stage, termed "Katayama fever" or, "toxemic schistosomiasis" is a febrile stage in which the infected patient may suffer from fever, malaise, headache, cough, arthralgia, hepatosplenomegaly, and marked eosinophilia. The fever can mimic malaria with alternating spikes and chills.

This early postinfection period is the stage at which the schistosomules mature into the adult form. The adult flukes mate and start to lay eggs. One theory postulates that, as the flukes begin to lay eggs, soluble antigens leak out from the eggs into the blood stream. At this stage, antibody production lags behind antigen release, and excess antigen prevails. This imbalance causes the immune complex disease, and because the antigen is soluble the effect is systemic. Recovery takes place after antigen–antibody balance is achieved (12). However, our and other data show clearly that this syndrome may occur well before oviposition takes place (10,13,14). Thus, the symptoms are probably the result of an immunological reaction to a variety of circulating antigens at different stages in the life cycle of the parasite. The clinical symptoms are a form of serum sickness or antigen–antibody complex disease (15).

This clinical phase is unique to nonimmune patients and rarely seen in the endogenous population; thus, it mainly affects travelers to endemic areas. The symptoms were originally described in Japan in the Katayama district and therefore it was first believed to occur only in *S. japonicum* infection. However, it was later observed in *S. mansoni* (13,16) and *S. hematobium* (10) infections as well.

The late stage, or chronic schistosomiasis, appears months to years after infection, and results from granuloma formation around the schistosome eggs retained in the tissues. *S. hematobium* infection affects the urinary system and may cause painless hematuria (usually terminal hematuria), dysuria, and later obstructive uropathy. It may even cause squamous cell carcinoma of the bladder.

S. mansoni and *S. japonicum* affect the gastrointestinal system; infection may cause chronic diarrhea, abdominal discomfort, and colonic polyposis. Severe and longstanding infection may cause hepatic fibrosis with portal hypertension and splenomegaly.

During the oviposition stage, ectopic migration of the eggs can occur through the veins to tissues out of their usual habitats, such as the brain (17), spinal cord (18), and lungs (19).

V. Pathophysiology of Lung Involvement in Schistosomiasis

Although the lungs are not an end organ in the life cycle of schistosome infection in humans, pulmonary pathology exists. For many years, pulmonary pathology was described mainly as a late complication of the infection. However, it has recently been recognized that pulmonary involvement may occur also in the early, acute stages (10,20). Early stage pulmonary involvement is unique to nonimmune patients, i.e., populations that had never previously been exposed to schistosome infection, usually travelers from developed countries to endemic areas. Thus, physicians practicing in Western countries who treat returning travelers are more likely to encounter pulmonary involvement in the early stages of infection rather with the later complications (21). Early and late pulmonary schistosomiasis are two different diseases with different clinical manifestations and different pathogenesis and pathology, not merely a difference in time of onset and therefore will be discussed separately.

VI. Early Pulmonary Schistosomiasis

A. Clinical Presentation

Early pulmonary manifestations occur usually 3–8 weeks after schistosome penetration (10,20). Patients with pulmonary schistosomiasis reported shortness of breath, wheezing, and dry cough, mainly while recumbent. Reports show that in some cases the pulmonary symptoms coincided with febrile illness (Katayama fever) (8). However, most patients presented several weeks after the fever had subsided. Almost all the patients could recall having febrile disease before the onset of pulmonary symptoms, but the pulmonary symptoms continued for weeks after the fever subsided (10,20). In this aspect, the clinical picture is different from that of the classical Katayama fever. The physical examination was usually unremarkable, although in some patients prolonged expirium was noted.

Based on our experience (22), pulmonary involvement can be divided into three types:

    a. Symptomatic cases with radiological findings (either chest X-ray or CT scan). The radiological findings may be evident at presentation, or, not uncommonly, may appear after anti-schistosomal treatment. In either case, cough may persist for several weeks, despite the treatment.

    b. Symptomatic cases without radiological findings. In some patients, the clinical course is similar to the one state above, but radiological findings (either chest X-ray or CT scan) are absent. This may be due either to the small dimensions of the findings, making them invisible by conventional methods, or to their transient nature.

    c. Asymptomatic cases with radiological findings. Cases in which there are pulmonary findings without a current history of pulmonary symptoms are rare. The incidence of these cases is unknown, since radiology is usually not performed for asymptomatic patients. However, we were able to identify such cases, since we performed chest X-rays as part of the evaluation of patients who were diagnosed with a suspicion of early schistosomiasis.

B. Pathogenesis

Pulmonary involvement in nonimmune patients occurs relatively early after infection, and is reversible. Symptoms begin about 1 month after exposure and, in our patients, the radiographic evaluations were performed even later, 4–12 weeks after exposure. The infiltrates can therefore not be attributed to schistosomule migration through the lungs, which occurs typically 5–7 days after penetration, nor can they be attributed to granuloma formation around schistosomal eggs, since this process starts before oviposition is expected to take place. Indeed, in the cases we and others saw, there was no correlation between clinical findings and egg burden, and eggs were not detected at the time patients presented with pulmonary symptoms (8,10,20). Furthermore, the pulmonary findings were completely reversible, which would not occur if the pathology were due to granuloma formation around the eggs. It is most likely that the pulmonary pathology is immunologically mediated, and similar to that seen in other forms of eosinophilic pneumonias, such as Loeffler's syndrome, where the inciting agent exists elsewhere in the body (e.g., intestine), but the eosinophils are sequestered in the pulmonary capillaries (23). Indeed, in cases in which transbronchial biopsy was done, eosinophilic infiltration of the air spaces and eosinophilic abscesses were found, but failed to reveal ova or parasite (10,12). Additional support to the immunological theory is the observation that some of the patients developed radiological findings only after anti-schistosomal treatment was initiated. Treatment is a known factor of antigenic stimulation (24), and may be accompanied by transient clinical deterioration, such as fever, skin rash, pulmonary function test abnormality, pleural effusion, and respiratory failure (12,25,26).

Katayama fever is also the result of an immunological process that occurs in nonimmune patients 3–8 weeks after infection, as a reaction to the circulating parasite antigen(s), just as in the afebrile pulmonary schistosomiasis described above. Thus, the whole range of symptoms occurring in nonimmune patients during the early stage of the infection, such as fever, urticaria, pulmonary manifestations, and eosinophilia, are all part of the same immunological process, and can be assembled under the term "schistosoma hyper-reactive syndrome."

Laboratory and Imaging

Laboratory findings reveal significant eosinophilia, usually in a range of 30–50%, with mild leukocytosis (10,12,20). Liver function tests are occasionally abnormal with elevated levels of the transaminases.

Radiography: The most common chest radiograph abnormalities observed were small, nodular lesions with ill-defined borders. Less common were reticulonodular patterns. Chest CT revealed more nodular lesions than had been apparent on the chest X rays. In rare cases a bilateral, diffuse, ground glass pattern was demonstrated, with ill-defined nodules. Neither pleural effusion nor lymphadenopathy was evident. In about 25% of our cases, the radiographic abnormalities appeared only after praziquantel therapy (10,20).

Diagnosis

In general, the diagnosis of early schistosomiasis in travelers still poses a challenge, and has to be based initially on clinical judgment. The traditional test, of examining stool and urine for parasite eggs, has low sensitivity. The sensitivity of stool or urine examinations, even when performed on three separate occasions is limited by the sporadic passage of eggs by the adult flukes, and the low fluke burden usually found in travelers. Rectal biopsy may, to some extent, increase the sensitivity of the test. However, it must be emphasized that nonimmune patients may be acutely ill with pulmonary manifestation well before oviposition by the adult flukes has begun, and thus stool or urine exams performed at this time will be unrevealing. PCR performed on feces and serum was recently shown to have high sensitivity and specificity when tested in endemic area of Brazil (27). This method is an attractive option for travelers in whom the burden of eggs is usually low and symptoms may appear before oviposition.

Serologic testing is potentially much more sensitive; however, it is not routinely used, and is mainly performed in research laboratories. In addition, the sensitivity and specificity of the tests vary according the antigen used. The parasite laboratory at the Center of Disease Control and Prevention (CDC, Atlanta, USA) uses FAST-ELISA as the initial step in diagnosis. Confirmation and speciation of positive ELISA results is performed with an enzyme-linked immunoelectrotransfer blot (EITB) that provides almost 100% specificity in confirming the presence of the *Schistosoma* species (3). This method has proved to be highly sensitive and specific, and usually becomes positive relatively early, 4–6 weeks after exposure. Other methods, in other laboratories, seem to be less sensitive and specific, becoming positive at a later date.

A major limitation of the serology test is that it stays positive for many years despite efficacious treatment, thus excluding it for use in confirming re-exposure, or for evaluating the success or failure of treatment.

For the clinician, the most important clue to obtain is a good travel history of the patient and especially to ask about exposure to freshwater in endemic areas. The high eosinophilic counts that occur during the acute stage of the disease may be a very useful indication for diagnosis.

Treatment

The drug of choice for treating all schistosome species is two doses of 20–30 mg/kg praziquantel given orally within 12 hours.

Praziquantel is an excellent and well-tolerated agent. However, it is known to be effective only against the adult fluke (28). Thus, its role in acute schistosomiasis has not been proved, since at that stage of the disease the fluke may not have fully matured. Despite this, many of our patients appeared to improve soon after receiving the drug. We cannot rule out the fact that this might have been due to the self-limiting nature of the process rather than to praziquantel treatment (29).

Acute schistosomiasis is immunological by nature, and thus corticosteroids may be effective therapy. Patients with severe manifestations either at presentation or following the treatment should get short course of steroids.

Some physicians recommend a repeat course of praziquantel several weeks following the first course, since the first course may have been given too early, when the fluke had not matured enough to be killed by the drug (8), or because the concomitant steroid may have reduced the blood levels of praziquantel (30).

Based on the pathophysiology of the disease at this stage, the treatment of early, acute schistosomiasis at presentation can be with corticosteroids alone, followed by praziquantel several weeks later, to ensure eradication of the adult flukes. Controlled studies comparing these options are very difficult to perform due to the small numbers of patients seen at each clinic, and due to the fact that we don't have a good tool to assess eradication of the flukes.

A new promising antischistosomal drugs are the artemisinin derivates. Artemether, a Chinese drug that originally was developed as an antimalaria agent, has been shown to have antischistosomal activity, that is by a different mechanism than that of praziquantel. Artemether acts on the juvenile forms of the schistosome (31), in contrast to praziquantel that acts on the mature form. Thus, artemether may play a roll in the future in treating the acute stage of *Schistosoma* infection.

VII. Chronic Pulmonary Disease

The chronic pulmonary disease is seen among the people of hyperendemic schistosome areas and it is the result of heavy and untreated infection.

A. Pathophysiology

The ectopic migration of schistosome eggs can reach the pulmonary beds. In the case of *S. hematobium* infection, the final station of the adult flukes is in the perivesical plexus. From there the eggs laid by the mature flukes can be swept by the systemic venous system that drains the venous plexus to reach the lungs. As for *S. mansoni* and *S. japonicum,* their ova are swept with the portal blood flow, and become lodged in the venules of the liver. There, the host immune system creates a granuloma around the eggs, which can eventually cause periportal hepatic fibrosis ("pipestem fibrosis") and portal hypertension. As a result of portal hypertension, portocaval shunts are opened. This enables the schistosome eggs to be swept along until they become lodged in the lungs. In such cases, pulmonary involvement follows portal hypertension. Although this is the accepted explanation, there have been reports documenting *S. mansoni* eggs in lungs of patients without evidence of hepatic fibrosis (32).

When the eggs reach the pulmonary beds, they either remain in the lumen or migrate to the lung tissue itself. Antigenic properties released by the eggs stimulate local lymphocytic reactions, causing granuloma formation. The resulting granuloma and the fibrosis following it may lead to obliterative arteritis, and, if extensive enough, to pulmonary hypertension, and subsequently to the development of cor pulmonale.

Lung histology shows dumbbell-shaped interarterial and perivascular granulomas with local angiogenesis, causing dilated and twisted vessels, named "angiomatoid" (33).

B. Clinical Presentation

The clinical expression of chronic pulmonary schistosomiasis can be divided into three groups (34): (a) asymptomatic cases with schistosomal eggs in the pulmonary beds, with or without granuloma formation; (b) granuloma formation with pulmonary hypertension; (c) granuloma formation with pulmonary hypertension and cor pulmonale.

Upon the patient develop symptoms, the clinical symptoms are similar to those of any patients with pulmonary hypertension and cor pulmonale: dyspnea, chest pain, fatigue, palpitation, and cough. As in cor pulmonale, signs of right heart failure are also evident. Pulmonary function tests may show some alterations, such as mild airway obstruction or decreased lung volumes, but these findings are nonspecific (35). Similarly, chest X-rays are not different from those of other patients with pulmonary hypertension and cor pulmonale, manifest as cardiomegaly and pulmonary arterial enlargement. Focal opacities in the lung parenchyma and radiographic findings mimicking tuberculosis or tumor have been reported (11).

In addition, hepatosplenomegaly may be found due to portal hypertension that is secondary to infection with *S. mansoni* or *S. japonicum*. Cirrhosis of the liver is not part of the disease, since it affects the presinusoidal areas.

It is still not clear whether all cases inevitably develop into cor pulmonale and whether such a progression is only a matter of time.

Other possibilities to explain why not all patients developed symptoms are:

a. eggs load: only high density of fluke eggs may cause the progression to occur.
b. rate at which eggs are released: if a low density of eggs is released over time, a less vigorous response from the immune system may result (34).
c. species-specific response: in a comparison of autopsy and clinical data, it was documented that although *S. hematobium* is found at significant percentages in pulmonary beds, it causes much less cor pulmonale compared to *S. mansoni* (11).

Diagnosis

Diagnosis should be based on demonstration of schistosome infection, i.e., demonstrating eggs in stool or urine by direct microscopy or rectal/bladder biopsy. Serology tests in these cases are not useful since they cannot differentiate between current infection and past exposure. Since most people with this pathology are from endemic areas (residents or immigrants), with a high probability of past exposure to schistosome, serology testing is not indicated.

Indirect evidence of infection can be found by demonstrating hepatosplenic or genitourinary schistosomiasis by means of ultrasound or CT scans (19). The usefulness of bronchoscopy and tissue biopsy for diagnosis has never been assessed systematically, but they are unlikely to be helpful, due to the small amount of tissue obtained and to the sporadic distribution of the granulomas (19). There have been case reports in which open lung biopsy revealed the diagnosis (36,37), but this should not be adopted as protocol.

Sputum analysis for ova has a very low yield. However, PCR of sputum, already tested for filariasis (38), is a method currently under investigation for schistosomiasis with promising results (J. Hamburger, personal communication).

Treatment

As mentioned, the drug of choice for schistosome infection is praziquantel; however, when dealing with chronic infection with fibrotic sequela to granuloma formation, one may assume that the changes are irreversible. Interestingly, several prospective studies have shown that praziquantel treatment reverses mild to moderate changes in the liver and urinary systems (39,40). There are no data regarding the effect of the drug on the pulmonary changes. Nonetheless, there are several reasons in favor of this treatment. First, pragmatically, since the spectrum of side effects to the drug is mild, it is worth trying it. In addition, the treatment is targeted at killing the adult flukes, thus stopping the egg shedding and halting the progression of the disease. We therefore recommend that chronic patients be given drug therapy, regardless of the severity of their symptoms. The dose should be the same as for early infection: two doses of 20–30 mg/kg over 12 hours. The physician should be aware that clinical deterioration may also occur after chronic infection and be vigilant (12), although this is much less common compared to the nonimmune population.

VIII. Prevention

Control and prevention of the disease in the endemic countries is beyond the scope of this manuscript. Among travelers to endemic areas, mainly

Africa, prevention of the disease is primarily by avoiding contact with fresh-water lakes or rivers (there is no risk of contracting schistosomiasis in salt water). Our experience with travelers shows that this advice is often not fol-lowed, as water entertainment (such as diving in lake Malawi or rafting on rivers in Africa) is too enticing.

There are studies that are searching for other protective measures. Using a repellent before swimming, such as DEET (*N,N*-diethyl-toluamide), the active ingredient for mosquito repelling, may give some protection (41).

A new direction in prevention of schistosomiasis is by using arte-mether, the Chinese antimalaria drug, which was found to be active against the juvenile forms of schistosome (31). It does not prevent the infection but by treating people soon after exposure, it may prevent the clinical symptoms of the acute stage, and by preventing the maturation of the worms, chronic schistosomiasis and the chain of infection may be ceased (31,42).

A controlled study was done in China during flood and showed that people exposed to schistome who were treated by artemether significantly had less episodes of acute schistosomiasis (43). Further studies in nonim-mune population are needed before reaching a conclusion about the role of this drug.

Table 1 Comparison Between Early and Late Pulmonary Schistosomiasis

	Acute pulmonary disease	Chronic pulmonary disease
Time of onset (after exposure)	Weeks (4–8)	Years
Population at risk	Nonimmune (mainly travelers)	Immune population residing in endemic areas
Pathogenesis	Immune-complex disease	Granuloma formation
Clinical manifestation	Cough, fever, eosinophilia	Pulmonary hypertension
Imaging	Pulmonary nodules	Pulmonary hypertension, cor pulmonale
Species specific	All species (most probably)	All species; *S. mansoni* more severe disease
Diagnosis	Mainly by means of serology. Ova in stool/urine may be found	Demonstrating ova in stool/urine or in lung tissue; serology is not helpful
Treatment: Steroid	Effective	Non-effective
Praziquantel	Effective+/−	Effective
Artemether	May play a role	Probably, not effective
Outcome	Reversible	May be partially reversible

Source: From Ref. 22.

IX. Conclusion

Pulmonary involvement in patients with schistosomiasis can be seen early after infection in nonimmune population such as travelers to endemic areas or in residents in areas where schistosomiasis is not hyperendemic.

Another form of pulmonary involvement is seen as a late consequence of chronic and heavy infection in population of endemic areas who are chronically exposed to the infection.

The clinical spectrum of these two manifestations, the pathophysiology, and treatment are all different and summarized in Table 1.

Clinicians in the Western countries have a higher chance of encountering the early (acute) form of the disease, although immigrants from endemic countries may present with late (chronic) schistosomiasis. In the differential diagnosis of pulmonary pathology, especially when accompanied by eosinophilia, schistosomal infection should be considered. The travel history of the patient is mandatory for an evaluation.

Acknowledgment

The author thanks Dr. Judith Rozenman, The Department of Radiology, Sheba Medical Center for her valuable assistance in preparing the radiology section.

References

1. Mahmoud AAF, Abdel Wahab MF. Schistosomiasis. In: Warren KS, Mahmoud AAF, eds. Tropical and Geographical Medicine. New York: McGraw-Hill, 1990:470–471.
2. Freedman DO, et al. GeoSentinel: the global emerging infections sentinel network of the International Society of Travel Medicine. J Travel Med 1999; 6(2):94–98.
3. Cetron MS, et al. Schistosomiasis in Lake Malawi. Lancet 1996; 348(9037): 1274–1278.
4. Chapman PJ, Wilkinson PR, Davidson RN. Acute schistosomiasis (Katayama fever) among British air crew. BMJ 1988; 297(6656):1101.
5. Anonymous. From the Centers for Disease Control. Acute schistosomiasis in US travelers returning from Africa. JAMA 1990; 263(16):2165–2166.
6. Pitkanen YT, et al. Acute schistosomiasis mansoni in Finnish hunters visiting Africa: need for appropriate diagnostic serology. Scand J Infect Dis 1990; 22(5):597–600.
7. Schwartz E, et al. Schistosome infection among rafters on the Omo River, Ethiopia. J Travel Med 2005; 12:3–8.
8. Doherty JF, Moody AH, Wright SG. Katayama fever: an acute manifestation of schistosomiasis. BMJ 1996; 313(7064):1071–1072.

9. Visser LG, Polderman AM, Stuiver PC. Outbreak of schistosomiasis among travelers returning from Mali, West Africa. Clin Infect Dis 1995; 20(2):280–285.
10. Schwartz E, Rozenman J, Perelman M. Pulmonary manifestations of early schistosome infection among nonimmune travelers. Am J Med 2000; 109(9): 718–722.
11. Morris W, Knauer CM. Cardiopulmonary manifestations of schistosomiasis. Semin Respir Infect 1997; 12(2):159–170.
12. Davidson BL, et al. The "lung shift" in treated schistosomiasis. Bronchoalveolar lavage evidence of eosinophilic pneumonia. Chest 1986; 89(3):455–457.
13. Hiatt RA, et al. Factors in the pathogenesis of acute schistosomiasis mansoni. J Infect Dis 1979; 139(6):659–666.
14. Walt F. The Katayama syndrome. South Afr Med J 1954; 28:89–93.
15. Hiatt RA, et al. Serial observations of circulating immune complexes in patients with acute schistosomiasis. J Infect Dis 1980; 142(5):665–670.
16. Diaz-Rivera E, et al. Acute Manson's schistosomiasis. Am J Med 1956; 18: 918–943.
17. Pittella JE. Neuroschistosomiasis. Brain Pathol 1997; 7(1):649–662.
18. Ferrari TC. Spinal cord schistosomiasis. A report of 2 cases and review emphasizing clinical aspects. Medicine 1999; 78(3):176–190.
19. Phillips JF, et al. Radiographic evaluation of patients with schistosomiasis. Radiology 1975; 114(1):31–37.
20. Cooke GS, et al. Acute pulmonary schistosomiasis in travelers returning from Lake Malawi, sub-Saharan Africa. Clin Infect Dis 1999; 29(4):836–839.
21. Schwartz E, Rozenman J. Schistosomiasis [comment]. N Engl J Med 2002; 347(10):766–768; author reply 766–768.
22. Schwartz E. Pulmonary schistosomiasis. Clin Chest Med 2002; 23(2):433–443.
23. Lucas SB, Schwartz DA, Hasleton PS. Parasitic lung disease. In: Spencer H, Hasleton PS, eds. Spencer's pathology of the lung. New York: McGraw-Hill, 1996:327–332.
24. Harnett W, Kusel JR. Increased exposure of parasite antigens at the surface of adult male *Schistosoma mansoni* exposed to praziquantel in vitro. Parasitology 1986; 93(Pt 2):401–405.
25. Azher M, et al. Exudative polyserositis and acute respiratory failure following praziquantel therapy. Chest 1990; 98(1):241–243.
26. Harries AD, Cook GC. Acute schistosomiasis (Katayama fever): clinical deterioration after chemotherapy. J Infect 1987; 14(2):159–161.
27. Pontes LA, Dias-Neto E, Rabello A. Detection by polymerase chain reaction of *Schistosoma mansoni* DNA in human serum, and feces. Am J Trop Med Hyg 2002; 66(2):157–162.
28. Xiao SH, Catto BA, Webster LT Jr. Effects of praziquantel on different developmental stages of *Schistosoma mansoni* in vitro and in vivo. J Infect Dis 1985; 151(6):1130–1137.
29. Nash TE, et al. Schistosome infections in humans: perspectives and recent findings. N1H conference. Ann Intern Med 1982; 97(5):740–754.
30. Vazquez ML, Jung H, Sotelo J. Plasma levels of praziquantel decrease when dexamethasone is given simultaneously. Neurology 1987; 37(9):1561–1562.

31. Xiao S, et al. Tegumental alterations in juvenile *Schistosoma haematobium* harboured in hamsters following artemether treatment. Parasitology Int 2001; 50(3):175–183.

32. Shaw AFB, Ghareb AA. The pathogenesis of pulmonary schistosomiasis in Egypt with special reference to Ayerza's disease. J Pathol Bacteriol 1938; 46:401–424.

33. Sadigursky M, Andrade ZA. Pulmonary changes in schistosomal cor pulmonale. Am J Trop Med Hyg 1982; 31(4):779–784.

34. Andrade ZA, Andrade SG. Pathogenesis of schistosomal pulmonary arteritis. Am J Trop Med Hyg 1970; 19(2):305–310.

35. Frayser R, De Alonso AE. Studies of pulmonary function in patients with *Schistosomiasis mansoni*. Am Rev Respir Dis 1967; 95(6):1036–1040.

36. Wessel HU, Sommers HM, Cugell DW. Variants of cardiopulmonary manifestations of Manson's schistosomiasis: report of two cases. Ann Intern Med 1965; 62:757–766.

37. Richter J, et al. Hepatosplenic schistosomiasis: comparison of sonographic findings in Brazilian and Sudanese patients—correlation of sonographic findings with clinical symptoms. Radiology 1992; 184(3):711–716.

38. Abbasi I, et al. Diagnosis of *Wuchereria bancrofti* infection by the polymerase chain reaction employing patients' sputum. Parasitology Res 1999; 85(10): 844–849.

39. Homeida MA, et al. Association of the therapeutic activity of praziquantel with the reversal of Symmers' fibrosis induced by *Schistosoma mansoni*. Am J Trop Med Hyg 1991; 45(3):360–365.

40. Ohmae H, et al. Improvement of ultrasonographic and serologic changes in *Schistosoma japonicum*-infected patients after treatment with praziquantel. Am J Trop Med Hyg 1992; 46(1):99–104.

41. Secor WE, Freeman GL Jr, Wirtz RA. Short report: prevention of *Schistosoma mansoni* infections in mice by the insect repellents AI3-3 7220 and *N,N*-diethyl-3-methylbenzamide. Am J Trop Med Hyg 1999; 60(6):1061–1062.

42. Utzinger J, et al. Oral artemether for prevention of *Schistosoma mansoni* infection: randomised controlled trial. Lancet 2000; 355(9212):1320–1325.

43. Song Y, et al. Preventive effect of artemether on schistosome infection. Chin Med J 1998; 111(2):123–127.

16

Pulmonary Manifestations in Familial Mediterranean Fever

NURIT TWEEZER-ZAKS, PNINA LANGEVITZ, and EINAT RABINOVICH

Internal Medicine "F" and the Heller Institute for Medical Research, Sheba Medical Center, Tel Hashomer, Israel

AVI LIVNEH

Tel Aviv University, Sackler School of Medicine, Tel Aviv, Israel

I. Introduction

Although probably existing since ancient times, familial Mediterranean fever (FMF) was not recognized as a unique entity until 1945, when Siegal (1) described 10 cases of "benign paroxysmal peritonitis." Since then, this condition has been given a variety of names (e.g., hereditary recurrent polyserositis, periodic disease, Armenian disease), emphasizing its genetic and episodic nature and the geographic distribution. FMF is characterized by recurrent episodes of fever and serositis, involving primarily the peritoneum (affecting 95% of patients), the pleura (40% of patients) and the synovial membrane of the joints (75% of patients). Typical febrile episodes of skin rash (erysipelas-like erythema), pericarditis, scrotal pain, and myalgia occur less frequently. The poorly understood leg pain, together with the rare manifestation of protracted febrile myalgia, the uncommon development of chronic arthritis and the nephropathic AA amyloidosis complete the clinical spectrum (2).

A single attack begins abruptly, attains its peak within 24–72 hours, and resolves spontaneously. It may involve one or several serosal sites and is generally accompanied by fever. FMF attacks are followed by symptom-free intervals varying in length, from days to years (3).

Acute phase response is the hallmark of an FMF attack, with marked elevation in the serum levels of erythrocyte sedimentation rates and acute phase proteins [i.e., fibrinogen, serum amyloid A protein (SAA—the AA amyloid precursor), C reactive protein]. Proinflammatory cytokine levels (IL1, IL6, IL8, TNF-alpha) are also elevated (4,5). Even between the attacks, some of the acute phase proteins and the transcript levels of some cytokines may still remain high (6–8).

Chest involvement, the subject of the present report, is frequent in FMF, with pleuritic chest pain being its pathognomonic feature. Uncommon thoracic presentations, including those associated with pericardial, myocardial, lung, and vascular abnormalities are recently being increasingly reported, and will be commented on in this paper.

II. Incidence and Epidemiology

FMF is most common among four ethnic groups: Jews, Armenians, Turks, and middle-eastern Arabs, populations residing in the Mediterranean basin, as indicated by the name of the disease (9). Among Jewish patients, the disease is most frequent in the Sephardi (North African origin and Iraqi) sub-populations, with a prevalence ranging from 1:250 to 1:1000. FMF is less common among Ashkenazi (of European descent) Jews, with a prevalence of about 1:73,000 (10). In Turkey, the frequency of the disorder may be as high as 1:1000, depending on the region where the study was performed (11). In Armenia, the prevalence of FMF is very high (12). According to a calculated carrier frequency, the estimated prevalence may be as high as in North African Jews (13). FMF attacks typically begin during the first decade of life, but late onset of FMF has also been reported (14). Even to date, a big diagnostic delay is frequently seen, despite the increasing knowledge and the multitude of reports on FMF in the medical literature.

III. Genetics

The gene causing FMF, *MEFV*, was cloned from the short arm of chromosome 16 in 1997 (15). So far, some 40 mutations have been identified, mostly in exon 10, including, in declining order of frequency, the *M694V* mutation (common in North African Jews and in most other ethnic groups), the *V726A* mutation (Iraqi Jews and Arabs), the *M694I* mutation (Arabs), and the *E148Q* mutation (all ethnicities).

Numerous studies on phenotype–genotype correlations have been published since the cloning of the gene, attributing both the severity and the different FMF manifestations to certain mutations or mutation combinations. The strongest genotype–phenotype association was formed between disease severity and homozygosity for *M694V* (16–18).

Because the mutations so far discovered recognize only about 60% of the patients, the diagnosis is still based on clinical criteria, which hold a sensitivity of 97% (19). Mutational analysis of the MEFV gene is therefore currently used only to aid the clinical diagnosis. Low sensitivity is also a problem in the genetic evaluation of the disease (20,21). A population screen revealed many unaffected individuals carrying two mutations. Surprisingly, the prevalence of such phenotype III subjects is several times higher than that of individuals with an overt disease (22).

The high gene frequency and high rate of carrier state in the affected populations suggest a possible biological advantage to heterozygotes. It is believed that carriage of the gene confers a protection against an already obliterated infectious agent. Yet, this possible increased "alertness" to infection works against a heterozygote, affected by an autoinflammatory or autoimmune disease, such as rheumatiod arthritis and multiple sclerosis, by increasing the severity of this disease (23,24).

IV. Pathophysiology

Pyrin protein, the *MEFV* gene product, expressed primarily in mature neutrophils, monocytes, and eosinophils, is thought to be a downregulator of inflammation. In neutrophils, pyrin is expressed in the cytoplasm, bound to the microtubules of neutrophil cytoskeleton, thus probably affecting neutrophil migration to the serosal tissues, where they play a major role in FMF attacks. Pyrin protein, deriving its name from the Greek word Pyrus (meaning fire or fever), is part of a large, structurally related family of proteins (including cryopyrin, ASC, PYPAF7, NOD, NALP1, and others), involved in apoptosis and inflammation via transcription factors (NFkB, IL1) and intracellular signal transduction, through protein–protein interactions. The specific role of pyrin in this complex molecular network is yet to be defined (25).

V. FMF as a Prototype of the Periodic Fever Syndromes

FMF is the prototype of an expanding number of disorders (the episodic febrile autoinflammatory diseases, or EFAIDs), defined by recurrent attacks of painful manifestations, fever, elevated serum levels of acute phase reactants, and spontaneous remissions (26). These include the hyper-IgD syndrome (HIDS), TNF receptor 1-associated periodic fever syndrome (TRAPS), Muckle Wells syndrome (MWS), chronic infantile neurological, cutaneous, and articular syndrome (CINCA), familial cold autoinflammatory syndrome (FCAS), periodic fever with aphthous stomatitis, pharyngitis and adenopathy (PFAPA), pyogenic arthritis with pyoderma gangrenosum and acne (PAPA), chronic recurrent multifocal osteomyelitis (CRMO) and other, yet undifferentiated EFAIDs. The term *autoinflammatory* differentiates these conditions from *autoimmune* diseases, in the absence of detectable auto-antibodies or involvement of antigen-specific T cells in the inflammatory attack.

VI. Treatment

Colchicine, introduced in 1972 (27) is the hallmark of therapy in FMF, reducing both the frequency and the severity of the FMF attacks. Colchicine administered at a dose of 1–2 mg/day, not only prevents the attacks but also protects the kidneys from AA amyloidosis (28). During the attacks, analgesics or nonsteroidal anti-inflammatory drugs are being used to alleviate the fever and the pain, because FMF attacks are unresponsive to an increase in colchicine dosage or corticosteroids.

Patients resistant to colchicine therapy may benefit from the addition of intravenous colchicine, thalidomide, or anti-TNF therapy to their regular oral colchicine treatment regimen (29,30). Allogeneic bone marrow transplantation, which was also reported successful in one FMF patient with concomitant diserythropoietic anemia, is at this point not considered an applicable alternative because it carries a high risk of morbidity and mortality (31). Recently, subcutaneous interferon-α administration just prior to the attack was suggested as a means of prevention of attack initiation and/or shortening of its duration (32).

VII. Chest Manifestations of FMF

A. Pleural Involvement

Pleural attacks have been commonly reported in FMF patients. Pleuritis is the most common thoracic manifestation of FMF, affecting roughly 70% of children and 40% of adult patients. The typical attacks last 24 to 72 hours and include symptoms and signs of pleuritis (unilateral, stabbing chest pain, aggravated by inspiration), associated with fever and laboratory evidence of acute phase response (leucocytosis, elevated erythrocyte sedimentation rate, C reactive protein, or other acute phase reactants). Physical examination is usually unrevealing, but diminished breath sounds or pleural friction rub may be evident. Evidence for a small amount of pleural fluid, or atelectasis can be detected on plain chest X-ray or echocardiography (33,34). It is remarkable that pleural adhesions are only rarely produced even after hundreds of attacks.

B. Lung Involvement

Involvement of lung parenchyma in FMF has rarely been reported and was mainly found in association with secondary (AA) amyloidosis and vasculitis. Pulmonary amyloidosis is extremely rare and is usually part of diffuse, multiorgan AA amyloidosis. Two case reports of diffuse and extensive amyloid depositions in lung parenchyma of FMF patients have so far been reported (35,36). In autopsies of 42 FMF patients, very fine amyloid deposits were reported in alveolar septa, in areas adjacent to the pleura. But these findings caused no symptoms.

In severely affected individuals, suffering of multiple chest attacks and homozygotes to the *M694V* mutation, the pulmonary function tests may demonstrate a restrictive pattern in between the FMF attacks. This finding suggests a development of chronic pleural disease and pleural thickening as a possible sequela of recurrent pleuritis in FMF (37,38).

Several vasculitides (including polyarteritis nodosa, Henoch Shoenlein purpura, Behçet's disease, protracted febrile myalgia) have been reported to be relatively frequent in FMF. Yet, only a single case of pulmonary vasculitis has so far been published (39). Also worth mentioning is a single case of superior vena cava thrombosis in an FMF patient, with no evidence of nephrotic syndrome or amyloidosis (40). The patient's brother was diagnosed with Behçet's disease and some form of FMF–Behçet's disease overlap was believed to exist in this patient.

Finally, the negative association between FMF and asthma, once thought to reflect a protective role of the FMF gene, is now considered false (41). The possible genetic and enzymatic links described in the past still remain to be established.

C. Pericardial Involvement

Pericarditis has uncommonly been reported in FMF. In a large, retrospective series of 4000 patients, merely 27 (< 0.7%) had evidence of pericarditis (per electrocardiogam, echocardiogram, or chest X-ray). In all of these patients, the course of the attack was typical for FMF, with respect to duration, physical signs and symptoms, and spontaneous remissions (42,43). We are aware of only a single FMF patient, with recurrent attacks of pericarditis as the sole clinical manifestation (44). Interestingly, an echocardiographic study in a series of 30 randomly selected FMF patients revealed echocardiographic evidence of pericardial disease (including pericardial effusions and/or pericardial thickening) in eight (27%) (45). One FMF patient with constrictive pericarditis has also been reported (46).

D. Heart Involvement

Cardiac involvement due to AA amyloidosis is a well-established feature of advanced, untreated, or poorly responsive FMF. Other forms of myocardial involvement are very uncommon. Cardiovascular autonomic dysfunction was evaluated in 40 asymptomatic FMF patients using tilt test. In 17% of the patients, but in none of the control group, the provocative head up tilt test demonstrated dysautonomia (47).

An Armenian study on a large cohort of 4167 untreated FMF patients reported an increased risk for coronary events, possibly due to the atherogenic effect of chronic inflammation. In contrast, we found that the prevalence of ischemic heart diseases in patients with colchicine-treated FMF was comparable to that of their healthy spouses, and to the matched controls from the general population, thus underscoring the importance of colchicine therapy in reducing ischemic heart disease in FMF (48,49). Other rare reports include a case of acute myocardial infarction due to vasculitis in the myocardium (50), and a possible increased susceptibility to cardiac involvement in rheumatic fever (51).

E. Thoracic Malignancy

Over the years, several case reports of peritoneal mesothelioma in patients with recurrent abdominal attacks have been published (52–55). In our large cohort of some 6000 FMF patients, only a single case of malignant pleural mesothelioma was observed. In addition, only one case of bronchoalveolar carcinoma in FMF patients was published (56). Furthermore, the Israeli Cancer Registry, which receives data on all patients with cancer in Israel, does not imply an increased or decreased incidence of malignancy in FMF patients.

VIII. Conclusions and Perspective

This report brings light to some of the recent advances in FMF research, including the demonstration of a pyrin domain in a family of apoptotic proteins, the presentation of a relatively large array of new therapies for FMF, the classification of FMF among the newly defined FMF-like entities, and the progress made in the elucidation of new thoracic associations of FMF. These undoubtedly predict a scientifically exciting future, in which it is expected that the specific role of pyrin in inflammation will be detailed, leading to a better understanding of the pathophysiology of FMF attack. Additionally, it is possible that the accumulating experience with new medications will establish an alternative safe treatment for colchicine failure. Finally, it is expected that further research will shed new light on the older, currently considered speculative links and define new thoracic associations of FMF.

References

1. Siegal S. Benign paraoxysmal peritonitis. Ann Intern Med 1945; 23:1–21.
2. Ben Chetrit E, Levy M. Familial Mediterranean fever. Lancet 1998; 351: 659–664.
3. Livneh A, Langevitz P, Zemer D, Padeh S, Migdal A, Sohar E, Pras M. The changing face of familial Mediterranean fever. Semin Arthritis Rheum 1996; 26:612–627.
4. Gang N, Drenth JP, Langevitz P, Zemer D, Brezniak N, Pras M, van der Meed JW, Livneh A. Activation of the cytokine network in familial Mediterranean fever. J Rheumatol 1999; 26:890–897.
5. Drenth JP, van Deuren M, van der Ven-Jongekrijg J, Schalkwijk CG, van der Meer JW. Cytokine activation during attacks of hyper immunoglobulin D syndrome and periodic fever. Blood 1995; 85:3586–3593.
6. Korkmaz C, Ozdogan H, Kasepcopur O, Yazici H. Acute phase response in familial Mediterranean fever. Ann Rheum Dis 2002; 61:79–81.
7. Duzova A, Bakkaloglu A, Besbas N, Topaloglu R, Ozen S, Ozaltin F, Bassoy Y, Yilmaz E. Role of A-SAA in monitoring subclinical inflammation and in colchicine dosage in familial Mediterranean fever. Clin Exp Rheumatol 2003; 21:509–514.
8. Notarnicola C, Didelot MN, Seguret F, Demaille J, Touitou I. Enhanced cytokine mRNA levels in attack free patients with familial Mediterranean fever. Genes Immun 2002; 3:43–45.
9. Brik R, Limanovitz D, Berkowitz D, Shamir R, Rosenthal E, Shinawi M, Gershoni-Baruch R. Incidence of familial Mediterranean fever mutations among children of Mediterranean extraction with functional abdominal pain. J Pediatr 2001; 138:759–762.
10. Gershoni-Baruch R, Shinawi M, Leah K, Badarnah K, Brik R. Familial Mediterranean fever: prevalence, penetrance and genetic drift. Eur J Hum Genet 2001; 9:634–637.
11. Yalchinkaya F, Cakar N, Misirlioglu M, Tumer N, Akar N, Tekin M, Tastan H, Kocak H, Oskaya N, Elhan AH. Genotype–phenotype correlation in a large group of Turkish patients with FMF: evidence for mutation independent amyloidosis. Rheumatology (Oxford) 2000; 39:67–72.
12. Cazeneuve C, Hovannesyan Z, Genevieve D, Hayrapetyan H, Rapin S, Girodon-Boulandet E, Boissier B, Feingold J, Atayan K, Sarkisian T, Amsalem S. Familial Mediterranean fever among patients from Karabakh and the diagnostic value of MEFV gene analysis in all classically affected populations. Arthritis Rheum 2003; 48:2324–2331.
13. Armenian HK, Sha'ar KH. Epidemiologic observations in familial paroxysmal polyserositis. Epidemiol Rev 1986; 8:106–116.
14. Tamir N, Langevitz P, Zemer D, Pras E, Shinar Y, Padeh S, Zaks N, Pras M, Livneh A. Late onset familial Mediterranean fever: a subset with distinct

clinical, demographic and molecular characteristics. Am J Med Genet 1999; 87:30–35.

15. The international FMF consortium. Ancient missense mutations in a new member of the RoRet gene family are likely to cause FMF. Cell 1997; 90: 797–807.

16. Livneh A, Langevitz P, Shinar Y, Zaks N, Kastner DL, Pras M. MEFV mutation analysis in patients suffering from amyloidosis of FMF. Amyloid 1999; 6:1–6.

17. Shinar Y, Livneh A, Langevitz P, Zaks N, Aksentijevich I, Koziol DE. Genotype–phenotype assessment of common genotypes among patients with FMF. J Rheumatol 2000; 27:1703–1707.

18. Sidi G, Shinar Y, Livneh A, Langevitz P, Pras M, Pras E. Protracted febrile myalgia of FMF—mutation analysis and clinical correlations. Scand J Rheumatol 2000; 29:174–176.

19. Livneh A, Langevitz P, Zemer D, Zaks N, Kees S, Lidar Z. Criteria for the diagnosis of FMF. Arthritis Rheum 1997; 40:1884–1890.

20. Livneh A, Langevitz P. Diagnosis and treatment concerns in familial Mediterranean fever. Baillieres Best Pract Res Clin Rheumatol 2000; 14:477–498.

21. Ben Chetrit E, Sagi M. Genetic counseling in familial Mediterranean fever: has the time come? Rheumatology (Oxford) 2001; 40:606–609.

22. Kogan A, Shinar Y, Lidar M, Revivo A, Langevitz P, Padeh S, Pras M, Livneh A. Common MEFV mutations among Jewish ethnic groups in Israel: high frequency of carrier and phenotype III state and absence of a perceptible advantage or the carrier state. Am J Med Genet 2001; 102:272–276.

23. Rabinovich E, Livneh A, Lagnevitz P, Shinar E, Zaks N, Shinar Y. Mediterranean fever gene (MEFV) mutations and rheumatoid arthritis: a severe combination. Clin Exp Rheumatol 2002; 20(s26):s–73.

24. Shinar Y, Livneh A, Villa Y, Pinhasov A, Zeitoun I, Kogan A, Achiron A. Common mutations in the familial Mediterranean fever gene associate with rapid progression to disability in non Ashkenazi Jewish multiple sclerosis patients. Genes Immun 2003; 4:197–203.

25. Gumucio D, Diaz A, Schaner P, Richards N, Babcock C, Schaller M, Cesena T. Fire and ice: the role of pyrin domain containing proteins in inflammation and apoptosis. Clin Exp Rheumatol 2002; 20(suppl 26):s45–s51.

26. Hull KM, Shoam N, Chae JJ, Aksentijevich I, Kastner DL. The expanding spectrum of systemic autoinflammatory disorders and their rheumatic manifestations. Curr Opin Rheumatol 2003; 15:61–69.

27. Goldfinger SE. Colchicine for FMF. N Engl J Med 1972; 287:302.

28. Zemer D, Revah M, Pras M, Schor S, Sohar E, Gafni J. A controlled trial of colchicine in preventing attacks of FMF. N Engl J Med 1974; 18:932–934.

29. Seyahi E, Ozdogan S, Masatlioglu S, Yazici H. Successful treatment of FMF attacks with thalidomide in a colchicine resistant patient. Clin Exp Rheum 2002; (suppl 26):s43–s44.

30. Ozylkan E, Simsek H, Teleter H. Tumor necrosis factor in FMF. Am J Med 1992; 92:579.

31. Milledge J, Shaw JP, Mansour A, Williamson S, Bennetts B, Roscioli T, Curtis J, Christodoulou J. Allogeneic bone marrow transplantation: cure for FMF. Blood 2002; 100:774–777.

32. Tankurt E, Tunka M, Akbaylar H. Resolving FMF attacks with interferon alpha. Br J Rheum 1996; 35:1188–1189.
33. Sohar E, Gafni J, Pras M, Heller H. Familial Mediterranean fever: a survey of 470 cases and review of the literature. Am J Med 1967; 43:227–253.
34. Siegal S. Familial paroxysmal peritonitis. Analysis of 50 cases. Am J Med 1964; 36:893–918.
35. Metaxas P, Madias NE. Familial Mediterranean fever and amyloidosis. Kidney Int 1981; 20:676–685.
36. Utz JP, Swensen SJ, Gerz MA. Pulmonary amyloidosis. The Mayo clinic experience from 1980 to 1993. Ann Intern Med 1996; 124:407–413.
37. Johnson WJ, Lie JT. Pulmonary hypertension and familial Mediterranean fever: a previously unrecognized association. Mayo Clin Proc 1991; 66:919–925.
38. Brick BR, Gershoni-Baruch GR, Bentur BL. Pulmonary function tests in patients diagnosed as having FMF. Pediatr Pulmonol 2003; 35:452–455.
39. Braun E, Schapira D, Guralnik L, Azzam ZS. Acute vasculitis in multiorgan involvement in a patient with familial Mediterranean fever. Am J Med Sci 2003; 325:363–364.
40. Ustundag Y, Bayrakta Y, Salih E. Superior vena cava thrombosis and obstructive sleep apnea in a patient with familial Mediterranean fever. Am J Med Sci 1998; 316:53–55.
41. Lidar M, Pras M, Langevitz P, Livneh A. Thoracic and lung involvement in familial Mediterranean fever. Clin Chest Med 2002; 23:505–511.
42. Kees S, Langevitz P, Zemer D, Padeh S, Pras M, Livneh A. Attacks of pericarditis as a manifestation of familial Mediterranean fever. Q J Med 1997; 36: 893–918.
43. Ercan-Tutar H, Imamoglu A, Atalay S. Recurrent pericarditis as a manifestation of familial Mediterranean fever. Circulation 2000; 101:E71–E72.
44. Tutar HE, Imamoglu A, Kendiri T, Akar E, Atalay S, Akar N. Isolated recurrent pericarditis in a patient with familial Mediterranean fever. Eur J Pediatr 2001; 160:264–265.
45. Dabetani A, Noble LM, Child JS, Krivokapich J, Schwabe AD. Pericardial disease in familial Mediterranean fever: an echocardiographic study. Chest 1982; 81:592–595.
46. Zemer D, Cabili S, Revach M, Shahin N. Constrictive pericarditis in familial Mediterranean fever. Isr J Med Sci 1997; 13:55–58.
47. Rosenbaum M, Naschitz JE, Yudashkin M, Rosner I, Sabo E, Shaviv N, Gaitini L, Zuckerman E, Yeshurun D. Cardiovascular autonomic dysfunction in familial Mediterranean fever. J Rheumatol 2002; 29:987–989.
48. Langevitz P, Livneh A, Neuman L, Buskila D, Shemer J, Amolsky D, Pras M. Prevalence of ischemic heart disease in patients with familial Mediterranean fever. Isr Med Assoc J 2001; 3:9–12.
49. Nazaretyan EY, Ayvazyan A. Familial Mediterranean fever as a risk factor for myocardial infarction. Clin Exp Rheumatol 2002; 20(suppl 26):s80.
50. Serrano R, Martinez MA, Andres A, Morales JM, Samartin R. Familial Mediterranean fever and acute myocardial infarction secondary to coronary vasculitis. Histopathology 1998; 33:163–167.

51. Tekin M, Yalcinkaya F, Tumer N, Cakar N, Kocak H. Familial Mediterranean fever and acute rheumatic fever: a pathogenetic relationship? Clin Rheumatol 1999; 18:446–449.
52. Belange G, Gompel H, Chaouat Y, Chaouat D. Malignant peritoneal mesothelioma occurring in periodic disease: apropos of a case. Rev Med Interne 1998; 19:427–430.
53. Chahinian AP, Pajak TF, Holland JF, Norton L, Ambinder RM, Mandel EM. Diffuse malignant mesothelioma. Prospective evaluation of 69 patients. Ann Intern Med 1982; 96:746–755.
54. Gentiloni N, Febrraro S, Barone C, Lemmo G, Neri G, Zannoni G. Perotoneal mesothelioma in recurrent familial peritonitis. J Clin Gastroenterol 1997; 24: 276–279.
55. Riddell RH, Goodman MJ, Moosa AR. Peritoneal malignant mesothelioma in a patient with recurrent peritonitis. Cancer 1981; 48:134–139.
56. Ariad S, Sandbank J, Lupu L. Bronchoalveolar carcinoma in a patient with recurrent familial Mediterranean fever attacks, fibrothorax, and treatment with colchicine. Isr Med Assoc J 1999; 1:121–122.

17

Pulmonary Complications of Behçet's Disease

AHMET GÜL

Division of Rheumatology, Department of
    Internal Medicine, Istanbul University,
Istanbul, Turkey

**ATADAN TUNACI and
ENSAR YEKELER**

Department of Radiology,
    Istanbul University,
Istanbul, Turkey

FEYZA ERKAN

Department of Chest Diseases,
    Istanbul University,
Istanbul, Turkey

I. Introduction

Behçet's disease (BD) is an inflammatory disorder of unknown etiology, which is characterized by recurring manifestations at certain body sites, which includes the respiratory system. It was originally described by Professor Hulusi Behçet, a Turkish dermatologist, as a triad of relapsing oral aphthous ulcers, genital ulcers, and uveitis (1). BD is later recognized as a multisystem disorder, also affecting skin, joints, blood vessels, heart, lungs, gastrointestinal and central nervous systems (2). Immune-mediated vascular and perivascular inflammatory changes are the hallmarks of underlying pathology.

II. Incidence and Epidemiology

Although there are reports of cases from all over the world, BD is quite prevalent in a region extending from the Mediterranean basin and Middle East to Eastern Asia. It has also been named as "silk route" disease because of its distinctive geographic distribution (3). The prevalence rate varies between 13.5 and 420/100,000 in this endemic region and reaches the highest level in Turkey (2,4). However, it is very rare in Northern Europe and North America (2).

BD usually starts in the third and forth decades. Juvenile and elderly BD patients have also been reported (2). The number of males usually equals to females in big series. However, BD runs a more severe course in males and in those with a younger age of onset (5). Involvement of vital organs, including pulmonary artery aneurysms, is seen mainly in men (5,6).

III. Genetics

Epidemiological studies suggest a complex genetic etiology for BD with important genetic and environmental contributions (7–9). Most of the BD cases are sporadic with unaffected parents. However, a familial aggregation has long been noted, which gives a λs value of 11.4–52.5 in Turkey (7). Most of these multicase families did not show a particular Mendelian inheritance pattern. Recently, a classical segregation analysis provided an evidence for autosomal recessive inheritance in a pediatric subgroup (10).

BD has been strongly associated with an HLA class I antigen, HLA-B51, and this association has been confirmed in different ethnic groups (9,11). The direct role of HLA-B51 in BD pathogenesis has been a matter of debate, and a putative susceptibility gene in linkage disequilibrium with HLA-B51 has been extensively investigated. Association studies covering a genomic segment between the HLA-B and the tumor necrosis factor (TNF) alpha gene in the class III major histocompatibility complex (MHC) identified a critical region of 46-kb between the HLA-B and another class I chain-related antigen (MIC-A) gene (9,12). Allelic association, genotypic differentiation, and stratification analyses in different ethnic groups have proved that HLA-B51 is showing the strongest association with BD among all candidates in this region (13). However, it is very hard to rule out additional contributions of the TNF and MIC-A gene polymorphisms on an HLA-B51 carrying haplotype because of strong linkage disequilibrium within the MHC (14).

Genetic studies using multicase families suggested that the contribution of the HLA-B locus to the overall genetic susceptibility to BD (λ_{HLA}) is less than 20%, even with an assumption of multiplicative interaction between the susceptibility loci (15). A novel BD susceptibility locus has been mapped to 6p22–23, and a whole genome screening of multicase families has provided evidences for several non-MHC susceptibility loci for BD (16,17).

IV. Clinical Presentation

A. Extrapulmonary Manifestations

BD is a multisystem disorder and a multidisciplinary approach is necessary for its management. Mucocutaneous lesions are the most frequently observed features of BD (Table 1). However, involvement of eyes, blood vessels, intestines, and central nervous system constitutes the major cause of morbidity and mortality (2,18). Characteristic BD manifestations are recurrent, which may last a few days to several weeks, some of them leaving permanent tissue damage and causing chronic manifestations or even death.

Oral aphthous ulcers, which are indistinguishable from simple aphthous stomatitis, are the most frequent BD manifestation both at presentation and during the course. Genital ulcers look quite similar to those in oral mucosa, occur mainly on the scrotum in men and vulva in women, and they usually heal with a scar.

Common skin manifestations include erythema nodosum-like vasculitic nodular lesions, acne-like lesions, papulopastular lesions and superficial thrombophlebitis. The skin pathergy reaction is a pathognomonic feature of BD and a very helpful diagnostic tool when it is positive. It demonstrates the skin hyper-reactivity to nonspecific trauma, and it is characterized by development of an erythematous papulopustular skin reaction at the needle prick site at 48 hours (19). A similar hyper-reactivity to trauma can be elicited at other body sites as well (2). The frequency of positive pathergy reaction has reported to be lower in Western countries.

Uveitis can be seen in about half of the patients, which can affect both anterior and posterior uveal tracts bilaterally. Recurrent attacks of posterior uveitis and retinal vasculitis can result in a decrease in visual acuity or even a total loss of vision.

Arthritis attacks usually involve lower extremities and rarely run a chronic course.

Vascular involvement is an important feature of BD, which characteristically affects both veins and arteries of all sizes with accompanying thrombotic tendency (9). Venous side of the vasculature has been affected

Table 1 Clinical Findings of Behçet's Disease

Manifestation	Frequency (%)
Oral ulcers	96–100
Genital ulcers	72–79
Eye lesions	48–75
Skin lesions	73–94
Positive pathergy test	30–75
Arthritis	47–59
Epididymitis	6–32
Gastrointestinal lesions	3–25
Central nervous system symptoms	8–20
Vascular lesions	7–38

Source: From Ref. 2.

predominantly in BD, most commonly as superficial thrombophlebitis and deep vein thrombosis of the lower extremities. The typical BD thrombus has been defined as sticky to the inflamed vessel wall, and hence pulmonary thromboembolism has been reported very rarely. Arterial involvement is seen less frequently, as true and/or false aneurysms or less frequently as a thrombotic occlusion. Endothelial dysfunction, which results from immune-mediated inflammatory infiltrate, is believed to be the basis of the observed thrombotic tendency in BD.

Parenchymal neurological involvement mainly affects the brainstem and indicates a bad prognosis. On the other hand, patients with cerebral sinus thrombosis and intracranial hypertension may have a better disease course.

Gastrointestinal ulcers mainly affect the ileocecal region and can cause colicky pain, diarrhea, bleeding, and even perforation. It is more frequent in patients from eastern Asia.

B. Pulmonary Manifestations

The prevalence of the pulmonary complications in previous studies ranges between 3% and 11.9% (20,21). Pulmonary artery aneurysms, arterial and venous thrombosis, pulmonary infarction, recurrent pneumonia, bronchiolitis obliterans organized pneumonia, and pleurisy are the main features of pulmonary involvement in BD (20–43).

Pulmonary artery aneurysms. Pulmonary arteries are the second most common site of arterial involvement, preceded by the aorta. The aneurysms are predominantly located in the right lower lobar arteries, followed by the right and left main pulmonary arteries (44,45). Pulmonary artery aneurysms affect mainly young men. Hemoptysis of varying degrees (up to 500 mL of blood in an individual patient) is the most common and predominant symptom. Rupture of an aneurysm with erosion into a bronchus and the development of in situ thrombosis due to active vasculitis have both been suggested as the causes of hemoptysis. Other clinical signs of aneurysms include cough, dyspnea, and chest pain.

Pulmonary parenchymal findings. Atelectasis, volume loss, wedge-shaped or linear shadows, ill-defined nodular or reticular opacities have also been described in BD with or without pulmonary artery aneurysms. These findings are generally accepted as foci of pulmonary hemorrhage and/or infarcts. However, the pathological correlation of the parenchymal opacities is documented in only a few cases (44,46). Recently, bronchiolitis obliterans organizing pneumonia (BOOP) associated with pulmonary artery aneurysms was reported in a male patient with prominent clinical, radiological, and pathological findings (39). In another patient with BD and peripheral nonsegmental pulmonary infiltrates, eosinophilic pneumonia was diagnosed by transbronchial biopsy (44).

Other thoracic manifestations in BD. The involvement of major veins, including the occlusion of the superior vena cava is a more prevalent finding than arteritis. One-third of patients with pulmonary complications of BD may have accompanying inferior or superior vena cava thrombosis, which develops either as in situ thrombus formation or propagation of a thrombus from a distal vein.

Thrombosis of the innominate and subclavian veins has been shown to accompany superior vena caval occlusion (47–49). Pseudoaneurysms of the aortic arch as well as the subclavian and coronary arteries have been described in BD (50,51). Mediastinal mass, mediastinitis, chyloptysis, and pleurisy are other associated conditions (52). Pleural effusion may result from vasculitis of the pleura or thrombosis of the superior vena cava (42).

V. Pathophysiology

The exact pathogenesis of BD has yet been unknown. Vascular and perivascular inflammatory changes are usually the main pathological findings (2). Immunological mechanisms have an important role in the development of BD manifestations, and BD-related aberrant immune response can be triggered by environmental agents, mainly microbial agents, in genetically susceptible individuals (8,9). Behçet himself suggested a viral etiology (1). The parts of *Herpes simplex* virus (HSV) type 1 genome were demonstrated using different methods within the peripheral blood lymphocytes and in the genital and gastrointestinal ulcers of patients with BD (8). An animal model was developed with the inoculation of HSV type 1 to the ICR mice, and about 30% of the mice showed various manifestations, some of them showing similarities to those of BD (53). However, none of the animal model findings were specific for BD, and no data could be obtained for HSV or another virus to support a direct causative role (8,9).

Triggering of BD manifestations with streptococcal antigens have also been claimed in the pathogenesis of BD. BD patients showed an increased reactivity to skin testing using streptococcal antigens, and some of them even developed systemic BD manifestations following skin challenge (54). Uncommon serotypes of *S. oralis* strains were detected in increased frequencies in the oral flora of BD patients, which can be an important source for microbial triggering (8). Flare of BD manifestations following dental treatment or extraction also supports this view (55).

Different microbial agents may share a quite similar group of proteins, heat shock proteins (hsp), and microbial hsp also show a significant homology with human mitochondrial hsp (8,9). Four epitopes from 65-kD mycobacterial hsp were shown as antigens triggering a specific immune response in BD patients, which may cross-react with their human homologous peptides (56). Increased immune reactivity was also observed against the homologous peptides from human 60-kD hsp by T-cell epitope mapping using short-term cell lines in BD (56,57). These hsp peptides also induced anterior uveitis in Lewis rats by subcutaneus immunization in complete Freund adjuvant with intraperitoneal *Bordatella pertussis* (58). The most uveitogenic peptide was the 336–351 from the human 60-kD hsp, and this pepdide elicited uveitis even by oral or nasal mucosal administration (59). However, none of the rats developed other findings in the mouth, skin, and external genitalia.

VI. Immunological Alterations

Immunological studies indicate involvement of both innate and adaptive immune systems with a dysregulated, enhanced, and even self-destructive inflammatory reactions in BD (8,9). The skin pathergy test is the typical example of nonspecific increased inflammatory reactions, and it can also be shown at the cellular level with an upregulated inflammatory response (60). Spontaneous or induced overexpression of proinflammatory and Th1-type cytokines from various cellular sources seems responsible for the enhanced inflammatory reaction in BD, and it may be associated with the genetic susceptibility (8,61,62).

Enhanced superoxide generation after fMLP stimulation suggests that neutrophils are primed in vivo in BD. Neutrophil hyperactivity, character-ized by increased chemotaxis, phagocytosis, superoxide generation, and myeloperoxidase levels as well as a higher expression of CD11a, CD10, and CD14 on the cell surface, has been suggested as one of the main patho-genic mechanisms in BD (62–67). Association of HLA-B51 with enhanced neutrophil functions is still a controversial issue (67).

An antigen-driven immune response superimposed on this activated innate immunity and induced by hsp peptides or other antigens from differ-ent strains of streptoccocci or other microbial agents was suggested to trig-ger BD manifestations (8). Recent studies have revealed the central role of T-cell-mediated immune response in the pathogenesis of BD, which involves both $\alpha\beta+$ and $\gamma\delta+$ T-cell subsets (8,9).

Intracytoplasmic cytokine expression patterns and T-bet expression indicates a strong Th1 polarization in BD (8,9,68,69). Oligoclonal T-cell expansions, which correlate with BD activity, have proved the contribution of the antigen-driven immune response to the pathogenesis (70). Antigens that have been found to stimulate T cells in BD included streptococcal anti-gens, hsp-derived peptides, and staphylococcal enterotoxins (8). Hasan and colleagues (71) reported a significant proliferative response to four myco-bacterial hsp-derived peptides in specifically $\gamma\delta$ subset of T cells, and also observed a correlation between disease activity and T-cell response.

Some abnormalities have been observed in both NK (CD16+CD56+) cells and CD56+ T cells (8,9), which may affect both innate and adaptive immune responses. Some findings suggest that interaction of NK cells and/or other cytotoxic T cells through KIR and/or CD94 receptors with class I HLA molecules may constitute the missing link between HLA-B51 and BD (72,73).

Increased inflammatory activity of BD also involves endothelial cells, and endothelial activation/injury and the resultant occlusive vasculopathy may also contribute to the tissue damage. The presence of procoagulant mutations, such as the factor V Leiden or the prothrombin gene mutation has been shown to contribute to the thrombotic tendency of BD (9,74,75).

VII. Biochemical and Laboratory Features

There is no diagnostic test for BD, and a set of criteria developed by the International Study Group has been widely used for the classification of patients (Table 2) (76). An acute phase response can be observed in some patients; however, no correlation with the clinical activity was documented.

Skin pathergy reaction has been regarded as specific when positive; however, its results are quite inconsistent. It can easily be tested by pricking the avascular antecubital skin with a sterile 20–22-gauge needle obliquely to

Table 2 International Study Group Criteria for the Diagnosis of Behçet's Disease

1. Recurrent oral ulceration	Minor aphthous, major aphthous, or herpetiform observed by the physician or patient, which have recurred at least three times over a 12-month period plus any two of the following clinical findings.
2. Recurrent genital ulceration	Aphthous ulceration or scarring observed by the physician or patient
3. Eye lesions	Anterior uveitis, posterior uveitis, or cells in the vitreous on slit-lamp examination; or retinal vasculitis detected by an ophthalmologist
4. Skin lesions	Erythema nodosum observed by the physician or patient, pseudofolliculitis, or papulopustular lesions; or acneiform nodules observed by the physician in a postadolescent patient who is not receiving corticosteroids
5. Positive pathergy test	Test interpreted as positive by the physician at 48 hr.

Source: From Ref. 76.

a depth of 5 mm, and development of a 2 mm erythematous papule or pustule at the needle insertion site at 48 hours indicates a positive response. Intradermal uric acid injection can also be used to test the skin hyperreactivity; however, it has not been standardized yet (77).

The presence of common prothrombotic mutations may indicate an increased risk for vascular complications. Recently, a strong association has been described between the prothrombin gene 3'-UTR mutation and pulmonary artery aneurysms (75).

A. Imaging of Pulmonary Findings

The aneurysms appear as round, lobulated opacities on chest radiography (35,43). Sudden hilar enlargement resembling enlarged lymph nodes may be a sign of pulmonary artery aneurysm. CT scan shows in detail the findings of vascular involvement such as lung mass due to aneurysm of the right or left pulmonary arteries, mediastinal widening due to thrombosis, or narrowing of the superior vena cava resulting from mediastinal edema or fibrosis (43,78).

Digital subtraction angiography has been used in the diagnosis of pulmonary artery aneurysms. But, it may be inadequate if the aneurysm or vessels are completely thrombosed, and this procedure may carry some risks for patients with BD. Venous puncture or rapid injection of a large amount of contrast material during the procedure may initiate a thrombus or aggravate an existing one in BD patients (27,44). Helical CT has been suggested as a safe method of investigation of vascular changes. Because helical CT reveals excellent vascular images with only a small amount of contrast material, and with the addition of recently developed multislice CT (MSCT) technology, it is currently the method of choice for the diagnosis of vascular lesions.

MSCT offers important advantages over more conventional imaging methods in the evaluation of the mediastinal and pulmonary vasculature. It allows faster scanning with less motion and breathing artifacts, thinner slice thickness, rapid intravenous administration of contrast material, excellent opacification of the mediastinal, and pulmonary vasculature. This improves the quality of the three-dimensional (3D) data sets, which in turn leads to improved 3D vascular maps and more accurate assessment of various thoracic conditions (79,80). This improvement in CT technology is especially important in the evaluation of pulmonary aneurysms or other vascular manifestations of BD.

MR angiography can also be used as a diagnostic tool for evaluating thoracic vascular involvement in BD (Fig. 1) (81). Although MR angiography is capable to demonstrate the lumen of the aneurysms well, CT angiography is superior to MR angiography in detection of mural thrombotic changes and much smaller aneurysms, and also adding more information

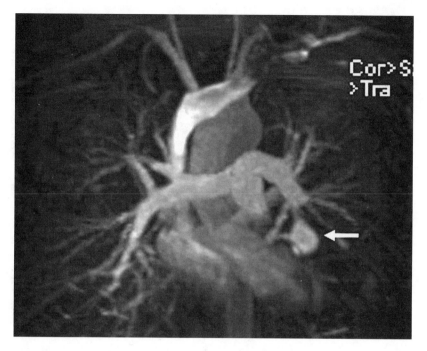

Figure 1 Twenty-eight-year-old patient with Behçet's disease and hemoptysis. MR angiography reveals aneurysm of the left lower lobe pulmonary artery (*arrow*).

about pulmonary parenchymal pathologies such as air-space nodules, cavities, and mosaic areas of lung attenuation (45,82)

Rarely, the lung opacities due to pulmonary artery aneurysms may be large enough to reach the pleural surface. Doppler ultrasonography is also a useful diagnostic tool in detecting and monitoring the response to the medical treatment for these aneurysms adjacent to the pleural surface (Fig. 2A, B) (83).

The size of the pulmonary artery aneurysms may decrease with treatment, and some of them may even disappear (Fig. 2C, D). Perianeurysmal consolidation and air-space nodules, and mosaic attenuation areas may also disappear during or after the treatment (45,46). Since the monitoring of the treatment needs serial imaging of the aneurysms, CT is the method of choice compared to digital subtraction angiography (84,85).

MSCT with its multiplanar and 3D image capabilities is the method of choice to detect superior caval vein thrombosis and to demonstrate collateral pathways (Fig. 3).

Radiographic features of the aortic involvement in BD are similar to those of Takayasu's arteritis and differential diagnosis must be made by clinical findings (37). A false aneurysm of the coronary artery that presented as a large mediastinal mass has also been reported (86).

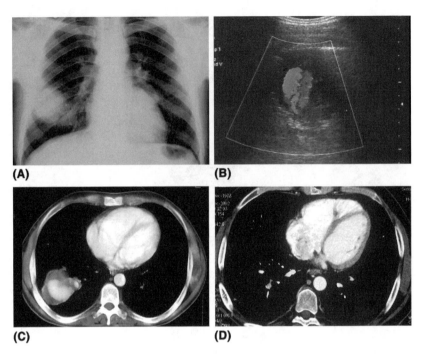

Figure 2 Disappearance of pulmonary artery aneurysm in a 25-year-old man with Behçet's disease. Chest roentgenogram (**A**) shows large nodular opacity with irregular contour in the right lobe. Thoracic Doppler US (**B**) and contrast-enhanced CT (**C**) detect a huge pulmonary artery aneurysm with peripheral thrombosis. Two months after the medical treatment, control CT examination (**D**) reveals disappearing of the aneurysm.

B. Scintigraphic Methods

Ventilation–perfusion lung scanning shows bilateral well-defined, mismatched areas (87). Although deep vein thrombosis of the lower extremities frequently accompanies pulmonary artery aneurysms, pulmonary thromboembolism is seen very rarely in BD, because of the strictly adherent thrombus in inflamed veins (32). In a case report, radionuclide angiography showed alterations in pulmonary artery blood flow as clearly as the subsequent contrast pulmonary angiography did (88). Prolonged lung retention of 123I-meta-iodobenzyl-guanidine is also reported to reflect the severity of the disease (89).

C. Pathology

The pathological examination of pulmonary artery aneurysms revealed perivascular infiltrates around the vasa vasorum, marked intimal thickening with degenerative changes in the elastic lamina, thrombotic occlusion and recanalization as well as fresh thrombi (29,39,90).

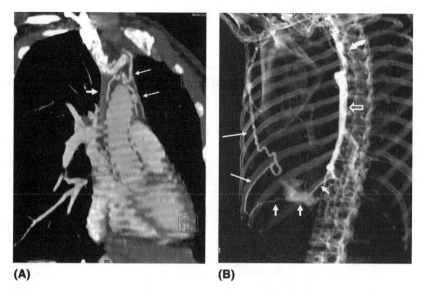

(A) **(B)**

Figure 3 Forty-one-year-old-woman with Behçet's disease and chronic occlusion of the superior vena cava (SVC). Coronal reconstructed contrast-enhanced MSCT image (**A**) shows no contrast medium filling of the SVC (short thick arrow) and collateral venous structures (long thin arrows). 3D volume rendering technique image (**B**) maps collateral vessels such as thoracic wall veins and intercostal veins (long thin arrows), diaphragmatic collaterals draining via hepatic parenchymal shunts to the inferior vena cava (*short thick arrow*), dilated azygos (*hollow arrow*) and left superior intercostal veins (*curved arrows*).

VIII. Natural History and Prognosis

Pulmonary artery aneurysms have a very poor prognosis and it is one of the leading causes of death in BD. About one-third of patients with this condition die within 2 years (29,32,34). The mean survival after the onset of hemoptysis was previously reported as around 10 months in a study of BD patients with pulmonary artery aneurysms (32). A more recent follow-up study of computed tomography findings of 13 patients receiving immunosuppressant treatment showed complete disappearance or regression of pulmonary artery aneurysms during the 3–42 months (mean 21 months) of treatment (45). Disappearance and regression of the aneurysm were both preceded by thrombus formation. After treatment, the thrombi regressed and pulmonary artery aneurysms disappeared. Massive bleeding was reported even in cases receiving immunosuppressant therapy, although a partial remission was achieved (32,39,45).

IX. Treatment

A. Immunosuppressant Therapy

Empiric anti-inflammatory and/or immunosuppressive drugs, which are tailored according to the severity of the disease, remain the mainstay of therapy (91–93). The combination of cyclophosphamide and methylprednisolone is the most frequently used treatment for patients with pulmonary artery aneurysms (93), although no controlled trial has assessed the efficacy of this combination by now. The suggested protocol consists of cyclophosphamide, as 1000 mg monthly intravenous pulses or 2 mg/kg/day orally, and methylprednisolone, as 1 mg/kg orally. For patients with severe hemoptysis, it has been suggested to start with 500–1000 mg methylprednisolone intravenous pulses for 3 days, along with cyclophosphamide pulse (94,95). The prednisone dose is suggested to be tapered depending on the clinical response, whereas the cyclophosphamide is continued for at least 1 year after complete remission and then frequently switched to azathioprine. Azathioprine has also been used instead of cyclophosphamide (96). Cyclosporine combined with coumarin was reported to be successful in a patient with a single pulmonary artery aneurysm (30). In another patient with pulmonary infiltrates, FK506 was used with good results (97).

B. Thrombolytic and Anticoagulant Therapy

Hemoptysis in BD frequently leads to the misdiagnosis of pulmonary thromboembolism due to the usual presence of associated peripheral deep vein thrombosis and abnormal ventilation and perfusion scans. Anticoagulation may carry significant risks in patients with pulmonary artery aneurysms and must be used cautiously and only after systemic immunosuppressant therapy (35). If thrombi are not extensive, antiplatelet therapy (e.g., low-dose aspirin) may probably be sufficient (31,35).

Thrombolytic therapy with urokinase was tried in one patient with a thrombosed pulmonary artery aneurysm (98) and with streptokinase in another patient with superior vena cava syndrome (48). In the follow-up period of 2 years, no evidence of new thrombotic episodes was observed (98). Since both patients were receiving immunosuppressant therapy simultaneously, the risks and efficacy of this method cannot be evaluated separately.

C. Embolization

The bleeding of pulmonary artery aneurysm is reported to be successfully treated with endovascular embolization using *n*-butyl cyanoacrylate (99–101). The size and the number of the aneurysms, the presence of superior or inferior vena caval occlusion, and severe bleeding as a potential complication are the main limitations to the use of embolization in BD.

D. Surgery

In cases of massive hemoptysis, urgent surgical resection may be required. The main problem facing the vascular surgeon is 25% incidence of recurrent, anastomotic aneurysms after both inlay graft repair, and patching (102–104). False aneurysms and arteriovenous fistula are also common at sites of previous iatrogenic trauma. Perioperative steroid covering has been suggested to reduce the risk of complications. The mainstay of the treatment in BD is immunosuppressant therapy as suggested in other severe vasculitides. Other treatment modalities should be used only in combination with this therapy and as palliative measures in special complications.

X. The Future

The preliminary results of genetic studies are promising, and some of the candidate polymorphisms may identify BD patients with an increased risk for pulmonary and other life-threatening manifestations. Early detection of high-risk patients may help to plan better management strategies. Future of the pharmacogenomics may enable us to develop better treatment modalities or tailor-made drugs for individual patients.

No data are available to assess the efficacy and long-term effects of currently used and new immunosuppressant drugs for pulmonary complications and the role of anticoagulant or antiplatelet therapies in management of thrombotic tendency in BD, and double-blind controlled trials are urgently needed.

Acknowledgments

Dr. Ahmet Gül's work was supported by Turkish Academy of Sciences, in the framework of the Young Scientist Award Program (EA-TUBA-GEBIP/ 2001-1-1).

References

1. Behçet H. Über rezidivierende aphthöse durch ein Virus verursachte Geschwüre am Mund am Auge und an den Genitalien. Dermatol Wochenschr 1937; 105:1152–1157.
2. Sakane T, Takeno M, Suzuki N, Inaba G. Behçet's disease. N Engl J Med 1999; 341:1284–1291.
3. Verity DH, Marr JE, Ohno S, Wallace GR, Stanford MR. Behçet's disease, the silk road and HLA-B51: historical and geographical perspectives. Tissue Antigens 1999; 54:213–220.

4. Azizlerli G, Akdağ Köse A, Sarica R, Gül A, Tugal Tutkun I, Kulaç M, Tunç R, Urgancioğlu M, Dişçi R. Prevalence of Behçet's disease in Istanbul, Turkey. Int J Dermatol 2003; 42:803–806.

5. Yazici H, Tuzun Y, Pazarli H, Yurdakul S, Ozyazgan Y, Ozdogan H, Serdaroglu S, Ersanli M, Ulku BY, Muftuoglu AU. Influence of age of onset and patient's sex on the prevalence and severity of manifestations of Behçet's syndrome. Ann Rheum Dis 1984; 43:783–789.

6. Dilsen N, Koniçe M, Aral O, Ocal L, Inanc M, Gül A. Risk factors for vital organ involvement in Behçet's disease. In: Wechsler B, Godeau P, eds. Behçet's Disease. Amsterdam: Excerpta Medica, 1993:165–169.

7. Gül A, Inanc M, Ocal L, Aral O, Konice M. Familial aggregation of Behcet's disease in Turkey. Ann Rheum Dis 2000; 59:622–625.

8. Gül A. Behçet's disease: an update on the pathogenesis. Clin Exp Rheum 2001; 19(suppl 24):S6–S12.

9. Zierhut M, Mizuki N, Ohno S, Inoko H, Gül A, Onoé K, Isogai E. Immunology and functional genomics of Behçet's disease. Cell Mol Life Sci 2003; 60: 1903–1922.

10. Molinari N, Paut IK, Manna R, Demaille J, Daures JP, Touitou I. Identification of an autosomal recessive mode of inheritance in paediatric Behçet's families by segregation analysis. Am J Med Genet 2003; 122A(2):115–118.

11. Ohno S, Ohguchi M, Hirose S, Matsuda H, Wakisaka A, Aizawa M. Close association of HLA-Bw51 with Behçet's disease. Arch Ophthalmol 1982; 100: 1445–1458.

12. Ota M, Mizuki N, Katsuyama Y, Tamiya G, Shiina T, Oka A, Ando H, Kimura M, Goto K, Ohno S, Inoko H. The critical region for Behçet's disease in the human major histocompatibility complex is reduced to a 46-kb segment centromeric of HLA-B, by association analysis using refined microsatellite mapping. Am J Hum Genet 1999; 64:1406–1410.

13. Mizuki N, Ota M, Yabuki K, Katsuyama Y, Ando H, Palimeris GD, Kaklamani E, Accorinti M, Pivetti-Pezzi P, Ohno S, Inoko H. Localization of the pathogenic gene of Behçet's disease by microsatellite analysis of three different populations. Invest Ophthalmol Vis Sci 2000; 41:3702–3708.

14. Ahmad T, Wallace GR, James T, Neville M, Bunce M, Mulcahy-Hawes K, Armuzzi A, Crawshaw J, Fortune F, Walton R, Stanford MR, Welsh KI, Marshall SE, Jewell DP. Mapping the HLA Association in Behçet's disease. A role for tumor necrosis factor polymorphisms? Arthritis Rheum 2003; 48: 807–813.

15. Gül A, Hajeer AH, Worthington J, Barrett JH, Ollier WER, Silman AJ. Evidence for linkage of the HLA-B locus in Behçet's disease, obtained using the transmission disequilibrium test. Arthritis Rheum 2001; 44:239–240.

16. Gül A, Hajeer AH, Worthington J, Ollier WER, Silman AJ. Linkage mapping of a novel susceptibility gene for Behçet's disease to chromosome 6p22–23. Arthritis Rheum 2001; 44:2693–2696.

17. Karasneh JA, Gül A, Ollier WE, Silman A, Worthington J. Whole-genome screening of multicase families for Behçet's disease susceptibility genes. Arthritis Rheum 2005; 52:1836–1842.

18. Shimizu T, Ehrlich GE, Inaba G, Hayashi K. Behcet disease (Behcet syndrome). Semin Arthritis Rheum 1979; 8:223–260.

19. Gül A, Esin S, Dilşen N, Koniçe M, Wigzell H, Biberfeld P. Immunohistology of skin pathergy reaction in Behçet's disease. Br J Dermatol 1995; 132: 901–907.

20. Tursen U, Gurler A, Boyvat A. Evaluation of clinical findings according to sex in 2313 Turkish patient with Behcet's disease. Int J Dermatol 2003; 42: 346–351.

21. Gunen H, Evereklioglu C, Kosar F, Er H, Kizkin O. Thoracic involvement in Behcet's disease and its correlation with multiple parameters. Lung 2000; 178: 161–170.

22. Davies JD. Behçet's syndrome with haemoptysis and pulmonary lesions. J Pathol 1973; 109:351–356.

23. Cadman EC, Lundberg WB, Mitchell MS. Pulmonary manifestations in Behçet syndrome. Arch Intern Med 1976; 136:944–947.

24. Petty TL, Scoggin CH, Good JD. Recurrent pneumonia in Behçet's syndrome. JAMA 1977; 238:2529–2530.

25. Durieux P, Bletry O, Huchon G, Wechsler B, Chretion J, Godeau P. Multiple pulmonary arterial aneurysms in Behçet's disease and Hughes–Stovin syndrome. Am J Med 1981; 71:736–741.

26. Grenier PH, Bletry O, Cornud F, Godeau P, Nahum H. Pulmonary involvement in Behçet disease. AJR 1981; 137:565–569.

27. Park JH, Han MC, Bettman MA. Arterial manifestations of Behçet disease. AJR 1984; 143:821–825.

28. Efthimiou J, Johnston C, Spiro SG, Turner Warwick M. Pulmonary disease in Behçet's syndrome. Q J Med 1986; 227:259–280.

29. Raz I, Okon E, Chajek-Shoul T. Pulmonary manifestations in Behçet's syndrome. Chest 1989; 95:585–589.

30. Vansteenkiste J, Van-Haecke P, Demedts M. Long term treatment with cyclosporin and coumarin in pulmonary thromboembolic Behçet's disease. Monaldi Arch Chest Dis 1998; 53:142–143.

31. Erkan F, Çavdar T. Pulmonary vasculitis in Behçet's disease. Am Rev Respir Dis 1992; 146:232–239.

32. Hamuryudan V, Yurdakul S, Moral F, Numan F, Tüzün H, Tüzüner N, Mat C, Tüzün Y, Özyazgan S, Yazici H. Pulmonary artery aneurysms in Behçet's syndrome: a report of 24 cases. Br J Rheumatol 1994; 33:48–51.

33. Malik KJ, Weber SL, Sohail S, Balaan MR. Hilar mass and papilledema on presentation. Chest 1998; 113:227–229.

34. Erkan F. Pulmonary involvement in Behçet disease. Curr Opin Pulm Med 1999; 5:314–318.

35. Erkan F, Gül A, Tasali E. Pulmonary manifestations of Behçet's disease. Thorax 2001; 56:572–578.

36. Stricker H, Malinverni R. Multiple, large aneurysms of pulmonary arteries in Behçet's disease. Arch Intern Med 1989; 149:925–927.

37. Sullivan EJ, Hoffman GS. Pulmonary vasculitis. Clin Chest Med 1998; 19: 759–776.

38. Huong DLT, deGennes C, Papo T, Wechsler B, Bletry O, Piette JC, Godeau P. Pleuropulmonary manifestations of systemic vasculitis. Rev Med Interne 1996; 17:640–652.

39. Gül A, Yilmazbayhan D, Büyükyabani N, Lie JT, Tunaci M, Tunaci A, Inanc M, Ocal L, Aral O, Konice M. Organizing pneumonia associated with pulmonary artery aneurysms in Behçet's disease. Rheumatology 1999; 38:1285–1289.

40. Cohle SD, Colby T. Fatal hemoptysis from Behcet's disease in a child. Cardiovasc Pathol 2002; 11:296–299.

41. Dikensoy O, Bayram NG, Filiz A. Massive haemoptysis in a young woman. Postgrad Med J 2002; 78:187–188.

42. Caterino U, Paciocco G, D'Auria D, Mazzarella G. Subpleural lung involvement in Behcet's disease: first localization of a systemic entity. Monaldi Arch Chest Dis 2000; 55:289–292.

43. Erkan F, Kiyan E, Tunaci A. Pulmonary complications of Behçet's disease. Clin Chest Med 2002; 23:493–503.

44. Tunaci A, Berkmen YM, Gokmen E. Thoracic involvement in Behcet's disease: pathologic, clinical, and imaging features. AJR 1995; 164:51–56.

45. Tunaci M, Ozkorkmaz B, Tunaci A, Gul A, Engin G, Acunas B. CT findings of pulmonary artery aneurysms during treatment for Behcet's disease. AJR 1999; 172:729–733.

46. Numan F, Islak C, Berkmen T, Tüzün H, Çokyüksel O. Behcet disease: pulmonary arterial involvement in 15 cases. Radiology 1994; 192:465–468.

47. Abid R, Hadj T, Abid F, Chaabane M, Boussen K, Robbana A, Bouhaouala H, Ber Maiz H, Hamza R. Superior caval syndrome, caused by chronic mediastinitis in Behçet's disease. J Radiol 1995; 76:155–157.

48. Kroger K, Ansasy M, Rudofsky G. Postoperative thrombosis of the superior caval vein in a patient with primary asymptomatic Behçet's disease. Angiology 1997; 48:649–653.

49. Terzioglu E, Kirmaz C, Uslu R, Sin A, Kokuludag A, Sagduyu A, Uzunel H, Sebik F, Kabakci T. Superior vena cava syndrome together with multiple venous thrombosis. Clin Rheumatol 1998; 17:176–177.

50. Okita Y, Ando M, Minatoya K, Kitamura S, Matsuo H. Multiple pseudoaneurysms of the aortic arch, right subclavian artery and abdominal aorta in a patient with Behçet's disease. J Vasc Surg 1998; 28:723–726.

51. Nonaka K, Makuuchi H, Naruse J, Kobayashi T, Goto M, Yamamoto T. Pseudoaneurysm of aortic arch and rupture into pericardium, a case report of successful surgical management. Jpn J Thorac Cardiovasc Surg 1998; 46: 772–776.

52. Abadoğlu O, Osma E, Uçan ES, Cavdar C, Akkoc N, Kupelioglu A, Akbaylar H. Behçet's disease with pulmonary involvement, superior vena cava syndrome, chyloptysis, and chylous ascites. Respir Med 1996; 90:429–431.

53. Sohn S, Lee ES, Bang D, Lee S. Behçet's disease-like symptoms induced by the Herpes simplex virus in ICR mice. Eur J Dermatol 1998; 8:21–23.

54. The Behçet's Disease Research Committee of Japan. Skin hypersensitivity to streptococcal antigens and the induction of systemic symptoms by the antigens in Behçet's disease—a multicenter study. J Rheumatol 1989; 16:506–511.

55. Mizushima Y, Matsuda T, Hoshi K, Ohno S. Induction of Behçet's disease symptoms following dental treatment and streptococcal antigen skin test. J Rheumatol 1988; 15:1029–1030.

56. Pervin K, Childerstone A, Shinnick T, Mizushima Y, van der Zee R, Hasan A, Vaughan R, Lehner T. T-cell epitope expression of mycobacterial and homologous human 65-kilodalton heat shock protein peptides in short term cell lines from patients with Behcet's disease. J Immunol 1993; 151:2273–2282.

57. Kaneko S, Suzuki N, Yamashita N, Nagafuchi H, Nakajima T, Wakisaka S, Yamamoto S, Sakane T. Characterization of T cells specific for an epitope of human 60-kD heat shock protein (hsp) in patients with Behçet's disease (BD) in Japan. Clin Exp Immunol 1997; 108:204–212.

58. Stanford MR, Kasp E, Whiston R, Hasan A, Todryk S, Shinnick T, Mizushima Y, Dumonde DC, van der Zee R, Lehner T. Heat shock protein peptides reactive in patients with Behçet's disease are uveitogenic in Lewis rats. Clin Exp Immunol 1994; 97:226–231.

59. Hu W, Hasan A, Wilson A, Stanford MR, Li-Yang Y, Todryk S, Whiston R, Shinnick T, Mizushima Y, van der Zee R, Lehner T. Experimental mucosal induction of uveitis with the 60-kDa heat shock protein-derived peptide 336–351. Eur J Immunol 1998; 28:2444–2455.

60. Hirohota S, Hashimoto T. Abnormal T cell responses to bacterial superantigens in Behçet's disease. Clin Exp Immunol 1998; 112:317–324.

61. Gül A. Cytokines in Behçet's disease. In: Zierhut M, Ohno S, eds. Immunology of Behçet's Disease. Lisse: Swets & Zeitlinger, 2003:73–79.

62. Mege J-L, Dilsen N, Sanguedolce V, Gül A, Bongrand P, Roux H, Ocal L, Inanç M, Capo C. Overproduction of monocyte derived tumor necrosis factor α, interleukin (IL) 6, IL-8 and increased neutrophil superoxide generation in Behçet's disease. A comparative study with familial Mediterranean fever and healthy subjects. J Rheumatol 1993; 20:1544–1549.

63. Sakane T, Suzuki N, Nagafuchi H. Etiopathology of Behcet's disease: immunological aspects. Yonsei Med J 1997; 38:350–358.

64. Niwa Y, Miyake S, Sakane T, Shingu M, Yokoyama M. Auto-oxidative damage in Behçet's disease-endothelial cell damage following the elevated oxygen radicals generated by stimulated neutrophils. Clin Exp Immunol 1982; 49: 247–255.

65. Accardo-Palumbo A, Triolo G, Carbone MC, Ferrante A, Ciccia F, Giardina E, Triolo G. Polymorphonuclear leukocyte myeloperoxidase levels in patients with Behçet's disease. Clin Exp Rheumatol 2000; 18:495–498.

66. Takeno M, Kariyone A, Yamashita N, Takiguchi M, Mizushima Y, Kaneoka H, Sakane T. Excessive function of peripheral blood neutrophils from patients with Behçet's disease and from HLA-B51 transgenic mice. Arthritis Rheum 1995; 38:426–433.

67. Takeno M, Shimoyama Y, Nagafuchi H, Suzuki N, Sakane T. Neutrophil hyperfunction in Behçet's disease. In: Zierhut M, Ohno S, eds. Immunology of Behçet's Disease. Lisse: Swets & Zeitlinger, 2003:96–101.

68. Frassanito MA, Dammacco R, Cafforio P, Dammacco F. Th1 polarization of the immune response in Behçet's disease. Arthritis Rheum 1999; 42: 1967–1974.

69. Li B, Yang P, Zhou H, Zhang Z, Xie C, Lin X, Huang X, Kijlstra A. T-bet expression is upregulated in active Behçet's disease. Br J Ophthalmol 2003; 87:1264–1267.

70. Esin S, Gül A, Hodara V, Jeddi-Tehrani M, Dilsen N, Koniçe M, Andersson R, Wigzell H. Peripheral blood T cell expansions in patients with Behçet's disease. Clin Exp Immunol 1997; 107:520–527.

71. Hasan A, Fortune F, Wilson A, Warr K, Shinnick T, Mizushima Y, van der Zee R, Stanford MR, Sanderson J, Lehner T. Role of $\gamma\delta$ T cells in the pathogenesis and diagnosis of Behçet's disease. Lancet 1996; 347:789–794.

72. Gul A, Uyar FA, Inanc M, Ocal L, Barrett JH, Aral O, Konice M, Saruhan-Direskeneli G. A weak association of HLA-B*2702 with Behcet's disease. Genes Immun 2002; 3:368–372.

73. Saruhan-Direskeneli G, Uyar FA, Cefle A, Onder SC, Eksioglu-Demiralp E, Kamali S, Inanc M, Ocal L, Gul A. Expression of KIR and C-type lectin receptors in Behçet's disease. Rheumatology (Oxford) 2004; 43:423–427.

74. Gül A, Aslantas AB, Tekinay T, Konice M, Ozcelik T. Procoagulant mutations and venous thrombosis in Behcet's disease. Rheumatology (Oxford) 1999; 38:1298–1299.

75. Çelebi-Önder S, Özbek U, Akman-Demir G, Kamali S, Inanç M, Öcal L, Aral O, Koniçe M, Gül A. The role of procoagulant mutations on the type and site of thrombosis in Behçet's disease [abstr]. Arthritis Rheum 2002; 45(suppl):S206.

76. International Study Group for Behcet's Disease. Criteria for diagnosis of Behçet's disease. Lancet 1990; 335:1078–1080.

77. Cakir N, Imeryuz N, Suna D, Gozukara Y, Serdaroglu S, Mert A, Yazici H. Urate crystal test in Behcet's syndrome. Br J Rheumatol 1993; 32:1112–1114.

78. Winer-Muram HT, Gavant ML. Pulmonary CT findings in Behcet disease. J Comput Assist Tomogr 1989; 13:346–347.

79. Schoepf UJ, Kessler MA, Rieger CT, Herzog P, Klotz E, Wiesgigl S, Becker CR, Exarhos DN, Reiser MF. Multislice CT imaging of pulmonary embolism. Eur Radiol 2001; 11:2278–2286.

80. Lawler LP, Fishman EK. Thoracic venous anatomy multidetector row CT evaluation. Radiol Clin North Am 2003; 41:545–550.

81. Berkmen T. MR Angiography of aneurysms in Behcet disease: a report of four cases. JCAT 1998; 22:202–206.

82. Ley S, Kauczor HU, Heussel CP, Kramm T, Mayer E, Thelen M, Kreitner KF. Value of contrast-enhanced MR angiography and helical CT angiography in chronic thromboembolic pulmonary hypertension. Eur Radiol 2003; 13: 2365–2371.

83. Ozcan H, Aytac SK, Yagmurlu B, Kaya A. Color Doppler examination of a regressing pulmonary artery pseudoaneurysm due to Behcet disease. J Ultrasound Med 2002; 21:697–700.

84. Tuzun H, Besirli K, Sayin A, Vural FS, Hamuryudan V, Hizli N, Yurdakul S, Yazici H. Management of aneurysms in Behcet's syndrome: an analysis of 24 patients. Surgery 1997; 121:150–156.

85. Celenk C, Celenk P, Akan H, Basoglu A. Pulmonary artery aneurysms due to Behçet's disease: MR imaging and digital subtraction angiography findings. AJR 1999; 172:844–845.

86. Kaseda S, Koiwaya Y, Tajimi T, Mitsutake A, Kanaide H, Takeshita A, Kikuchi Y, Nakamura M, Mayumi H, Komori M, Tokunaga K. Huge false aneurysm due to rupture of the right coronary artery in Behcet's syndrome. Am Heart J 1982; 103:569–571.

87. Caglar M, Ergun E, Emri S. 99Tcm-MAA lung scintigraphy in patients with Behcet's disease. Its value and correlation with clinical course and other diagnostic modalities. Nucl Med Commun 2000; 1:171–179.

88. Basoglu T, Canbaz F, Bernay I, Danaci M. Bilateral pulmonary artery aneurysms in a patient with Behçet syndrome: evaluation with radionuclide angiography and V/Q lung scanning. Clin Nucl Med 1998; 23:735–738.

89. Unlu M, Akincioglu C, Yamac K, Onder M. Pulmonary involvement in Behcet's disease: evaluation of 123 I-MIBC retention. Nucl Med Commun 2001; 22:1083–1088.

90. Ota G, Nishino T, Onchi K, Tsumura G, Ooe K. An autopsy case of Behçet's syndrome associated with pulmonary arteritis and tuberculosis. Jpn Circ J 1974; 38:35–45.

91. Singer NG, McCune WJ. Update on immunosuppressive therapy. Curr Opin Rheumatol 1998; 10:169–173.

92. Gross WL. New concepts in treatment protocols for severe systemic vasculitis. Curr Opin Rheumatol 1999; 11:41–46.

93. Fresko I, Yurdakul S, Hamuryudan V, Ozyazgan Y, Mat C, Tanverdi MM, Yazici H. The management of Behçet's syndrome. Ann Med Interne 1999; 150:576–581.

94. Duzgun N, Anil C, Ozer F, Acican T. The disappearance of pulmonary artery aneurysms and intracardiac thrombus with immunosupressive treatment in a patient with Behcet's disease. Clin Exp Rheumatol 2002; 20(suppl 26): S56–S57.

95. Aktogu S, Erer OF, Urpek G, Soy O, Tibet G. Multiple pulmonary arterial aneurysms in Behcet's disease: clinical and radiologic remission after cyclophosphamide and corticosteroid therapy. Respiration 2002; 69:178–181.

96. Acican T, Gurkan OU. Azathiopine–steroid combination therapy for pulmonary arterial aneurysms in Behcet's disease. Rheumatol Int 2001; 20:171–174.

97. Koga T, Yano T, Ichikawa Y, Oizumi K, Mochizuki M. Pulmonary infiltrates recovered by FK506 in a patient with Behçet's disease. Chest 1993; 104: 309–311.

98. Sanchez-Burson J, Corzo JE, Marenco JL, Rejon-Gieb E. Thrombolytic therapy in pulmonary embolism of Behcet's disease. Acta Hematol 1996; 96: 181–183.

99. Mouas H, Lortholary O, Lacombe P, Cohen P, Bourezak SE, Deloche A, Azorin J, Guillevin L. Embolization of multiple pulmonary arterial aneurysms in Behcet's disease. Scand J Rheumotol 1996; 25:58–60.

100. Bozkurt AK. Embolisation in Behcet's disease. Thorax 2002; 57:469–470.

101. Cantasdemir M, Kantarci F, Mihmanli I, Akman C, Numan F, Islak C, Bozkurt AK. Emergency endovascular management of pulmonary artery

aneurisms in Behcet's disease: report of two cases and a review of the literature. Cardiovasc Intervent Radiol 2002; 25:533–537.

102. Bradbury AW, Milne AA, Murie JA. Surgical aspects of Behçet's disease. Br J Surg 1994; 81:1712–1721.

103. Tuzun H, Hamuryudan V, Yildirim S, Besirli K, Yoruk Y, Yurdakul S, Yazici H. Surgical therapy of pulmonary arterial aneurysms in Behcet's syndrome. Ann Thorac Surg 1996; 61:733–735.

104. de Montpreville VT, Macchiarini P, Dartevelle PG, Dulmet EM. Large bilateral pulmonary artery aneurysms in Behcet's disease: rupture of the contralateral lesion after aneurysmorrhaphy. Respiration 1996; 63:49–51.

18

Endemic Mycosis

CHADI A. HAGE and GEORGE A. SAROSI

Indiana University-School of Medicine, and Roudebush VA Medical Center, Indianapolis, Indiana, U.S.A.

I. Introduction

Histoplasmosis, blastomycosis, and coccidioidomycosis are the three major endemic fungi in North America. Paracoccidioidomycosis is endemic in South America (1). Although histoplasmosis is found in all continents except Antarctica, coccidioidomycosis in South America, and blastomycosis in Africa, only in North America are these illnesses common.

These fungal diseases share many characteristics. The causative agents are mycelial soil organisms. Illness is acquired by inhaling aerosolized spores. In the infected host, the organisms change their form, a characteristic called dimorphism. *Histoplasma capsulatum* and *Blastomyces dermatitidis* convert to a yeast form at 37°C (thermal dimorphism), whereas *Coccidioides immitis* converts in tissue to a spherule that replicates by forming endospores (tissue dimorphism).

The endemic areas are large. Most of the mid-west and south Central United States is endemic for both histoplasmosis (2) and blastomycosis (3), and a large area in the Southwest United States and an adjacent area of Mexico are endemic for coccidioidomycosis (4). All three illnesses occur in normal hosts, although histoplasmosis and coccidioidomycosis are also major opportunistic mycoses in patients with depressed cell-mediated immunity, and especially in patients with acquired immunodeficiency syndrome (AIDS) (5,6).

Histoplasmosis, blastomycosis, and coccidioidomycosis are major T-cell opportunistic infections, as demonstrated by the very aggressive course seen in patients with AIDS, in whom T-cell deficiency is most severe.

II. Histoplasmosis

In the United States, *H. capsulatum* var. *capsulatum* is responsible for the majority of the cases of histoplasmosis. *H. capsulatum* var. *duboisii* is predominantly found in South Africa and Europe (7). The spectrum of disease ranges from the asymptomatic acquisition of a positive histoplasmin skin test reaction to a rapidly fatal pulmonary or disseminated illness. It is the balance between the net immune status of the subject and the load of the infecting inoculum that determines the severity of the illness. During the past two decades, histoplasmosis has emerged as a common opportunistic infection in patients with AIDS, especially those residing in endemic areas. Most of our current knowledge about this disease is derived from outbreak investigation in the midwestern United States.

A. The Pathogen and Epidemiology

Histoplasma is a thermally dimorphic fungus. It has two forms; a mycelial phase and a yeast phase. Mycelia are the forms found in the environment, they are considered to be the infectious form. Mycelia display macro- and microconidia. Yeasts are what is found in the infected individuals. In the laboratory, these two forms are interconvertible by altering the temperatures and nutrients of the growth medium. The disease is highly endemic in the Midwestern and southeastern parts of the United States. It is estimated that 50–80% of people living in the Ohio and Mississippi river valleys have evidence of remote infection with histoplasma (8).

Human and animal infections occurred after inhalation of aerosolized microconidia, the infecting particle, which can reach the alveolar space due to its very small size of 2–5 μm. Extensive skin test surveys suggest that as many as 50 million people in the United States have been infected by *H. capsulatum* and that there are up to 500,000 new infections yearly (9).

For decades most outbreaks have occurred in urban settings. Most are associated with construction projects that disturbed contaminated soil. The most recent (and largest ever) outbreak occurred in Indianapolis, Indiana (10), associated with downtown construction of a swimming pool complex.

Mini-outbreaks also still occur. Activities such as cutting up fallen trees or cleaning large bushes have been linked to smaller outbreaks.

Histoplasmosis occurs in 2–5% of patients with AIDS who reside in endemic areas and up to 25% in selected areas during periods of outbreaks (11).

Pathogenesis

The lung is the portal of entry in almost every case. Due to their small size, microconidia can reach the alveolar space where they convert to the yeast form, a key step in the pathogenesis. The initial tissue response to the organism is predominantly neutrophilic, followed by an increase in alveolar macrophages (12). After being phagocytosed, the yeast survives and actually proliferates inside the macrophages, which serve then as a carrier throughout the reticuloendothelial system. Shortly after infection, the yeast forms can be identified in the mediastinal lymph nodes. The fungus then gains access to the circulation. It is likely that transient self-limited fungemia occurs in most, if not all, patients. Later, the yeast disseminates throughout the body to establish foci of infection in many organs, such as the liver, spleen, and the adrenal glands (6).

About 2 weeks after infection, specific cellular immunity begins to develop. Activated lymphocytes secrete cytokines that stimulate macrophages in an attempt to boost their fungicidal activity. In mice, interleukin-12 is an important signal, leading to increased interferon-gamma production that confers protection against primary infection (13–15). Tumor necrosis factor-alpha seems to be an important element in this scheme. Inhibition of TNF-α has been shown to alter the adaptive immune response to histoplasma infection and may predispose patients' disseminated infection (13,16,17).

With the advent of T-lymphocyte-mediated cellular immunity, fungal replication is checked and granuloma formation begins. Healing of these lesions is accompanied by peripheral fibrosis. Central areas of encapsulated, necrotic material frequently calcify. These calcified foci manifest on chest roentgenogram as single or multiple calcified nodules. Calcified lesions are often seen in the liver and the spleen (18).

If the cell-mediated immune response is poor, the yeast continues to multiply. More macrophages are recruited, which in turn become parasitized and eventually disrupted, perpetuating the cycle (6). A severe systemic illness develops, which invariably leads to death unless treated promptly and aggressively.

B. Clinical Manifestations

Most normal persons who are infected by the fungus remain asymptomatic. When present, symptoms vary widely from brief periods of malaise to severe, life-threatening illness. The incubation time of acute histoplasmosis in previously nonimmune individuals ranges between 9 and 17 days. It is classically a flu-like illness with abrupt onset of fever, chills, and substernal chest discomfort. A harsh, nonproductive cough develops along with head-ache, arthralgias, and myalgias. Normal hosts usually recover uneventfully from primary pulmonary infection.

Acute pulmonary histoplasmosis is characterized by a single (or occa-sionally multiple) area of pneumonitis, usually in the lower lung zones, with enlarged ipsilateral hilar and mediastinal lymph nodes. Healing of the pneu-monitis may lead to the formation of pulmonary nodule with central necro-sis and concentric fibrosis, which may later become calcified. Hilar lymph nodes are often similarly calcified.

A complex of arthralgia–erythema nodosum–erythema multiforme is occasionally seen during acute illness. Arthralgias may be severe enough to interfere with walking and other activities of daily living. Arthralgias usually resolve within several days but may last a week or more. In several large outbreaks, erythema nodosum and erythema multiforme were noted, usually in patients with arthralgias (19).

A hallmark of histoplasmosis is mediastinal lymphadenopathy. Mark-edly enlarged paratracheal lymph nodes may compress the trachea or one of the main stem bronchi, causing an irritative cough and/or dyspnea. Enlarged mediastinal lymph nodes may impinge on the esophagus (causing dysphagia) or on the superior vena cava (causing edema of the head and upper extremities) (20). These complications are encompassed within the term "mediastinal granuloma".

Lymph nodes that calcify during healing may also impinge on adjacent structures or may even erode into various tissues. Erosion through the wall of the trachea or bronchi may cause broncholithiasis. Patients present with obstructive pneumonia, with expectoration of stones, or with hemoptysis. Rarely, calcified nodes may create tracheoesophageal fistulas when they erode into both adjacent structures.

Another rare manifestation of histoplasmosis is mediastinal fibrosis (21), which accompanies the healing of involved mediastinal lymph nodes, entrapping contiguous mediastinal structures. Bronchi may be entrapped, as may branches of pulmonary arteries and veins. In extreme cases, progres-sive obliteration of pulmonary vessels leads to pulmonary hypertension and death from cor pulmonale. Unfortunately, a surgical approach to diffuse mediastinal fibrosis is risky and not usually helpful, even though the course of illness is progressive. There have been anecdotal reports of endovascular stenting of focally narrowed arteries and pulmonary veins with some symp-tomatic improvement.

Chronic pulmonary (cavitary) histoplasmosis is seen in individuals with structurally abnormal lungs, such as heavy smokers with established emphysema (22). The infection often involves the upper lobes, which are most abnormal. Radiographically, the infection frequently mimics reinfec-tion tuberculosis. The lung parenchyma between the emphysematous air spaces develops an infiltrate, which sharply outlines the abnormal air spaces and mimics cavitary disease.

Clinically as well as radiographically, the symptoms of this progressive form of upper lobe histoplasmosis mimic those of tuberculosis. Low-grade fever and anorexia with weight loss are common. Most patients develop a productive cough, with variable amounts of mucopurulent sputum. Night sweats also occur, but are not as prominent as in tuberculosis. The chest roentgenographic findings are usually similar to those of reinfection tuberculosis, showing fibrocavitary disease, sometimes with volume loss.

In immunocompetent individuals severe pulmonary illness develops rarely, only when the infective dose is unusually high. It may progress rapidly to the acute respiratory distress syndrome, and may lead to death from respiratory insufficiency if not treated promptly (2).

Immunocompromised individuals are more likely to progress to disseminated disease even after an infection with a smaller inoculom. The vast majority of progressive disseminated histoplasmosis (PDH) is seen in patients with advanced AIDS with CD4 counts below 200 cells/mL (11).

Most patients with progressive disseminated histoplasmsosis present with fever, chills, weight loss, cough, and progressive dyspnea (23). On physical examination, patients are febrile and acutely ill. Hepatosplenomegaly may be present. Laboratory evaluation shows anemia, leukopenia, and thrombocytopenia. In extremely ill patients, the syndrome of disseminated intravascular coagulation may be seen. Occasionally, patients present with severe septic shock, respiratory failure, and progress to multiorgan failure. This syndrome represents an advanced stage of the illness and is usually seen when diagnosis and appropriate therapy were delayed. Mortality is very high with this scenario.

Chest roentgenographic findings are variable, ranging from normal to diffusely abnormal, with reticulonodular pattern being the most frequently reported finding. Pleural effusions are rarely seen (24). The radiographic findings are very similar to those seen with *Pneumocystis carinii* pneumonia (5) (Fig. 1).

Peripheral blood smear may show phagocytized yeast in patients with severe disease. Biopsy material from the bone marrow and other involved tissue shows collections of macrophages full of intracellular yeast or, in the most severe instances, widespread necrosis with large numbers of organisms lying loose in the extracellular debris. There is little, if any, evidence of granuloma formation (25). Virtually, all patients with this form of the illness have some degree of T-cell defect. Before the modern era of widespread use of cytotoxic agents and glucocorticoids, many patients had underlying Hodgkin's disease, a well-known example of naturally occurring T-cell immune deficiency (5,6).

The most severe form of PDH occurs in patients with AIDS with profound T-cell dysfunction (26). In fact, most cases of PDH now occur in

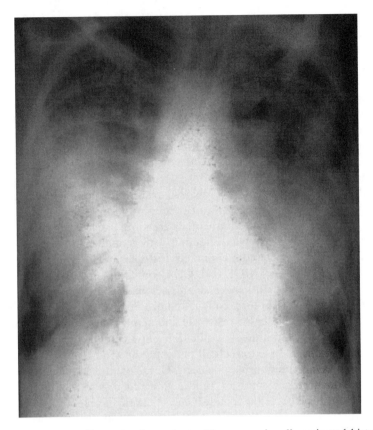

Figure 1 Chest radiograph of a patient with progressive disseminated histoplasmosis showing bilateral reticulonodular infiltrates and ground glass opacifications.

AIDS patients, and most occur in highly endemic areas (27,28). Newer biological therapies, such as TNF-α blocking agents, have added a new pool of immunosuppressed patients at risk for tuberculosis and also histoplasmosis and other T-cell opportunistic fungal infections.

In most instances, exposure of an immunosuppressed person to an infected aerosol is the antecedent event preceding PDH. In the recent large outbreak in Indianapolis, most patients who were immunocompromised when they developed primary histoplasmosis progressed to PDH (28). In particular, patients with AIDS nearly always progressed to PDH (11).

In other cases, the onset of PDH is temporally related to intense immunosuppression, most commonly progression of AIDS or therapy with high doses of glucocorticoids. In some of these cases, reactivation of dormant histoplasmosis may be the mechanism of infection (5). Patients with AIDS who develop PDH after long residence in New York City or

San Francisco are clear examples of such endogenous reactivation because primary infections are never seen in these cities.

Some patients with PDH present with a subacute to chronic illness. They may have a chronic wasting disease with anorexia, weight loss, and low-grade fever. Mucosal and mucocutaneous junction ulcers may occur in the mouth, oral pharynx, rectum, and glans penis. Adrenal involvement may cause Addison's disease (29). Biopsy material from involved tissues shows well-formed epithelioid granulomas, and only a diligent search will reveal rare organisms. Demonstration of organisms almost always requires special stains (6,25). The disease may be systemic or involve only one organ. This more chronic form of PDH generally occurs in patients who are less immunosuppressed than the patients who develop more fulminant PDH.

Central nervous system histoplasmosis is rare and may present as chronic meningitis or intracranial histoplasmoma (30). Endocarditis can also occur, involving either the aortic or mitral valves. Vegetations are usually large, and emboli are common. Endocarditis may occur on prosthetic or previously normal valves. Recently, histoplasma involvement of abdominal aortic aneurysms has been reported in a few patients with the chronic form of PDH (31).

C. Diagnosis

The gold standard of diagnosis is culture of the fungus from biologic material. Cultures are time consuming and one cannot wait for them in the management of cases with severe PDH. Delay in diagnosis while awaiting results of fungal cultures may lead to a fatal outcome in more severe cases. Isolation of *H. capsulatum* may occur within 1 week in a minority of patients but usually takes several weeks.

Serologic Studies

Serologic tests are extremely important in the setting of acute histoplasmosis (32). Two standard tests are available for the serodiagnosis of histoplasmosis. The first and most important is the complement fixation test. The result becomes positive 3 or more weeks after the exposure and remains positive for months or occasionally years in diminishing titer. A fourfold rise in titer or a single determination of 1:32 or higher to the yeast phase is suggestive of recent infection. When the clinical picture strongly suggests acute pulmonary histoplasmosis, then a titer of 1:8 or higher has strong positive predictive value. Unfortunately, the complement fixation test is negative in about 30% of patients with acute histoplasmosis and in up to 50% of patients with PDH. Patients with chronic pulmonary histoplasmosis frequently have titers of 1:8 or 1:16 that do not rise during the period of observation.

The second test is immunodiffusion testing for precipitating antibodies to the M and H antigens, which produce separate M and H bands

(M band is more common and more important; the H band almost never occurs alone). The test is easy to perform and has more specificity than a low-titer complement fixation test. Regrettably, immunodiffusion fails to identify up to 50% of patients with acute histoplasmosis and usually does not reach maximum positivity for 4 to 6 weeks after exposure (33).

Serologic studies of histoplasmsosis are seldom useful in the management of PDH. Positive serology does not predict development of PDH in patients undergoing bone marrow transplantation (34). The complement fixation test is negative in up to 50% of patients with PDH. Immunodiffusion fails to identify up to 50% of patients with acute histoplasmosis and usually does not reach maximum positivity for 4 to 6 weeks after exposure (33). Their main drawbacks are imperfect sensitivity and lack of timeliness. Several weeks must pass before they become positive. By that time, most patients have either recovered or have required other more invasive methods of diagnosis because of rapidly worsening disease.

There are two ways to make a rapid diagnosis of PDH, sampling and examination of likely infected tissue with the use of special stains and the use of the ultrasensitive assay for fungal antigens.

D. Mycologic Studies

Bronchoscopy is an important diagnostic tool, especially for PDH. Specimens obtained from bronchoscopy have a high but poorly defined yield in severe primary histoplasmosis with progressive ARDS and especially in PDH in AIDS, when diffuse infiltrates are one of the clinical features. In highly selected series, the diagnostic yield of bronchoscopy for diagnosis of histoplasmosis in an endemic area is about 60% in patients with infiltrates (35). In a strictly AIDS population in Indianapolis, Indiana, fungal stains performed on bronchoalveolar lavage fluid provided a rapid diagnosis in 70% of patients; diagnostic yield increased to 89% when culture results were included. In that series, 22% of patients had coinfections or alternative diagnoses that were detected by BAL and would not have been detected if *Histoplasma* antigen testing had been the sole diagnostic test (36). Use of cytologic examination without special fungal staining (silver, PAS) may explain the lower yield of BAL reported in series from nonendemic areas (37). It is likely best to do a battery of stains including a silver stain. Although transbronchial biopsy is not mandatory at the time of bronchoscopy and BAL, histopathology does appear to enhance the diagnostic yield (37). The fungus is difficult to see on standard hematoxylin and eosin stains; special stains (usually a silver stain) are needed. Special stains are particularly important when well-formed granulomas are present because of the paucity of organisms in such cases.

In patients with suspected PDH, sampling of the reticuloendothelial system is often effective for diagnosis. Bone marrow biopsy is likely the best and safest method (25). In heavily parasitized samples, a direct smear of the bone marrow, stained with a supravital stain such as the Giemsa stain, usually gives a rapid diagnosis (Fig. 2). On permanent histologic sections, the fungus is difficult to see on standard slides prepared with hematoxylin and eosin stain. It is best to go directly to special stains, usually one of several modifications of the silver stain or the PAS stain.

Recently, the role of blood cultures in diagnosis of PDH has expanded. The lysis-centrifugation system increases sensitivity. In AIDS patients with PDH, the density of organisms is higher than in other immunosuppressed patients, and blood cultures are particularly useful, yielding a diagnosis in up to 90% of cases. In fact, in AIDS patients with PDH, typical intracellular organisms can be seen directly on peripheral blood smears (buffy coat preparations) up to 50% of the time. Bronchoalveolar lavage also has a very high yield, both by direct smear and by culture in AIDS patients with high burden of organisms. Bronchoalveolar lavage offers the additional advantage of

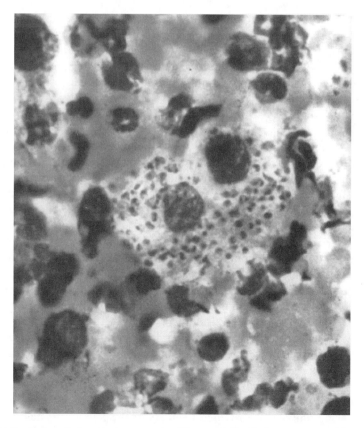

Figure 2   Intracellular yeasts seen on a Giemsa stain of a bone marrow biopsy of a patient with progressive disseminated histoplasmosis.

ready diagnosis of other opportunistic infections that are usually in the differential diagnosis, including *P. carinii* pneumonia.

E. Antigen Detection

Another approach to diagnosis of fungal infections is the use of the ultrasensitive assays for fungal antigens. This test is very useful when the burden of the infection is high. Detection of the histoplasma antigen in body fluids permits rapid diagnosis of PDH. The specificity of antigen detection is greater than 98%. There is, however, known cross-reactivity with the other endemic fungi such as African histoplasmosis, blastomycosis, paracoccidioidomycosis, and *Penicillium marneffii* infection (38). Sensitivity is lower in patients who are moderately immunosuppressed. However, the high density of organisms in AIDS patients with PDH makes antigen testing extremely useful in that setting.

Antigen testing is more sensitive on urine than serum. It is positive in either urine or serum in up to 95% of patients with PDH complicating AIDS (36). Levels of histoplasma polysaccharide antigen in urine and serum also are useful for following the course of treatment and for predicting relapses (39,40). The test is done reliably in a single reference laboratory in Indianapolis, which makes it a "send out" for many institutions.

F. Treatment

The overwhelming majority of patients with acute histoplasmosis are either asymptomatic or have rapidly resolving, self-limited disease that requires no treatment. Progressive cavitary upper-lobe pulmonary disease can be treated successfully with 200 mg twice a day of itraconazole (41). Alternatively, amphotericin B in a total dose of 35 mg/kg may be used over a 12–16-week treatment course with excellent results (42).

Severe cases of PDH in non-AIDS patients are best treated promptly and aggressively with amphotericin B to a total dose of 40 mg/kg. Itraconazole (200 mg twice daily) can be used successfully for patients with mild to moderate disease (41). Sequential therapy for severely ill patients with amphotericin B to clinical improvement followed by 6 months of itraconazole is also being used but is not well studied.

AIDS patients are treated differently from other PDH cases. Relapse is expected if treatment is stopped. All patients require induction therapy to control symptoms and then maintenance therapy. Amphotericin B is used initially for all moderately and severely ill patients. After clinical response, treatment is changed to itraconazole (400 mg daily for 6 or more weeks, then 200 mg daily until sustained recovery of the immune system) (43,44). There are emerging data that support the discontinuation of maintenance itraconazole in patients with HIV who recover their immune system (45).

Itraconazole can be used from onset for mild cases (46). Other maintenance strategies for those intolerant of itraconazole include weekly amphotericin B infusions or fluconazole at doses of at least 400 mg/day. Ketoconazole therapy is ineffective for maintenance therapy, and fluconazole even at high daily doses (400–800 mg) is less effective than itraconazole (47). In a recent double-blind, randomized trial, liposomal amphotericin B (L-AMB) was somewhat more effective than AMB in both time of response and survival, although the differences were not statistically significant (48).

In this study, both types of AMB were used for 14 days before switching to oral itraconazole therapy.

III. Blastomycosis

Blastomycosis is an illness caused by the thermal dimorphic fungus *Blastomyces dermatitidis*. The spectrum of disease ranges from the asymptomatic acquisition of the fungus to a rapidly progressive and life-threatening respiratory or disseminated illness.

A. Epidemiology

Blastomycosis is most common in the central and south-central United States (49). The proposed endemic area includes much of the central, south-central, and southeastern United States, beginning near the Minnesota–North Dakota border to west Texas and extending eastward and southward. The southeastern limit extends to South Carolina but not to Florida. This area overlaps most of the endemic area of histoplasmosis (2). The northern limit, however, extends further. Northern Minnesota and northern Wisconsin and also the adjacent Canadian provinces of Ontario and Manitoba are endemic for blastomycosis but are free of histoplasmosis (50,51).

Similar to *H. capsulatum*, *B. dermatitidis* is a soil-dwelling fungus. Infection occurs by inhalation of airborne spores. As with histoplasmosis, isolated microfoci of high infectivity exist in a large endemic area. Outbreaks often occur during activities such as hunting, camping, or canoeing in wooded or swampy environments (52); these are most common when soil temperatures have been increasing for several days and when there is rain on the day of exposure. For sporadic cases, residence close to water in a highly endemic area and recent excavation activity are risk factors (53). Dogs are also susceptible to blastomycosis. Canine blastomycosis is a well-recognized entity in veterinary practice in the endemic areas. The recognition of canine cases in a community should alert physicians that human blastomycosis might be present in their geographic area (54).

B. Pathogenesis

At ambient temperatures, the fungus grows as an aerial mycelium. When foci of actively growing blastomyces are disturbed, small 2–5 μm spores become airborne and an infective aerosol is formed. These infecting particles then may be inhaled by humans or by other mammals disturbing the site. Some spores may escape the nonspecific defenses of the lung and reach the alveoli.

The initial inflammatory response is neutrophilic. As the organism converts to the parasitic yeast form and begins to multiply, large numbers of yeast are seen, surrounded by neutrophils. Following this macrophages increase in number. Eventually, as specific cellular immunity develops, there are giant cells and well-formed epithelioid granulomas. In contrast to histoplasmosis, the neutrophilic component of the inflammatory response does not disappear completely, and the histopathologic examination often shows a mixed pyogenic and granulomatous response, even in chronic cases (3).

It would be misleading, however, to think that there is a "characteristic" tissue response in blastomycosis. Occasionally, the neutrophilic component is minimal and the granulomas are noncaseating, producing a picture similar to that of sarcoidosis. In contrast, granulomas are sometimes entirely absent in overwhelming infections. The entire inflammatory reaction consists of neutrophils, and the histopathologic picture mimics that of bacterial infection.

The histopathologic response in cutaneous blastomycosis is striking. The stratified squamous epithelium becomes markedly hyperplastic, with exaggerated downgrowth of the rete pegs. Within these fingerlike projections are a number of microabscesses. The same hypertrophic tissue response is seen when the disease involves the oropharynx or the larynx. The histopathologic appearance may superficially resemble carcinoma. The characteristic organisms, seen best with special stains, provide a diagnosis.

The initial inflammatory and immune response may confine the infection to the lungs and the hilar lymph nodes. It is likely (but not proven) that self-limited early fungemia does not occur as often as it does in histoplasmosis. In some instances, however, the organism spreads beyond lung and the hilar nodes. Dissemination is usually to skin, bones, prostate, and meninges but can be seen in any organ (3,55).

The incubation time for blastomycosis is longer than for histoplasmosis and more variable. In the Eagle River outbreak, in which time of exposure was short and precisely defined, the median incubation period was 45 days, with a range of 21–106 days (56,57).

C. Clinical Manifestations

The portal of entry is almost always the lung, and the primary illness is a lower respiratory infection. Some patients have an acute illness that resembles bacterial pneumonia, in contrast to acute pulmonary histoplasmosis, which more closely mimics influenza. The onset of symptoms is abrupt, with high fever and chills, followed by cough that rapidly becomes productive of large amounts of mucopurulent sputum. Pleuritic chest pain may occur.

This acute onset is common in an outbreak setting, but also may be seen in sporadic cases. In most sporadic cases, however, the onset of clinical symptoms is more gradual. The patient presents with a low-grade fever, productive cough, and weight loss (55,58). Lung cancer or tuberculosis are highest in the differential diagnosis, rather than bacterial pneumonia, depending on the roentgenographic findings.

Physical examination is usually unremarkable except for fever. Auscultation of the chest in patients who have segmental or lobar infiltrates may show crackles and focal consolidation; more often the physical examination is negative. Skin lesions are highly variable in appearance, ranging from subcutaneous nodules and abscesses to papules to ulcers with heaped up borders mimicking squamous cell cancers. Perhaps, the most characteristic lesion has irregular borders and a crusted surface, varying in size from 1 to 10 or more centimeters. Skin lesions may be single or multiple and may occur in crops of several new lesions daily or every few days if the disease is rapidly disseminating.

Routine laboratory tests are seldom helpful. In cases resembling acute bacterial pneumonia, the white blood cell count is elevated, and frequently there is a shift to the left toward earlier forms in the granulocyte series.

There is no "characteristic" chest roentgenographic pattern in blastomycosis (59). Lesions may vary from single or multiple round densities throughout both lung fields to segmental or lobar consolidation. Severe pulmonary infections can present with diffuse infiltrates, nodular, interstitial, or even alveolar (Fig. 3). The diffuse alveolar infiltrates are identical to acute lung injury (as in acute respiratory distress syndrome) of diverse cause. Mass-like perihilar infiltrates, especially on the right side, are common and are often misinterpreted as neoplastic. On the lateral chest roentgenogram, the mass-like infiltrate is usually behind the hilum, in the apical-posterior segment of the lower lobe. Hilar lymph node involvement may occur but is not nearly as common as in histoplasmosis. Cavities may occur during the acute phase of the illness and usually close during successful treatment. Unlike histoplasmosis, calcification due to healed blastomycosis is rare.

Extrapulmonary spread of the fungus may occur during the acute, symptomatic phase of the illness. In some instances, only the distant lesion (usually skin or bone) is symptomatic.

The skin and the bony skeleton are the most common sites of symptomatic extrapulmonary spread. The prostate gland, meninges, oral pharynx, larynx, and abdominal viscera, including the liver and the adrenal glands, are involved less frequently (3).

Blastomycosis can present as a progressive infection in patients with T-cell defects, including organ transplant recipients and other patients

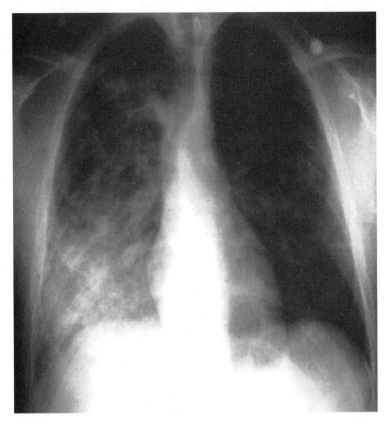

Figure 3 Pulmonary blastomycosis presenting as a lobar community acquired pneumonia.

being treated with high-dose glucocorticoids and other immunosuppressive therapy for malignant and nonmalignant disorders. As with histoplasmosis, the disease can often be cured with amphotericin B in patients with intermediate degrees of immunosuppression.

Blastomycosis is much less common in AIDS and other T-cell-deficient conditions than are histoplasmosis and coccidioidomycosis. This is probably because exposure to this fungus, while immunosuppressed, is less common and because there is a smaller reservoir of patients with remote healed infection waiting to relapse should T-cell function markedly decline (60).

Blastomycosis can also occur in AIDS, usually with a CD4 count below 200/μL. Infection is particularly severe, and cure is not likely. Maintenance therapy is required for those who respond to initial treatment. Patients with AIDS are likely to progress with widespread dissemination of the infection with multiorgan involvement. Patients may present with sepsis-like picture. Meningitis or brain abscess are common in this setting and it is associated with a high early mortality (61).

D. Diagnosis

The easiest and most rapid method of diagnosis is examination of expectorated sputum or aspirated pus after 10% potassium hydroxide digestion (3). The characteristic large (8–20 μm) organism is easily identified. The yeast is single budding, with a broad neck of attachment between the parent and the daughter cells. The wall is thick and is double refractile, and there are multiple nuclei. Other direct fungal stains including periodic acid Schiff (PAS), calcoflour white, and silver stains are commonly used. Another sensitive technique for rapid diagnosis of blastomycosis on direct sputum smears is cytologic analysis with the standard Papanicolaou stain (Fig. 4). The direct

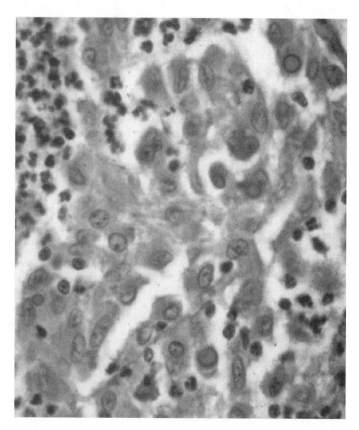

Figure 4   Yeasts of blastomyces shown on a PAS stain of a pulmonary specimen (450×).

techniques are probably complementary and examining multiple sputum samples increases diagnostic yield (62).

Bronchoscopy is useful when patients are unable to expectorate adequate sputum, and when urgent diagnosis is needed because of rapid pace of the illness. In one study, bronchoscopy [specimens obtained included bronchoalveolar lavage (BAL) in 64% and bronchial washings in all] was diagnostic in 92% of patients when culture results were included in the final analysis (63).

For patients who are acutely ill or have an ARDS-like picture, rapid diagnosis is crucial and can only be achieved by direct examination of respiratory secretions. If direct sputum smears are negative or not possible, then bronchoscopy should be done urgently with BAL and bronchial washings sent for both direct fungal stains (some combination of KOH, calcofluor white, and silver stain) and for culture (64). The cytology laboratory should be informed whenever there is high clinical suspicion of infection. Cellblocks of concentrated BAL fluid can be done to maximize the yield of the submitted specimens.

Histopathologic examination of biopsy material is also an excellent way to establish the diagnosis. The decision whether or not to perform transbronchial biopsies at the time of initial bronchoscopy will likely depend on contraindications in any given patient that give added risk beyond risk of BAL. This is particularly true in critically ill patients. If blastomycosis is being considered in this setting, bronchoscopy with BAL can be the initial procedure, reserving transbronchial biopsy for cases with no diagnosis from a safer and easier first procedure. Standard hematoxylin and eosin stains do not stain the fungus and special stains are required. The periodic acid Schiff stain preserves morphological detail, but silver stains are more commonly used.

Identification of the fungus by culture is not difficult, but it is slower. Growth may occur as early as 5 to 7 days but often takes several weeks. Exoantigen testing can provide positive identification as soon as good growth is established. Formerly, positive identification required conversion of the mycelial culture to the yeast phase of growth, adding 1 or more weeks of delay.

Serologic testing is of limited value in diagnosis of blastomycosis. They are positive in about a quarter of cases. Most cases of blastomycosis are diagnosed by smear, culture, and histopathology rather than by serological tests.

E. Treatment

Severely ill patients with pulmonary blastomycosis require immediate and aggressive treatment with amphotericin B.

Itraconazole is highly effective for blastomycosis and is the treatment of choice for most patients with pulmonary and nonmeningeal disseminated disease; oral therapy with 200 mg twice daily for 6 months successfully treats most patients with mild to moderate pulmonary disease, skin disease, and bone disease.

Amphotericin B (dosing as described for histoplasmosis; total cumulative dose of 2000 mg) is preferred for a small minority of severely ill patients, including all patients with diffuse infiltrates and severe gas exchange abnormalities. Patients with edematous lobar pneumonia (bulging fissures), extremely toxic patients, and patients who are rapidly disseminating should all receive AMB. For these severe infections, sequential therapy with AMB to clinical improvement (usually 500–1000 mg total dose) followed by 6 months of oral itraconazole is often used and is effective though not well studied. This approach is also used for AIDS patients. Patients with AIDS and blastomycosis are not permanently cured. Life-long maintenance therapy is needed after induction therapy to improve symptoms.

Meningeal blastomycosis is always treated with systemic amphotericin B therapy in standard doses. L-AMB achieves higher brain tissue levels in animals and may be preferred. Fluconazole is overall less potent for blastomycocis than itraconazole but penetrates CNS much better. High-dose fluconazole (often in combination with L-AMB) has been used for central nervous system blastomycosis. Voriconazole is theoretically attractive but has not been studied. Intracisternal amphotericin B has been used anecdotally in addition to systemic therapy for selected patients, but it is uncertain whether there is additional benefit (65,66). Intracisternal therapy is used less often now, as there is a wider range of therapy.

IV. Coccidioidomycosis

Coccidioidomycosis is the illness caused by the tissue-dimorphic fungus *Coccidioides immitis.* Although most infections are mild and self-limited, the spectrum of illness includes life-threatening pulmonary disease and widely disseminated systemic disease with a high mortality rate. Differences between it and histoplasmosis and blastomycosis include different endemic areas, higher frequency of meningeal infections, and poorer response to all antifungal therapy, including amphotericin B.

A. Epidemiology

The endemic area for coccidioidomycosis in North America is the southwestern United States and the contiguous areas of northern Mexico. The endemic area of the United States includes central and southern California and extends eastward to Arizona, New Mexico, and western Texas.

In nature, the fungus grows as an aerial mycelium with septate hyphae. Alternating cells form thick-walled barrel-shaped structures called *arthroconidia*, with empty cells in between. When a natural site is disturbed, the mature arthrospores easily detach and become airborne, producing an infective aerosol.

The risk of infection is greatest during the hot dry summers. Strong winds can carry the arthrospores for long distances. A huge windstorm that blew north from the San Joaquin Valley in 1977 caused a major outbreak of coccidioidomycosis in Sacramento, far north of the usual endemic area (67). Not surprisingly, occupations and activities with exposure to the soil carry the greatest risk for infection, including construction work, farm labor, and working on archeological digs (68).

B. Pathogenesis

After inhalation, some arthrospores evade the nonspecific lung defenses and reach the alveoli, where germination begins. The arthrospores develop into spherules, the tissue phase of the fungus. Spherules are large, round, thick-walled structures that vary in diameter between 10 and 80 µm. Reproduction of the fungus occurs within the spherule. The cytoplasm of the spherule undergoes progressive cleavage, forming numerous endospores within the spherule. Once a spherule matures, it bursts and releases the endospores into the surrounding tissues. Each endospore can become a new spherule and thus repeat the process.

The initial inflammatory response to inhaled arthrospores is neutrophilic. Resident alveolar macrophages also phagocytose the arthrospores and prime specific T lymphocytes, which multiply, recruit more macrophages, and arm the macrophages, engaging specific cell-mediated immunity. Even though many well-formed granulomas are seen, the neutrophilic inflammatory exudate does not disappear. Histopathologically, there is a mixed granulomatous and suppurative reaction more similar to blastomycosis than to histoplasmosis. Granuloma formation is important for successful limitation of the infection. Good outcome correlates with preponderance of well-formed granulomas.

Most primary infections are asymptomatic or relatively mild. The fungus usually remains localized to the lung and hilar lymph nodes. Dissemination occurs in less than 1% of patients. Hematogenous spread can affect many tissues, including the skin, bones, lymph nodes, visceral organs, and meninges (69). Meningitis is the most feared clinical syndrome with an ominous prognosis (70).

C. Clinical Manifestations

Except for rare instances of inoculation coccidioidomycosis, the portal of entry is the lung. About 60% of individuals with primary pulmonary infection remain totally asymptomatic. In the remaining 40%, the spectrum of disease ranges from a mild, influenza-like respiratory illness to a severe, life-threatening pneumonia (69).

The clinical symptoms and their severity are variable. Common symptoms include cough, fever, and pleuritic chest pain. Cough may be nonproductive, or there may be small amounts of mucopurulent sputum. True rigors are not common. Headache, common during the acute phase of the illness, is nonspecific. Severe headache is always worrisome, however, because coccidioidal meningitis often becomes clinically apparent during the early part of the illness. If meningitis is suspected, a lumbar puncture should be performed immediately.

Several dermatologic aspects of acute coccidioidomycosis are important. A mild nonspecific so-called toxic rash occurs in many patients (68,71). It is an erythematous macular rash that occurs early during the illness, before the skin test turns positive. Erythema nodosum and rarely erythema multiforme are other skin manifestations of primary coccidioidal infection. Together with fever and arthralgias, these skin lesions are part of a variable symptom complex first recognized by locals in the San Joaquin valley of south central California and labeled "valley fever."

More than 75% of patients with primary coccidioidomycosis have an abnormal chest roentgenogram. The most common roentgenographic abnormality is single or multiple areas of patchy pneumonitis. The ipsilateral hilar nodes are enlarged in about 25% of patients (72). Hilar adenopathy may also be seen without recognizable parenchymal disease (Fig. 5).

This primary complex usually heals rapidly. Necrosis in the center of a pneumonic lesion may produce cavitation (73). This is often accompanied by minor hemoptysis, which may be alarming but is seldom life-threatening. Hemoptysis as a late complication is uncommon but can be life-threatening, in contrast to the minimal bleeding that is often seen as the cavity forms. Another complication is rupture of the cavity with development of a pyopneumothorax.

In rare instances, primary pulmonary coccidioidomycosis is not self-limited but progresses within the lung. Symptoms are fever, cough, and weight loss. The chest roentgenogram shows progression of the infiltrate and variable involvement of the hilar nodes (72). This form of pulmonary coccidioidomycosis is dangerous and augers impending dissemination. Most of the patients with progressive pulmonary disease are either immunosuppressed or belong to groups at high risk for dissemination.

The primary pulmonary infection usually either resolves completely or stabilizes. Rarely does a patient die when the disease is restricted to the lung. In some individuals, however, the fungus spreads widely throughout the body, resulting in a systemic infection known as disseminated coccidioidomycosis.

Patients receiving glucocorticoid or cytotoxic or newer immune modulating therapy for malignant or nonmalignant diseases are at risk of dissemination. This is especially true for recipients of renal and other organ transplants and patients with AIDS (74,75). The excess risk of coccidiodomycosis in organ transplant recipients in highly endemic areas has led to targeted

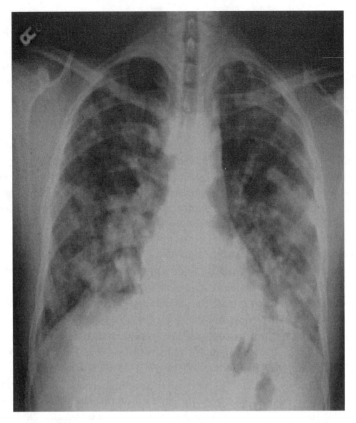

Figure 5   Chest radiograph of a patient with severe pulmonary coccidioidomycosis showing bilateral alveolar infiltrates.

prophylaxis to prevent reactivation whenever there is a history of coccidiodal infection or positive serologic results on pretransplant screening (76). There are other well-recognized risk factors for dissemination. Race and ethnicity are important. Disseminated coccidioidomycosis is more likely in Blacks, Filipinos, and native Americans than in Whites. Male gender is also a risk factor, as is diabetes mellitus. The very young and the very old are more likely to have dissemination (69). There is much anecdotal information suggesting that coccidioidomycosis during the third trimester of pregnancy may be a severe illness with rapid dissemination.

Dissemination from the primary pulmonary focus tends to occur early, usually within a few months after a symptomatic pulmonary infection. In some patients, however, the findings of disseminated disease are the first manifestations of coccidioidomycosis, presumably because the preceding pulmonary infection was subclinical.

Dissemination may involve any organ in the body. The skin is one of the most common sites of dissemination and is involved in most patients some time in the course of the disease. Involvement of the bones is the next most common manifestation of disseminated coccidioidomycosis. Osteomyelitis may be either the sole evidence of extrapulmonary spread or part of a more widespread dissemination. Bone disease is usually restricted to one or two sites, but occasionally as many as eight separate lesions may be present.

Meningitis is the most dreaded complication of coccidioidal dissemination. Between one-third and one-half of all patients with disseminated disease have meningitis, frequently as the only obvious extrapulmonary site. The onset of meningitis may be subtle, with only mild headache and minimal alteration of mental functions. Striking board-like nuchal rigidity, as in purulent meningitis, is seldom seen (70). In fact, the findings of meningitis can be so minimal that all patients with dissemination at other sites should have a diagnostic lumbar puncture to exclude meningitis. Involvement of the base of the brain is characteristic. As the disease progresses, an exudate frequently obstructs the aqueduct of Sylvius and the foramina of the fourth ventricle, producing hydrocephalus. When obstruction occurs, the patient's clinical condition suddenly worsens, with diminished level of consciousness and the development of papilledema. The cerebrospinal fluid shows characteristics of chronic meningitis: predominantly mononuclear cell pleocytosis, increased protein, and decreased glucose. Occasionally, eosinophils are present in the cerebrospinal fluid. If present, they are a valuable clue to the possible coccidioidal nature of the chronic meningitis.

When coccidioidomycosis complicates HIV infection, the severity depends on the residual immune competence of the host.

With near-normal CD4 lymphocyte counts, coccidioidomycosis is not significantly different from the disease seen in normal hosts. When the CD4 count falls below 250 cells/μL, disseminated disease tends to be severe and rapidly progressive. Patients usually have high fever, complain of dyspnea, and are hypoxemic; chest roentgenograms often show diffuse reticulonodular infiltrates with nodules 5 mm or greater in diameter. Diffuse macronodular pulmonary infiltrates are present in less than 1% of non-AIDS patients with disseminated coccidioidomycosis, but in up to 50% of advanced AIDS patients with this condition. Meningeal disease is present in up to 25% of the patients (77,78).

D. Diagnosis

Mycologic Studies

Direct examination of sputum and other respiratory specimens (or pus from a nonpulmonary site) may reveal the diagnostic spherules. Direct smears have highest utility in patients who produce copious sputum or have multilobar infiltrates (79). Bronchoscopy is often performed in selected cases.

In one study, bronchoscopy was diagnostic in 69% of patients (compared to 32% for sputum stains and cultures) when patients with solitary pulmonary nodules on chest radiograph were excluded from analysis (80). This study also showed usefulness of a postbronchoscopy sputum and equivalent sensitivity for Papanicolaou and silver staining. The airway can be examined at the time of bronchoscopy and may be abnormal, providing clues to the diagnosis (81).

Bronchoscopy is typically performed in patients who are immunosuppressed and severely ill, especially if they have diffuse infiltrates on chest radiograph. Multiple infections often coexist, adding additional value to diagnostic bronchoscopy early in the course of illness (82,83). Bronchial washings and bronchoalveolar lavage fluid should be sent for cytology, fungal stains, and culture. In a recent study of an AIDS patient in Phoenix, Arizona, the Papanicolaou stain was the most useful direct test (when compared to KOH and calcofluor white) for rapid diagnosis of pulmonary coccidioidomycosis and was even positive in two patients with negative cultures (84). Histopathologic examination of biopsy material is extremely helpful. When mature spherules (visible on standard hematoxylin- and eosin-stained tissue sections) are seen, the diagnosis is secure. More commonly, only endospores, immature spherules, or spherule fragments are present. Therefore, fungal stains such as a silver stain should always be used in addition to hematoxylin and eosin staining. In one study, transbronchial biopsy yielded a specific tissue diagnosis of coccidioidomycosis in eight of eight patients.

Cultural identification of the fungus is not difficult but is hazardous to laboratory personnel. Isolation should be attempted only under rigid biohazard protection. Traditional laboratory methods for identifying culture isolates require conversion of mycelial-phase cultures to the tissue phase either by animal inoculation or directly by the use of slide cultures. Now immunodiffusion tests are performed directly on the supernatants of liquid mycelial-phase cultures. This method of identification (called exoantigen testing) is safer, simpler, and faster (85). Positive identification of a coccidioidal isolate can sometimes be made by day 5, although it usually takes longer.

Serologic Studies

Because cultural identification is slow and even somewhat dangerous, serologic tests have been developed that facilitate rapid diagnosis (4,86). A tube precipitin tests for detection of IgM antibodies is positive in 90% of patients by the third week (negative only in very mild infections). Because the test usually reverts to negative within 3 months, it is quite specific for recent infection (4). Currently, an immunodiffusion test for IgM has largely replaced the tube precipitin test. The immunodiffusion test measures the same antibodies, but it is easier to perform.

The most important serodiagnostic test is the complement fixation (CF) test.

CF antibodies are of the IgG class and appear later than IgM antibodies. In most symptomatic patients, the CF test is positive by 2 months and remains positive for several months or longer (86). The test is highly specific but is not sensitive. Most asymptomatic skin test converters never have CF titers over 1:8, which is the threshold for a positive result. Most symptomatic patients have titers of 1:8 or 1:16. Titers of 1:32 or higher are generally associated with more severe infections and poorer prognosis. It appears that these serological studies are most reliable when they are performed in few selected laboratories using specific antigens. In the classic studies of Smith and colleagues (86), many patients with these high titers either had already undergone or were about to undergo dissemination. However, other patients with disseminated coccidioidomycosis did not have high titers. Also the cutoff of a 1:32 CF titer as a harbinger of dissemination never transferred perfectly to other laboratories that did not use the same method or the same antigen. A single CF titer, no matter how high, should never be used to make a diagnosis of disseminated coccidioidomycosis. Nonetheless, a steadily rising titer should raise the suspicion of disseminated coccidioidomycosis and prompt further tests (including bone scan, spinal tap, or both when appropriate) to better define the extent of disease.

E. Treatment

Because dissemination is more likely in immunosuppressed patients, in diabetics, and in certain racial and ethnic groups, it may be prudent to treat patients in high-risk groups during the primary infection, before dissemination takes place. In the past, some authorities recommended a treatment course to a total dose of 500–2000 mg of amphotericin B (87). Similarly, many experts believed that all patients with pulmonary disease that is severe or persists beyond a few weeks should receive amphotericin B to approximately the same total dose to prevent local pulmonary progression and to prevent dissemination. In current practice, many such patients (and also less symptomatic patients with pulmonary coccidioidomycosis of shorter duration) are often given fluconazole for 3–6 months, reserving AMB for patients with diffuse infiltrates and women in the third trimester of pregnancy. These recommendations are based on expert opinion and observational studies.

Amphotericin B is likely the best treatment for persistent pulmonary coccidioidomycosis. Because of their lesser toxicity, oral azoles are often tried. About two-thirds of patients have clinical improvement with azole therapy, but many relapse when the course of treatment is finished. Ketoconazole was used first. Currently, fluconazole and itraconazole are being used. Voriconazole will likely be evaluated in the future.

Disseminated coccidioidomycosis requires prompt and aggressive treatment. Unfortunately, amphotericin B is not as effective for disseminated coccidioidomycosis as it is for disseminated histoplasmosis or blastomycosis. The standard dose of amphotericin B is 2500–3000 mg given over many weeks or months. If necessary, much larger total doses may be given (88). Daily doses of amphotericin B (usually 40–50 mg) are given while the patient is acutely ill. When the patient stabilizes, frequency should be reduced to three times weekly. Currently, disseminated disease without CNS involvement should be treated with fluconazole or itraconazole first, especially in mild to moderate cases. AMB should be reserved for severe disease or treatment failure.

Fluconazole and itraconazole are now azoles of choice for nonmeningeal disseminated coccidioidomycosis. Neither is perfect for difficult cases for which even amphotericin B is often only suppressive. Long-term therapy is often required, extending to years or even indefinitely. Fluconazole has the advantage of better absorption, less gastrointestinal upset, and better penetration of the central nervous system. In a recently published randomized controlled trial, oral fluconazole and itraconazole were compared for treatment of nonmeningeal coccidioidomycosis. Soft-tissue dissemination responded best. Overall, itraconazole was somewhat more effective than fluconazole, producing response in 63% of the patients versus 50% response in fluconazole treated patients ($p = 0.08$). Among patients with skeletal infections, itraconazole was clearly superior ($p = 0.05$) (89). Some difficult cases of bone, lymph node, and soft-tissue coccidioidomycosis may be best managed with surgical drainage of focal abscesses, a 1000–2000 mg course of amphotericin B, and a prolonged course of itraconazole or fluconazole.

As might be expected, the treatment of disseminated coccidioidomycosis in AIDS is particularly difficult. Because of the rapid tempo of the disease, amphotericin B should be used initially, especially if the patient is severely ill. If the clinical course stabilizes, it is reasonable to switch to fluconazole for long-term suppression. Prognosis is poor. Even with prompt diagnosis and treatment, up to 40% of severely immunosuppressed patients die during the initial hospitalization. Other patients, usually with lesser degrees of immunosuppression, respond well to treatment (77,78).

Meningeal coccidioidomycosis is a major therapeutic challenge. The standard therapy in the past included a course of 2000–3000 mg systemic amphotericin therapy plus intensive and lengthy intrathecal (by lumbar or cisternal route) AMB therapy (70). Intrathecal [or, less commonly, intraventricular via surgically placed reservoir (90)] AMB in doses between 0.25 and 1 mg was injected two to three times weekly until symptoms and cerebrospinal fluid pleocytosis resolve. Even after the patient had apparently recovered fully and cerebrospinal fluid pleocytosis had resolved, most authorities recommended continued injections of amphotericin to prevent relapse, first weekly and then at longer intervals. Relapses were common, but, with careful management, lengthy remissions could be obtained.

Because of the toxicity of this once standard approach to coccidioidomycotic meningitis, fluconazole has been evaluated as primary therapy for stable patients and as suppressive therapy after initial response to amphotericin B for more severely ill patients. Most patients respond favorably to fluconazole and maintain good clinical function. Dosage is 400–600 mg/day or even higher. Therapy has to be continued long term, likely indefinitely (91). Recently, anecdotal reports have shown favorable response to voriconazole and this agent will undoubtedly be tried in various forms of coccidioidomycosis, including meningitis. A drug with potency and wide spectrum of itraconazole but with tissue penetration like fluconazole seems especially attractive for a treatment-resistant illness with high incidence of meningeal spread. However, clinical data are sparse.

Severely ill patients with both nonmeningeal and meningeal disease were previously treated with intravenous and intrathecal amphotericin B. Now they are sometimes treated with intravenous amphotericin B for faster, more effective initial therapy of the nonmeningeal disease and with fluconazole to control the central nervous system infection. Amphotericin B is continued to clinical improvement and fluconazole indefinitely.

Newer antifungal agents are being developed; their potential role in coccidioidomycosis is uncertain. As mentioned, voriconazole has some promise because it has better CNS penetration than itraconazole—and yet may retain the potency advantage of itraconazole over fluconazole, which has been demonstrated in nonmeningeal disseminated disease.

V. Paracoccidioidomycosis

Paracoccidioidomycosis is the illness caused by the thermal dimorphic fungus *Paracoccidioides brasiliensis.* The spectrum of illness ranges from asymptomatic skin-test conversion to widespread disseminated disease.

A. Epidemiology

The fungus is endemic in South America, Central America, and southern Mexico (92). Although it is undoubtedly a soil organism, it has been difficult to isolate from the soil (similar to *B. dermatitidis*). As with other respiratory mycoses, inhalation of the infective spores is the usual method of infection. Most patients with the disease are male agricultural workers in close daily contact with the soil.

Although 13 patients with paracoccidioidomycosis have been reported in the United States, all previously resided in areas of known endemicity. The United States is not in the endemic area for this fungus (93).

B. Pathogenesis

After inhalation of the infective particles, an area of alveolitis occurs. The initial inflammatory exudate contains predominantly neutrophils. Later, macrophages are recruited, and granuloma formation occurs in immunologically intact patients. Cell-mediated immunity is important to limit the infection (94). After the initial episode of pneumonitis, the organism may disseminate throughout the body. The most common sites of distant spread include skin, mucous membranes, lymph nodes, adrenal glands, liver, and spleen (95).

C. Clinical Manifestations

In many patients, the primary infection is mild, self-limited, and never diagnosed. In some cases, there are residual pulmonary nodules. Calcifications are rare. In the endemic area, single nodules surgically removed primarily to rule out lung cancer often prove to be paracoccidiodal granulomas. Many of these patients have no past history of any symptomatic pneumonia.

Many patients currently diagnosed with paracoccidioidomycosis have pulmonary symptoms at the time of diagnosis. Up to one-third of diagnosed patients have only pulmonary disease (96), which is clinically similar to most other subacute or chronic pulmonary infections, with fever, weight loss, and chronic cough. Chest radiographs are variable with infiltrates, nodules, cavities, and sometimes impressive intrathoracic lymphadenopathy (even to the point of mimicking lymphoma).

The findings on high-resolution computed tomography (CT) often show more extensive involvement than suspected from plain films (97). In immunocompromised patients, paracoccidioidomycosis can present as a severe, rapidly progressive pneumonia. Such patients often have high fever and are acutely ill and toxic. As with the other endemic mycoses, particularly severe disease has been reported in patients with AIDS (98).

Currently, the majority of paracoccidioidomycosis cases have disseminated disease. This is probably because skin involvement is obvious and dramatic and causes most patients to quickly seek medical attention. Patients usually present with lesions on the skin or in the oropharynx. There may be prominent cervical adenopathy, a feature not seen in the other endemic mycoses. Some patients have concomitant pulmonary disease. In other cases, the lungs are clear when extrapulmonary spread is recognized. Presumably initial asymptomatic or minimally symptomatic pulmonary lesions have already healed, and disseminated disease presents months or even years later, as in blastomycosis.

The clinical appearance of the oropharyngeal lesions is somewhat characteristic (99). Ulcers are infiltrated and show multiple hemorrhagic spots. The oral mucosal lesions commonly extend to adjacent skin. Similarly, lesions involving the rectal mucosa often extend to the perianal skin.

Organs of the reticuloendothelial system are frequently involved. Hepatosplenomegaly is common, and lymph nodes may be involved. Cervical adenopathy commonly accompanies mucosal lesions of the mouth and oral pharynx. Necrosis occurs within the nodes, and draining fistulas may extend from infected nodes to the skin. The adrenal glands are often involved; roughly half of autopsied cases show some involvement of the adrenal glands. Clinically significant hypoadrenalism, however, is considerably less common. Other sites of dissemination include the kidneys, the male genital tract, and the meninges.

D. Diagnosis

Direct examination of tissue or sputum after 10% potassium hydroxide digestion frequently shows the characteristic "pilot wheel" yeast. The organism is large (6–30 μm in diameter) and shows multiple buds circling the parent cell, each with a narrow neck of attachment. Histopathologic examination of biopsy material is also useful. The fungus can be seen on routine sections stained with hematoxylin and eosin. Silver stains increase diagnostic yield.

The fungus is readily cultured from biological material. It grows slowly, and a positive identification usually takes 3 to 4 weeks. Specimens cultured at room temperature grow as a mycelium. Specimens cultured at 37°C grow in the yeast form.

A skin test is available for the diagnosis of paracoccidioidomycosis. There is some cross-reactivity with histoplasmin. The diagnostic accuracy of the skin test is low. Up to 60% of patients tested have a negative skin-test reaction at the time of diagnosis. Skin-test reactivity is low because most patients have widely disseminated disease. It is not certain whether the skin test is useful in diagnosing primary pulmonary paracoccidioidomycosis because the sensitivity of the test and the background positivity in endemic areas are not known.

Serologic tests are useful (100). The CF test with a yeast-derived antigen yields a positive result in 80% of cases. Titers of 1:64 or higher are considered diagnostic. A rising CF titer suggests progressive disease or a relapse following initial treatment. Low titers may persist for years, even after successful treatment. An immunodiffusion test is positive in 95% of cases. Cross-reactions are rare, and most patients convert to negative after successful treatment.

E. Treatment

In the past, long courses (often for several years) of sulfadiazine were used successfully for treatment of paracoccidioidomycosis. Two-thirds of the patients had a good clinical response. Amphotericin B was used for patients who did not respond to sulfadiazine and for those who relapsed after treatment was stopped. The usual total dose ranged from 1000 to 1500 mg. After a course of amphotericin B, sulfonamide therapy was resumed and continued long term.

Treatment options have expanded with the availability of oral azoles. Ketoconazole is very effective and now, with itraconazole, is one of two preferred treatments (92,100). A daily dose of 200 mg of ketoconazole usually produces clinical remission in 6 to 8 weeks. Treatment should be continued for a minimum of 12 months. The risk of relapse following keto-conazole treatment is not well defined, but is relatively low. Itraconazole 100 mg/day for 12 months is also highly effective, curing more than 90% of patients. Amphotericin B is used only for critically ill patients and for patients who fail oral azole therapy. Only a small number of patients meet these criteria.

References

1. Greer DA, Restrepo A. The epidemiology of paracoccidioidomycosis. In: Al-Doory Y, ed. The Epidemiology of Human Mycotic Diseases. Springfield, IL: Charles C Thomas, 1978:117–141.
2. Goodwin RA Jr, Des Prez RM. State of the art: histoplasmosis. Am Rev Respir Dis 1978; 117(5):929–956.
3. Sarosi GA, Davies SF. Blastomycosis. Am Rev Respir Dis 1979; 120(4):911–938.
4. Drutz DJ, Catanzaro A. Coccidioidomycosis. Part I. Am Rev Respir Dis 1978; 117(3):559–585.
5. Davies SF, Khan M, Sarosi GA. Disseminated histoplasmosis in immunologically suppressed patients. Occurrence in a nonendemic area. Am J Med 1978; 64(1):94–100.
6. Goodwin RA Jr, et al. Disseminated histoplasmosis: clinical and pathologic correlations. Medicine (Baltimore) 1980; 59(1):1–33.
7. Manfredi R, et al. *Histoplasmosis capsulati* and *duboisii* in Europe: the impact of the HIV pandemic, travel and immigration. Eur J Epidemiol 1994; 10(6):675–681.
8. Edwards LB, et al. An atlas of sensitivity to tuberculin, PPD-B, and histoplasmin in the United States. Am Rev Respir Dis 1969; 99(4)(suppl):1–132.
9. Hammerman KJ, Powell KE, Tosh FE. The incidence of hospitalized cases of systemic mycotic infections. Sabouraudia 1974; 12(1):33–45.
10. Wheat LJ, et al. A large urban outbreak of histoplasmosis: clinical features. Ann Intern Med 1981; 94(3):331–337.
11. Wheat LJ, et al. Disseminated histoplasmosis in the acquired immune deficiency syndrome: clinical findings, diagnosis and treatment, and review of the literature. Medicine (Baltimore) 1990; 69(6):361–374.
12. Procknow JJ, Page MI, Loosli CG. Early pathogenesis of experimental histoplasmosis. Arch Pathol 1960; 69:413–426.

13. Zhou P, Miller G, Seder RA. Factors involved in regulating primary and secondary immunity to infection with *Histoplasma capsulatum*. TNF-alpha plays a critical role in maintaining secondary immunity in the absence of IFN-gamma. J Immunol 1998; 160(3):1359–1368.
14. Allendoerfer R, Biovin GP, Deepe GS Jr. Modulation of immune responses in murine pulmonary histoplasmosis. J Infect Dis 1997; 175(4):905–914.
15. Allendorfer R, Brunner GD, Deepe GS Jr. Complex requirements for nascent and memory immunity in pulmonary histoplasmosis. J Immunol 1999; 162(12):7389–7396.
16. Allendoerfer R, Deepe GS Jr. Intrapulmonary response to *Histoplasma capsulatum* in gamma interferon knockout mice. Infect Immun 1997; 65(7):2564–2569.
17. Wood KL, et al. Histoplasmosis after treatment with anti-tumor necrosis factor-alpha therapy. Am J Respir Crit Care Med 2003; 167(9):1279–1282.
18. Straub M, Schwarz J. The healed primary complex in histoplasmosis. Am J Clin Pathol 1955; 25(7):727–741.
19. Medeiros AA, et al. Erythema nodosum and erythema multiforme as clinical manifestations of histoplasmosis in a community outbreak. N Engl J Med 1966; 274(8):415–420.
20. Goodwin RA, Loyd JE, Des Prez RM. Histoplasmosis in normal hosts. Medicine (Baltimore) 1981; 60(4):231–266.
21. Goodwin RA, Nickell JA, Des Prez RM. Mediastinal fibrosis complicating healed primary histoplasmosis and tuberculosis. Medicine (Baltimore) 1972; 51(3):227–246.
22. Goodwin RA Jr, et al. Chronic pulmonary histoplasmosis. Medicine (Baltimore) 1976; 55(6):413–452.
23. Wheat J. Histoplasmosis. Experience during outbreaks in Indianapolis and review of the literature. Medicine (Baltimore) 1997; 76(5):339–354.
24. Conces, DJ, Jr, et al. Disseminated histoplasmosis in AIDS: findings on chest radiographs. AJR Am J Roentgenol 1993; 160(1):15–19.
25. Davies SF, McKenna RW, Sarosi GA. Trephine biopsy of the bone marrow in disseminated histoplasmosis. Am J Med 1979; 67(4):617–622.
26. Wheat LJ, Slama TG, Zeckel ML. Histoplasmosis in the acquired immune deficiency syndrome. Am J Med 1985; 78(2):203–210.
27. Johnson PC, Hamill RJ, Sarosi GA. Clinical review: progressive disseminated histoplasmosis in the AIDS patient. Semin Respir Infect 1989; 4(2):139–146.
28. Wheat LJ, et al. Risk factors for disseminated or fatal histoplasmosis. Analysis of a large urban outbreak. Ann Intern Med 1982; 96(2):159–163.
29. Sarosi GA, et al. Disseminated histoplasmosis: results of long-term follow-up. A center for disease control cooperative mycoses study. Ann Intern Med 1971; 75(4):511–516.
30. Wheat LJ, Batteiger BE. Sathapatayavongs. *Histoplasma capsulatum* infections of the central nervous system. A clinical review. Medicine (Baltimore) 1990; 69(4):244–260.
31. Hawkins SS, Gregory DW, Alford RH. Progressive disseminated histoplasmosis; favorable response to ketoconazole. Ann Intern Med 1981; 95(4):446–449.

32. Wheat J, et al. The diagnostic laboratory tests for histoplasmosis: analysis of experience in a large urban outbreak. Ann Intern Med 1982; 97(5):680–685.
33. Davies SF. Serodiagnosis of histoplasmosis. Semin Respir Infect 1986; 1(1): 9–15.
34. Vail GM, et al. Incidence of histoplasmosis following allogeneic bone marrow transplant or solid organ transplant in a hyperendemic area. Transpl Infect Dis 2002; 4(3):148–151.
35. Prechter GC, Prakash UB. Bronchoscopy in the diagnosis of pulmonary histoplasmosis. Chest 1989; 95(5):1033–1036.
36. Wheat LJ, et al. Diagnosis of histoplasmosis in patients with the acquired immunodeficiency syndrome by detection of *Histoplasma capsulatum* polysaccharide antigen in bronchoalveolar lavage fluid. Am Rev Respir Dis 1992; 145(6):1421–1424.
37. Salzman SH, Smith RL, Aranda CP. Histoplasmosis in patients at risk for the acquired immunodeficiency syndrome in a nonendemic setting. Chest 1988; 93(5):916–921.
38. Wheat J, et al. Cross-reactivity in *Histoplasma capsulatum* variety capsulatum antigen assays of urine samples from patients with endemic mycoses. Clin Infect Dis 1997; 24(6):1169–1171.
39. Wheat LJ, et al. Histoplasmosis relapse in patients with AIDS: detection using *Histoplasma capsulatum* variety capsulatum antigen levels. Ann Intern Med 1991; 115(12):936–941.
40. Wheat LJ, et al. Effect of successful treatment with amphotericin B on *Histoplasma capsulatum* variety capsulatum polysaccharide antigen levels in patients with AIDS and histoplasmosis. Am J Med 1992; 92(2):153–160.
41. Dismukes WE, et al. Itraconazole therapy for blastomycosis and histoplasmosis. NIAID Mycoses Study Group. Am J Med 1992; 93(5):489–497.
42. Parker JD, et al. Treatment of chronic pulmonary histoplasmosis. N Engl J Med 1970; 283(5):225–229.
43. Wheat J, et al. Prevention of relapse of histoplasmosis with itraconazole in patients with the acquired immunodeficiency syndrome. The National Institute of Allergy and Infectious Diseases Clinical Trials and Mycoses Study Group Collaborators. Ann Intern Med 1993; 118(8):610–616.
44. Hecht FM, et al. Itraconazole maintenance treatment for histoplasmosis in AIDS: a prospective, multicenter trial. J Acquir Immune Defic Syndr Hum Retrovirol 1997; 16(2):100–107.
45. Goldman M, et al. Discontinuation of antifungal therapy for disseminated histoplasmosis (DH) following immunologic response to antiretroviral therapy (ART) is safe: AIDS Clinical Trials Group Study A5038. Abstracts of the 43rd Interscience Conference on Antimicrobial Agents and Chemotherapy Chicago, IL, 2003. 2003:Abstract# M-1761a.
46. Wheat J, et al. Itraconazole treatment of disseminated histoplasmosis in patients with the acquired immunodeficiency syndrome. AIDS Clinical Trial Group. Am J Med 1995; 98(4):336–342.
47. Wheat J, et al. Treatment of histoplasmosis with fluconazole in patients with acquired immunodeficiency syndrome. National Institute of Allergy and

Infectious Diseases Acquired Immunodeficiency Syndrome Clinical Trials Group and Mycoses Study Group. Am J Med 1997; 103(3):223–232.

48. Johnson PC, et al. Safety and efficacy of liposomal amphotericin B compared with conventional amphotericin B for induction therapy of histoplasmosis in patients with AIDS. Ann Intern Med 2002; 137(2):105–109.

49. Furcolow ML, et al. Prevalence and incidence studies of human and canine blastomycosis. 1. Cases in the United States, 1885–1968. Am Rev Respir Dis 1970; 102(1):60–67.

50. Kepron MW, et al. North American blastomycosis in Central Canada. A review of 36 cases. Can Med Assoc J 1972; 106(3):243–246.

51. Tosh FE, et al. A common source epidemic of North American blastomycosis. Am Rev Respir Dis 1974; 109(5):525–529.

52. Greenberg SB. Serious waterborne and wilderness infections. Crit Care Clin 1999; 15(2):387–414.

53. Baumgardner DJ, Brockman K. Epidemiology of human blastomycosis in Vilas County, Wisconsin. II: 1991–1996. WMJ 1998; 97(5):44–47.

54. Sarosi GA, et al. Canine blastomycosis as a harbinger of human disease. Ann Intern Med 1979; 91(5):733–735.

55. Witorsch P, Utz JP. North American blastomycosis: a study of 40 patients. Medicine (Baltimore) 1968; 47(3):169–200.

56. Klein BS, et al. Isolation of *Blastomyces dermatitidis* in soil associated with a large outbreak of blastomycosis in Wisconsin. N Engl J Med 1986; 314(9): 529–534.

57. Klein BS, Vergeront JM, Davis JP. Epidemiologic aspects of blastomycosis, the enigmatic systemic mycosis. Semin Respir Infect 1986; 1(1):29–39.

58. Abernathy RS. Clinical manifestations of pulmonary blastomycosis. Ann Intern Med 1959; 51:707–727.

59. Laskey W, Sarosi GA. The radiological appearance of pulmonary blastomycosis. Radiology 1978; 126(2):351–357.

60. Davies S, Sarosi G. Clinical manifestations and management of blastomycosis in the compromised patient. In: Warnock DW, Richard MD, eds. Fungal Infection in the Compromised Patient. New York: John Wiley & Sons, 1982:215–229.

61. Pappas PG, et al. Blastomycosis in patients with the acquired immunodeficiency syndrome. Ann Intern Med 1992; 116(10):847–853.

62. Trumbull ML, Chesney TM. The cytological diagnosis of pulmonary blastomycosis. JAMA 1981; 245(8):836–838.

63. Martynowicz MA, Prakash UB. Pulmonary blastomycosis: an appraisal of diagnostic techniques. Chest 2002; 121(3):768–773.

64. Lemos LB, Guo M, Baliga M. Blastomycosis: organ involvement and etiologic diagnosis. A review of 123 patients from Mississippi. Ann Diagn Pathol 2000; 4(6):391–406.

65. Gonyea EF. The spectrum of primary blastomycotic meningitis: a review of central nervous system blastomycosis. Ann Neurol 1978; 3(1):26–39.

66. Kravitz GR, et al. Chronic blastomycotic meningitis. Am J Med 1981; 71(3): 501–505.

67. Flynn NM, et al. An unusual outbreak of windborne coccidioidomycosis. N Engl J Med 1979; 301(7):358–361.
68. Werner SB, et al. An epidemic of coccidioidomycosis among archeology students in northern California. N Engl J Med 1972; 286(10):507–512.
69. Drutz DJ, Catanzaro A. Coccidioidomycosis. Part II. Am Rev Respir Dis 1978; 117(4):727–771.
70. Bouza E, et al. Coccidioidal meningitis. An analysis of thirty-one cases and review of the literature. Medicine (Baltimore) 1981; 60(3):139–172.
71. Bayer AS, et al. Unusual syndromes of coccidioidomycosis: diagnostic and therapeutic considerations; a report of 10 cases and review of the English literature. Medicine (Baltimore) 1976; 55(2):131–152.
72. Bayer AS. Fungal pneumonias; pulmonary coccidioidal syndromes (Part I). Primary and progressive primary coccidioidal pneumonias—diagnostic, therapeutic, and prognostic considerations. Chest 1981; 79(5):575–583.
73. Winn WA. A long term study of 300 patients with cavitary-abscess lesions of the lung of coccidioidal origin. An analytical study with special reference to treatment. Dis Chest 1968; 54(suppl 1):268+.
74. Rutala PJ, Smith JW. Coccidioidomycosis in potentially compromised hosts: the effect of immunosuppressive therapy in dissemination. Am J Med Sci 1978; 275(3):283–295.
75. Cohen IM, et al. Coccidioidomycosis in renal replacement therapy. Arch Intern Med 1982; 142(3):489–494.
76. Blair JE, Douglas DD, Mulligan DC. Early results of targeted prophylaxis for coccidioidomycosis in patients undergoing orthotopic liver transplantation within an endemic area. Transpl Infect Dis 2003; 5(1):3–8.
77. Bronnimann DA, et al. Coccidioidomycosis in the acquired immunodeficiency syndrome. Ann Intern Med 1987; 106(3):372–379.
78. Fish DG, et al. Coccidioidomycosis during human immunodeficiency virus infection. A review of 77 patients. Medicine (Baltimore) 1990; 69(6):384–391.
79. Warlick MA, Quan SF, Sobonya RE. Rapid diagnosis of pulmonary coccidioidomycosis. Cytologic v potassium hydroxide preparations. Arch Intern Med 1983; 143(4):723–725.
80. Wallace JM, et al. Flexible fiberoptic bronchoscopy for diagnosing pulmonary coccidioidomycosis. Am Rev Respir Dis 1981; 123(3):286–290.
81. Polesky A, et al. Airway coccidioidomycosis—report of cases and review. Clin Infect Dis 1999; 28(6):1273–1280.
82. Mahaffey KW, et al. Unrecognized coccidioidomycosis complicating *Pneumocystis carinii* pneumonia in patients infected with the human immunodeficiency virus and treated with corticosteroids. A report of two cases. Arch Intern Med 1993; 153(12):1496–1498.
83. Sobonya RE, et al. Detection of fungi and other pathogens in immunocompromised patients by bronchoalveolar lavage in an area endemic for coccidioidomycosis. Chest 1990; 97(6):1349–1355.
84. Sarosi GA, et al. Rapid diagnostic evaluation of bronchial washings in patients with suspected coccidioidomycosis. Semin Respir Infect 2001; 16(4):238–241.

85. Standard PG, Kaufman L. Immunological procedure for the rapid and specific identification of *Coccidioides immitis* cultures. J Clin Microbiol 1977; 5(2): 149–153.
86. Smith CE, Saito MT, Simons SA. Pattern of 39,500 serologic tests in coccidioidomycosis. J Am Med Assoc 1956; 160(7):546–552.
87. Galgiani JN, et al. Practice guideline for the treatment of coccidioidomycosis. Infectious Diseases Society of America. Clin Infect Dis 2000; 30(4):658–661.
88. Bennett JE. Chemotherapy of systemic mycoses (first of two parts). N Engl J Med 1974; 290(1):30–32.
89. Galgiani JN, et al. Comparison of oral fluconazole and itraconazole for progressive, nonmeningeal coccidioidomycosis. A randomized, double-blind trial. Mycoses Study Group. Ann Intern Med 2000; 133(9):676–686.
90. Diamond RD, Bennett JE. A subcutaneous reservoir for intrathecal therapy of fungal meningitis. N Engl J Med 1973; 288(4):186–188.
91. Dewsnup DH, et al. Is it ever safe to stop azole therapy for *Coccidioides immitis* meningitis? Ann Intern Med 1996; 124(3):305–310.
92. Restrepo-Moreno A, DL G. Paracoccidioidomycosis. In: AF D, ed. Occupational Mycoses. Philadelphia: Lea & Febiger, 1983:43–64.
93. Joseph E, Mare E, IW. Oral South American blastomycosis in the United States. Oral Surg 1966; 21:732–737.
94. Robledo MA, et al. Host defense against experimental paracoccidioidomycosis. Am Rev Respir Dis 1982; 125(5):563–567.
95. Londero AT, Ramos CD. Paracoccidioidomycosis. A clinical and mycologic study of forty-one cases observed in Santa Maria, RS, Brazil. Am J Med 1972; 52(6):771–775.
96. Londero AT, Severo LC. The gamut of progressive pulmonary paracoccidioidomycosis. Mycopathologia 1981; 75(2):65–74.
97. Funari M, et al. Chronic pulmonary paracoccidioidomycosis (South American blastomycosis): high-resolution CT findings in 41 patients. AJR Am J Roentgenol 1999; 173(1):59–64.
98. Silva-Vergara ML, et al. Paracoccidioidomycosis associated with human immunodeficiency virus infection. Report of 10 cases. Med Mycol 2003; 41(3):259–263.
99. Restrepo A, et al. The gamut of paracoccidioidomycosis. Am J Med 1976; 61(1):33–42.
100. Cuce LC, Wroclawski EL, Sampaio SA. Treatment of paracoccidioidomycosis with ketoconazole. Rev Inst Med Trop Sao Paulo 1981; 23(2):82–85.

19

Pulmonary Leptospirosis: Lung Biology in Health and Diseases

EDUARDO P. BETHLEM

Division of Pulmonary Medicine,
Federal University of Rio de Janeiro
State—UNI-RIO,
Rio de Janeiro, Brazil

**CARLOS ROBERTO
RIBEIRO CARVALHO**

Division of Respiratory Diseases—
Heart Institute (InCor), University of
São Paulo Medical School,
São Paulo, Brazil

I. Introduction

Leptospirosis is a re-emerging infectious disease with large outbreaks all around the world. It is a worldwide distributed zoonosis caused by a spirochete called *Leptospira interrogans*. The disease has a broad clinical spectrum that ranges from subclinical benign illness to fatal respiratory failure. The disease is prevalent in tropical regions where its etiologic agent survives under favorable environmental conditions.

Leptospirosis is an acute febrile illness characterized by a generalized vascular injury and capillary damage in the affected organs. Generally, virulence does not correlate with specific serovars, but the different strains can cause different clinical manifestations (1,2).

In 1882, Lancereaux (3) from France described seven cases of a systemic fever and jaundice. One year later, Landouzy reported two benign cases; one of "Fièvre bilieuse ou hépatique" (4) and one of "Typhus hépatique" (5) in two drain workers. The first detailed description of leptospirosis is attributed to Weil (6) in 1886. The term Weil's disease is used to describe the severe form of leptospirosis associated with high fever, intense jaundice, bleeding, renal and pulmonary dysfunction, neurologic alterations, and cardiovascular collapse. In the same year, Mathieu (7) presented a case of "hepatic typhus" and emphasized differences with typhus. Stimson in 1907, demonstrated by silver staining, the presence of spirochetes in the kidney tubules of a patient who reportedly died of yellow fever. The author observed that the spirochetes had hooked ends, then the author named them *Spirochaeta interrogans* because of their question mark appearance (8). Leptospirosis was most often misdiagnosed as yellow fever, malaria, and typhus until its spirochetal cause was demonstrated independently in Japan and Germany, in 1916. In Germany, two different groups, Uhlenhuth & Fromme and Hübener & Reiter, detected spirochetes in the blood of guinea pigs inoculated with blood of infected German soldiers afflicted by "French disease" in the trenches of northeast France (9). Inada and Ido (10), studied coal mine workers with Weil's disease in Japan and postulated that systemic manifestations of the disease were preceded by cutaneous portal of entry. They isolated a spirochete and named it *Spirochaeta icterohaemorragiae*.

Ido et al. (11) also observed spirochetes in the kidneys of almost half of the drain rats studied emphasizing the importance of this animal in the disease dissemination. Wadsworth in 1922, however, was the first one to relate that Weil's disease was associated with rat contact. Later in the 1940s, it was established that *Leptospira* was the agent of this disease (6,12,13).

II. Etiology

The agent is a pathogenic spirochete of the genus *Leptospira*. Leptospires are thin, flexible, finely coiled, gram-negative bacteria 0.1 μm in diameter, 6–12 μm in length, with a coil amplitude of 0.1–0.15 μm. Motility is achieved via paired axial flagella, one at each end. Leptospires are slow growing obligates aerobes, with nutritional requirements for long-chain fatty acids or long-chain alcohol as a primary energy source. An outer envelope rich in lipopolysaccharide (LPS) surrounds their cell walls. The variation in LPS antigens determines the specificity of host immune responses against *Leptospira* spp., and this variation is the basis for the serologic classification scheme that differentiates serologic variants into serovars (2,14).

Classification of the genus *Leptospira* has undergone substantial revision. The traditional classification system is based on the serovar, defined by agglutination after cross-absorption with homologous antigen. The genus contains two species: the pathogenic species *Leptospira interrogans* with at least 218 serovars, and the saprophytic, free-living, nonpathogenic species *Leptospira biflexa* with a minimum of 60 serovars. Within each species, serovars are organized into serogroups based on shared antigenicity (15). *L. interrogans* contains 23 serogroups with strains pathogenic for amphibians, reptiles, and mammals including humans. *L. biflexa* contains

28 serogroups with strains found in fresh water and soils of high moisture and organic matter content and is a saprophytic strain. *L. biflexa* was differentiated from the *L. interrogans* by the growth of the former at 13°C and growth in the presence of 8-azaguanine and by the failure of *L. biflexa* to form spherical cells in 1 M NaCl.

More recently, evidences based on DNA sequencing and DNA–DNA homology techniques have revealed that taxonomy of the genus *Leptospira* may be more complex than traditionally thought. At least eight distinct pathogenic species and five nonpathogenic species are differentiated; however, for practical purposes, the serovars classification continues to be widely used (16). Serovars classifications can be useful epidemiologically to identify common-source outbreaks. The serogroup most frequently found is the icterohaemorrhagie and the serotype also is icterohaemorrhagie, but others also found are the grippotyphosa, panama, canicola, pomona, andamana, wolfii, batavae, and australis. Recently, a complete genomic sequence of a representative virulent serovar-type strain (Lai) of *L. interrogans* serogroup icterohaemorrhagie consisting of a 4.33-megabase large chromosome and a 359-kilobase small chromosome, with a total of 4768 predicted genes has been reported (17).

III. Epidemiology

Leptospirosis is an ubiquitous disease with wild and domestic mammals serving as primary hosts. These mammals, while remaining asymptomatic, can harbor *L. interrogans* for months in the proximal convoluted tubules of the kidneys. The great disseminators of the disease all over the world are rodents, particularly rats, although many others animals like dogs, livestock (cattle and swine), wild mammals and cats can be infected with *Leptospira*. These animals seldom get sick but eliminate *Leptospira* in their urine. Under favorable conditions such as a temperature of 28–32°C and a neutral or slightly alkaline pH, the spirochete may survive for months in the environment after urine excretion (18). As the organisms proliferate in surface water, human transmission is facilitated by indirect contact between infected material (water or soil) and abraded skin, exposed mucous membranes and/or conjunctiva. Although the most common mode of transmission is by indirect exposure, direct exposure to infectious urine can infect pet owners, farms workers, and veterinarians.

Indirect transmission takes place through contact with ground or water contaminated with urine of infected animals. Artificial or natural collection of free water, with little flow, such as small brooks, ponds, river branches, dams, and marshes are preferred habitat. Leptospirosis epidemics are related to floods caused by summer rainstorms (1,13,19–21).

Leptospirosis incidence may be related to geographic location, occupation, and seasonal conditions. It is most frequently encountered in tropical and subtropical areas. The traditionally most common occupational hazards involved include farmers, ranchers, rice field workers, veterinarians, miners, abattoir workers, and military personnel. Until 1970, it was almost an occupational disease. After this time, there was more evidence of urban, homes, and recreational settings transmission. With globalization and the increasing travel facilities, some practices such as hiking, swimming, fishing, hunting, kayaking/canoeing, and riding trail bikes through puddles need also to be considered as risk factors (22,23). Between 1987 and 1991, 14% of the confirmed cases of leptospirosis reported in the Netherlands were associated with foreign travel. In 1991, an outbreak occurred among five boys who had been swimming in a small pond in rural Illinois, United States. The creek that emptied into the pond drained two cattle pastures. In Costa Rica, 1996, 35% of a group of American whitewater rafters fall ill after return to the United States meeting the case definition for leptospirosis. In the summer of 1998, an outbreak occurred among 9% of 110 triathlon participants from 44 states and eight different countries that swan in Lake Springfield, Illinois, United States (22,23). In Malaysian Borneo, in the year 2000, some cases of leptospirosis were diagnosed in the "Eco-Challenge" multisport race athletes (24).

The true incidence and prevalence of leptospirosis in the United States is not known but the pattern is predominantly sporadic. The highest reported incidences have been in the South Atlantic Gulf and the Pacific coastal states. About 40–120 cases of leptospirosis have been annually reported to the Center for Disease Control and Prevention (CDC) (25) since 1970. Hawaii has one of the great incidences with 30 out of 54 in 1992, and 24 out of 51 cases in 1993 of leptospirosis related to the CDC (26,27). The average annual reported incidence in the United States as a whole is 0.05 cases per 100,000 population, while in Hawaii is 1.08 per 100,000 population. Active, as opposed to passive, surveillance for the infection results in a fivefold increase in the incidence of the disease (22,28).

The incidence of leptospirosis has been estimated low and stable in metropolitan France, with an average of 290 new cases per year between 1984 and 2000—268 cases in 2000, incidence of 0.44 cases per 100,000 inhabitants (29), and some clustered cases of leptospirosis in Rochefort (30). Recently, there has been reported an increase in incidence during the last few years in France (31).

Leptospirosis is more common in rural populations in Latin America although in some big cities epidemics have occurred after rainstorms. Men are more frequently involved than women. A high rate of infection has been found among garbage collectors (46.7%), farm workers (25.9%), butchers (24.6%), domestic employees (22.2%), and children (17.2%) (2), especially during rainy seasons. It is endemic in most Caribbean countries (32).

The annual morbidity rate for leptospirosis in Venezuela has ranged between 0.21 and 0.42 per 100,000 inhabitants with a mortality rate of 0.005 to 0.03 per 100,000 inhabitants and a lethality of 2.2–6.9% among the patients (2).

Leptospirosis was responsible for an epidemic of "hemorrhagic fever," without jaundice or renal involvement, in 1995, in rural Nicaragua. Some patients died due to pulmonary hemorrhage. Case-control studies demonstrated that the patients were more likely than controls to have ever walked in creeks (odds radio—OR—15.0), have household rodents (OR 10.4), or own dogs with high titers (>400) to *Leptospira* species (OR 23.4). This epidemic resulted from exposure to flood waters contaminated by urine from infected animals, particularly the dogs (21).

In Brazil, there is a great incidence in the summer days as a consequence of heavy rains and flood in urban areas. The Brazilian government officially reported 2634 new hospitalized cases (range 2396–4138) per year and 448 deaths (range 265–425) per year (33), during 1990 and 1995. In São Paulo, the Central Institute of the Hospital das Clínicas, a tertiary University Hospital, with about 950 beds (being 150, ICU beds), admitted 264 patients with leptospirosis between January 1991 and June 2001. This population presented the median age of 33 years old (9–77 years), 223 being men (85.4%), and a lethality rate of 10.0% (26 patients died). The median duration of stay at the hospital was 10 days (0–42 days). About 60% of these patients were admitted to the ICU for at least 1 day and 10% needed mechanical ventilation (34).

In the State of Rio de Janeiro (not only the Rio de Janeiro city), there was a notification of 3336 cases of leptospirosis between 1995 and 1999 (Tables 1–3). From 2000 to 2002, there were 2600 cases with an overall mortality of 165 cases (6.4%). Sixty-six (40.0%) of the cases had pulmonary involvement as a possible or contributive cause of death (Table 4).

The pulmonary involvement that used to be incidental and mild in the course of the disease seems to be getting serious and progressive resulting in an increased mortality (35–38).

Table 1 Notification of Leptospirosis Cases and Incidence (Cases/100,000 hab.) in Rio de Janeiro, Brazil from 1995 to 1999

	1995	1996	1997	1998	1999
No. of cases informed	157	1952	428	342	457
Incidence	1.18	14.56	3.16	2.49	3.31

Table 2 Age Distribution of Leptospirosis Cases Informed from 1995 to 1999 in Rio de Janeiro, Brazil

Age (yr)	1995 No.	1995 %	1996 No.	1996 %	1997 No.	1997 %	1998 No.	1998 %	1999 No.	1999 %
00–04	12	7.6	218	11.2	19	4.4	11	3.2	7	1.5
05–09	1	0.6	62	3.2	7	1.6	11	3.2	17	3.7
10–14	6	3.8	118	6.0	19	4.4	17	5.0	19	4.2
15–24	22	14.0	412	21.1	86	20.1	60	17.5	104	22.8
25–34	42	26.8	473	24.2	73	17.1	62	18.1	63	13.8
35–44	28	17.8	332	17.0	95	22.2	73	21.3	102	22.3
45+	46	29.3	337	17.3	129	30.1	108	31.6	145	31.7
Total	157	100	1952	100	428	100	342	100	457	100

Table 3 Sex Distribution of Leptospirosis Cases Informed from 1995 to 1999 in Rio de Janeiro, Brazil

Sex	1995 No.	1995 %	1996 No.	1996 %	1997 No.	1997 %	1998 No.	1998 %	1999 No.	1999 %
Male	135	86	1262	64.7	334	78.1	247	72.2	344	75.3
Female	22	14.0	690	35.3	94	21.9	95	27.8	113	24.7

Table 4 Notification of Leptospirosis Cases, Lethality, and Pulmonary Involvement in Lethal Cases in 2000, 2001, and 2002 in Rio de Janeiro, Brazil

Year	Notification N	Lethality		Lethality with pulmonary involvement	
		N	%	N	%
2000	992	52	05.2	16	30.8
2001	827	51	06.2	20	39.2
2002	781	62	07.9	30	48.4
Total	2600	165	06.4	66	40.0

Severe leptospirosis may present with pulmonary hemorrhage, which is usually massive and leads to respiratory insufficiency and death by asphyxiation. In a prospective study from Thailand, four independent risk factors were associated with high mortality. They were hypotension [relative risk (RR), 10.3; 95% CI, 1.3–83.2; $P < 0.05$]; oliguria (RR, 8.8; 95% CI, 2.4–31.8; $P < 0.01$); hyperkalemia (RR, 5.9; 95% CI, 1.7–21; $P < 0.01$), and the presence of pulmonary rales (RR, 5.2; 95% CI, 1.4–19.9; $P < 0.05$) (39).

IV. Clinical Presentation

The clinical spectrum of leptospirosis ranges from a subclinical illness only detected by seroconversion to two different clinically recognizable syndromes: a self-limited systemic illness seen in roughly 90% of infections, with flu-like symptoms with mild fever, headache, myalgias, and gastrointestinal complaints; and a potentially fatal multisystem disease (Weil's syndrome) with kidney and liver failure, pulmonary hemorrhage, and acute respiratory distress syndrome (ARDS).

The clinical presentation of leptospirosis is biphasic. The first one, also called septicemic stage, is characterized by a sudden onset of intense symptomatology lasting around a week. After an almost asymptomatic period of 24–48 hours, a posterior variable immunologic stage develops with the appearance of antileptospira IgM antibodies in the serum, excretion of leptospira in urine, and return of symptoms during 7 and 20 days. Aseptic meningitis and a reduction of fever and constitutional symptoms may be found at this stage (1,40). Most complication of leptospirosis is associated with the localization of leptospira within the tissues during the immune phase.

The disease has two classical forms of presentation: the icteric and anicteric form. The anicteric form seems to be more common and less severe (41), with more than 90% of the patients having a clinically mild anicteric illness that resolves spontaneously, although this does not mean that it is not associated with severe renal and pulmonary compromise (40). Anicteric cases with severe hemoptysis frequently fatal were related in China with an association with *L. icterohaemorrhagiae* serovar Lai and pulmonary involvement, but it was not confirmed by Singh et al. (37). The incidence of pulmonary involvement in the icteric and anicteric form is still a controversial issue (40,42,43). The icteric form tends to have a more severe clinical presentation with a mortality rate that range from 5% to 15%. The jaundice is usually deep with conjunctival congestion, and is generally not associated with hepatocellular necrosis, with liver function returning to normal after recovery. The jaundice is almost always associated with intense myalgias especially in the calves. The multisystemic nature of the disease can lead to several complications with an overall mortality rate of about 5% (44), but Weil's syndrome has a high one. Death in severe leptospirosis often results from acute renal failure or, eventually, from irreversible myocardial failure. Myocardiopathy probably occurs more frequently than recognized, once it is almost only diagnosed after the correction of the renal failure. Cardiomyosistis is completely independent of the existence of peripheral myositis. Metabolic disturbances, such as hypokalemia, may aggravate this condition. Patients who survive these complications usually recover within 6 to 12 weeks. Although hepatic dysfunction is not directly a major cause of death, it is associated with higher incidence of complications and higher mortality. Hemorrhagic phenomena are relatively common in Weil's syndrome, and they may occur in the skin, mucosa, or internal organs. Hemoptysis may vary from a blood-tinged sputum to massive pulmonary bleed (2,22,45). The presence of pulmonary signs and symptoms may be associated with a poor prognosis (38,46,47); whereas, the patients with normal renal function usually have no pulmonary complication. Occasionally, pulmonary hemorrhage may occur without any renal failure or jaundice (21). A recent outbreak of leptospirosis in Mumbai, India (39), reported an association of mortality with pulmonary signs and symptoms (46).

Severe pulmonary form of leptospirosis manifests itself by pulmonary hemorrhage (Fig. 1), which is usually massive and leads to respiratory insufficiency and death by asphyxiation (42,48).

Alveolar hemorrhage seems to be a common finding probably secondary to capillary endothelium damage with different grades of interstitial and alveolar hemorrhage. Interestingly, significant inflammation is absent in the areas of hemorrhage (49–51). Du Couedic and coworkers (52), performing bronchoalveolar lavage, found that alveolar hemorrhage was present in all patients with signs of pulmonary involvement and in seven of 10 with no respiratory symptoms (52). Once established, the respiratory picture may have a rapid and severe course, with mortality rates as high as 30–60% (53,54).

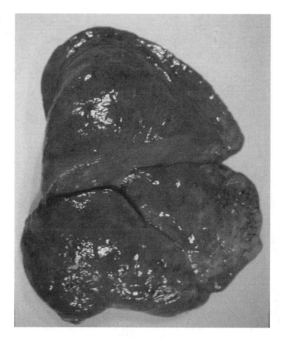

Figure 1 Lung macroscopy showing pulmonary hemorrhage. Leptospirosis.
Source: Courtesy of Prof. Carlos Alberto Basílio de Oliveira.

The first publication of lung involvement in leptospirosis is attributed
to Moeschlin in 1943. This involvement usually has a large spectrum of
presentation ranging from cough (either dry or productive of bloodstained
sputum), different grades of dyspnea, and hemoptysis (which may be mild
or severe) to adult respiratory distress syndrome. These symptoms may
have no correlation with the intensity of the radiograph involvement
(1,14,40,42,43,55). Pulmonary examination may be normal or reveal the
presence of fine crackles at the bases and/or dyspnea. Dyspnea is often
found in association with significant hemoptysis and extensive pulmonary
involvement whether associated or not with cyanosis (40). With a good evolution most patients are asymptomatic in 15 days, but patients with severe
pulmonary involvement and major hemoptysis can die in less than 24 hours.
The radiographic pattern is similar to those of other pulmonary hemorrhagic syndromes with a patchy alveolar infiltration that can conglomerate in
evolution, especially in those cases with severe pulmonary hemorrhage with
massive hemoptysis (42,51). These shadows are common at the bases and
lung periphery (40) (Fig. 2), the involvement of apices and hilar areas being
less frequent (42,43,51). Accentuated marking of the lungs can also be
found (51) but other patterns like interstitial infiltration, ground glass

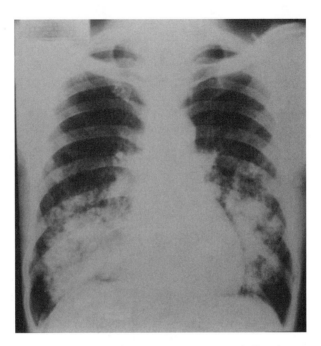

Figure 2 Thorax X-ray showing bilateral alveolar infiltration secondary to pulmonary hemorrhage. Leptospirosis.

appearance (Fig. 3), and pleural effusion are not so commonly reported (40,42). The pulmonary infiltration is almost always bilateral, although sporadic unilateral manifestation can be found (56). The radiographic manifestation may be seen as early as the first 24 hours, during the septicemic stage of the disease. Although in a speticemic phase, leptospira are only occasionally identified in lung tissues (50,52) or in the bronchoalveolar lavage fluid (57). Acute respiratory failure (ARF, ARDS) has also been reported (25,58–62). This may indicate a different pathogenesis of organ injury (61).

The pulmonary involvement in leptospirosis seems to be changing from mild to a severe one in the last 25 years in many places like Brazil (34,35), Nicaragua (63), Andaman Islands—India (37,64), Seychelles (65), and North Queensland, Australia (66). It used to be a sign of mild disease but it seems more likely in our days to have an association with mortality. Pulmonary signs and symptoms need to be analyzed in the global clinical context but almost always with caution. Leptospirosis severity as a hole may also be increasing with more severe cases. The reason for such a case may be the different virulence of the infecting serovar but also the intensity of the reaction in the immune phase. The more severe signs and symptoms of leptospirosis appear in the immune phase when specific agglutinins are

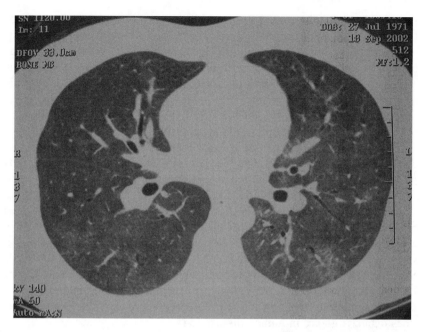

Figure 3 Thorax TCAR showing a ground glass opacity secondary to pulmonary hemorrhage in leptospirosis. *Source*: Courtesy of Dr. Domenico Capone.

detected (67). Similar immune reaction is found in other infectious diseases like dengue (68). Abdulkader et al. (69) recently studied 35 hospitalized patients with Weil's diseases, from the 15th day to the 12th month of symptoms, with five blood samples drawn for ELISA-IgM, -IgG, and -IgA specific antibody detection. According their first IgG, 13 had a titer > 1:400 (group 1) and 22 titers ≤1:400 (group 2). Early IgG antibodies in group 1 showed high avidity which may indicate reinfection. Group 1 also had worse pulmonary and renal function, and fever for a long period than group 2. They concluded that the severity of Weil's disease might be associated with the intensity of humoral immune response to leptospire.

V. Pathophysiology

The pathophysiology associated with leptospirosis is poorly understood. The incubation period of leptospirosis is around 7 to 14 days. Spirochetes can adhere to epithelial cells but rarely cause any direct injury during penetration. This adherence capacity may explain the persistence of the microorganism in tissues, such as the kidney, leading to a carrier state (70). After gaining entry into the bloodstream, the leptospira disseminate to different organs, specially the liver, kidneys, muscles, and lungs. With leptospiremia, the organism may be recovered from blood, cerebrospinal fluid, and most tissues. In the liver, it normally concentrates and reproduces (71) in experimental animals, although it is not verified in humans. Vascular injury, mainly capillary damage, and hemorrhagic diathesis are prominent features in the affected organs. Once a focus of tissue infection has developed, bacterial multiplication rapidly begins (2,72,73). The lesion considered characteristic in leptospirosis' tissue alteration is a hemorrhagic phenomenon attributed to severe vasculitis with endothelial damage, resulting in capillary injury. Lipids of the bacterial cell wall interact with similar substances of the cell membrane during the adherence of *Leptospira* organism to the cell membranes. Leptospiral phospholipases can metabolize host's cell membrane fatty acids enhancing cell membrane permeability (74,75). It seems that toxins and enzymes produced by *Leptospira* may contribute to their pathogenicity, and although clinical and pathological features of infection suggest the presence of an endotoxin, these substances have not yet been isolated (22). Depletion of serum prothrombin or thrombocytopenia seems not to be the cause of the hemorrhagic diathesis seen in severe cases. Also there is no clinical, laboratory, or histopathologic evidence for the occurrence of disseminated intravascular coagulation (DIC) in human leptospirosis, and if this phenomenon does occur, it is rare in human disease (54).

The jaundice mechanism in leptospirosis seems to be similar to that of other septicemic syndromes and toxins may be involved in hepatic lesions. Pathological and histochemical studies suggest that the fundamental hepatic lesion is due to subcellular effect on enzyme systems (22) showing only slight or focal hepatocellular necrosis.

Tubular damage frequently in the absence of interstitial inflammation seems to be the cause of acute renal failure in leptospirosis. In fatal cases, acute tubular necrosis and focal interstitial nephritis can be found (1,22,54). Renal ischemia leading to hypoxia is a fundamental alteration in leptospirosis' nephropathy. A hypokalemic renal failure, secondary to a urine potassium waste, is a characteristic feature of this illness (76). Leptospires can be initially detected in capillary lumen and later in the interstitium causing edema and inflammatory infiltrate. A prerenal component due to dehydration, hypovolemia, hypotension, eventual hemorrhages, and low cardiac output (myocarditis and/or plasma sequestration) may also play a role in renal insufficiency.

The hemorrhagic phenomenon seen in pulmonary lesion of leptospirosis seems to be done by endothelial lesion although not completely understood. There are two principal hypotheses. The first one says that a direct interaction with the parenchymal cells membrane, initially caused by the intact leptospires and latter by their macrophage-degraded granular products, could lead to functional disorders and latter to necrosis of these membranes. Vascular damage may be due to the same process that occurs in endothelial cells (54). Leptospiral antigen detection by immunoperoxidase has been detected in lung tissues of severe pulmonary form of leptospirosis, suggesting that the microorganism exerts a local direct destructive action (77).

The second one says that the pulmonary endothelial capillaries damage leading to increased permeability is related to an undefined leptospiral toxin (78). Significant higher levels of circulating tumor-necrosis factor alpha (TNF-α) is associated with severe leptospiral infection with kidney, liver, and lung involvement as compared with patients without these complications (49,54,71–73,78,79).

VI. Immunological Alterations and Diagnosis

Innate and adaptive immune responses induced by leptospirosis have not yet been well characterized. The human humoral immune response is directed to the outer envelope LPS side-chain epitopes, the same epitopes used to serotype leptospires. LPS antigens elicit the production of immunoglobulin M (IgM) and later IgG antibodies that specifically bind LPS epitopes of the serovar, or cross-reacting serovar or serovars, causing infection. After opsonization and subsequent phagocytosis in tissues, the spirochetes are cleared from the circulation by the reticuloendothelial system. The rapidity of leptospiral clearance seems to be of prognostic importance. Among survivors, long-lasting immunity is believed to be serovar specific. The duration of detectable IgM and IgG antibody, however, is not completely known. The ELISA technique has been used to study the behavior of specific IgM, IgG, and IgA class antibodies in human leptospirosis. IgM class antibodies can be detected early in the course of the disease and up to the 12th month. IgG class antibodies are usually detected around the 7th day of symptoms with a maximum reactivity between the 2nd and 3rd month, but some patients can have it for long periods. IgA class antibodies can also be detected early in the disease (around the 5th day of symptoms) almost in every patient till up to the 9th month of follow-up and can also be detected in 80% of patients at the 12th month of follow-up (80). Recently, Klimpel et al. (81) showed that *L. interrogans* could activate gamma–delta T cells and alpha–beta T cells resulting in cell proliferation and the production of IFN-gamma, IL-12, and TNF-α. This different cell activation seems to be related to the number of *Leptospira* causing the infection. Cell proliferation was highest when using high numbers of *Leptospira* and these T cells were predominantly gamma–delta. On the other hand, alpha–beta T-cell proliferation were seen with a low number of *Leptospira*. This is an important issue and will guide further investigations into the roles of these T-cell populations in host defense and/or the pathology of leptospirosis.

The definitive diagnosis of leptospirosis is based in the finding of *Leptospira*, but it takes time for the organism to develop in culture and growth is unreliable needing special culture media (Fletcher, Stuart, and Tween 80), so diagnosis usually depends on clinical assessment and serologic tests. *Leptospira* can be isolated from the blood and cerebrospinal fluid during the first week of illness and from the urine in the immune phase. Hemocultures should be done until the 7th day and the elimination of *Leptospira* in the urine is intermittent and it is advisable to take several samples. *Leptospira* identification in such material by dark field microscopy has a low sensibility (1). *Leptospira* can also be occasionally detected by direct examination with dark-field methods in bronchoalveolar lavage fluid in the screening for nosocomial infection in suspected cases mechanically ventilated (48). In recent years, PCR methods have been developed for the rapid detection of *Leptospira* DNA in human specimens like serum, urine, aqueous humor, and CSF (82,83).

Serology with macro- or microscopic agglutination is the most common way of doing the diagnosis of leptospirosis. The microscopic agglutination test (MAT), in which live antigen suspensions are titrated with patients' sera and then inspected microscopically for agglutination, is considered the definitive serologic diagnosis. However, this assay requires significant expertise to perform and interpret as well as the laboratory maintenance of a battery of live culture antigens. Other serologic approaches have been developed, including the use of an ELISA for both IgM and IgG antibodies (84,85). Agglutinating antibodies can be detected for a prolonged period after recovery and it is usual to examine paired (acute-phase and convalescent) sera. A fourfold increase in titer between these paired sera is usually accepted in confirming a current case of leptospirosis. A presumptive diagnosis of leptospirosis can also be reasonably made in the presence of clinical suggestive symptoms and a single elevated titer. The cut-off used for this presumptive diagnosis depends on the prevalence of the disease in such an area. It may be as low as 1:200 (86) or as high as 1:800 (87). It is noted that high MAT titers may be retained for several months after acute infection (88). Individuals who have had leptospirosis can retain high levels of IgM and IgG and agglutinating antibodies detectable for months and even years (80,89,90). Cumberland et al. (91) related that more than 20% of cases with evidence of infection with serogroup *Autumnalis* retained titers of >800, 4 years after the acute illness, and in one case a titer of 800 was detected 11 years after infection. Persistence of agglutinating antibody titers can create problems in interpretation of serological results and make it impossible to estimate the time of infection, given a specific titer. In endemic areas where seroprevalence is high, the use of a single elevated titer is not reliable to define a current infection.

Detection of specific IgM antibodies by ELISA (84,92) has been shown to be more sensitive than the detection of agglutinating antibodies (93,94). Recently, Levett and Branch (95) evaluated two commercially available Kits for IgM-ELISA (InDx IVD Microwell ELISA—Integrated Diagnostics, Baltimore, Maryland, U.S.A. and PanBio Leptospira IgM ELISA—Pan-Bio, Queensland, Australia), showing that the sensitivity of the two assays was 89.6% and 97.5%, respectively, and specificities were 92.7% and 96.4%, respectively. The positive predictive values were 87.8% and 95.5%, and the negative predictive values were 90.7% and 89.5%, respectively. Either of these assays can be used for early diagnosis of leptospirosis, particularly in laboratories that cannot perform more specialized leptospiral serology. Others simplified methodologies have also been studied showing goods results (96,97), especially in the early diagnosis of the disease.

VII. Biochemical and Laboratory Features

Routine laboratory tests in leptospirosis are nonspecific. Urinalysis may reveal mild proteinuria, pyuria, hematuria, and hyaline or granular casts. Serum bilirubin levels, if elevated, is normally below 20 mg/dL. Conjugate serum bilirubin may rise up to 80 mg/dL with modest elevation of alkaline phostatase levels with progression to severe disease. Alanine aminotransferase and aspartate aminotransferase rarely exceed 200 U/L (45,98). The observation of a high level of the MM fraction of the creatine phosphokinase usually out of proportion to elevation in serum transaminases can help the distinction of leptospirosis from other causes of acute hepatitis (99). During the acute phase of illness, there are usually urea nitrogen levels below 100 mg/dL and serum creatinine below 2–8 mg/dL, but it also may exceed 300 and 18 mg/dL, respectively (22,45,98).

Intrapulmonary shunt, hypoxemia, hyperventilation with hypocarbia, and normal steady-state diffusion capacity of carbon monoxide are some abnormalities found in lung function tests, which is consistent with intra-alveolar hemorrhage (100).

VIII. Treatment

Once the great majority of patients recover spontaneously, there is usually no need for a specific treatment, although symptomatic medications can be relied.

Since the late 1940s, there are many reports of efficacy of different antibiotic in experimental in vitro and animal models against leptospirosis. However, placebo-controlled trials comparing penicillin, tetracycline, chloramphenicol, and other antibiotics in the 1950s failed to demonstrate a beneficial effect. Most authorities agree that if antibiotics are not started early in the disease (up to the 4th day), they do not change the course of the illness. At this early time, the specific diagnosis may be difficult and therefore antibiotics end up not being used very frequently. On the other hand, some more recent studies show clinical efficacy for intravenous penicillin therapy, oral amoxicillin, ampicillin, tetracycline, or doxycycline for severe and mild infections even in the immunologic stage of the disease (2,13,18,101).

Therefore, the use of antibiotics in leptospirosis is a controvertible issue. The currently recommended antimicrobial agents for leptospirosis are based on the severity of the disease. Mild infections can be treated with oral doxycycline (100 mg PO bid), or ampicillin (500–750 mg q6h), or amoxicillin (500 mg q6h). Moderate-to-severe disease requiring hospitalization can be treated with intravenous penicillin (1.5 million U IV q6h), or ampicillin (0.5–1 g IV q6h).

Recently, a systematic review from the Cochrane Foundation was presented that was based on randomized clinical trials (RCT) evaluating the effectiveness and safety of antibiotics versus placebo or other antibiotic regimens in treating leptospirosis. Only three studies met the inclusion criteria. Of the patients enrolled, 75 were treated with placebo and 75 with antibiotics: 61 (81.3%) with penicillin and 14 (18.6%) with doxycycline. Despite the absence of RCTs that compared each antibiotic regimen to other antibiotic regimens, the reviewers concluded that there is insufficient evidence to provide clear guidelines for administration of an antibiotic regimen for the treatment of leptospirosis. The randomized trials suggest that antibiotics (penicillin and doxycycline) could be useful, causing more good than harm, although the indication for general use of these antibiotics is uncertain (102).

Intravenous hydration and symptomatic therapy should be provided to patients with mild and moderate forms of the illness. In the most severe forms, patients must be admitted to the ICU in order to undergo respiratory, hemodynamic, and renal assistance or other life-supporting measures.

Lung involvement can be one of the most fatal conditions in leptospirosis. Pulmonary hemorrhage and ARDS are the main cause of death in the most recent cases presented (25,54,58,60,61,65,103–105). A significant reduction in mortality has been achieved in the use of mechanical ventilation in ARDS patients applying lung-protective strategies, based on the use of low tidal volumes (58,106,107). In a prospective randomized study conducted in Brazil, the use of high levels of positive end-expiratory pressure, according to the inflection point of the pressure $\times$ volume curve of the respiratory system, associated with small tidal volumes demonstrated very good results. In this trial, comparing two different modes of mechanical ventilation (conventional $\times$ lung protective strategy), the authors described eight patients with leptospirosis associated with ARDS. Four patients were treated in a conventional method with high tidal volume and a positive end-expiratory pressure level high enough to maintain inspired oxygen function of less than 60%; all patients died. Four other patients were ventilated in a protected strategy with small tidal volumes (≤ 6 mL/kg) and high positive end-expiratory pressure levels (> 15 cmH$_2$O); only one patient died, because of central nervous system bleeding (58,108). In spite of the permissive hypercapnia and the high mean airway pressure observed, due to the high positive end-expiratory pressure applied, no deleterious hemodynamic compromise occurred, demonstrating a safety of this strategy (109).

Massive hemoptysis in the patients with severe leptospirosis is often resistant to conventional therapies and can rapidly become fatal. Other forms of treatment in order to have a successful strategy have been tried like nitric oxide inhalation and hemofiltration (110). Recently, Pea et al. (111) related good results using desmopressin infusions to treat massive pulmonary hemorrhage in six leptospirosis patients with respiratory failure, shock, and multiple organ dysfunction. These and new forms of management of pulmonary involvement have to be tested in the future to get better control of this fatal complication of leptospirosis.

IX. Prophylaxis

Prophylaxis for leptospirosis is a difficult task. Good sanitary measures and special recommendations about some specific professional activities may be useful. Animal and human vaccination is still under study. In certain special circumstances, chemoprophylaxis may be used (1).

In clinical practice, doxycycline is used as a prophylactic agent in leptospirosis. Recently, a systematic review performed by the Cochrane Foundation evaluated all RCTs, but only two satisfied all the inclusion criteria. Both compared doxycycline with placebo. The number of the patients enrolled were 1022; 509 received doxycycline and 513 were given a placebo. Another trial included 940 soldiers. Both trials suggested that prophylaxis of leptospirosis could be achieved by administrating doxycycline to individuals in endemic areas with a high risk of exposure to *Leptospira*. Whether these findings will apply to other situations remains uninvestigated (44).

X. The Future

Leptospirosis is a re-emerging zoonosis with a worldwide distribution. In some areas, the disease has become more virulent. The pulmonary involvement in the past used to be infrequent and mild. Now many more cases of severe pneumonia with respiratory failure and poor prognosis have been reported. A better understanding of the immune response and the knowledge of the genetic pattern of *Leptospira* will bring progress in vaccination and treatment. One day we may be able to eradicate the illness.

Acknowledgments

We would like to thank Prof. Om P. Sharma for the invitation and review of the manuscript. I am also in debt with Dr. Paulo Francisco de Almeida

Lopes, Dr. Gualberto Teixeira dos Santos Jr, and Dr. Tereza Cravo de Almeida for the help with the manuscript and the data from the SES-RJ.

References

1. Bethlem N, Lemle A, Pereira NG. Leptospirosis. Semin Respir Med 1991; 12:58–67.
2. Lomar AV, Diament D, Torres JR. Leptospirosis in Latin America. Infect Dis Clin North Am 2000; 14:23–39.
3. Lancereaux E. Des icteres graves et des hepatites parenchymateuses. Rev Med 1882; 2:605–624.
4. Landouzy M. Fièvre bilieuse ou hépatique. Gaz Hôpital 1883; 56:809.
5. Landouzy M. Typhus hépatique. Gaz Hôpital 1883; 56:913.
6. Weil A. Veber eine eigenthumliche, milmilztumor, icterus and nephritis einhergehende, acute infectionskrankheit. Deutsches Archiv fur Klinische Medizin 1886; 39:209.
7. Mathieu A. Typhus hepatique bénin. Rechute-Guérison. Ver Med 1886; 6:633–639.
8. Stimson AM. Note on an organism found in yellow-fever tissue. Public Health Rep 1907; 22:541.
9. Levett PN. Leptospirosis. Clin Microbiol Ver 2001; 14:296–326.
10. Inada R, Ido Y, Hoki R, Kaneko R, Ito H. The etiology, mode of infection, and specific therapy of Weil's disease (Spirochaetosis icterohaemorrhagica). J Exp Med 1916; 28:377–402.
11. Ido Y, Hoki R, Ito H, Wani H. The rat as a carrier of *Spirochaeta icterohaemorragiae*, the causative agent of Weil's disease (Spirochaetosis icterohaemorrhagica). J Exp Med 1917; 26:341–353.
12. Appud Pereira MM. Leptospirose em área urbana do Município do Rio de Janeiro. Rio de Janeiro: Fundação Oswaldo Cruz, 1985:158. Tese de Mestrado em Medicina Tropical.
13. Bethlem EP, Carvalho CRR. Pulmonary leptospirosis. Curr Opin Pulm Med 2000; 6:436–441.
14. Farrar WE. Leptospira species. In: Mandell GL, Douglas RG Jr, Bennett JE, eds. Principles and Practice of Infectious Diseases. 2nd ed. New York: John Wiley and Sons, 1985:1338–1341.
15. Kmety E, Dikken H. Classification of the Species *L. interrogans* and History of Its Serovars. Groningen, The Netherlands: University Press Groningen, 1993.
16. Zuerner RL, Bolin CA. Differentiation of *Leptospira interrogans* isolates by IS1500 hybridization and PCR assays. J Clin Microbiol 1997; 35:2612–2617.
17. Ren SX, Fu G, Jiang XG, Zeng R, Miao YG, Xu H, et al. Unique physiological and pathogenic features of *Leptospira interrogans* revealed by whole-genome sequencing. Nature 2003; 422(6934):888–893.
18. Watt G, Padre LP, Tuazon ML. Placebo-controlled trial intravenous penicillin for severe and late leptospirosis. Lancet 1988; 1:433–435.

19. Andrade J, Brandão AP. Contribuição ao conhecimento da epidemiologia da leptospirose humana com especial referência ao Grande Rio, Brasil, de 1970 a 1982. Mem Inst Oswaldo Cruz 1987; 82:91.

20. Feigin RD, Anderson DC. Leptospirosis. In: Feigin RD, Cherry JD, eds. Textbook of Pediatrics Infectious Disease. 2nd ed. Philadelphia: WB Sounders, 1987:1190.

21. Trevejo RT, Rigau-Pérez JG, Ashford DA, McClure EM, Jarquin-González C, Amador JJ, et al. Epidemic leptospirosis associated with pulmonary hemorrhage—Nicaragua, 1995. J Infect Dis 1998; 178:1457–1463.

22. Farr RW. Leptospirosis. Clin Infect Dis 1995; 21:1–8.

23. Freedman DO, Woodall J. Emerging infectious diseases and risk to the traveler. Med Clin North Am 1999; 83:865–883.

24. Sejvar J, Bancroft E, Winthrop K, Bettinger J, Bajani M, Bragg S, Shutt K, Kaiser R, Marano N, Popovic T, Tappero J Ashford D, Mascola L, Vugia D, Perkins B, Rosenstein N, and the Eco-Challenge Investigation Team. Leptospirosis in "eco-challenge" athletes, Malaysian Borneo, 2000. Emerg Infect Dis 2003; 9(6):702–707.

25. Carvalho JEM, Marchiori ES, Silva JBG, Souza Neto BA, Tavares W, Paula AV. Comprometimento pulmonar na leptospirose. Rev Soc Brasil Med Trop 1992; 25:21–30.

26. Center for Disease Control and Prevention. Graphs and maps for selected notifiable diseases in the United States, 1993. MMWR Morb Mortal Wkly Rep 1994; 42:1–12.

27. Cinco M, Banfi E, Soranzo MR. Studies on the interactions between macrophages and leptospires. J Gen Microbiol 1981; 124:409–413.

28. Sasaki DM, Pang L, Minette HP. Active surveillance and risk factors for leptospirosis in Hawaii. Am J Trop Med Hyg 1993; 48:35–43.

29. Baranton G, Postic D. Rapport Annuels d'Activité 2000, Centre National de Référence des Leptospiroses, Institut Pasteur.

30. Perra A, Servas V, Terrier G, Postic D, Baranton G, André-Fontaine G, Vaillant V, Capek I. Surveillance report—clustered cases of leptospirosis in Rochefort, France, June 2001. Eurosurveillance 2002; 7(10):131–136.

31. Estavoyer JM, Tran TA, Hoen B. Leptospiroses. Rev Prat 2001; 51(19): 2086–2090.

32. Everard JD, Everard COR. Leptospirosis in the Caribbean. Rev Med Microbiol 1993; 4:114–122.

33. DATASUS. Ministério da Saúde. Sistema Único de Saúde (SUS). Sistema de Informação Hospitalar, 1998 (www.datasus.gov.br).

34. Carvalho CRR, Bethlem EP. Pulmonary complications of leptospirosis. Clin Chest Med 2002; 23:469–478.

35. Daher E, Zanetta DMT, Cavalcante MB, Abdulkader RC. Risk factors for death and changing patterns in leptospirosis acute renal failure. Am J Trop Med Hyg 1999; 61:630–634.

36. Rios-Gonçalves AJ, Capone D, Paz NA, et al. Leptospirose. Observações sobre as mudanças dos padrões clínicos no Rio de Janeiro após a grande epidemia de 1988. Arq Bras Med 1990; 64:389–397.

37. Singh SS, Vijayachari P, Sinha A, Sugunan AP, Rasheed MA, Sehgal SC. Clinical-epidemiological study of hospitalized cases of severe leptospirosis. Indian J Med Res 1999; 109:94–99.

38. Niwattayakul K, Homvijitkul J, Niwattayakul S, Khow O, Sitprija V. Hypotension, renal failure, and pulmonary complications in leptospirosis. Ren Fail 2002; 24(3):297–305.

39. Panaphut T, Domrongkitchaiporn S, Thinkamrop B. Prognostic factors of death in leptospirosis: a prospective cohort study in Khon Kaen, Thailand. Int J Infect Dis 2002; 6(1):52–59.

40. O'Neil KM, Rickman LS, Lazarus AA. Pulmonary manifestations of leptospirosis. Rev Infect Dis 1991; 13:705–709.

41. Vieira A, Barros MS, Valente C, Trindade L, Faria MJ, Freitas F. Leptospirose humana. Breves considerações a propósito de uma casuística. Acta Med Portuguesa 1999; 12:331–340.

42. Im JG, Yeon KM, Han MC, Kim CW, Webb WR, Lee JS, et al. Leptospirosis of the lung: radiographic findings in 58 patients. Am J Roentgenol 1989; 152:955–959.

43. Lee REJ, Terry SI, Walker TM, Urquhart AE. The chest radiograph in leptospirosis in Jamaica. Br J Radiol 1981; 54:939–943.

44. Guidugli F, Castro AA, Atallah NA. Antibiotics for Preventing Leptospirosis (Cochrane Review). The Cochrane Library, Issue 3. Oxford. Update Software, 2001b.

45. Feigin RD, Anderson DC. Human leptospirosis. Crit Rev Clin Lab Sci 1975; 5:413–465.

46. Bharadwaj R, Bal AM, Joshi S A, Kagal A, Pol SS, Garad G, Arjunwadkar V, Katti R. An outbreak of leptospirosis in Mumbai, India. Jpn J Infect Dis 2002; 55:194–196.

47. Divate SA, Chaturvedi R, Jadhav NN, Vaideeswar P. Leptospirosis associated with diffuse alveolar haemorrhage. J Postgrad Med 2002; 48(2):131–132.

48. Carvalho JEM, Oliveira JMC, Nicol AF, Dalston MO, Vilar EAG, Rodrigues CC, Santos PRN, Pereira, MM, Pereira da Silva JJ. Identificação da leptospira em tecido pulmonar por broncofibroscopia e biópsia brônquica. Pulmão RJ 1999; 8:377–381.

49. Edwards G, Domm BM. Human leptospirosis. Medicine (Baltimore) 1960; 39:117–156.

50. Silverstein CM. Pulmonary manifestations of leptospirosis. Radiology 1953; 61:327–334.

51. Wang CP, Chi CW, Lu FL. Studies on anicteric leptospirosis. III. Roentgenologic observations of pulmonary changes. Chin Med J (Engl) 1965; 84: 298–306.

52. Du Couedic L, Courtin JP, Poubeau P, Tanguy B, Di Francia M, Arvin-Berod C. Patent and occult intra-alveolar hemorrhage in leptospirosis. Rev Mal Respir 1998; 15:61–67.

53. Friedland JS, Warrell DA. The Jarisch–Herxheimer reaction in leptospirosis: possible pathogenesis and review. Rev Infect Dis 1991; 13:207–210.

54. Nicodemo AC, Duarte MIS, Alves AF, Takamura CFH, Santos RTM, Nicodemo EL. Lung lesions in human leptospirosis: microscopic, immuno-

histochemical, and ultrastructural features related to thrombocytopenia. Am J Trop Med Hyg 1997; 56:181–187.

55. Poh SC, Soh CS. Lung manifestations in leptospirosis. Thorax 1970; 25: 751–755.
56. Bowsher B, Callaham CW, Pearson DA, Ruess L. Unilateral leptospiral pneumonia and cold agglutinin disease. Chest 1999; 116:830–832.
57. Paganin F, Gauzere BA, Lugagne N, Blanc P, Robin X. Bronchoalveolar lavage in rapid diagnosis of leptospirosis. Lancet 1996; 347:1483–1484.
58. Amato MBP, Barbas CSV, Medeiros DM, Magaldi RB, Schetino GPP, Lorenzi-Filho G, et al. Effect of a lung protective approach on mortality in the acute respiratory distress syndrome. N Engl J Med 1998; 338:347–354.
59. Chee HD, Ossenkoppele GJ, Bronsveld W, Thijs LG. Adult respiratory distress syndrome in *Leptospira icterohaemorrhagiae* infection. Intens Care Med 1985; 11:254–256.
60. Gonçalves AJR, Carvalho JEM, Silva JBG, Rozembaum R, Vieira ARM. Hemoptises e síndrome de angústia respiratória do adulto como causas de morte na leptospirose. Mudanças de padrões clínicos e anatomopatológicos. Rev Soc Bras Med Trop 1992; 25:261–270.
61. Kiatboonsri S, Vathesatogit P, Charoenpan P. Adult respiratory distress syndrome in Thai medical patients. Southeast Asian J Trop Med Public Health 1995; 26:774–780.
62. Zaltzman M, Kallenbach JM, Goss GD, Lewis M, Zwi S, Gear JHS. Adult respiratory distress syndrome in *Leptospira canicola* infection. BMJ 1981; 283:519–520.
63. Zaki SR, Shieh WJ. Leptospirosis associated with outbreak of acute febrile illness and pulmonary haemorrhage, Nicaragua 1995. The Epidemic Working Group at Ministry of Health in Nicaragua.. Lancet 1996; 347:535–536.
64. Sehgal SC, Vijayachari P, Smythe L D, Norris M, Symmonds M, Dount M, et al. Lai-like leptospira from Andaman Islands. Indian J Med Res 2000; 112:135–139.
65. Yersin C, Bovet P, Merien F, Clement J, Laille M, VanRaust M, et al. Pulmonary haemorrhage as a predominant cause of death in leptospirosis in Seychelles. Trans R Soc Trop Med Hyg 2000; 94:71–76.
66. Simpson FG, Green KA, Hang GJ, Brookes DL. Leptospirosis associated with severe pulmonary haemorrhage in Far North Queensland. Med J Aust 1998; 169:151–153.
67. Fainer S, Adler B, Perolat P, Bolin C. *Leptospira* and Leptospirosis. 2nd ed. Melbourne: MediSci, 1999.
68. Branch SL, Levett PN. Evaluation of four methods for detection of immunoglobulin M antibodies to dengue virus. Clin Diag Lab Immunol 1999; 6: 555–557.
69. Abdulkader RCRM, Daher EF, Camargo ED, Spinosa C, Silva MV. Leptospirosis severity may be associated with the intensity of humoral immune response. Ver Inst Med Trop S Paulo 2002; 44(2):79–83.
70. Vihn T, Adler B, Faine S. Glycolipoprotein cytotoxin from *Leptospira interrogans* serovar copenhageni. J Gen Microbiol 1984; 18:73–85.

71. DeBrito T, Bohm GM, Yasuda PH. Vascular damage in acute experimental leptospirosis of the guinea pig. J Pathol 1979; 128:177–182.
72. Arean VM, Sarasin G, Green JH. The pathogenesis of leptospirosis: toxin productions by *Leptospira icterohaemorrhagiae*. Am J Vet Res 1964; 25:836–843.
73. DeBrito T, Morais CF, Yasuda PH, Lancelloti CP, Shimizu S, Yamashiro E, et al. Cardiovascular involvement in human and experimental leptospirosis: pathologic findings and immunohistochemical detection of leptospiral antigen. Ann Trop Med Parasitol 1987; 81:207–214.
74. Alves VAF, Gayotto LCC, Yasuda PH. Leptospiral antigen in the kidney of experimentally infected guinea pigs and their relation to the pathogenesis of renal injury. Exp Pathol 1991; 42:81–93.
75. Volina EG, Levina LF, Soboleva GL. Phospholipase activity and virulence of pathogenic leptospirae. J Hyg Epidemiol Microbiol Immunol 1986; 2:163–169.
76. Seguro AC, Lomar AV, Rocha AS. Acute renal failure of leptospirosis: nonoliguric and hypokalemic forms. Nephron 1990; 55(2):146–151.
77. Silva JJP, Dalston MO, Carvalho JEM, Setúbal S, Oliveira JMC, Pereira MM. Clinicopathological and immunohistochemical features of the severe pulmonary form of leptospirosis. Rev Soc Bras Med Trop 2002; 35(4):395–399.
78. Emmanouilides CE, Kohn OF, Garibaldi R. Leptospirosis complicated by a Jarisch–Herxheimer reaction and adult respiratory distress syndrome: case report. Clin Infect Dis 1994; 18:1004–1006.
79. Pereira MM, Andrade J, Marchevsky RS, Ribeiro dos Santos R. Morphological characterization of lung and kidney lesions in C3H/HeJ mice infected with *Leptospira interrogans* serovar icterohaemorrhagiae: defect of CD4+and and CD8+ T-cells are prognosticators of the disease progression. Exp Toxicol Pathol 1998; 50:191–198.
80. Silva MV, Camargo ED, Batista L, Vaz AJ, Brandao AP, Nakamura PM, Negrao JM. Behaviour of specific IgM, IgG and IgA class antibodies in human leptospirosis during the acute phase of the disease and during convalescence. J Trop Med Hyg 1995; 98(4):268–272.
81. Klimpel GR, Matthias MA, Vinetz JM. *Leptospira interrogans* activation of human peripheral blood mononuclear cells: preferential expansion of TCR gamma delta+ T cells vs TCR alpha beta+ T cells. J Immunol 2003; 171(3): 1447–1455.
82. Merien F, Baranton G, Perolat P. Comparison of polymerase chain reaction with microagglutination test and culture for diagnosis of leptospirosis. J Infect Dis 1995; 172(1):281–285.
83. Brown PD, Gravekamp C, Carrington DG, van de Kemp H, Hartskeerl RA, Edwards CN, Everard CO, Terpstra WJ, Levett PN. Evaluation of the polymerase chain reaction for early diagnosis of leptospirosis. J Med Microbiol 1995; 43(2):110–114.
84. Adler B, Murphy AM, Locarnini SA, Faine S. Detection of specific anti-leptospiral immunoglobulins M and G in human serum by solid-phase enzyme-linked immunoabsorbent assay. J Clin Microbiol 1980; 11:452–457.
85. Terpstra WJ, Ligthart GS, Schoone GJ. Serodiagnosis of human leptospirosis by enzyme-linked-immunoabsorbent-assay (ELISA). Zentralbl Bakteriol Microbiol Hyg 1980; [A] 247:400–405.

86. Centers for Disease Control and Prevention. Case definitions for infectious conditions under public health surveillance. MMWR Morb Mortal Wkly Rep 1997; 46:49.

87. Faine S. Guidelines for the Control of Leptospirosis. Geneva: World Health Organization, 1982.

88. Romero EC, Caly CR, Yasuda PH. The persistence of leptospiral agglutinins titers in human sera diagnosed by the microscopic agglutination test. Rev Inst Med Trop Sao Paulo 1998; 40:183–184.

89. Adler B, Faine S. The antibodies involved in the human immune response to leptospiral infection. J Med Microbiol 1978; 11:387–400.

90. Blackmore DK. The magnitude and duration of titers of leptospiral agglutinins in human sera. N Z Med J 1984; 97:83–86.

91. Cumberland P, Everard CO, Wheeler JG, Levett PN. Persistence of anti-leptospiral IgM, IgG and agglutinating antibodies in patients presenting with acute febrile illness in Barbados 1979–1989. Eur J Epidemiol 2001; 17(7): 601–608.

92. Terpstra WJ, Ligthart GS, Schoone GJ. ELISA for the detection of specific IgM and IgG in human leptospirosis. J Gen Microbiol 1985; 131:377–385.

93. Levett PN, Whittington CU. Evaluation of the indirect hemagglutination assay for diagnosis of acute leptospirosis. J Clin Microbiol 1998; 36:11–14.

94. Cumberland P, Everard COR, Levett PN. Assessment of the efficacy of an IgM-Elisa and microscopic agglutination test (MAT) in the diagnosis of acute leptospirosis. Am Soc Trop Med Hyg 1999; 61:731–734.

95. Levett PN, Branch SL. Evaluation of two enzyme-linked immunosorbent assay methods for detection of immunoglobulin M antibodies in acute leptospirosis. Am J Trop Med Hyg 2002; 66(6):745–748.

96. Gussenhoven GC, Van der Hoorn MAWG, Goris MGA, Terpstra WJ, Hartskeerl RA, Mol BW, van Ingen CW, Smits HL. LEPTO dipstick, a dipstick assay for detection of leptospira-specific immunoglobulin M antibodies in human sera. J Clin Microbiol 1997; 35(1):92–97.

97. Brandão AP, Camargo ED, da Silva ED, Silva MV, Abrão RV. Macroscopic agglutination test for rapid diagnosis of human leptospirosis. J Clin Microbiol 1998; 36(11):3138–3142.

98. Health CW, Alexander AD, Galton MM. Leptospirosis in the United States: analysis of 483 cases in man, 1949–1961. N Engl J Med 1965; 273:1–15.

99. Johnson WD, Silva IC, Rocha H. Serum creatinine phosphokinase in leptospirosis. JAMA 1975; 233:981–982.

100. Nery LE, De Paula AB, Nakatani J, dos Santos ML, Ratto OR. Clinical, radiological and functional pulmonary manifestations in patients with leptospirosis. Rev Inst Med Trop São Paulo 1977; 19:366–373.

101. Klein NC, Cunha BA. New uses of older antibiotics. Med Clin North Am 2001; 85:125–132.

102. Guidugli F, Castro AA, Atallah NA. Antibiotics for Leptospirosis (Cochrane Review). The Cochrane Library. Issue 3. Update SoftwareOxford2001a.

103. Coutin JP, Di Francia M, Du Couedic L, Poubeau P, Mahe C, Bapteste J, et al. Respiratory manifestations of leptospirosis. A retrospective study of 91 cases (1978–1984). Rev Pneumol Clin 1998; 54:382–392.

104. Martinez-García MA. Pulmonary involvement in leptospirosis. Eur J Clin Microbiol Infect Dis 2000; 19:471–474.

105. Shieh WJ, Greer P, Ferebee T, Goldsmith C, Guarner J, Zali SR. The role of pathology in studies of emerging infectious diseases associated with acute respiratory distress syndrome. Int Conf Emerg Infect Dis 1998; 75:8–11.

106. Amato MBP, Barbas CSV, Carvalho CRR. Protective ventilation for the acute respiratory distress syndrome. N Engl J Med 1998; 339:196–199.

107. The Acute Respiratory Distress Syndrome Network. Ventilation with lower tidal volumes as compared with traditional tidal volumes for acute lung injury and the acute respiratory distress syndrome. N Engl J Med 2000; 342: 1301–1308.

108. Amato MBP, Barbas CSV, Medeiros RB, Schettino GPP, Lorenzi-Filho G, Kairalla RA, et al. Beneficial effects of the "open lung approach" with low distending pressures in acute respiratory distress syndrome. Am J Respir Crit Care Med 1995; 152:1835–1846.

109. Carvalho CRR, Barbas CV, Medeiros DM, Magaldi RB, Lorenzi-Filho G, Kairalla RA, et al. Temporal hemodynamic effects of permissive hypercapnia associated with "ideal PEEP" in ARDS. Am J Respir Crit Care Med 1997; 156:1458–1466.

110. Borer A, Metz I, Gilad J, Riesenberg K, Weksler N, Weber G, et al. Massive pulmonary haemorrhage caused by leptospirosis successfully treated with nitric oxide inhalation and haemofiltration. J Infect 1999; 38:42–45.

111. Pea L, Roda L, Boussaud V, Lonjon B. Desmopressin therapy for massive hemoptysis associated with severe leptospirosis. Am J Respir Crit Care Med 2003; 167(5):726–728.

20

Diffuse Panbronchiolitis

SONOKO NAGAI

Department of Respiratory Medicine,
    Kyoto University,
Kyoto, Japan

MASANORI KITAICHI

Department of Anatomical Pathology,
    Kyoto University Hospital,
Kyoto, Japan

TAKATERU IZUMI

Central Clinic in Kyoto,
Kyoto, Japan

I. Introduction

Diffuse panbronchiolitis (DPB), an inflammatory airway disease of the lungs, predominantly involves respiratory bronchioles. It causes chronic cough, copious sputum (chronic infectious disease), and exertional dyspnea with airflow limitation (obstructive airway disease). DPB is a distinct clinico-pathologic disease that involves the upper and lower respiratory tracts. Chest roentgenograms typically show small nodular shadows and hyperinflation involving both lungs. Computed Tomography (CT) scans reveal characteristic small nodular shadows localized in a centrilobular distribution with or without bronchioloectasis.

DPB was first described by Takizawa in 1963 in Japan. In 1969, Yamanaka proposed the name of DPB to distinguish it from chronic bronchitis. "Diffuse" refers to the diffuse distribution of the lesion through both lungs, and "pan" refers to the involvement of the inflammation in all layers of the respiratory bronchiole (1,2). Homma et al. (3) provided the clinical definition of DPB in 1971 based on their evaluation of Japanese patients as shown in Table 1.

Table 1 Clinical Diagnostic Criteria for DPB

1. Symptoms	Chronic cough, sputum, and dyspnea on exertion
2. Physical signs	Rales and rhonchi
3. Chest radiograph	Diffuse diseminated fine nodular shadows, mainly in the lower lung fields with hyperinflation of the lungs
4. Lung function studies	At least 3 of the 4 abnormalities listed
	(a) FEV1.0% < 70%
	(b) %VC < 80%
	(c) %RV > 150% or RV/TLC > 4.5%
	(d) $PaO_2 < 80\,mmHg$

II. Incidence and Epidemiology

The two nationwide surveys on DPB, funded by the Ministry of Health and Welfare, have been carried out in Japan. In the first survey (1980–1982), 319 clinically diagnosed patients and 82 histopathologically confirmed patients were reported. The second survey (1988–1991) consisted of 229 clinically diagnosed patients. These surveys have clarified clinical and pathological features of DPB (1,4).

III. Pathological Features of DPB (Table 2)

Macroscopically, conducting airways were usually dilated cylindrically throughout the lungs. In some cases, peribronchiolar fibrosis or perifibrotic emphysema was found. Necrotizing or non-necrotizing granulomas, vasculitic, or marked tissue eosinophilia were not observed.

Microscopically, centrilobular inflammatory response consisted of interstitial accumulation of foamy cells and lymphoid cells in the wall of

Table 2 A Summary of Histopathologic Features of DPB

Bronchus membranous bronchiole	Chronic mural inflammation and dilatation in the late stage
Respiratory bronchiole alveolar duct	Mural and luminal inflammation with foamy cells in the wall
Alveolus	Accumulation of foamy cells in the interstitium and air spaces

NB: Sometimes positive for focal denudation of bronchiolar epithelial layer elastolysis in the lamina propria of bronchioles, peribronchiolar fibrotic changes, and perifibrotic emphysematous changes.
Negative for neoplastic features, formation of granulomas, necrotizing vasculitic features, marked tissue eosinophiia.
Source: From Ref. 5.

a respiratory bronchiole, adjacent alveolar ducts, and alveoli (unit lesion of panbronchiolitis/PB unit lesion) was noted in all cases (Fig. 1A, B) (5).

The PB unit lesion was absent in patients with asthma, chronic bronchitis, cystic fibrosis, cryptogenic organizing pneumonia, follicular bronchiolitis, and small airway disease. Five percent of the patients with localized bronchiectasis also demonstrated the DPB unit (5). Iwata et al., on the other hand, reported seven cases of DPB and 20 examples of histologically similar lesions (PB-like lesion) in a large review of cases of bronchiolitis, cystic fibrosis, bronchiectasis, aspiration pneumonia, extrinsic allergic alveolitis, Wegener's granulomatosis, bronchocentric granulomatosis, and malignant lymphoma. The results indicated that the PB-like lesion in itself is a nonspecific histologic finding (6).

Pathologic diagnostic criteria for DPB are as follows:

1. The pulmonary inflammation is chronic and involves airways diffusely in both lungs.
2. The predominant sites of chronic inflammation are the walls of membranous and respiratory bronchioles and the centrilobular regions.
3. The lesions consist of one or more unit lesions of PB (an interstitial accumulation of foamy cells with lymphoid cells in the walls of a respiratory bronchiole and adjacent alveolar ducts and alveoli) (5).

IV. DPB: Is it an Illness Limited Only to Japan?

It has been claimed that DPB is a unique disease found only in Japan. However, there are many cases of DPB reported from outside of Japan (Table 3). An association with chronic sinusitis was reported in the studies from Korea (7), Thailand (8), Turkey (9), Brazil (10,11), United States (12), and Spain (13). In some cases, diagnosis was based on the typical histological appearance (10,11,14), whereas, in others only clinical and radiological features were used (13,15–18).

Treatment with erythromycin was effective in most of the cases (10,11,14–16,18,19).

The first European DPB case was described in 1990. Over the next 10-year period, four additional DPB patients were identified. In one study of five Caucasians cases of "idiopathic" bronchiolitis that had both clinical symptoms and HRCT findings indistinguishable from those of DPB, the typical histological changes were absent (20). Randhawa et al. (21) reported two white patients with DPB. Homer et al. (13) reported DPB in a Hispanic patient who had an extensive travel history to the Far East, including Japan. This case raised the possibility of a transmissible infectious agent responsible for the disease. Fitzgerald et al. (12) have identified DPB in five citizens

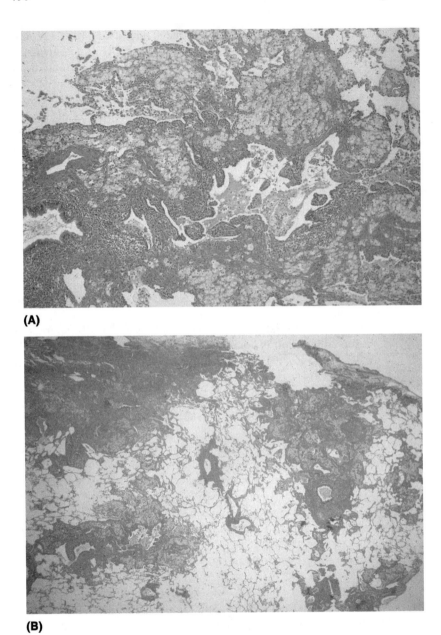

(A)

(B)

Figure 1 (A) Histopathological features of DPB. Microscopically, centrilobular inflammatory changes with interstitial accumulation of foamy cells and lymphoid cells in the wall of a respiratory bronchiole, adjacent alveolar ducts and alveoli can be found diffusely (5). (B) Histopathological PB-unit lesion. Microscopically, centrilobular inflammatory changes with interstitial accumulation of foamy cells and lymphoid cells in the wall of a respiratory bronchiole, adjacent alveolar ducts and alveoli (unit lesion of panbronchiolitis/PB unit lesion) was noted (5).

Table 3 DPB: Case Reports from Various Countries Outside Japan

Authors	Ref. no.	Year of publication	Country	No. of cases with DPB	Population	Age and sex	Biopsy proven	Chronic sinusitis
Randhawa et al.	20	1991	USA	3	2 White, 1 Asian			
Kim et al.	7	1992	Korea	5	Korean	3 men/2 women, 27–59	2SLB	100%
Chu et al.	15	1992	Taiwan	1	Chinese	Man 33 yr	SLB	
Homer etal.	21	1995	Spain	1	Hispanic			
Fitzgerald et al.	12	1996	USA	5	Caucasian			100%
Zainudin et al.	17	1996	Malaysia	3	Malaysian		TBLB	
Brugiere et al.	16	1996	France	1	Asian immigrant	Man, 32	SLB	Present
Tsang et al.	13	1998	China	7	Chinese	3 women, 48 yr	2SLB	
Chantarotom et al.	8	1999	Thailand	3	Thai	2 women/1 man, 60 yr	1SLB	Present
Gulhan et al.	9	2000	Turkey	18	Turkish			Present
Martinez et al.	11	2000	Brazil	1	Non-Asian			Present
Souza et al.	10	2002	Brazil	4	3 Japanese, Black		TBLB	Present
Poletti et al.	19	2003	Italy	5	Caucasian			Present

Source: Adapted from Refs. 7–21.

of the United States, three with histologic confirmation, who have never traveled to the Far East.

In summary, it appears that DPB is a disease that is not exclusive to the Asian population. Further epidemiologic studies will increase the number of patients with DPB-like bronchiolar diseases all over the world (5).

A. Genetics

Familial cases of DPB have been reported in Japan. Most of the patients with DPB and their first-degree relatives have chronic sinusitis. DPB tends to occur in younger patients. These features suggest that there may be a genetic background for DPB.

HLA class I and class II antigens became a first focus of genetic studies in patients with DPB and their siblings with chronic sinusitis. HLA-B54 antigen is increased in frequency and might be directly involved in the pathogenesis of DPB (22,23). Not only Bw54 and its related haplotype exist only in Japanese, Chinese, and Korean populations, the prevalence of DPB is also increased among these populations. Among 76 Japanese DPB patients, 37% possessed HLA-B*5401 allele conserved predominantly in East Asians, as compared with 15% of 110 healthy volunteers (24). Based on the screening of HLA-A, -B, and -C antigens by the conventional typing method, a distinctive molecular structure of HLA-B alleles appears to contribute to genetic predisposition in DPB (25).

HLA-DRB1 class II gene does not demonstrate strong positive association with the disease (25). In a study of class I molecules that may cause a syndrome resembling DPB, TAP1, TAP2, and LMP2, that are located in the HLA region of the sixth chromosome were analyzed in 76 patients with DPB and 120 healthy subjects (26). The combination of Ala-665 and Gln-687 in exon 11 of the TAP2 gene was associated with the disease. This positive association might be independent of linkage disequilibrium with HLA-B*5401, as this TAP2 variation was associated with the disease even in the B*5401-negative subgroup. On the other hand, the His-60 substitution within the LMP2 gene exhibited a negative association with the disease due to a strong linkage disequilibrium with HLA-B44, which showed a negative association with the disease in the previous study. Thus, DPB may be influenced by genetic factors in the HLA region. Besides the class I gene, genes relevant to the class I antigen presenting system might also contribute to its genetic predisposition.

It was reported that an HLA-associated major susceptibility gene for DPB is probably located within the 200 kb in the class I region 300 kb telomeric of the HLA-B locus on the chromosome 6p (13,27,28).

A candidate gene for DPB from the gene localized in the HLA class I region was studied using refined microsatellite-based association mapping (29). The gene was C6orf37 (chromosome 6 open reading frame 37), sharing homology with the mucin-like domain of human zonadhesin. Unexpectedly, RT-PCR analysis detected transcripts from the antisense DNA strand of this C6orf37 locus. The gene designated as C6orf37OS (C6orf37 opposite strand) and represented by these antisense transcripts contained no open reading frame. The transcripts from C6orf37 and C6orf37OS were observed in numerous tissues, with most abundant expression in lung, kidney, and testis. These genes may be candidate genes for DPB28.

In a study of 82 Japanese patients with intractable chronic sinusitis, which is similar to DPB in terms of chronic mucous inflammatory process, B54 antigen was significantly increased when compared with 176 healthy subjects by conventional microcytotoxicity assays (30). For class II antigens, no antigens were significantly increased (30).

Genes other than those of the HLA system may also contribute to a genetic predisposition to DPB as there are some studies regarding genes different from HLA antigens. The association was investigated between genetic variation that codes for the 416th and 420th amino acid of Gc-globulin, reported to be associated with chemotaxis of neutrophils. The proportion of GC*1F homozygotes was significantly higher in the COPD patients than the control subjects. Though the GC*IF gene polymorphism of Gc-globulin may be one of the risk factors for COPD, no association was found between this polymorphism of Gc-globulin and susceptibility to diffuse panbronchiolitis (31).

In one study, specific allele at the IL-8 locus was associated with the DPB, although further studies are needed to examine whether neutrophil accumulation in the airways of patients with DPB is controlled by a possible genetic variation of IL-8 or other chemokine genes (32).

Presence of HTLV-I proviral DNA was examined using polymerase chain reaction (PCR) for the region of env or the two-step PCR for the pX region of this virus (28). The presence of the pX region was found in the lung tissue of DPB patients (27.3%). None of other subjects were positive for HTLV-I proviral DNA.

Genetic similarities or differences are warranted to investigate between cystic fibrosis and DPB, as both clinical features are similar except for difference in prevalence among ethnicity in the two diseases. There may be a possibility of a variant of cystic fibrosis, as some of the patients with DPB showed a gene expression of cystic fibrosis transmembrane conductance regulator gene (CFTR), though abnormalities of exocrine function and sweat eletrolytes were not shown (Yoshimura et al., personal communication).

V. Pathophysiology and Immunological Alterations

There is an interesting report of a case of DPB in an African-American patient who underwent bilateral sequential lung transplantation (33). Ten weeks after transplantation, DPB recurred in the lung allograft, with rapid and significant deterioration in graft function. Allograft function improved after beginning treatment with erythromycin.

In the patients with DPB, the chronic inflammatory process is usually complicated with infectious modification and increase in immunoglobulin level. A marked elevation of the serum secretary IgA level in DPB patients may be due to extensive, chronic infection of the airways of the lungs, especially the peripheral airways (34).

The titer of myeloperoxidase antineutrophil cytoplasmic antibodies (MPO-ANCA) was positive in serum samples from four of 30 patients with DPB and in none of 57 patients with other pulmonary diseases (35). It remains to be solved whether this autoantibody is associated with DPB or incidental phenomenon, as no positive features of vasculitis were found in DPB patients (5).

Immune alteration can be induced by enhancing the antigenic presentation capacity. Dendritic cells are found in both the bronchiolar epithelium and submucosal tissues of patients with DPB, compared with control subjects with normal lungs, using immunohistochemical methods (36). The most striking increase occurred in the dendritic cells in the submucosal tissues of patients with DPB. Furthermore, a pathogenesis of DPB was examined in the context with T-cell activation. The interaction between activated $CD8^+$ T cells and MIP-1alpha in BALF may contribute to the pathogenesis of DPB (37). In another study, soluble CD44 concentration in BALF was significantly lower and percentages of alveolar macrophages expressing low CD44 were higher in the patients with DPB compared with healthy volunteers (38). Furthermore, macrolide therapy normalized CD44 expression in BALF from DPB patients. Alveolar macrophage dysfunction could result from abnormalities of CD44 expression in patients with DPB and that these events could contribute to the pathogenesis of DPB (38).

Patients with DPB suffer from chronic airway infections resulting from mucociliary dysfunction. A high concentration of nasal nitric oxide (NO) has been documented in healthy subjects. Only two diseases are known to reduce nasal NO, primary ciliary dyskinesia syndrome and cystic fibrosis. Nasal NO was 88% lower in DPB patients than in the age-matched control subjects (39).

In one study, a link has been suggested between the macrolide transmembrane carrier system and the P-glycoprotein family, which comprises multiple drug resistance and CFTR (cystic fibrosis transmembrane conductance regulator), which are involved in the genesis of cystic fibrosis (40). This finding suggests one mechanism of effectiveness of macrolide in the patients with DPB.

VI. Biochemical and Laboratory Features Relevant to Disease Activity or Progression

Disease progression with diffuse bronchiectasis may relate to prominent neutrophils that are able to enhance lung injuries. Neurtophila was found in BAL fluid of patients with DPB, when compared with chronic bronchitis, and normal controls (41). Several cytokines such as IL8 may be involved in a prominent increase in neutrophils. The relative amounts of IL-1beta and IL-1Ra or IL-8 may contribute, at least in part, to the neutrophil-mediated chronic airway inflammation in the patients with chronic airway disease. Long-term erythromycin therapy may downregulate the vicious cycle between the cytokine network and neutrophil accumulation, with resultant reduction of neutrophil-mediated inflammatory response (42).

BALF from DPB patients contains a higher percentage of neutrophils than that from patients with bronchiectasis or healthy volunteers, whereas the percentage of lymphocytes is similar in the three groups (43).

In the serum and BALF of the patients with DPB, markedly high levels of the tumor-associated carbohydrate antigens sialyl SSEA-1 (SLX) and sialyl Lewis (a) (CA19-9) were demonstrated in the serum and BALF (44). An immunohistochemical study of open-lung biopsy specimens from patients with DPB indicated that these antigens were selectively expressed on the bronchiolar epithelial cells and mucinous exudates in airspaces (45).

There is extensive literature on the subject of macrolide-induced modulation of immune and inflammatory responses (46). Several inflammatory cytokines and oxidant production by phagocytes may be downregulated by macrolide, but as other possible targets, bacterial virulence factors, bronchial and epithelial cells may be included.

VII. Clinical Presentation

Patients with DPB have chronic cough, copious sputa, and exertional dyspnea and airflow limitation (Table 1). These symptoms are nonspecific. The most prominent clinical feature of DPB is copious sputum containing mostly neutrophils. Radiological features are typical (1,3,4,7). Changes in pathologic flora from *Hemophilus influenzae* to *Pseudomonas aeruginosa* is usually found during the clinical course of DPB. Chronic sinusitis is frequently present. There is no definite pattern of inheritance.

Regarding the radiological features of chest CT, centrilobularly distributed, small nodular opacities, branched linear opacities, contiguous with the small rounded areas, dilated airways with thick walls, and decreased lung attenuation in peripheral have been pointed out to be characteristic (47). Akira et al. classified CT findings of DPB into four types: (1) small nodules around the end of bronchovascular branching, (2) small nodules in the centrilobular area connected with small branching linear opacities, (3) nodules accompanied by dilated bronchovascular bundles, (4) large cystic opacities accompanied by dilated proximal bronchi (Fig. 2) (48). The classification of chest CT findings reflects the clinical stages and pathologic processes of DPB. The selective injury to the bronchioles in the peripheral parts can be demonstrated by using CT and positron emission tomography (PET) (49).

A. Case Presentation

A 47-year-old housewife, nonsmoker, presented with a 10-year history of productive cough and a 5-year history of exertional dyspnea. The patient was not exposed to any kind of industrial dust. The paranasal sinusitis was diagnosed and a right sinusotomy was performed. Elder brother of the patient also had sinusitis but no chest diseases. The patient began to cough up sputa at the age of 38, and felt exertional dyspnea at the age of 42. At the age of 44, a chest radiographic abnormality was found during a routine check up. Dyspnea and productive cough worsened gradually and the patient was admitted to our hospital. The patient expectorated sputa about 30 times a day. At admission the body temperature of the patient was 36.4°C, and the respiratory rate was 18/min. Auscultation

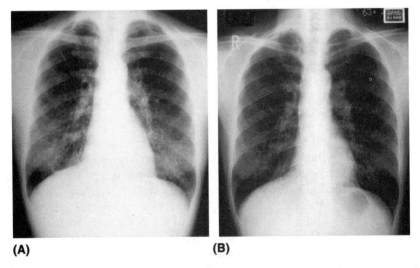

(A)   **(B)**

Figure 2 (A) Chest radiologic findings in a DPB case. Her chest radiograph showed small nodular shadows in bilateral lungs, predominantly in the lower lung fields. (B) Oral administration of low-dose erythromycin (600 mg/day) was initiated on hospital day 35 and continued for 2 years. Her chest radiograph after the initiation of the therapy showed marked improvement.

revealed bilateral inspiratory coarse crackles and inspiratory wheezes. The fingers were not clubbed.

Complete blood count and blood chemistry were normal. C-reactive protein was negative and erythrocyte sedimentation rate was 22 mm/hr. Cold hemagglutination test titer was elevated, at 256-fold, while antibody to *Mycoplasma pneumoniae* was within normal limits. Serum IgG was slightly elevated to 2131 mg/dL. Sputum culture yielded *P. aeruginosa*, repeatedly. Cytology of sputa showed no malignant cells, and the sputa contained abundant neutrophils. Arterial blood gas analysis revealed PaO_2 62 mmHg and $PaCO_2$ 40 mmHg. In the pulmonary function test, VC was 2.25 L (88%), FEV1 1.25 L (57% of the predicted value). FEV1/FVC and DLCO were 65% and 74% of the predicted values, respectively. The chest radiograph of the patient showed small nodular shadows in bilateral lungs, predominantly in the lower lung fields (Fig. 2A). Chest HRCT scan showed multiple centrilobular shadows smaller than 5 mm in diameter in all lung lobes with small branching structures (Fig. 3). To obtain the diagnosis, open lung biopsy was performed. Bacteriological examinations revealed *P. aeruginosa* cultured from the fresh biopsy samples. The lesions were located in centrilobular regions and 2–3 mm apart from the pleura. PB-unit lesions and a dilatation of membranous bronchiole were seen in the specimens. According to the diagnostic criteria, the patient was diagnosed not

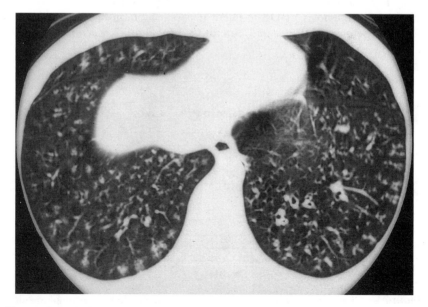

Figure 3 Findings on chest HRCT scan. Chest HRCT scan showed multiple centrilobular shadows smaller than 5 mm in diameter in all lung lobes with small branching structures.

having DPB. Oral administration of low-dose erythromycin (600 mg/day) was initiated on hospital day 35 and continued for 2 years. The chest radiograph of the patient and CT after the initiation of the therapy showed marked improvement (Fig. 2B). A pulmonary function test 30 months after the initiation of the therapy also showed an improvement, as shown in Figure 4. The patient remained in good health at the 12 years after the diagnosis and therapy.

B. Differential Diagnosis

Clinicoradiological features of DPB should be differentiated from other lung diseases. Major differential diagnoses are discussed below.

Pulmonary disease in adult T-cell leukemia (ATL) and chronic HTLV-I infection is one of the major differential diagnoses. In one study, among 43 cases with ATL, three patients were found to be complicated with DPB. It remains to be solved whether DPB-like lesion is due to a pathophysiologic process of ATL (50). In another report, a 45-year-old male was found to have a DPB-like lesion in association with an increase in lymphocytes and neutrophils in BAL fluid. The DPB-like lesion in the biopsied lung was associated with a positive human T-cell lymphotropic virus type I (HTLV-I) antibody in the serum, and a past history of uveitis and ulcerative colitis (51).

Lung disease associated with rheumatoid arthritis is another major differential diagnosis of DPB. There is a considerable overlap in clinical features between DPB and obliterative bronchiolitis secondary to the

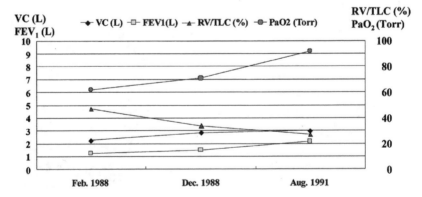

Figure 4 Effectiveness of low-dose erythromycin. Oral administration of low-dose erythromycin (600 mg/day) was initiated on hospital day 35 and continued for 2 years. A pulmonary function test 30 months after the initiation of the therapy also showed an improvement.

rheumatoid process (52). The differentiation between these two diseases is important in making therapeutic decisions. Sugiyama et al. (53) analyzed the HLA antigens in two patients with rheumatoid arthritis accompanied by DPB and found the presence of B54 and DR4 alleles.

Not only rheumatoid arthritis but also other diseases such as ulcerative colitis tend to be associated with DPB (54). In one report, DPB preceded several years prior to bowel manifestation and partial resolved following colectomy (54).

Other diffuse bronchiolar diseases, sinobronchial syndromes, and diffuse bronchiectasis are also included in the differential diagnosis of DPB. Aspiration pneumonia, hypersensitivity pneumonitis, Wegener's granulomatosis, bronchocentric granulomatosis, malignant lymphoma, lymphoproliferative diseases, immotile cilia syndrome, cystic fibrosis, and immunodeficiency syndrome should also be included (5).

The presence of chronic sinusitis, age of onset, amount of sputum, and HRCT findings, and some genetic investigations are useful for evaluating DPB patients.

VIII. Treatment and Clinical Course

A copious sputum production and recurrent infections of lower respiratory tract are two critical problems that demand therapeutic intervention. A therapeutic clue emerged when a Japanese physician treated DPB patients with erythromycin by chance in Japan. Kudoh et al. (55) evaluated the effects of treatment with erythromycin on the survival rate of 498 patients with DPB, after dividing them into three groups according to the date of their first medical examination (Group A: 1970–1979, Group B: 1980–1984, Group C: 1985–1990) in Japan (55). The survival rate of Group C was significantly higher than that of Groups A and B. In Group C, eight of 87 patients died; five died from 24 patients not treated with erythromycin (EM), and three died from 63 EM-treated patients. Thus, low-dose treatment with EM was associated with a significant improvement in the rate of survival of patients with DPB (55).

The long-term effect of erythromycin was examined retrospectively in a group of patients with DPB, with and without *P. aeruginosa* infection. The drug-induced bacterial clearance and clinical improvement may be due to anti-inflammatory effect, independent of *P. aeruginosa* infection or bacterial clearance (56).

The long-term effect of low-dose administration of macrolide antibiotics has been examined for sinusitis, DPB, asthma, bronchiectasis, and cystic fibrosis. It is associated with downregulation of nonspecific host inflammatory response to injury and promotion of tissue repair. So far, the prolonged use of these drugs has not been associated with emergence of clinically significant bacterial resistance or immunosuppression. Long-term, low-dose administration of 14- and 15-membered ring macrolide anti-biotics may represent an important adjunct in the treatment of chronic inflammatory sinopulmonary diseases in humans (57).

Effects of erythromycin on the DPB patients have been examined not only in survival rates but also other indexes such as radiology and pulmon-ary function tests. In one study, after initial CT examination, 12 patients were randomly assigned to receive long-term low-dose erythromycin ther-apy and seven patients received no treatment (58). Follow-up CT scans revealed that centrilobular areas of high attenuation observed initially had progressed to dilatation of the proximal airway in some patients in the untreated group. In the treated group, the centrilobular and branched linear areas of high attenuation were decreased in number and size, although the airway dilatation and decreased lung attenuation in the peripheral areas remained unchanged or were slightly increased. Based on these results, CT examination seems to be valuable for evaluating the disease process and the response to therapy in DPB (58). Another study demonstrated the positive correlation of improved scores of centrilobular nodules on CT scan with improvement of %VC and RV/TLC%. A decreased air trap-ping in DPB patients correlated with an improvement of centrilobular nodules during therapy (58).

The methacholine challenge studies, carried out in the patients with COPD and DPB, showed fixed airflow limitation as a result of structural bronchiolar lesions in the DPB patients (59). The 14-member macrolides has inhibitory effect on IL-8 expression in human bronchial epithelial cells. This may be another mode of action of the drug and may have some rele-vance to their clinical effectiveness in airway disease (60).

Erythromycin therapy significantly reduced the accumulation of neutrophils in BAL fluid, in parallel with an improvement in clinical symptoms (61).

In addition to erythromycin, therapeutic effectiveness of other macro-lides such as clarithromycin and azithromycin has been investigated recently. In one prospective open trial of long-term (4 years) treatment with clarithromycin (200 mg once a day), pulmonary function improved in most of the patients within 6 months and maintained a stable condition with con-tinued therapy. No side effects of clarithromycin were observed during the study (62).

In another 3-month prospective randomized double-blind, placebo-controlled study in adults, 60 of patients with cystic fibrosis, FEV1%, and forced vital capacity (FVC)% predicted were maintained in the azithromi-cin (250 mg/day) group, while in the placebo group there was a decline of both tests (63). The long-term azythromycin may have a significant impact on morbidity and mortality in patients with cystic fibrosis. Similar results may be expected in patients with DPB.

A. The Future

The recognition of the differences amongst the bronchiolar airflow disorders is essential to further understanding the pathogenesis and developing new therapeutic agents (64). DPB has emerged from Japan as a unique disease that has been identified in other parts of Asia, America, and Europe. Genetic studies suggest a presence of a disease susceptibility of DPB in Asian (mainly Japanese) population. Further comparative studies between cystic fibrosis, other inflammatory bronchiolar lesions, and DPB, because of their clinical similarities, are needed. These studies should focus on detecting similarities, which connect these common destructive bronchiolar diseases.

Acknowledgment

The authors thank Professor Om P. Sharma for reviewing our manuscript, and Dr. Koichi Nishimura, who managed the patients, and Dr. Isao Ito, who kindly introduces the case of DPB.

References

1. Izumi T. Diffuse panbronchiolitis. Chest 1991; 100:596–597.
2. Maeda M, Saiki S, Yamanaka A. Serial section analysis of the lesions in diffuse panbronchiolitis. Acta Pathol Jpn 1987; 37:693–704.
3. Homma H, Yamanaka A, Tanimoto S, Tamura M, Chijimatsu Y, Kira S, Izumi T. Diffuse panbronchiolitis. A disease of the transitional zone of the lung. Chest 1983; 83:63–69.
4. Izumi T. A nation-wide survey of diffuse panbronchiolitis and the high incidence of diffuse panbronchiolitis seen in Japanese respiratory clinics. In: Grassi C, Rizzato G, Pozzi E, eds. Sarcoidosis and Other Granulomatous Disorders. New York: Elsevier Science Publishers, 1988:853.
5. Kitaichi M, Nishimura K, Izumi T. Diffuse panbronchiolitis. In: Sharma OP, ed. Lung Disease in the Tropics. Lung Biology in Health and Disease 51. New York: Marcel Dekker, 1991:479–509.
6. Iwata M, Colby TV, Kitaichi M. Diffuse panbronchiolitis: diagnosis and distinction from various pulmonary diseases with centrilobular interstitial foam cell accumulations. Hum Pathol 1994; 25(4):357–363.
7. Kim YW, Han SK, Shim YS, Kim KY, Han YC, Seo JW, Im JG. The first report of diffuse panbronchiolitis in Korea: five case reports. Intern Med 1992; 31:695–701.
8. Chantarotorn S, Palwatwichai A, Vattanathum A, Tantamacharik D. Diffuse panbronchiolitis, the first case reports in Thailand. J Med Assoc Thai 1999; 82(8):833–838.

9. Gulhan M, Erturk A, Kurt B, Gulhan E, Ergul G, Unal P, Capan N. Diffuse panbronchiolitis observed in a white man in Turkey. Sarcoidosis Vasc Diffuse Lung Dis 2000; 17(3):292–296.

10. Souza R, Kairalla RA, Santos Ud Ude P, Takagaki TY, Capelozzi VL, Carvalho CR. Diffuse panbronchiolitis: an underdiagnosed disease? Study of 4 cases in Brazil. Rev Hosp Clin Fac Med Sao Paulo 2002; 57(4):167–174.

11. Martinez JA, Guimaraes SM, Ferreira RG, Pereira CA. Diffuse panbronchiolitis in Latin America. Am J Med Sci 2000; 319(3):183–185.

12. Fitzgerald JE, King TE Jr, Lynch DA, Tuder RM, Schwarz MI. Diffuse panbronchiolitis in the United States. Am J Respir Crit Care Med 1996; 154(2 Pt 1):497–503.

13. Homer RJ, Khoo L, Smith GJ. Diffuse panbronchiolitis in a Hispanic man with travel history to Japan. Chest 1995; 107(4):1176–1178.

14. Zainudin BM, Roslina AM, Fadilah SA, Samad SA, Sufarlan AW, Isa MR. A report of the first three cases of diffuse panbronchiolitis in Malaysia. Med J Malaysia 1996; 51(1):136–140.

15. Tsang KW, Ooi CG, Ip MS, Lam WK, Ngan H, Chan EY, Hawkins B, Ho CS, Amitani R, Tanaka E, Itoh H. Clinical profiles of Chinese patients with diffuse panbronchiolitis. Thorax 1998; 53:274–280.

16. Wang H, Sun T, Miao J, Li Y. A definite case of diffuse panbronchiolitis diagnosed by open lung biopsy. Chin Med J (Engl) 1998; 111(9):864.

17. Chu YC, Yeh SZ, Chen CL, Chen CY, Chang CY, Chiang CD. Diffuse panbronchiolitis: report of a case. J Formos Med Assoc 1992; 91(9):912–915.

18. Brugiere O, Milleron B, Antoine M, Carette MF, Philippe C, Mayaud C. Diffuse panbronchiolitis in an Asian immigrant. Thorax 1996; 51(10): 1065–1067.

19. Krishnan P, Thachil R, Gillego V. Diffuse panbronchitis. A treatable sinobronchial disease in need of recognition in the United States. Chest 2002; 121: 659–661.

20. Poletti V, Chilosi M, Trisolini R, Cancellieri A, Zompatori M, Agli LL, Boaron M, Schulte W, Theegarten D, Guzman J, Costabel U. Idiopathic bronchiolitis mimicking diffuse panbronchiolitis. Sarcoidosis Vasc Diffuse Lung Dis 2003; 20(1):62–68.

21. Randhawa P, Hoagland MH, Yousem SA. Diffuse panbronchiolitis in North America. Report of three cases and review of the literature. Am J Surg Pathol 1991; 15:43–47.

22. Sugiyama Y, Kudoh S, Maeda H, Suzaki H, Takaku F. Analysis of HLA antigens in patients with diffuse panbronchiolitis. Am Rev Respir Dis 1990; 141:1459–1462.

23. Tomita Y, Hashimoto S, Shimizu T, Son K, Azuma A, Kudoh S, Horie T. Restriction fragment length polymorphism analysis in the HLA class III genes of patients with diffuse panbronchiolitis. Intern Med 1996; 35(9):693–697.

24. Keicho N, Tokunaga K, Nakata K, Taguchi Y, Azuma A, Bannai M, Emi M, Ohishi N, Yazaki Y, Kudoh S. Contribution of HLA genes to genetic predisposition in diffuse panbronchiolitis. Am J Respir Crit Care Med 1998; 158(3):846–850.

25. Park MH, Kim YW, Yoon HI, Yoo CG, Han SK, Shim YS, Kim WD. Association of HLA class I antigens with diffuse panbronchiolitis in Korean patients. Am J Respir Crit Care Med 1999; 159(2):526–529.
26. Keicho N, Tokunaga K, Nakata K, Taguchi Y, Azuma A, Tanabe K, Matsushita M, Emi M, Ohishi N, Kudoh S. Contribution of TAP genes to genetic predisposition for diffuse panbronchiolitis. Tissue Antigens 1999; 53(4 Pt 1):366–373.
27. Keicho N, Ohashi J, Tamiya G, Nakata K, Taguchi Y, Azuma A, Ohishi N, Emi M, Park MH, Inoko H, Tokunaga K, Kudoh S. Fine localization of a major disease-susceptibility locus for diffuse panbronchiolitis. Am J Hum Genet 2000; 66(2):501–507.
28. Matsuse T, Fukuchi Y, Hsu CY, Nagase T, Higashimoto N, Teramoto S, Matsui H, Sudo E, Kida K, Morinari H, Fukayama M, Ouchi Y, Orimo H. Detection of human T lymphotropic virus type I proviral DNA in patients with diffuse panbronchiolitis. Respirology 1996; 1(2):139–144.
29. Matsuzaka Y, Tounai K, Denda A, Tomizawa M, Makino S, Okamoto K, Keicho N, Oka A, Kulski JK, Tamiya G, Inoko H. Identification of novel candidate genes in the diffuse panbronchiolitis critical region of the class I human MHC. Immunogenetics 2002; 54(5):301–309.
30. Takeuchi K, Majima Y, Shimizu T, Ukai K, Sakakura Y. Analysis of HLA antigens in Japanese patients with chronic sinusitis. Laryngoscope 1999; 109(2 Pt 1):275–278.
31. Ishii T, Keicho N, Teramoto S, Azuma A, Kudoh S, Fukuchi Y, Ouchi Y, Matsuse T. Association of Gc-globulin variation with susceptibility to COPD and diffuse panbronchiolitis. Eur Respir J 2001; 18(5):753–757.
32. Emi M, Keicho N, Tokunaga K, Katsumata H, Souma S, Nakata K, Taguchi Y, Ohishi N, Azuma A, Kudoh S. Association of diffuse panbronchiolitis with microsatellite polymorphism of the human interleukin-8 (IL-8) gene. J Hum Genet 1999; 44(3):169–172.
33. Baz MA, Kussin PS, Van Trigt P, Davis RD, Roggli VL, Tapson VF. Recurrence of diffuse panbronchiolitis after lung transplantation. Am J Respir Crit Care Med 1995; 151(3 Pt 1):895–898.
34. Noda Y, Yasuoka S, Tani K, Ogura T, Ogawara M, Kitatani F. Secretary IgA levels in sera from patients with diffuse panbronchiolitis. Jpn J Med 1989; 28:189–195.
35. Sugiyama Y, Kitamura S. Antineutrophil cytoplasmic antibodies in diffuse panbronchiolitis. Respiration 1999; 66(3):233–235.
36. Todate A, Chida K, Suda T, Imokawa S, Sato J, Ide K, Tsuchiya T, Inui N, Nakamura Y, Asada K, Hayakawa H, Nakamura H. Increased numbers of dendritic cells in the bronchiolar tissues of diffuse panbronchiolitis. Am J Respir Crit Care Med 2000; 162(1):148–153.
37. Kadota J, Mukae H, Tomono K, Kohno S. High concentrations of beta-chemokines in BAL fluid of patients with diffuse panbronchiolitis. Chest 2001; 120(2):602–607.
38. Katoh S, Matsubara Y, Taniguchi H, Fukushima K, Mukae H, Kadota J, Matsukura S, Kohno S. Characterization of CD44 expressed on alveolar

macrophages in patients with diffuse panbronchiolitis. Clin Exp Immunol 2001; 126(3):545–550.

39. Nakano H, Ide H, Imada M, Osanai S, Takahashi T, Kikuchi K, Iwamoto. Reduced nasal nitric oxide in diffuse panbronchiolitis. Am J Respir Crit Care Med 2000; 162(6):2218–2220.

40. Kadota J, Sakito O, Kohno S, Sawa H, Mukae H, Oda H, Kawakami K, Fukushima K, Hiratani K, Hara K. A mechanism of erythromycin treatment in patients with diffuse panbronchiolitis. Am Rev Respir Dis 1993; 147(1): 153–159.

41. Ichikawa Y, Koga H, Tanaka M, Nakamura M, Tokunaga N, Kaji M. Neurtophila in bronchoalveolar lavage fluid of diffuse panbronchilitis. Chest 1990; 98:917–923.

42. Kadota J, Matsubara Y, Ishimatsu Y, Ashida M, Abe K, Shirai R, Iida K, Kawakami K, Taniguchi H, Fujii T, Kaseda M, Kawamoto S, Kohno S. Significance of IL-1beta and IL-1 receptor antagonist (IL-1Ra) in bronchoalveolar lavage fluid (BALF) in patients with diffuse panbronchiolitis (DPB). Clin Exp Immunol 1996; 103(3):461–466.

43. Mukae H, Kadota J, Kohno S, Kusano S, Morikawa T, Matsukura S, Hara K. Increase in activated CD8+ cells in bronchoalveolar lavage fluid in patients with diffuse panbronchiolitis. Am J Respir Crit Care Med 1995; 152(2): 613–618.

44. Mukae H, Hirota M, Kohno S, Komori K, Fukushima K, Hiratani K, Kadota J, Hara K. Elevation of tumor-associated carbohydrate antigens in patients with diffuse panbronchiolitis. Am Rev Respir Dis 1993; 148(3):744–751.

45. Nakamura H, Abe S, Shibata Y, Yuki H, Suzuki H, Saito H, Sata M, Kato S, Tomoike H. Elevated levels of cytokeratin 19 in the bronchoalveolar lavage fluid of patients with chronic airway inflammatory diseases—a specific marker for bronchial epithelial injury. Am J Respir Crit Care Med 1997; 155(4): 1217–1221.

46. Labro MT, Abdelghaffar H. Immunomodulation by macrolide antibiotics. J Chemother 2001; 13(1):3–8.

47. Nishimura K, Kitaichi M, Izumi T, Itoh H. Diffuse panbronchiolitis: correlation of high-resolution CT and pathologic findings. Radiology 1992; 184(3): 779–785.

48. Akira M, Kitatani F, Lee YS, Kita N, Yamamoto S, Higashihara T, Morimoto S, Ikezoe J, Kozuka T. Diffuse panbronchilotis: evaluation with high resolution CT. Radiology 1988; 168:433–438.

49. Murata K, Itoh H, Senda M, Yonekura Y, Nishimura K, Izumi T, Oshima S, Torizuka K. Stratified impairment of pulmonary ventilation in "diffuse panbronchiolitis": PET and CT studies. J Comput Assist Tomogr 1989; 13:48–53.

50. Ono K, Shimamoto Y, Matsuzaki M, Sano M, Yamaguchi T, Kato O, Yamada H, Yamaguchi M. Diffuse panbronchilotis as a pulmonary complication in patients with adult T cell leukemia. Am J Hematol 1989; 30:86–90.

51. Kikuchi T, Saijo Y, Sakai T, Abe T, Ohnuma K, Tezuka F, Terunuma H, Ogata K, Nukiwa T. Human T-cell lymphotropic virus type I (HTLV-I) carrier with clinical manifestations characteristic of diffuse panbronchiolitis. Intern Med 1996; 35(4):305–309.

52. Homma S, Kawabata M, Kishi K, Tsuboi E, Narui K, Nakatani T, Uekusa T, Saiki S, Nakata K. Diffuse panbronchiolitis in rheumatoid arthritis. Eur Respir J 1998; 12(2):444–452.

53. Sugiyama Y, Ohno S, Kano S, Maeda H, Kitamura S. Diffuse panbronchiolitis and rheumatoid arthritis: a possible correlation with HLA-B54. Intern Med 1994; 33(10):612–614.

54. Desai SJ, Gephardt GN, Stoller JK. Diffuse panbronchiolitis and ulcerative collitis. Chest 1989; 95:1342–1344.

55. Kudoh S, Azuma A, Yamamoto M, Izumi T, Ando M. Improvement of survival in patients with diffuse panbronchiolitis treated with low-dose erythromycin. Am J Respir Crit Care Med 1998; 157(6 Pt 1):1829–1832.

56. Fujii T, Kadota J, Kawakami K, Iida K, Shirai R, Kaseda M, Kawamoto S, Kohno S. Long term effect of erythromycin therapy in patients with chronic *Pseudomonas aeruginosa* infection. Thorax 1995; 50(12):1246–1252.

57. Garey KW, Alwani A, Danziger LH, Rubinstein I. Tissue reparative effects of macrolide antibiotics in chronic inflammatory sinopulmonary diseases. Chest 2003; 123(1):261–265.

58. Akira M, Higashihara T, Sakatani M, Hara H. Diffuse panbronchiolitis: follow-up CT examination. Radiology 1993; 189(2):559–562.

59. Koyama H, Nishimura K, Mio T, Ikeda A, Sugiura N, Izumi T. Bronchial responsiveness and acute bronchodilator-response in chronic obstructive pulmonary disease and diffuse panbronchiolitis. Thorax 1994; 49(6):540–544.

60. Takizawa H, Desaki M, Ohtoshi T, Kawasaki S, Kohyama T, Sato M, Tanaka M, Kasama T, Kobayashi K, Nakajima J, Ito K. Erythromycin modulates IL-8 expression in normal and inflamed human bronchial epithelial cells. Am J Respir Crit Care Med 1997; 156(1):266–271.

61. Oda H, Kadota J, Kohno S, Hara K. Erythromycin inhibits neutrophil chemotaxis in bronchoalveoli of diffuse panbronchiolitis. Chest 1994; 106(4):1116–1123.

62. Kadota J, Mukae H, Ishii H, Nagata T, Kaida H, Tomono K, Kohno S. Long-term efficacy and safety of clarithromycin treatment in patients with diffuse panbronchiolitis. Respir Med 2003; 97(7):844–850.

63. Wolter J, Seeney S, Bell S, Bowler S, Masel P, McCormack J. Effect of long term treatment with azithromycin on disease parameters in cystic fibrosis: a randomised trial. Thorax 2002; 57(3):212–216.

64. Epler GR. Bronchiolar disorders with airflow obstruction. Curr Opin Pulm Med 1996; 2(2):134–140.

21

Pulmonary Complications of Sickle Cell Diseases: The Acute Chest Syndrome

CAGE S. JOHNSON

Comprehensive Sickle Cell Center, Keck School of Medicine,
University of Southern California,
Los Angeles, California, U.S.A.

I. Introduction

Sickle cell anemia and its variants are inherited disorders of hemoglobin (Hb) structure due to the substitution of valine for glutamic acid at position 6 of the beta globin chain. Upon deoxygenation of the erythrocyte, Hb S undergoes intracellular polymerization with morphologic transformation to the sickled shape. Repetitive sickling cycles induce a complex series of abnormalities in the erythrocyte, including cytoplasmic and membrane rigidity, dehydration, and an increase in intracellular Hb concentration. The circulating erythrocyte population is thus comprised of a heterogeneous population of cells including low-density reticulocytes, very dense discocytes, and irreversibly sickled cells. These dense, poorly deformable cells are ultimately responsible for the elevated whole blood viscosity and microvascular occlusion in this disease (1,2). The clinical features of the disease are the direct result of the beta 6 substitution and consist of chronic hemolytic anemia, frequent infections, and microvascular obstruction producing acute and chronic ischemia and ultimately resulting in organ damage from infarction and fibrosis (3).

Sickle cell anemia is the term applied to the homozygous form of the disease (Hb SS); it is the most common variant and generally has the most severe clinical manifestations. Other variants are due to the simultaneous inheritance of compound heterozygous states for Hb S and another hemoglobin that interacts with Hb S and participates in polymer formation causing disease. Heterozygosity for both Hb S and Hb C results in sickle-C disease, while combinations of Hb S with beta^0 or beta$^+$ thalassemia are known as sickle-thalassemia. Fractionation and quantification of hemoglobin using electrophoresis, isoelectric focusing, or liquid chromatography, and correlation with the CBC and blood smear (Table 1) will establish the specific diagnosis. Combinations of Hb S with other variants (such as D, E, O-Arab, etc.) are relatively rare. The variable clinical severity seen in the variant syndromes is partially explained by differences in polymer formation as the result of differences in amino acid composition of the second hemoglobin at the critical residues responsible for molecular aggregation, which promote or retard the ability of the second hemoglobin to participate in polymer formation.

Acute pulmonary disease is a common complication of the sickling disorders, with a frequency estimated at several hundred times that of the general population (4). Second only to pain as a cause of hospital admission, acute febrile illnesses associated with a pulmonary infiltrate cause considerable morbidity and mortality in the sickling diseases (5). Half of all patients will have at least one episode, and a subset will have multiple events. The term "acute chest syndrome" was introduced by Charache and colleagues (6), reflecting the difficulty in establishing a definitive etiology for these acute pulmonary episodes particularly in distinguishing infection from pulmonary infarction by microvascular occlusion. The terminology is potentially misleading since it includes those with a relatively benign course, as well as those cases that develop progressive disease with florid pulmonary infiltrates and an ARDS-like picture.

The acute chest syndrome (ACS) in sickle cell disease (SCD) is currently defined as a new infiltrate on chest X-ray associated with one or more symptoms, such as fever, cough, sputum production, tachypnea, dyspnea, or new onset hypoxia (7). The illness clinically and radiographically resembles bacterial pneumonia with fever, leucocytosis, pleuritic chest pain, pleural effusion, and cough with purulent sputum. However, the clinical course in SCD is considerably different from that in hematologically normal individuals. Multiple lobe involvement and recurrent infiltrates are more common in SCD. The duration of clinical illness and of radiological clearing of infiltrates is prolonged to 10 to 12 days (5,7–9).

Table 1 Examples of Typical Hemoglobin Analysis and Blood Counts in Various Conditions

Condition	Hb A (%)	Hb A$_2$ (%)	Hb F (%)	Hb S (%)	Hb C (%)	Hgb (g/dL)	MCV (fL)	Reticulocytes (%)
Normal adult	96	3	<2	0	0	13–15	90 ± 9	1.0
Sickle cell trait (Hb AS)	58	3	<2	38	0	13–15	90 ± 9	1.0
Sickle cell anemia (Hb SS)	0	3	2–15	80–95	0	7–9	89 ± 9	6–12
Sickle-C disease (Hb SC)	0	3	3	47	47	11–14	82 ± 9	2–4
Sickle β^0 thalassemia	0	5	5–20	70–85	0	8–10	68 ± 9	5–8
Sickle β$^+$ thalassemia	10–30	5	5–20	50–70	0	9–12	72 ± 9	3–6

II. Epidemiology

In the seminal reports by Barrett-Connor (4,10), 84 of 169 episodes of ACS had evidence of bacterial infection on culture of blood or sputum. As there was no difference in the clinical course between culture-positive and culture-negative cases, the author concluded that all cases were likely due to infection, most commonly *S. pneumoniae*. The author's conclusion was supported by the known propensity for bacterial infection in SCD and was widely accepted. However, numerous epidemiological studies in those with normal hemoglobin type indicate a changing epidemiology for pneumonia in recent years. For example, studies (11) in armed forces personnel indicate that the attack rate of pneumonia in the 1990s (77.6/100,000/year) is one-fourth that of the 1970s (307.6/100,000/year). Furthermore, the frequency of *S. pneumoniae* has declined substantially, while that of *Mycoplasma pneumoniae* has increased so that the two are nearly equal in frequency. Moreover, a definite etiology is not established by culture in 65–75% of cases. Thus, the epidemiology of pneumonia in the general population has undergone secular changes, and the spectrum of pulmonary microbial infection is likely to undergo further changes with time in both these populations.

Subsequent studies in SCD showed similar findings. Poncz et al. (12) studied 102 episodes of ACS in 70 patients with careful culture techniques and found that they could document bacterial infection in only 12 episodes; the single most common cause found was mycoplasma (16%), and viral disease at 8% was almost as frequent as the common bacterial agents. In 66% of the episodes, no etiology was established. Nearly identical findings were seen by Sprinkle et al. (13) in their study of 100 episodes of the ACS in 57 patients. On the other hand, in Curacao (14), 43% of sputum cultures were positive in 81 episodes seen in 53 patients. The most common bacterium was *H. influenza*. Both *S. Aureus* and *Klebsiella* were more common than *S. pneumoniae*. Other reports have stressed the evolving importance of *Chlamydiae pneumoniae* and *legionella*. Viral agents causing ACS include influenza, respiratory syncytial virus, CMV, parvovirus, adenovirus, and para influenza virus.

The Cooperative Study of Sickle Cell Disease (CSSCD) reported on patients with a new infiltrate on chest X-ray; data from this study indicate that this complication occurs with an overall incidence of 10.5 per 100 patient-years (5,9). ACS occurs most often as a single episode, but certain patients have multiple episodes. A past history of an ACS is associated with early mortality compared to those who have never had an episode. The disorder is most common in the 2- to 4-year age group with a peak incidence of 25.3 per 100 patient-years and gradually declines in incidence with age to 8.8 per 100 patient-years in those over 20 years of age. It is believed that the slower decline of Hb F concentration than normal exerts a protective effect on those patients less than 2 years of age. The decline in the incidence of ACS observed in older age groups is believed to be related to at least two other factors: (a) excess mortality in the group, which had an ACS and (b) fewer viral episodes in adults due to acquired immunity. The incidence of ACS is related to genotype, where the frequency in Hb SS is slightly greater than that in Hb S beta^0 thalassemia but is much less frequent in Hb SC and Hb S beta$^+$ thalassemia. Additional data showed that a lower hematocrit or a higher Hb F was associated with a reduced incidence of the ACS, whereas a high WBC was associated with a higher incidence.

The National Acute Chest Syndrome Study Group (NACSSG) employed a more stringent definition of the ACS; its inclusion criteria were a new infiltrate plus one or more pulmonary signs or symptoms, such as fever, cough, sputum production, tachypnea, dyspnea, or new onset hypoxia (7). Viral culture techniques and acute and convalescent serologies were employed, as well as careful examination of deep sputum cytology for fat-laden macrophages indicative of fat embolism. In this study, there were 671 episodes of ACS in 538 patients. In 48% of the episodes, ACS developed during hospitalization for acute pain or other cause. A definitive etiology was established in 256 (38%) of these episodes but incomplete data precluded full assessment in 306 episodes (46%). Of the 27 pathogens identified, the most common infectious agents were chlamydia (7.2%), mycoplasma (6.6%), and viruses (6.4%), particularly respiratory syncytial virus. Pulmonary infarction was diagnosed by exclusion and found in 16.1% of episodes, while fat embolism was found in 8.8%. *S. pneumoniae* was recovered in only 11 episodes. A variety of bacterial and viral agents were identified in the remainder of cases. Mechanical ventilation was required in 13% of patients and was associated with extensive lobar involvement, a platelet count less than 200,000/μL or a preceding history of cardiac disease. There were 18 deaths (2.7%) primarily as the consequence of pulmonary embolism with bone marrow, fat, or thrombi.

III. Clinical Presentation

The clinical characteristics of ACS in both children and adults have been more clearly defined by these large clinical studies in recent years. The CSSCD reported on 1732 episodes of ACS in 939 subjects (9), and the NACSSG study (7) described the findings in 671 cases of ACS in 537 subjects (Table 2). Fever >38.5° and cough were the most common presenting symptoms and were significantly more common in children. Tachypnea and bronchospasm, particularly in children, were the common physical findings; however, a normal physical examination was found in 35% of the cases, and additional data support the unreliability of the physical examination in the detection of the ACS (15). Chest, rib, and extremity pain were more

Table 2 Age-Related Clinical Features at Presentation of the Acute Chest Syndrome in the CSSCD and NACSSG Studies

	Age < 10 years		Age > 10 years	
	CSSCD $n = 483$	NACSSG $n = 264$	CSSCD $n = 454$	NACSSG $n = 273$
Fever	90	86	70	74
Cough	81	69	66	56
Chest Pain	26	27	81	61
Rib Pain	na	14	na	27
Extremity pain	na	22	na	51
Dyspnea	17	31	38	50
Temperature >39°C	44	86	12	74
Respiratory rate >40/min	28	na	7	na
Pulse >140/min	27	na	7	na
Reactive airway disease	na	17	na	9

The differences between young children and adolescents/adults were significantly different at $p \leq 0.006$.
Abbreviation: na, not available.
Source: Adapted from Refs. 7, 9, with permission.

common in adults. Isolated upper and middle lobe involvement were more common in children, with isolated lower lobe disease more common in adults. Pleural effusions were more common in adults. Bacteremia was more common in children aged 2 to 4 years; *S. pneumoniae* was detected in 78% of those children but found in only 25% of adults with bacteremia. Moreover, in nearly half the cases, the ACS developed several days after hospitalization for another reason. In both series, the hospital stay was longer for adults than for children. Adolescents behaved more like adults. The longer duration of hospital stay for the NACSSG study reflects the enrollment of a more acutely ill population because of more stringent inclusion criteria comprising a new pulmonary infiltrate involving at least one complete lung segment, excluding atelectasis, and with at least one of the following: chest pain, fever >38.50, tachypnea, wheezing, or cough. Additional data supporting the greater severity of the clinical illness in the NACSSG study were the more frequent use of transfusions and the higher mortality. Mortality in both studies was four- to nine-fold greater in adults than in children and was due to respiratory failure, cor pulmonale, hypovolemic shock, or sepsis.

These features of the ACS indicate that infection is most often the cause of ACS in young children. In adults, the strong association with bone pain and less frequent identification of microbial infection suggest that vascular occlusion is the etiology of ACS in most cases.

IV. Pathophysiology

The pathophysiology of acute lung injury in the sickling disorders is complex. The pulmonary microcirculation with its low oxygen tension, low pressure and slow flow is ideally suited to promote the polymerization of Hb S. In addition to the erythrocyte rheologic abnormalities induced by Hb S polymerization and the resulting increased blood viscosity, there are perturbations of erythrocyte membrane proteins and of endothelial cell biology that play a prominent role in the resulting microvascular obstruction. Polymerization of Hb S within the erythrocyte is caused by oxygen desaturation, which is modulated by pH balance, temperature, and intracellular dehydration and their effects upon oxygen affinity (16,17). Following deoxygenation, there is a variable delay of milliseconds to seconds that precedes the appearance of polymer; this delay time is inversely dependent upon the intracellular hemoglobin concentration by a factor of 30–50-fold (18). Once a critical mass has formed, polymer rapidly forms and eventually deforms the cell into the classic sickled shape. Sickling induces a host of erythrocyte abnormalities, including progressive erythrocyte dehydration via loss of K^+ and H_2O, increased membrane rigidity via oxidation of lipids and proteins, phospholipid asymmetry with exposure of phosphatidyl serine on the exterior, and coclustering of hemichromes with the erythrocyte membrane protein, band 3, with its resultant generation of reactive oxygen species (19,20).

Interaction with microvascular endothelium and/or endothelial matrix occurs through a variety of adhesive proteins expressed on the erythrocyte and corresponding molecules on the endothelial cell; these interactions are mediated by plasma ligands, such as thrombospondin and von Willebrand factor (21,22). Multiple studies have shown that sickle erythrocytes, especially reticulocytes, have an increased tendency to adhere to vascular endothelium and that, in the exchanged-transfused rodent model, adhesion occurred in the immediate postcapillary and collecting venules (23). Adhesogenic molecules on the sickle reticulocyte include the integrin, $\alpha_4\beta_1$ (very late activation antigen-4 or VLA-4), CD36, CD47, phosphatidyl serine, basal cell adhesion molecule, Lutheran blood group, and sulfated glycans. Other endothelial cell receptors, such as the integrin, $\alpha_v\beta_3$, and P-selectin, may also play substantial roles. Matrix components participating in adhesion include fibronectin, thrombospondin, vWF, and laminin (21,22,24).

Sickle erythrocytes have been shown to produce oxygen radicals via auto-oxidation at a rate nearly two-fold that of normal erythrocytes (20), with the resultant lipid peroxidation of the erythrocyte membrane (19). The sickle erythrocyte also has reduced ability to metabolize oxidants because of its lower levels of superoxide dismutase, catalase, and glutathione peroxidase (25,26). Adherence of sickle cells to endothelium induces lipid peroxidation of endothelium and endothelial transmigration of monocytes

(27). The decreased capacity for clearance of free radicals renders sickle patients more susceptible to oxidant lung damage and contributes to micro-vascular occlusion. Furthermore, oxygen radicals activate the transcription factor, NFκB, which upregulates expression of the adhesion molecules VCAM-1, on endothelium, which facilitates the endothelial adhesion of sickle erythrocytes via erythrocyte $\alpha_4\beta_1$ (22,28,29). VCAM-1 is upregulated by hypoxia, oxygen radicals, and by inflammatory cytokines such as inter-leukin-1 and tumor necrosis factor-α, both of which are elevated in ACS over the steady-state levels (22).

Endothelin-1 (ET-1) is a polypeptide and a potent vasoconstrictor of the pulmonary vascular bed; its levels are increased with hypoxemia (30). In patients with sickle cell disease, ET-1 levels are increased during the steady state and rise sharply just before and during ACS (31). Nitric oxide (NO) is a potent vasodilator, which is generated from the amino acid, L-arginine, via NO synthase (32). When administered by inhalation in low concentration, NO causes selective pulmonary vasodilatation, improving ventilation: perfusion ratios. Systemic vasodilatation does not occur as NO is rapidly inactivated by hemoglobin binding. Inhaled NO decreases PAP and PVR in acute lung injury and improves oxygenation in neonates with pulmonary hypertension (33,34). L-arginine levels are low in adults with sickle cell dis-ease and decrease during acute pain episodes and in the ACS (35,36), while NO metabolites (37,38) are increased, suggesting accelerated metabolism and possible depletion of NO in these acute illnesses. NO is important in counteracting the upregulation of VCAM-1. It has been shown to reduce cytokine-induced endothelial cell activation via repression of VCAM-1 gene transcription (39). Furthermore, NO inhibits the adherence of normal and sickle erythrocytes to vascular endothelium and prolongs survival in a transgenic mouse model of sickle cell disease exposed to hypoxia (39–41). Alterations in the balance between ET-1 vasoconstriction and NO vaso-dilatation can affect capillary transit time, endothelial cell expression of VCAM-1, and its attendant adherence characteristics, altering intrapulmo-nary flow and enhancing microvascular obstruction.

There is a growing body of evidence that granulocytes and monocytes play an important role in microvascular occlusion. Elevated leucocyte counts are associated with an increased risk of mortality and with cerebral infarction (42,43). In addition, leucocyte counts are indicative of overall disease severity (44,45). Reduction in leucocyte counts on hydroxyurea cor-related with the improvement in frequency of both acute painful events and of ACS (46). Elevated levels of IL-8 and G-CSF have been found in the bronchoalveolar lavage fluid in patients with the ACS (47). IL-8 mediates granulocyte chemotaxis and induces production of reactive oxygen species via the respiratory burst (48) and may participate in granulocyte-mediated lung injury. Finally, several recent reports appear to establish a link between severe vaso-occlusive events and the administration of G-CSF for hematopoietic stem cell mobilization, including apparent induction of an ACS (49–51). Granulocytes have been shown to adhere to sickle erythrocytes, preferentially to the dense cell fractions containing irreversibly sickled cells rather than the low density, reticulocyte-rich fractions that adhere to endothelium (52). Moreover, intravital microscopy of a transgenic sickle mouse model demonstrated adherence of circulating sickle erythrocytes to granulocytes already adherent to venular endothelium (53). This interaction increased after administration of TNF-α and resulted in complete vaso-occlusion. However, trapping of dense erythrocytes may occur on a mechanical basis in areas of hypoxic lung aside from the mechanisms of cellular adhesion (54,55).

Thus, microvascular occlusion in the sickling diseases may occur as the result of a complex series of reactions involving activation of the endothelium by oxygen radicals from the erythrocytes or by infectious processes that induce the secretion of inflammatory cytokines. Adherence of sickle erythrocytes or of leucocytes to endothelium and adherence of dense sickle erythrocytes to leucocytes follows, leading to partial obstruction to microcirculatory flow. Prolonged transit time allows extensive polymerization of Hb S with its resultant erythrocyte rigidity. Trapping of poorly deformable sickle erythrocytes results in transient or prolonged obstruction of microvascular flow. The subsequent ischemia further induces endothelial activation, leading to a vicious cycle of adherence, trapping and prolonged ischemia responsible for the signs and symptoms of ACS in this disease.

V. Immunology

The reasons for the pronounced susceptibility to infection in SCD are not fully understood. A number of abnormalities in host defense mechanisms have been described, which may play a role in the development of the ACS. The progressive splenic autoinfarction characteristic of Hb SS is associated with variable loss of antibody production and of phagocytic function. The enlarged spleen found in the sickle variant syndromes also has reduced immune function, rendering these patients susceptible to bloodstream infections with encapsulated bacteria, such as *S. pneumoniae*, *H. influenza* and the salmonella species (56). Splenic hypofunction, either anatomic or functional, has been correlated with the increased susceptibility to infection and with reduced concentrations of tuftsin, a serum protein that stimulates phagocytosis (57,58).

Defective opsonization of pneumcocci, salmonella and yeast has been repeatedly demonstrated (59–65). Recognition that the defect was due to a heat labile serum factor and that immunoglobulin levels are normal or elevated lead to investigations of the complement pathway in which the classic activation pathway was shown to be normal, but deficient activation of the alternate pathway was demonstrated (64–66). Total hemolytic complement is normal (59,60,63), but functional levels of factor B and of C3b are low, and there is evidence for accelerated catabolism of factor B (64,65). The levels of C3 activity cannot be correlated with the opsonization defect, leading to the conclusion that factor B deficiency may be responsible for the reduced opsonization and for the susceptibility to certain infections via deficient activation of C3b (61,62). Constant intravascular hemolysis with its release of red cell stroma into the circulation may activate the alternate pathway causing consumption of factor B (61,67). This same defect in alternate pathway activation has been described in Hb sickle-C disease, presumably extends to the other sickle variants, and serial studies show that the defect is persistent for at least 1 year (63). Defective opsonization has clinical relevance, as it correlated with a past history of pneumococcal infection (68).

The leucocyte count in SCD is elevated during the steady state and is another factor associated with overall clinical disease severity, with the risk of stroke and with increased mortality (42,45). Granulocytes are increased in number and have relatively low intracellular alkaline phosphatase and have subnormal phagocytic activity (42,69–71). The demonstration that sickle cells adhere to granulocytes and initiate the respiratory burst (52) suggests that granulocyte function may be impaired overall because of "relative exhaustion."

There is an absolute lymphocytosis in SCD with an increase in both T and B cells. There is conflicting data on the proportion of helper and suppressor subsets; the data favor an increase in T8 cells so that the T4:T8 ratio is near 1:1 (72–74). Studies of lymphocyte transformation have also shown variable results (75–77) but it appears that there is no significant abnormality in lymphocyte function. Moreover, the spectrum of infectious diseases in SCD does not suggest impairment of cell-mediated immunity.

Immunoglobulin levels are generally elevated (66), especially IgA, which is likely secondary to splenic hypofunction (78). Serotype-specific IgG antibody responses to pneumococcal reimmunization in general were mediocre or poor and were not affected by continued penicillin prophylaxis. This relatively poor response is not surprising, since pneumococcal polysaccharides are T lymphocyte-independent antigens (79) and are not thought to induce immunologic memory in either children or adults (80–82). The occurrence of pneumococcal bacteremia was associated with low IgG antibody concentrations to the infecting serotype. The most prevalent pneumococcal serotypes causing disease in this era of prophylactic antibiotics and vaccination include types 6, 14, 18, 19, and 23; these same serotypes are most frequently involved in previously reported "vaccine failures" (83). Aside from evidence supporting an immune defect related to pneumococcal infections and the phagocytic defect, there is little evidence to suggest that impaired immunity has substantial clinical relevance to the spectrum of the ACS, but recent evidence for impaired lymphocyte blasto-genic response and γ-interferon production in patients with the ACS suggest that these immunological abnormalities may contribute to the clinical severity of acute pulmonary disease in this patient population (84).

VI. Biochemical/Laboratory Features

The radiographic findings include segmental, lobar, or multilobar consolidation. In nearly half the cases, the initial chest radiograph shows only the characteristic findings of cardiomegaly with redistribution of blood flow to the upper lobes consequent to the chronic anemia, and the infiltrates appear 2 or 3 days later (7,9,15,85). The chest X-ray findings vary by age; children have isolated upper or middle lobe disease significantly more commonly than adults, while adults have lower lobe or multilobe disease more often (7,9). Pleural effusions are seen in more than half of the episodes and are more common in adults (7,9,85). The chest radiograph underestimates the degree of pulmonary involvement as has been shown by simultaneous high-resolution CT scan or perfusion scintigraphy. Thin section (3 mm) CT scans have shown consolidation, hypoperfusion, a paucity of arterioles, and venules and areas of ground-glass attenuation in areas both involved and not involved on plain radiograph (86). Perfusion lung scan has also shown defects in areas that were normal on X-ray (87,88). These imaging findings are consistent with vascular occlusion of large vessels as an important component of the ACS.

The hemoglobin declines by 0.7 g/dL, and the WBC increases by 70% on average (5,7,9). Bacteremia is more common in children, with *S. pneumoniae* and *H. influenza* found most commonly.

Sputum and blood cultures are relatively insensitive means of detecting bacterial pneumonia and likely underestimate its frequency. There is a growing trend towards the use of bronchoscopy to obtain high-quality material for culture. In one study, bacterial disease was detected by broncho-alveolar lavage in 20% of adult cases (89), a substantially higher frequency than that reported in the multi-institutional group studies despite an aggressive approach in obtaining deep sputum for culture. Bronchoscopy has been extremely successful in detecting lipid-laden macrophages for the diagnosis of fat embolism (90,91). Bronchoscopy has the additional advantage of detecting plastic bronchitis, a complication with branching bronchial cast formation that can produce worsening hypoxemia from ventilation/perfusion mismatch (92). Plastic bronchitis was detected in 21 of 29 (72%) episodes of the ACS in one study, where bronchoscopy was performed in patients with worsening lung consolidation and progressive hypoxemia (92) and was associated with improvement in chest X-ray findings after the procedure. This high frequency of plastic bronchitis may not be representative of all cases of the ACS, as the procedure tends to be performed in the sickest group of patients (90,92).

Secretory phospholipase A₂ (sPLA₂) is a potent inflammatory mediator that has been implicated in the pathophysiology of multiple conditions, including sepsis, multiorgan failure, and arthritis (93,94). sPLA₂ hydrolyzes phospholipids to produce free fatty acids and lysophospholipids, both of which result in acute lung injury. Additional inflammatory hydrolysis products, such as leukotrienes, thromboxanes, and prostaglandins, are produced when arachadonic acid is the fatty acid product of sPLA₂ (93). Elevation of sPLA₂ is found in acute respiratory distress syndrome (95). sPLA₂ is modestly elevated in sickle cell patients at baseline and increases dramatically with the ACS; the degree of elevation correlates with measures of the severity of the lung injury, such as A-a gradient (96,97). Nearly half of the ACS episodes occur in patients presenting with VOC, and sPLA₂ rises 24 to 48 hours before the onset of ACS in preliminary studies (96,97). Thus, sPLA₂ in combination with fever has predictive value for the development of ACS in patients presenting with pain and may indicate the fat embolism syndrome, where free fatty acids and eicosanoids may be generated from the fat particles lodged in the pulmonary circulation.

Measurement of oxygen saturation in Hb S disorders is confounded by the lower oxygen affinity of Hb S (Fig. 1) and by elevations of

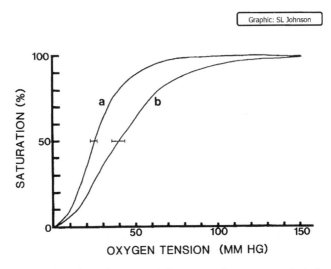

Figure 1   Representative oxygen saturation curves (by oxygen association) in (**a**) 41 normals (mean p50 = 26.3 ± 1.1 SEM mmHg) and in (**b**) 53 subjects with sickle cell anemia (mean p50 = 37.8 ± 4.1 SEM mmHg). Note that for any given PO₂, the saturation for Hb SS cells is less than that for normal erythrocytes. *Source*: Modified from Ref. 98, with permission.

carboxyhemoglobin and methemoglobin consequent to the hemolytic anemia. The oxygen saturation as assessed by automated blood gas analyzers calculates the saturation from the measured PO_2 against a standard oxygen dissociation curve for Hb A; consequently this method overestimates the saturation for samples containing Hb S (99). Co-oximetry uses multiple wavelengths to distinguish oxyhemoglobin from deoxyhemoglobin, carboxyhemoglobin, and methemoglobin, and is the most accurate method (100,101). Pulse oximetry measurements may overestimate the oxygen saturation by including methemoglobin and carboxyhemoglobin, which are often slightly increased in Hb S disorders; pulse oximetry is further affected by conditions that reduce the pulse amplitude such as hypotension, hypothermia, and vasoconstriction (101). In one study comparing the three methods, the co-oximetry and pulse oximetry showed near agreement (pulse oximetry only 2% greater than co-oximetry), but the calculated saturation overestimated the co-oximetry measurement by nearly 7% on average (99). A subsequent study confirmed that pulse oximetry overestimates co-oximetry by only 1.1% (102).

VII. Differential Diagnosis

The causes of the ACS are multiple (Table 3), including disorders directly or indirectly related to the sickling process, as well as causes distinct from sickling. Chlamydia, mycoplasma, and viral infections are now the most common agents identified (7,12,13). Sputum and blood culture should continue to be done despite the historically low yield so as to identify bacterial agents when present. Cultures positive for nonrespiratory pathogens must be carefully interpreted (103). Negative cultures are often explained by problems in contamination, collection or storage, handling, and prior antibiotic administration (104,105). Serologic studies for mycoplasma, chlamydia, and parvovirus are helpful in the diagnosis of these infections. Nasopharyngeal samples for viral cultures should be included, especially in children. Recent data indicate that fiber optic bronchoscopy and bronchoalveolar lavage (BAL) provide higher-quality specimens for culture and microscopic examination and a higher yield, thus improving confidence in a negative result (89–91).

However, all studies stress the fact that the majority of ACS episodes cannot be proved to be of infectious origin, and noninfectious causes must be sought for carefully. Vichinsky et al. (106) published a study in which 12 of 27 episodes of ACS had evidence for fat embolism as the cause; subsequent reports indicate an even higher prevalence of fat embolism in the ACS (90,91). Subsequent data from the NACSSG indicate that fat embolism at 8.8% was the most common diagnosis established (7). Fat and bone marrow elements within the circulation, released from necrotic marrow

Table 3   Etiologies of the Acute Chest Syndrome

---

1. Hemoglobin S related
    A. Direct consequences of Hb S
        Pulmonary vaso-occlusion (16.1%)
        Fat embolism syndrome (8.8%)
        Hypoventilation 2° to rib/sternal bone infarction
        Hypoventilation 2° to narcotic administration
        Pulmonary edema induced by narcotics or fluid overload
    B. Indirect consequences of Hb S
        Infections
        Atypical bacterial
            Chlamydia pneumoniae (7.2%)
            Mycoplasma pneumoniae (6.6 %)
            Mycoplasma hominis (1.5%)
        Bacterial
            Staphyloccus aureus, coagulase-positive (1.8%)
            Streptococcus pneumoniae (1.6%)
            Haemophilus influenzae (0.7%)
        Viral
            Respiratory syncytial virus (3.9%)
            Parvovirus B19 (1.5%)
            Rhinovirus (1.2%)
2. Unrelated to Hb S
        Fibrin thromboembolism
        Foreign body/intrinsic bronchial obstruction
        Other common pulmonary diseases, i.e., aspiration, trauma, asthma, etc.

The specific organisms are listed in the percentage detected in the NACSSG.
Source: Adapted from Refs. 7, 98, with permission.

sites of ischemic vaso-occlusion, can produce embolic phenomena involving the lungs and other tissues. The spectrum of disease in fat embolism varies widely to include a fulminant syndrome with high fever, severe tachypnea, hypoxemia, bilateral alveolar infiltrates, tachycardia, neurologic changes, thrombocytopenia, worsening anemia, and altered renal or liver function (107). Laboratory findings in the FES include a dramatic rise in LDH, uric acid, and nRBC and a decline in serum Ca^{2+}. Serum lipase and sPLA$_2$ increase. None of these biochemical tests are specific for the diagnosis so that clinical suspicion remains the mainstay of diagnosis. Examination of deep sputum and/or BAL specimens for fat-laden macrophages (90,91) is useful in the diagnosis of the fat embolism syndrome as is examination for trunkal petechiae and lipemia retinalis; fat globules may be found in the blood and urine (107). Severe bone pain and relative thrombocytopenia may provide clues to this diagnosis in sickle cell patients.

Vascular occlusion by sickle cells and pulmonary infarction as important causes of the ACS are suggested by the lack of positive bacterial or viral cultures in carefully studied patients and by the data indicating that antibiotic therapy produces no faster resolution than those treated with supportive care alone (6,7,9,103). The results from the Multi-Institutional Study of Hydroxyurea in SCD indicating a significant reduction in ACS in those on hydroxyurea further suggests that a substantial number of ACS episodes are secondary to vascular obstruction (46). Thus, our focus on infection as the most prevalent etiology may have been misplaced.

Fibrin thromboembolism occurs at a rate similar to that in the general population (108), but distinguishing thromboemboli from sickle cell vaso-occlusion by chest tomography or scintigraphy is extremely difficult, as recent data indicate nearly identical findings with these modalities (86,88). Evidence for concomitant venous thrombosis, comparison of current lung scintigraphy with baseline data, and angiography may be needed to help establish a diagnosis (109). In those cases of the ACS where pulmonary angiography has been performed, the findings were most consistent with vascular occlusion (110). Exchange transfusion prior to angiography is necessary to prevent vaso-occlusion due to sickling induced by hyperosmolar contrast media (111).

Hypoventilation can lead to regional pulmonary hypoxia and initiate the sequence of events that lead to adhesion-related vascular occlusion. The recognition that splinting due to the pain of rib infarction was frequently associated with atelectasis and evolved into the ACS led to the utilization of incentive spirometry for prevention (112,113). More recently, patients receiving oral sustained-release morphine for pain control during a VOC developed an ACS at a rate three-fold that of patients randomized to continuous-intravenous morphine (114). The difference was attributed to an area under the curve (AUC) for sustained-release morphine that was 2–3-fold greater than that for intravenous morphine and was associated with a significant decrease in SaO_2 for those on oral morphine related to hypoventilation.

VIII. Management

A. Prophylaxis

In the absence of a definitive etiologic diagnosis, treatment of the ACS is primarily supportive and can be approached from three general aspects: prophylaxis, standard management, and treatment of evolving respiratory failure. The advent of the polyvalent pneumococcal vaccine has had a favorable impact upon infections with this organism (115). Prophylactic penicillin and the use of the pneumococcal and *H. influenza* vaccines may have had a role in the changing epidemiology of ACS in SCD. Although specific studies of vaccine impact upon the frequency of pneumococcal pneumonia have not been reported, the reduced frequency of this organism in the ACS as reported in recent studies can be extrapolated from vaccine use and from the effect of prophylactic penicillin on the frequency of pneumococcal sepsis (116). The HiB vaccine may have had a similar effect upon the previously reported high frequency of pulmonary infection with this organism in SCD. Parvovirus B19 infection has been associated with a particularly severe form of the ACS, so vaccination for this virus, as well as influenza and respiratory syncytial virus, should be considered depending upon future availability (117). Treatment with hydroxyurea has been shown to reduce the incidence of the ACS by approximately 40% and is indicated for those with two or more episodes of the ACS, independent of its indication for recurrent VOC (46). Because of the relationship between ACS and premature mortality, prevention of ACS episodes and its associated complications with hydroxyurea is a possible factor in the reduction of mortality recently reported for hydroxyurea-treated patients (118).

B. Supportive Care

In an episode of ACS, the immediate goals of therapy are prevention of alveolar collapse, maintenance of gas exchange, and prevention of further pulmonary injury leading to a progressive downhill course. Serial determination of arterial blood gas can be quite useful in assessing progress. Charache et al. first noted that an increase in PO_2 occurs as the first sign of improvement prior to a change in chest X ray and that a PO_2 less than 75 mmHg (approximately equal to an SaO_2 of 85–90%, Fig. 1) was associated with a poor prognosis (6).

The chest X-ray lags the physiologic changes by a substantial margin and is not as useful for prognostication, although Davies and colleagues (102) noted that the duration of fever and degree of tachycardia were related to the extent of chest X-ray involvement, Charache et al. (6) did not find a difference in PO_2 between patients with more extensive radiographic changes. The arterial blood gas data should be carefully interpreted relative to the degree of FiO_2 required to achieve adequate oxygenation (119) and in view of the reduced oxygen affinity of Hb S (Fig. 1). SaO_2 should be maintained with supplemental oxygen at 92% or greater, since the effect of moderate arterial desaturation on the microvascular rheology of sickle erythrocyte is adversely affected by partial polymerization of intracellular hemoglobin S (16,17) with its attendant risk for pulmonary trapping of poorly deformable erythrocyte (54,55). In patients with partial nasal obstruction, oxygen by mask may provide superior efficacy over nasal cannula.

Serial chest X-rays are needed to assess the extent and course of the pulmonary changes. However, serial arterial blood gas determinations on an FiO_2 of 0.21 provide a clearer picture of ongoing pulmonary function as the chest X-ray often lags physiologic events. Arterial blood gas measurements can be replaced by continuous pulse oximetry monitoring, especially if there have been simultaneous determinations in the patient so as to establish the correlation between the two. Oxygen saturation and/or the alveolar–arterial oxygen gradient rather than oxygen tension provide more relevant information (120). Careful attention to clinical parameters—vital signs, respiratory effort, and overall status—is a key ingredient in overall assessment.

Antibiotics are generally given although the studies of Charache et al. (6) and Davies et al. (103) indicate that antibiotic treatment may not shorten the clinical course. The choice of antibiotic coverage must be made on clinical grounds, considering the well-described secular changes in microbial flora as well as geographic differences in the spectrum of flora (7,11,14). In view of the current epidemiology studies, the current recommendation is a third- or fourth-generation cephalosporin and a macrolide (7), but the decision should be guided by knowledge of local bacterial patterns and by the results of sputum smear analysis and modified as culture results become available. Alternate regimens include a quinolone or a macrolide plus a beta-lactam. Progression of disease should prompt a reassessment of antibiotic coverage because of the occasional gram-negative organism and the high frequency of viral agents.

Pain management usually requires narcotic analgesia, which can produce respiratory depression with its attendant risk of hypoxia and potential for acceleration of pulmonary vaso-occlusion. Pleuritic chest pain is a particular problem because splinting reduces ventilation and may predispose to atelectasis. Intercostal nerve block with a long-acting local anesthetic, such as bupivacaine, can alleviate chest wall pain and splinting and has the additional advantage of reducing the amount of systemic analgesia needed to control pain and lessening the consequent risks of respiratory depression, hypoxia, and atelectasis. A nerve block may provide relief for 18 to 24 hours and can be repeated as needed to control symptoms (98).

Intravenous fluid management at a rate of 1.5–2.0 times maintenance is the standard recommendation, since aggressive hydration, as well as opioid administration, can lead to pulmonary edema and cause the ACS (13,121). It seems unlikely that fluid overload alone would be a common cause of ACS in view of the large numbers of patients treated with this modality unless those affected had a subtle underlying cardiopulmonary pathologic condition that is uncovered by high-volume saline administration. Since the objective is rehydration of erythrocytes (17), a hypotonic infusion such as half-normal saline (0.25 normal for children) with or without dextrose is preferred over normal saline, which might be responsible for those cases of pulmonary edema reported (13,121).

Incentive spirometry (10 maximum inspirations every 2 hours while awake) has been shown to significantly reduce the development of atelectasis and the risk of ACS and should be instituted with all hospitalizations for pain as well as for those with ACS (122). The high frequency of reactive airway disease and wheezing reported in sickle cell disease supports the universal use of bronchodilators as an important adjunctive therapy (7,9,123,124). Mechanical ventilation is indicated as for other causes of progressive respiratory insufficiency. Both high-frequency ventilation and extracorporeal membrane oxygenation have been successfully employed in severe cases of respiratory failure in the ACS (125–129).

C. Transfusion

The role of transfusion support is not clearly defined, although there are sporadic case reports of rapid reversal of chest X-ray findings and symptoms immediately post transfusion (103,130,131). It seems clear that there are at least two broad indications for transfusion. Simple transfusion of one or two units can be given to raise the hemoglobin level whenever there is a need for an increase in oxygen-carrying capacity. The therapeutic objectives are to make the patient more comfortable and to reduce the cardiac workload, and the indications include moderately severe anemia, high cardiac output, tachypnea, and easy fatigability. Whenever the clinical situation suggests that mechanical ventilation might be required, exchange transfusion should be considered on an urgent basis. Exchange transfusion should be used early, at the first hint of difficulty, rather than late, when the situation may no longer be reversible. Exchange transfusion may produce rapid resolution of the ACS, which justifies its early use and suggests that vascular occlusion is readily reversible, at least in the early stages (103,130,131). This rapid improvement after transfusion is further evidence for microvascular occlusion as a part of the ACS, but could also indicate another reversible lung disease, such as fat embolism.

The indications for exchange transfusion in the ACS have not been fully defined (Table 4) but include worsening pulmonary function as evidenced by a progressive decrease in SaO_2, a decrease in PO_2 or increase in $A\text{-}aO_2$ gradient, worsening infiltrates on chest X ray or increasing tachycardia and increased work of breathing, such as increasing tachypnea for age, nasal flaring, intercostals retractions. In addition to these indications, exchange transfusion may have a specific therapeutic action in the FES where normal red cells may bind the free fatty acids, preventing further pulmonary damage. Finally, exchange should be considered whenever there is general clinical evidence of a declining course or when indicators of poor prognosis are present. Exchange transfusion dilutes the proportion of sickle cells, improves the blood rheology and flow and reduces the risk of further organ damage from either intrapulmonary or peripheral sickle vaso-occlusion (132). The objective of transfusion in these situations is life saving, since progressive worsening of clinical status is associated with high mortality.

Transfusion carries two risks that are particularly relevant to the sickle cell patient: allo-immunization and acute hyperviscosity. Allo-immunization

Table 4 Indications for Exchange Transfusion in the ACS

Clinical parameters:
  Unstable and/or worsening vital signs
  Persistent tachypnea and/or other signs of labored breathing
  Persistent acute neurologic findings
  Serial decline in pulse oximetry
Laboratory measures:
  Arterial oxygen saturation persistently <88%, despite aggressive ventilatory
    support
  Increasing A-a gradient
  Hemoglobin concentration falling by 2 g/dL or more
  Platelet count <200,000/μL
  Evidence for multiorgan failure
  Progression to multilobe infiltrates

---

data from the preoperative transfusion study indicate a 10% rate of new alloantibody formation from a transfusion intervention (133). Subsequent transfusion therapy has an increased risk of delayed hemolytic transfusion reaction (134); such reactions are extremely difficult to treat since further transfusion is usually ineffective in maintaining the hematocrit. An extended phenotype match can reduce the incidence of allo-immunization (135,136) and should include Rh, C, E, and Kell antigens at a minimum (136). The hyperviscosity syndrome may occur with mixtures of A and S cells at near normal hematocrits (137,138). The syndrome is characterized by hypertension and altered mental status and/or seizure activity. Screening donor units for sickle cell trait and maintaining the post-transfusion hematocrit at levels less than 35% may prevent this syndrome. It is widely believed that a post-transfusion level of hemoglobin S less than 10% is therapeutically superior to one of 20% or 30%. Data in support of this contention are lacking. However, the hypothesis is intuitively attractive. The simplest method of monitoring the post-transfusion hemoglobin S level is by determining the percentage of sickled cells in a meta-bisulfite preparation. Alternatively, hemoglobin S can be measured by one of the common column chromatography methods.

Recurrent episodes of the ACS can lead to sickle cell lung disease, characterized by diffuse interstitial fibrosis on chest X-ray, abnormal pulmonary function tests, symptomatic hypoxia, pulmonary hypertension, and sudden death (139–141). The further association of recurrent ACS with premature mortality in the CSSCD (5) provides justification for aggressive secondary prevention approaches in patients with recurrent episodes, including hydroxyurea, chronic transfusion therapy, and stem cell transplantation (142).

IX. Future Considerations

Despite the recent advances in our understanding of the pathophysiology and epidemiology of the ACS, there are still needs for better methods of distinguishing vaso-occlusion from fibrin or fat embolism, for rapid diagnostic tests to positively identify microbial infection, for adjunctive therapies that would affect prognosis and for identification of factors that influence prognosis and might predict which patients will recover with supportive care alone and which will progress to pulmonary failure. Documentation of the clinical utility of sPLA$_2$ for the ACS and its relationship to the fat embolism syndrome would be useful as an early marker for the ACS and, perhaps, for clinical severity. Potential therapies for sPLA$_2$ inhibition are under development, and clinical trials examining the predictive capability of sPLA$_2$ are underway (143).

In a recent study, dexamethasone 0.3 mg/kg was administered to patients with the ACS at 12-hour intervals for four doses and showed significant reductions in the treated group versus placebo with respect to duration of fever, analgesic use, supplemental oxygen therapy, transfusion requirements, and a 40% reduction in hospital stay (144). The beneficial effect was attributed to inhibition of sPLA$_2$and the inhibition of inflammation; however, this steroid also prevents cytokine induction of VCAM-1 on endothelial cells and could ameliorate the course of ACS via this mechanism as well (145). There was an apparent "rebound" effect with readmission to the hospital following discontinuation of steroids, suggesting that the dose duration or dose tapering needs further study. In addition, beneficial effects of high-dose steroid in the fat embolism syndrome have been reported in small controlled trials in trauma patients (146,147) and could have produced benefit in sickle ACS, where fat embolism is common, due to inhibition of inflammation. Dexamethasone has also shown a beneficial effect on VOC (148,149), and further studies of this agent in both VOC and ACS are warranted.

A beneficial effect of nitric oxide (NO) has been reported in small numbers of patients with the ACS, where inhaled NO at 80 ppm for 47 to 92 hours rapidly improved A-a gradient, reduced PAP and PVR and was felt to have accelerated recovery (150–152). Inhaled NO could benefit patients with the ACS by pulmonary vascular dilation, reducing pulmonary vascular resistance, and improving intrapulmonary blood flow. Further studies are needed to better define the therapeutic utility and potential for methemoglobin toxicity for this agent, but its use has the potential to reduce the need for more aggressive therapies and improve prognosis.

Purified polaxamer 188 is a non-ionic surfactant that reduces blood viscosity and inhibits erythrocyte adhesion to endothelium (153). A recent clinical trial of this agent showed a modest effect on the duration of VOC (154). The results of the polaxamer 188 study suggest that blocking sickle cell adhesion to endothelium may be beneficial for vascular occlusive events in SCD, such as the ACS. A further step in this process is the development of a recombinant P-selectin glycoprotein ligand that binds to P-selectin and to a lesser degree E- and L-selectin (155). Recent studies using monoclonal antibodies and knockout mice have shown that P-selectin mediates the initial interaction of sickle erythrocytes, and leucocytes with activated endothelial cells (156,157). Thus, blockade of P-selectin using this fusion protein could provide clinical benefit in the ACS via inhibition of the adhesion of leucocytes and sickle erythrocytes to pulmonary endothelium in the vaso-occlusive process; a phase II study of this agent is planned. Additional agents that inhibit other adhesogenic proteins involved in the vaso-occlusive process, such as the integrin, $\alpha_V\beta_3$, or VLA-4 are under study (158–160).

X. Conclusions

The difference in clinical course and severity between children and adults supports the results of current studies indicating multiple etiologies for the ACS. Infectious causes are more common in children, as suggested by the shorter and milder course, seasonal variation, upper lobe disease, and higher rate of bacteremia. In adults, severe bone pain and lower lobe or multilobe disease point to vascular occlusion as the common cause of ACS, much as Barrett-Connor indicated in her initial reports (4,10). The mainstay of successful treatment is high-quality supportive care. Consultation with pulmonary, infectious disease and intensive care specialists is a necessary part of management. Fluid management, oxygenation, chest physiotherapy, bronchodilators, intermittent incentive spirometry are essential elements of management in the absence of a specific therapy that consistently ameliorates clinical course.

References

1. Kaul DK, Fabry ME, Nagel RL. The pathophysiology of vascular obstruction in the sickle syndromes. Blood Rev 1996; 10:29–44.
2. Steinberg MH, Rodgers GP. Pathophysiology of sickle cell disease: role of cellular and genetic modifiers. Semin Hematol 2001; 38:299–306.
3. Serjeant GR. Sickle Cell Disease. 3rd ed. Oxford: Oxford University Press, 2001.
4. Barrett-Connor E. Acute pulmonary disease and sickle cell anemia. Am Rev Resp Dis 1971; 104:155–165.
5. Castro O, Brambilla DJ, Thorington B, Reindorf CA, Scott RB, Gillette P, Vera JC, Levy PS. The Cooperative Study of Sickle Cell Disease. The acute chest syndrome in sickle cell disease: incidence and risk factors. Blood 1994; 84:643–649.

6.   Charache S, Scott JC, Charache P. Acute chest syndrome in adults with sickle cell anemia: microbiology, treatment and prevention. Arch Intern Med 1979; 139:67–69.

7.   Vichinsky EP, Neumayr LD, Earles AN, Williams R, Lennette ET, Dean D, Nickerson B, Orringer E, McKie V, Bellevue R, Daeschner C, Manci EA. Causes and outcomes of the acute chest syndrome in sickle cell disease. National Acute Chest Syndrome Study Group. N Engl J Med 2000; 342: 1855–1865.

8.   Petch MC, Serjeant GR. Clinical features of pulmonary lesions in sickle-cell anaemia. Br Med J 1970; 3:31.

9.   Vichinsky EP, Styles LA, Colangelo LH, Wright EC, Castro O, Nickerson B. The Cooperative Study of Sickle Cell Disease. Acute chest syndrome in sickle cell disease: clinical presentation and course. Blood 1997; 89:1787–1792.

10.   Barrett-Connor E. Pneumonia and pulmonary infarction in sickle cell anemia. JAMA 1973; 224:997–1000.

11.   Gray GC, Mitchell BS, Tueller JE, Cross ER, Amundson DE. Pneumonia hospitalizations in the US Navy and Marine Corps: rates and risk factors for 6,522 admissions, 1981–1991. Amer J Epidemiol 1994; 139:793–802.

12.   Poncz M, Kane E, Gill FM. Acute chest syndrome in sickle cell disease: etiology and clinical correlates. J Pediatr 1985; 107:861–866.

13.   Sprinkle RH, Cole T, Smith S, Buchanan GR. Acute chest syndrome in children with sickle cell disease: a retrospective analysis of 100 hospitalized cases. Am J Pediatr Hematol/Oncol 1986; 8:105–110.

14.   van Agtmael MA, Cheng JD, Nassent HC. Acute chest syndrome in adult Afro-Caribbean patients with sickle cell disease. Arch Intern Med 1994; 154:557–561.

15.   Morris C, Vichinsky E, Styles L. Clinician assessment for acute chest syndrome in febrile patients with sickle cell disease: is it accurate enough? Ann Emerg Med 1999; 34:64–69.

16.   Stuart J, Johnson CS. Rheology of the sickle cell disorders. In: GDO Rowe, ed. Blood Rheology and Hyperviscosity Syndromes. Ballieŕe's Clin Haematol. Vol. 1. 1987:747–775.

17.   Sowter MC, Green MA, Keidan AJ, Johnson CS, Stuart J. Filtration of sickle cells is sensitive to factors that enhance polymerization of haemoglobin S. Clin Hemorheol 1988; 8:223–236.

18.   Hofrichter J, Ross PD, Eaton WA. Kinetics and mechanism of deoxyhemoglobin S gelation: a new approach to understanding sickle cell disease. Proc Natl Acad Sci USA 1974; 71:4864–4868.

19.   Chui D, Lubin B. Oxidative hemoglobin denaturation and RBC destruction: the effect of heme on red cell membranes. Semin Hematol 1989; 26: 128–135.

20.   Browne P, Shalev O, Hebbel RP. The molecular pathobiology of cell membrane iron: the sickle red cell as a model. Free Radic Biol Med 1998; 24: 1040–1048.

21.   Frenette P. Sickle cell vaso-occlusion: multistep and multicellular paradigm. Curr Opin Hematol 2002; 9:101–106.

22. Setty BNY, Stuart MJ. Vascular cell adhesion molecule-1 is involved in mediating hypoxia induced sickle red blood cell adherence to endothelium: potential role in sickle cell disease. Blood 1996; 88:2311–2320.

23. Kaul DK, Fabry ME, Nagel RL. Microvascular sites and characteristics of sickle cell adhesion to vascular endothelium in shear flow conditions: pathophysiologic implications. Proc Natl Acad Sci USA 1989; 86:3356–3360.

24. Stuart MJ, Setty BNY. Acute chest syndrome of sickle cell disease: new light on an old problem. Curr Opin Hematol 2001; 8:111–122.

25. Schacter L, Warth JA, Gordon EM, Prasad A, Klein BL. Altered amount and activity of superoxide dismutase in sickle cell anemia. FASEB J 1988; 2:237–243.

26. Chui D, Lubin B. Abnormal vitamin E and glutathione peroxidase levels in sickle cell anemia. J Clin Med 1979; 94:542–548.

27. Sultana C, Shen Y, Rattan V, Johnson C, Kalra VK. Interaction of sickle erythrocytes with endothelial cells in the presence of endothelial cell conditioned medium induces oxidant stress leading to transendothelial migration of monocytes. Blood 1998; 92:3924–3935.

28. Shiu Y-T, Udden MM, McIntire LV. Perfusion with sickle erythrocytes upregulates ICAM-1 and VCAM-1 gene expression in cultured human endothelial cells. Blood 2000; 95:3232–3241.

29. Kunsch C, Medford RM. Oxidative stress as a regulator of gene expression in the vasculature. Circ Res 1999; 85:753–766.

30. Yuan X-J, Wang J, Juhaszova M, Gaine SP, Rubin LJ. Attenuated K+ channel gene transcription in primary pulmonary hypertension. Lancet 1998; 351: 726–727.

31. Hammerman SI, Kourembanas S, Conca TJ Tucci M, Brauer M, Farber HW. Endothelin-1 production during the acute chest syndrome in sickle cell disease. Am J Respir Crit Care Med 1997; 156:280–285.

32. Moncada S, Higgs A. Mechanisms of disease: the L-arginine-nitric oxide pathway. N Engl J Med 1993; 329:2002–2012.

33. Rossaint R, Falke KJ, Lopez F, Slama K, Pison U, Zapol WM. Inhaled nitric oxide for the adult respiratory distress syndrome. N Engl J Med 1993; 328: 399–405.

34. Clark RH, Kueser TJ, Walker MW, Southgate M, Huckaby JL, Perez JA, Ray BJ, Keszler M, Kinsella JP. The Clinical Inhaled Nitric Oxide Research Group. Low-dose nitric oxide therapy for persistent pulmonary hypertension of the newborn. N Engl J Med 2000; 342:469–474.

35. Enwonwu CO. Increased metabolic demand for arginine in sickle cell anemia. Med Sci Res 1989; 17:997–998.

36. Morris CR, Kuypers FA, Larkin S, Styles LA. Patterns of arginine and nitric oxide in patients with sickle cell disease with vaso-occlusive crisis and acute chest syndrome. J Pediatr Hematol Oncol 2000; 22:515–520.

37. Morris CR, Kuypers FA, Larkin S, Sweeters N, Simon J, Vichinsky EP, Styles LA. Arginine therapy: a novel strategy to induce nitric oxide production in sickle cell disease. Br J Haematol 2000; 111:498–500.

38. Rees DC, Cervi P, Grimwade D, O'Driscoll A, Hamilton M, Parker NE, Porter JB. The metabolites of nitric oxide in sickle-cell disease. Br J Haematol 1995; 91:834–837.

39. De Caterina R, Libby P, Peng H, Thannickal VJ, Rajavashisth TB, Gimbrone MA Jr, Shin WS, Liao JK. Nitric oxide decreases cytokine-induced endothelial activation: nitric oxide selectively reduces endothelial expression of adhesion molecules and proinflammatory cytokines. J Clin Invest 1995; 96: 60–68.

40. Space SL, Lane PA, Pickett CK, Weil JV. Nitric oxide attenuates normal and sickle red blood cell adherence to pulmonary endothelium. Am J Hematol 2000; 63:200–204.

41. Martinez-Ruiz R, Montero-Huerta P, Hromi J, Head CA. Inhaled nitric oxide improves survival rates during hypoxia in a sickle cell (SAD) mouse model. Anesthesiology 2001; 94:1113–1118.

42. Platt OS, Brambilla DJ, Rosse WF, Milner PF, Castro O, Steinberg MH, Klug PP. Mortality in sickle cell disease. Life expectancy and risk factors for early death. N Engl J Med 1994; 330:1639–1644.

43. Kinney TR, Sleeper LA, Wang WC, Zimmerman RA, Pegelow CH, Ohene-Frempong K, Wethers DL, Bello JA, Vichinsky EP, Moser FG, Gallagher DM, DeBaun MR, Platt OS, Miller ST. Silent cerebral infarcts in sickle cell anemia: a risk factor analysis. The Cooperative Study of Sickle Cell Disease. Pediatrics 1999; 103:640–645.

44. Miller ST, Sleeper LA, Pegelow CH, Enos LE, Wang WC, Weiner SJ, Wethers DL, Smith J, Kinney TR. Prediction of adverse outcomes in children with sickle cell disease. N Engl J Med 2000; 342:83–89.

45. Anyaegbu CC, Okplal IE, Aken'Ova AY, Salimonu LS. Peripheral blood neutrophil count and candicidal activity correlate with the clinical severity in sickle cell anaemia. Eur J Hematol 1998; 60:267–268.

46. Charache S, Terrin ML, Moore RD, Dover GJ, Barton FB, Eckert SV, McMahon RP, Bonds DR. Effect of hydroxyurea on the frequency of painful crises in sickle cell anemia. N Engl J Med 1995; 332:1317–1322.

47. Abboud MR, Taylor EC, Habib D, Dantzler-Johnson T, Jackson SM, Xu F, Laver J, Ballas SK. Elevated serum and bronchoalveolar lavage fluid levels of interleukin 8 and granulocyte colony-stimulating factor associated with the acute chest syndrome in patients with sickle cell disease. Br J Haematol 2000; 111:482–490.

48. Baggiolini M, MoSeries B, Clark-Lewis I. Interleukin-8 and related chemotactic cytokines. Chest 1994; 105:95s–98s.

49. Abgboud M, Laver J, Blau CA. Granulocytosis causing sickle-cell crisis. Lancet 1998; 351:959.

50. Adler BK, Salzman DE, Carabasi MH, Vaughan WP, Reddy VV, Prchal JT. Fatal sickle cell crisis after granulocyte colony-stimulating factor administration. Blood 2001; 97:3313–3314.

51. Grigg AP. Granulocyte colony-stimulating factor-induced sickle cell crisis and multiorgan dysfunction in a patient with compound heterozygous sickle cell/ beta+ thalassemia. Blood 2001; 97:3998–3999.

52. Hofstra TC, Kalra VK, Meiselman HJ, Coates TD. Sickle erythrocytes adhere to polymorphonuclear neutrophils and activate the neutrophil respiratory burst. Blood 1996; 87:4440–4447.

53. Turhan A, Weiss LA, Mohandas N, Coller BS, Frenette PS. Primary role for adherent leukocytes in sickle cell vascular occlusion: a new paradigm. Proc Natl Acad Sci USA 2002; 99:3047–3051.

54. Aldrich TK, Dhuper SK, Patwa NS, Makolo E, Suzuka SM, Najeebi SA, Santhanakrishnan S, Nagel RL, Fabry ME. Pulmonary entrapment of sickle cells: the role of regional alveolar hypoxia. J Appl Physiol 1996; 80:531–539.

55. Haynes J Jr, Taylor AE, Dixon D, Voelkel N. Microvascular hemodynamics in the sickle red blood cell perfused isolated rat lung. Am J Physiol 1993; 264: H484–H489.

56. Pearson HA, McIntosh S, Ritchey AK, Lobel JS, Rooks Y, Johnston D. Developmental aspects of splenic function in sickle cell diseases. Blood 1979; 53:358–365.

57. Falter ML, Robinson MG, Kim OS, GO SC, Taubkin SP. Splenic function and infection in sickle cell anemia. Acta Hematol 1973; 59:154–161.

58. Spirer Z, Weisman Y, Zakuth V, Firdkin M, Bogair M. Decreased tuftsin concentration in sickle cell disease. Arch Dis Child 1980; 55:566–567.

59. Winkelstein JA, Drachman RH. Deficiency of pneumococcal serum opsonizing activity in sickle-cell disease. N Engl J Med 1968; 279:459–466.

60. Johnston RB, Newman SL, Struth AG. An abnormality of the alternate pathway of complement activation in sickle-cell disease. N Engl J Med 1973; 288: 803–808.

61. Koethe SM, Casper JT, Rodey GE. Alternative complement pathway activity in sera from patients with sickle cell disease. Clin Exp Immunol 1976; 23: 56–60.

62. Hand WL, King NL. Serum opsonization of salmonella in sickle cell anemia. Am J Med 1978; 64:388–395.

63. Bjornson AB, Lobel JS. Direct evidence that decreased serum opsonization of *Streptococcus pneumoniae* via the alternative complement pathway in sickle cell disease is related to antibody deficiency. J Clin Invest 1987; 79:388–398.

64. Wilson WA, Thomas EJ, Sissons JGP. Complement activation in asymptomatic patients with sickle cell anaemia. Clin Exp Immunol 1979; 36:130–139.

65. Larcher VF, Wyke RJ, Davies LR, Stroud CE, Williams R. Defective yeast opsonisation and functional deficiency of complement in sickle cell disease. Arch Dis Child 1982; 57:343–346.

66. Millard D, De Ceulaer K, Vaidya S, Serjeant GR. Serum immunoglobulin levels in children with homozygous sickle cell disease. Clin Chim Acta 1982; 125: 81–87.

67. Poskitt TR, Fortwengler HP Jr, Lunkskis BJ. Activation of the alternate complement pathway by autologous red cell stroma. J Exp Med 1973; 138:715–722.

68. Bjornson AB, Lobel JS, Harr KS. Relation between serum opsonic activity for *Streptococcus pneumoniae* and complement function in sickle cell disease. J Infect Dis 1985; 152:701–709.

69. Rosner F, Karayalcin G. Decreased leucocyte alkaline phosphatase activity in sickle-cell anemia. Ann Intern Med 1974; 80:668–669.

70. Carpentieri U, Smith L, Daeschner CW, Haggard ME. Neutrophils and zinc in infection-prone children with sickle cell disease. Pediatrics 1983; 72:88–92.

71. Hernandez DE, Gonzales N, Rios R, Merchan L, Wuani H. Phagocytosis in patients with sickle cell disease. J Clin Lab Immunol 1983; 12:137–140.

72. Ades EW, Hinson A, Morgan SK. Immunological studies in sickle cell disease. I. Analysis of circulating T-lymphocyte subpopulations. Clin Immunol Immunopathol 1980; 17:459–462.

73. Adedji MO. Lymphocyte subpopulations in homozygous sickle cell disease in Nigeria. Acta Haematol 1985; 74:10–13.

74. Venkataraman M, Westerman MP. B-cell changes in patients with sickle cell anemia. Am J Clin Pathol 1985; 84:153–158.

75. Glassman AB, Deas DV, Berlinsky FS, Bennett CE. Lymphocyte blast transformation and peripheral lymphocyte percentages in patients with sickle cell disease. Ann Clin Lab Sci 1980; 10:9–12.

76. Hernandez DE, Cruz C, Santos MN, Ballester JM. Immunologic dysfunction in sickle cell anaemia. Acta Hematol 1980; 63:156–161.

77. Hendriks J, De Ceulaer K, Williams E, Serjeant GR. Mononuclear cells in sickle cell disease: subpopulations and in vitro response to mitogens. J Clin Lab Immunol 1984; 13:129–132.

78. Schumacher MJ. Serum immunoglobulin and transferrin levels after childhood splenectomy. Arch Dis Child 1970; 45:114–117.

79. Bjornson AB, Falletta JM, Verter JI, Buchanan GR, Miller ST, Pegelow CH, Iyer RV, Johnstone HS, DeBaun MR, Wethers DL, et al. Serotype-specific immunoglobulin G antibody responses to pneumococcal polysaccharide vaccine in children with sickle cell anemia: effects of continued penicillin prophylaxis. J Pediatr 1996; 129:828–835.

80. Siber GR. Pneumococcal disease: prospects for a new generation of vaccines. Science 1994; 265:1385–1387.

81. Austrian R. Pneumococcal polysaccharide vaccines. Rev Infect Dis 1989; 11:S598–S602.

82. Musher DM, Watson DA, Dominguez EA. Pneumococcal vaccination: work to date and future prospects. Am J Med Sci 1990; 300:45–57.

83. Wang WC, Wong WY, Rogers ZA, Wilimas JA, Buchanan GR, Powars DR. Antibiotic-resistant pneumococcal infection in children with sickle cell disease in the United States. J Pediatr Hematol/Oncol 1996; 18:140–144.

84. Taylor SC, Shacks SJ, Mitchell RA. In vitro lymphocyte blastogenic responses and cytokine production in sickle cell disease patients with acute pneumonia. Pediatr Infect Dis J 1996; 15:340–344.

85. Martin L, Buonomo C. Acute chest syndrome of sickle cell disease: radiographic and clinical analysis of 70 cases. Pediatr Radiol 1997; 27:637–641.

86. Bhalla M, Abboud MR, McLoud TC, Shepard JO, Munden MM, Jackson SM, Beaty JR, Laver JH. Acute chest syndrome in sickle cell disease: CT evidence of microvascular occlusion. Radiology 1993; 187:45–49.

87. Lisbona R, Derbekyan V, Novales-Diaz JA. Scintigraphic evidence of pulmonary vascular occlusion in sickle cell disease. J Nucl Med 1997; 38:1151–1153.

88. Babiker MA, Obeid HA, Ashong EF. Acute reversible pulmonary ischemia. A cause of the acute chest syndrome in sickle cell disease. Clin Pediatr 1985; 24:716–718.

89. Kirkpatrick MB, Haynes J, Bass JB Jr. Results of brochoscopically obtained lower airway cultures from adult sickle cell disease patients with the acute chest syndrome. Am J Med 1991; 90:206–210.

90. Godeau B, Schaeffer A, Bachir D Fleury-Feith J, Galacteros F, Verra F, Escudier E, Vaillant JN, Brun-Buisson C, Rahmoni A, Allaoui AS, Lebargy F. Bronchoalveolar lavage in adult sickle cell patients with the acute chest syndrome: value for diagnostic assessment of fat embolism. Am J Respir Crit Care Med 1996; 153:1691–1696.

91. Maitre B, Habibi A, Roudot-Thoraval F, Bachir D, Belghtti DD, Galacteros F, Godeau B. Acute chest syndrome in adults with sickle cell disease: therapeutic approach, outcome, and results of BAL in a monocentric series of 107 episodes. Chest 2000; 117:1386–1392.

92. Moser C, Nussbaum E, Cooper DM. Plastic bronchitis and the role of bronchoscopy in the acute chest syndrome of sickle cell disease. Chest 2001; 120:608–613.

93. Schuster DP. ARDS: clinical lessons from the oleic acid model of acute lung injury. Am J Respir Crit Care Med 1994; 149:245–260.

94. Green J-A, Smith GM, Buchta R, Lee R, Ho KY, Rajkovic IA, Scott KF. Circulating phospholipase A_2 activity associated with sepsis and septic shock is indistinguishable from that associated with rheumatoid arthritis. Inflammation 1991; 15:355–367.

95. Rae D, Porter J, Beechey-Newman N, Sumar N, Bennett D, Herman-Taylor J. Type I phospholipase A_2 propeptide in acute lung injury. Lancet 1994; 344: 1472–1473.

96. Styles LA, Schalkwijk CG, Aarsman AJ, Vichinsky EP, Lubin BH, Kuypers FA. Phospholipase A_2 levels in acute chest syndrome of sickle cell disease. Blood 1996; 87:2573–2578.

97. Styles LA, Aarsman AJ, Vichinsky EP, Kuypers FA. Secretory phospholipase A_2 predicts impending acute chest syndrome in sickle cell disease. Blood 2000; 96:3276–3278.

98. Johnson CS, Verdegem TV. Pulmonary complications of sickle cell disease. Semin Respir Med 1988; 9:287–293.

99. Kress JP, Pohlman AS, Hall JB. Determination of hemoglobin saturation in patients with acute sickle chest syndrome: a comparison of arterial blood gases and pulse oximetry. Chest 1999; 115:1316–1320.

100. Forte VA Jr, Malconian MK, Burse RL, Rock PB, Young PM, Trad LA, Ruscio BA, Sutton JR, Houston CS, Cymerman A. Operation Everest II: comparison of four instruments for measuring blood O_2 saturation. J Appl Physiol 1989; 67:2135–2140.

101. Barker SJ, Tremper KK. Pulse oximetry: applications and limitations. Int Anesthesiol Clin 1987; 25:155–175.

102. Ortiz FO, Aldrich TK, Nagel RL, Benjamin LJ. Accuracy of pulse oximetry in sickle cell disease. Am J Respir Crit Care Med 1999; 159:447–451.

103. Davies SC, Luce PJ, Win AA, Riordan JF, Brozovic M. Acute chest syndrome in sickle-cell disease. Lancet 1984; I:36–38.

104. Barrett-Connor E. The nonvalue of sputum culture in the diagnosis of pneumococcal pneumonia. Am Rev Respir Dis 1971; 103:845–848.

105. Dean D, Neumayr L, Kelly DM, Ballas SK, Kleman K, Robertson S, Iyer RV, Ware RE, Koshy M, Rackoff WR, Pegelow CH, Waldron P, Benjamin L, Vichinsky E. Acute Chest Syndrome Study Group. *Chlamydia pneumoniae* and acute chest syndrome in patients with sickle cell disease. J Pediatr Hematol/Oncol 2003; 25:46–55.
106. Vichinsky E, Williams R, Das M, Earles AN, Lewis N, Adler A, McQuitty J. Pulmonary fat embolism: a distinct cause of severe acute chest syndrome in sickle cell anemia. Blood 1994; 83:3107–3112.
107. Mellor A, Soni N. Fat embolism. Anaesthesia 2001; 56:145–154.
108. Haupt HM, Moore GW, Bauer TW, Hutchins GM. The lung in sickle cell disease. Chest 1982; 81:332–337.
109. Walker BK, Ballas SK, Burka ER. The diagnosis of pulmonary thromboembolism in sickle cell disease. Am J Hematol 1979; 7:219–232.
110. Bashour TT, Lindsay J Jr. Hemoglobin S-C disease presenting as acute pneumonitis with pulmonary angiographic findings in two patients. Am J Med 1975; 58:559.
111. Richards D, Nulsen FE. Angiographic media and the sickling phenomenon. Surg Forum 1971; 22:403–404.
112. Rucknagel DL, Kalinyak KA, Gelfand MJ. Rib infarcts and acute chest syndrome in sickle cell diseases. Lancet 1991; 337:831–833.
113. Gelfand MJ, Daya SA, Rucknagel DL, Kalinyak KA, Paltiel HJ. Simultaneous occurrence of rib infarction and pulmonary infiltrates in sickle cell disease patients with acute chest syndrome. J Nucl Med 1993; 34:614–618.
114. Kopecky EA, Jacobson S, Joshi P, Koren G. Systemic exposure to morphine and the risk of acute chest syndrome in sickle cell disease. Clin Pharmacol Ther 2004; 75:140–146.
115. Ammann AJ, Addiego J, Wara DW, Lubin B, Smith WB, Mentzer WC. Polyvalent pneumococcal-polysaccharide immunization of patients with sickle-cell anemia and patients with splenectomy. N Engl J Med 1977; 297:897–900.
116. Gaston MH, Verter JI, Woods G, Pegelow C, Kelleher J, Presbury G, Zarkowsky H, Vichinsky E, Iyer R, Lobel JS, Diamond S, Holbrook CT, Gill FM, Ritchey K, Falletta JM. The Prophylactic Penicillin Study Group. Prophylaxis with oral penicillin in children with sickle cell anemia. A randomized trial. N Engl J Med 1986; 314:1593–1599.
117. Lowenthal EA, Wells A, Emanuel PD, Player R, Prchal JT. Sickle cell acute chest syndrome associated with parvovirus B19 infection: case series and review. Am J Hematol 1996; 51:207–213.
118. Steinberg MH, Barton F, Castro O, Pegelow CH, Ballas SK, Kutlar A, Orringer E, Bellevue R, Olivieri N, Eckman J, et al. Effect of hydroxyurea on mortality and morbidity in adult sickle cell anemia: risks and benefits up to 9 years of treatment. JAMA 2003; 289:1645–1651.
119. Gilbert R, Keighley JF. The arterial/alveolar oxygen tension ratio: an index of gas exchange applicable to varying inspired oxygen concentrations. Am Rev Resp Dis 1974; 109:142–145.
120. Emre U, Miller ST, Rao SP, Rao M. Alveolar-arterial oxygen gradient in acute chest syndrome of sickle cell disease. J Pediatr 1993; 123:272–275.

121. Haynes J Jr, Allison RC. Pulmonary edema: complication of the management of sickle cell pain crisis. Am J Med 1986; 80:833–840.

122. Bellet PS, Kalinyak KA, Shukla R, Gelfand MJ, Rucknagel DL. Incentive spirometry to prevent acute pulmonary complications in sickle cell diseases. N Engl J Med 1995; 333:699–703.

123. Leong MA, Dampier C, Varlotta L, Allen JL. Airway hyperreactivity in children with sickle cell disease. J Pediatr 1997; 131:278–283.

124. Koumbourlis AC, Zar HJ, Hurlet-Jensen A, Goldberg MR. Prevalence and reversibility of lower airway obstruction in children with sickle cell disease. J Pediatr 2001; 138:188–192.

125. Wratney AT, Gentile MA, Hamel DS, Cheifetz IM. Successful treatment of acute chest syndrome with high-frequency oscillatory ventilation in pediatric patients. Respir Care 2004; 49:263–269.

126. Baird JS, Johnson JL, Escudero J, Powars DR. Combined pressure control/high frequency ventilation in adult respiratory distress syndrome and sickle cell anemia. Chest 1994; 106:1913–1916.

127. Pelidis MA, Kato GJ, Resar LM, Dover GJ, Nichols DG, Walker LK, Casella JF. Successful treatment of life-threatening acute chest syndrome of sickle cell disease with venovenous extracorporeal membrane oxygenation. J Pediatr Hematol/Oncol 1997; 19:459–461.

128. Trant CA Jr, Casey JR, Hansell D, Cheifetz I, Meliones JN, Ungerleider RM, Browning I, Greeley WJ. Successful use of extracorporeal membrane oxygenation in the treatment of acute chest syndrome in a child with severe sickle cell anemia. ASAIO J 1996; 42:236–239.

129. Gillett DS, Gunning KE, Sawicka EH, Bellingham AJ, Ware RJ. Life threatening sickle chest syndrome treated with extracorporeal membrane oxygenation. Br Med J (Clin Res Ed) 1987; 294:81–82.

130. Emre U, Miller ST, Gutierez M, Steiner P, Rao SP, Rao M. Effect of transfusion in acute chest syndrome of sickle cell disease. J Pediatr 1995; 127:901–904.

131. Mallouh AA, Asha M. Beneficial effect of blood transfusions in children with sickle cell disease. Am J Dis Child 1988; 142:178–182.

132. Wayne AS, Kevy SV, Nathan DG. Transfusion management of sickle cell disease. Blood 1993; 81:1109–1123.

133. Vichinsky EP, Haberkern CM, Neumayr L, Earles AN, Black D, Koshy M, Pegelow C, Abboud M, Ohene-Frempong K, Iyer RV. A comparison of conservative and aggressive transfusion regimens in the perioperative management of sickle cell disease. The Preoperative Transfusion in Sickle Cell Disease Study Group. N Engl J Med 1995; 333:206–213.

134. Petz LD, Calhoun L, Shulman I, Johnson CS, Herron CM. The sickle cell hemolytic transfusion reaction syndrome. Transfusion 1997; 37:382–392.

135. Sosler SD, Jilly BJ, Saporito C, Koshy M. A simple, practical method for reducing alloimmunization in patients with sickle cell disease. Am J Hematol 1993; 43:103–106.

136. Rosse WF, Gallagher D, Kinney TR, Castro O, Dosik H, Moohr J, Wang W, Levy PS. Transfusion and alloimmunization in sickle cell disease. The Cooperative Study of Sickle Cell Disease. Blood 1990; 76:1431–1437.

137. Rackoff WR, Ohene-Frempong K, Month S, Scott JP, Neahring B, Cohen AR. Neurologic events after partial exchange transfusion for priapism in sickle cell disease. J Pediatr 1992; 120:882–885.

138. Schmalzer EA, Lee JO, Brown AK, Usami S, Chien S. Viscosity of mixtures of sickle and normal red cells at varying hematocrit levels, implications for transfusion. Transfusion 1987; 27:228–233.

139. Powars D, Weidman JA, Odom T, Niland J, Johnson C. Sickle cell chronic lung disease: prior morbidity and the risk of pulmonary failure. Medicine (Baltimore) 1988; 67:66–76.

140. Castro O, Hoque M, Brown BD. Pulmonary hypertension in sickle cell disease: cardiac catheterization results and survival. Blood 2003; 101:1257–1261.

141. Gladwin MT, Sachdev V, Jison ML, Shizukuda Y, Plehn JF, Minter K, Brown B, Coles WA, Nichols JS, Ernst I, et al. Pulmonary hypertension as a risk factor for death in patients with sickle cell disease. N Engl J Med 2004; 350:886–895.

142. Walters MC, Patience M, Leisenring W, Rogers ZR, Aquino VM, Buchanan GR, Roberts IA, Yeager AM, Hsu L, Adamkiewicz T, Kurtzberg J, Vichinsky E, Storer B, Storb R, Sullivan KM. Multicenter investigation of bone marrow transplantation for sickle cell disease. Stable mixed hematopoietic chimerism after bone marrow transplantation for sickle cell anemia. Biol Blood Marrow Transplant 2001; 7:665–673.

143. Franson RC, Rosenthal MD. PX-52, A novel inhibitor of 14 kDa secretory and 85 kDa cytosolic phospholipases A2. Adv Exp Med Biol 1997; 400A: 365–373.

144. Bernini JC, Rogers ZR, Sandler ES, Reisch JS, Quinn CT, Buchanan GR. Beneficial effect of intravenous dexamethasone in children with mild to moderately severe acute chest syndrome complicating sickle cell disease. Blood 1998; 92:3082–3089.

145. Aziz KE, Wakefield D. Modulation of endothelial cell expression of ICAM-1, E-selectin and VCAM-1 by β-estradiol, progesterone, and dexamethasone. Cell Immunol 1996; 167:79–85.

146. Lindeque BG, Schoerman HS, Dommisse GF, Boeyens MC, Vlok AL. Fat embolism and the fat embolism syndrome: a double-blind therapeutic study. J Bone Joint Surg Br 1987; 69:128–131.

147. Schonfeld SA, Ploysongsang Y, DiLisio R, Crissman JD, Miller E, Hammerschmidt DE, Jacob HS. Fat embolism prophylaxis with corticosteroids. A prospective study in high-risk patients. Ann Intern Med 1983; 99: 438–443.

148. Griffin TC, McIntire D, Buchanan GR. High-dose intravenous methylprednisolone therapy for pain in children and adolescents with sickle cell disease. N Engl J Med 1994; 330:733.

149. Isaacs WA, Effiong CE, Ayeni O. Steroid in the prevention of painful episodes in sickle-cell disease. Lancet 1995; I:570–571.

150. Sullivan KJ, Goodwin SR, Evangelist J, Moore RD, Mehta P. Nitric oxide successfully used to treat acute chest syndrome of sickle cell disease in a young adolescent. Crit Care Med 1999; 27:2563–2568.

151. Atz AM, Wessel DL. Inhaled nitric oxide in sickle cell disease with acute chest syndrome. Anesthesiology 1997; 87:988–990.

152. Oppert M, Jorres A, Barckow D, Eckardt KU, Frei U, Kaisers U. Inhaled nitric oxide for ARDS due to sickle cell disease. Swiss Med Wkly 2004; 134: 165–167.

153. Carter C, Fisher TC, Hamai H, Johnson CS, Meiselman HJ, Nash GB, Stuart J. Hemorheological effects of a nonionic copolymer surfactant (poloxamer 188). Clin Hemorheol 1992; 12:109–120.

154. Orringer EP, Casella JF, Ataga KI, Koshy M, Adams-Graves P, Luchtman-Jones L, Wun T, Watanabe M, Shafer F, Kutlar A, et al. Purified poloxamer 188 for treatment of acute vaso-occlusive crisis of sickle cell disease: a randomized controlled trial. JAMA 2001; 286:2099–2106.

155. Khor SP, McCarthy K, Dupont M, Murray K, Timony G. Pharmacokinetics, pharmacodynamics, allometry, and dose selection of rPSGL-Ig for phase I trial. J Pharmacol Exp Ther 2000; 293:618–624.

156. Matsui NM, Borsig L, Rosen SD, Yaghmai M, Embury SH. P-selectin mediates the adhesion of sickle serythrocytes to the endothelium. Blood 2001; 98:1955–1962.

157. Hicks AER, Nolan SL, Ridger VC, Hellewell PG, Norman KE. Recombinant P-selectin glycoprotein ligand-1 directly inhibits leucocyte rolling by all 3 selectins in vivo: complete inhibition of rolling is not required for anti-inflammatory effect. Blood 2003; 101:3249–3256.

158. Kumar A, Eckman JR, Wick TM. Inhibition of plasma-mediated adherence of sickle erythrocytes to microvascular endothelium by conformationally constrained RGD-containing peptides. Am J Hematol 1996; 53:92–98.

159. Kaul DK, Tsai HM, Liu XD, Nakada MT, Nagel RL, Coller BS. Monoclonal antibodies to $\alpha_V\beta_3$(7E3 and LM609) inhibit sickle red blood cell-endothelium interactions induced by platelet-activating factor. Blood 2000; 95:368–374.

160. Lutty GA, Taomoto M, Cao J, McLeod DS, Vanderslice P, McIntyre BW, Fabry ME, Nagel RL. Inhibition of TNF-alpha-induced sickle RBC retention in retina by a VLA-4 antagonist. Invest Ophthalmol Vis Sci 2001; 42: 1349–1355.

22

Treatment of Tuberculosis in the Tropics:
An Evidence-based Review

PATRICIO ESCALANTE

Division of Pulmonary and Critical Care
   Medicine, Keck School of Medicine,
   University of Southern California,
Los Angeles, California, U.S.A.

BRENDA E. JONES

Division of Infectious Diseases, Keck
   School of Medicine, University of
   Southern California,
Los Angeles, California, U.S.A.

I. Introduction

A. Epidemiology of TB in the Tropics

Cases of tuberculosis have been increasing globally despite declining incidence rates in developed countries. The World Health Organization (WHO) reported approximately 8 million new cases of tuberculosis (TB) per year in the late 1990s (1). An estimated 1.8 million people died with TB each year worldwide, the global fatality rate is about 23%, but this figure doubles in some African countries with high prevalence of HIV and TB coinfection. Eighty percent of all new TB cases annually originated in 23 high-burden countries, located in South East Asia, the Western Pacific, Africa, and the Americas (2). This chapter will address the treatment of TB in those high-burden countries, most of them located in tropical areas.

B. Impact of the HIV Epidemics on TB Epidemics in the Tropics

The worldwide HIV epidemics worsen the TB epidemic situation, and both are concentrated most heavily in the developing world, and especially in tropical areas. Of the 36.1 million people estimated to be infected with

HIV, approximately 90% live in tropical regions of sub-Saharan Africa, South East Asia and the Americas (3). In 1999, 23 out of 24 countries with an HIV seroprevalence greater than 5% were located in sub-Saharan Africa, the other one was Haiti in the Americas (4). Other countries in tropical areas such as Myanmar, Thailand, Cambodia (South East Asia), and Surinam, Guyana, Panama, Belize, Guatemala, and Honduras also have high HIV seroprevalence in their populations (4).

C. HIV and TB Coinfection

There is evidence of increasing rates of TB cases in many countries of sub-Saharan Africa and South East Asia attributable to the effect of the HIV epidemic (5). In addition, the proportion of TB cases coinfected with HIV is rising; about 8% of all TB cases have also HIV coinfection world-wide in 1999. TB+HIV coinfection proportion is as high as 32% in the sub-Saharan Africa, but the largest number of TB+HIV coinfection is in India (1). HIV coinfection affects negatively patients infected with TB in different ways; HIV infection increases the rate of progression to active TB disease in latent TB infection (LTBI) and recently acquired TB. The rate of progression to active TB in patients with LTBI coinfected with HIV range between 5% and 15% per year, a much higher rate compared to seronegative HIV subjects (6). Recurrent TB is more frequent in HIV coinfected individuals, either by exogenous reinfection (7), especially in high TB prevalent areas, and by increasing the rate of endogenous reactiva-tion (8). TB infection is also associated with increases in the HIV viral load and lower CD4+ lymphocyte count (9). There is a higher fatality rate in TB cases in areas of high prevalence of HIV infection due to other HIV-related illnesses, and misdiagnosis of smear-negative and extrapulmonary TB cases (10). In addition, highly active antiretroviral therapy (highly active ART), the treatment of choice for HIV in developed countries, is not readily available in many areas of the tropics, and the use of highly active ART can be problematic with the concomitant use of rifampin (R), one of the main first-line TB treatment agents (11).

D. Drug Resistance in TB

Another challenge for global control of the TB epidemic is the emergence of drug resistance (DR) in a significant proportion of patients in several of the high-burden countries, including some tropical areas in South East Asia, Africa, and the Americas (12). DR is associated with poor outcomes to TB treatment, such as higher relapse rate, higher treatment failure rate, and development of multidrug-resistant TB (MDR-TB) (13). Treatment of MDR-TB and chronic forms of TB is more expensive, and less effective compared to much better outcomes in treatment of pansensitive TB cases, even in well-run TB control programs using directly observed therapy

(DOT) (14–16). The treatment of MDR-TB is also associated with more frequent and more severe side effects to second-line agents (16,17).

II. Preventive Treatment and Measurements

A. Tuberculosis Vaccination

The effectiveness of preventing TB cases by BCG vaccination varied widely worldwide; unfortunately, results of BCG trials in tropical countries have been disappointing, despite the fact that BCG vaccination can prevent disseminated forms of TB such as TB meningitis and miliary TB in children (18). Variation on BCG trials efficacy could have been related to BCG strain differences over decades (19); however, BCG study sites with a greater distance from the equator were associated with a higher efficacy; other factors directly and indirectly related to latitude such as population characteristics, environmental conditions, and vaccination quality are also suspected to account with the discrepancy among the result of the studies (20). Although complications of BCG vaccination have been described uncommonly ranging from local mild forms (21) to disseminated BCG disease, especially in children with AIDS (22), BCG vaccination has been recommended to HIV-seronegative children, and to newborn infants of HIV-seropositive mothers (23,24). However, it is estimated that TB skin testing followed by isoniazid (H) therapy for LTBI in HIV-infected individuals could be more effective than BCG vaccination (25). Nevertheless, it is postulated that a future new and highly effective TB vaccine will make a great impact in the global control of TB (25,26).

B. Treatment of Latent Tuberculosis Infection

LTBI treatment is recommended for tuberculosis prevention in high-risk groups, such as children in close contact with TB, recent PPD converters, immunosupressive conditions among others; LTBI treatment in children is not always carried out, particularly in high incidence areas in tropical countries (27,28). LTBI treatment is also indicated in HIV-infected subjects; a prospective trial in Uganda showed a risk reduction in TB cases in HIV individuals with PPD reactions of ≥ 5 mm by taking H daily for 6 months, R and H daily for 3 months, and R, H, and pyrazinamide (Z) daily for 3 months. There was no TB risk reduction with LTBI treatment in anergic PPD HIV cases (29). More side effects were noted in patients taking the multidrug regimens, particularly with Z. Further meta-analysis and decision model studies confirmed the improvement in survival and the cost effectiveness of LTBI treatment in HIV-infected individuals in sub-Saharan Africa (30,31). Concomitant anergy (i.e., candida) skin testing in addition to PPD testing is not recommended due to the variability in the results over time of both tests (32). A prospective trial found a similar treatment efficacy with the use of R and Z daily for 2 months for LTBI in comparison to H daily treatment for 12 months in HIV-infected subjects from Mexico, Haiti, Brazil, and the United States (33); however, the recommendation for treatment of LTBI with R and Z for 2 months was significantly downgraded after reports of severe liver injury in U.S. cases associated to the use of R and Z in LTBI treatments (34). Protective effect of LTBI treatment with H for 6 months lasts for at least 2.5 years in HIV-infected African individuals, but appears to have no effect on HIV progression or mortality (35). Local HIV/AIDS clinics can successfully implement LTBI treatment with H. Difficulties in excluding active tuberculosis and the costs of running the programs may limit its widespread implementation in tropical low-income areas (36).

C. Other Preventive Measurements

Nosocomial TB transmission and TB outbreaks have been described in developing countries, and sometimes associated with MDR-TB transmission (37–40). TB skin test conversion in health workers associated with nosocomial TB transmission is not uncommon in high-burden countries (41,42). Simple measurements to prevent TB nosocomial transmission in high-burden TB countries have been proposed and implemented successfully (43,44).

III. Treatment of Active Pulmonary Tuberculosis Infection

A. International Recommendations and DOT

New comprehensive guidelines for the treatment of TB have been issued by the American Thoracic Society (ATS), Centers for Disease Control (CDC), and the Infectious Disease Society of North America (ISDA) in the United States (45). These new ATS/CDC/ISDA guidelines target mostly high-income, low-incidence countries and settings where relatively well-funded public and private health infrastructure and resources are available to treat TB, which usually includes a widely implemented DOT system. The International Union Against Tuberculosis and Lung Diseases (IUATLD) and the WHO have also published guidelines for the treatment of TB (46,47), but those target low-income, high-incidence countries and settings where mycobacterial cultures, drug-susceptibility testing, chest X rays, and second-line drugs may not be available. The IUATLD and the WHO recommend the treatment of TB in the context of DOTS (directly observed treatment, short course) strategy, which implies the organization of a national TB control program or geographical organizations alike that must have the following components: government or organization commitment to sustained TB control activities; case detection by sputum smear microscopy among symptomatic patients self-reported to health services; standardized treatment regimens of 6–8 months for at least all confirmed sputum smear-positive cases with DOT; a regular uninterrupted supply of medications, and a standardized recording and reporting system that allows assessment of treatment results for each patient and the TB control program overall. Despite several exceptions in the Americas, Asia, Oceania, and Africa, most of the tropical countries, especially the ones in the sub-Saharan Africa, fall into the low-income, high-incidence category. Regardless of the setting, it is essential that treatment be planned and supervision be based on each patient's clinical and social circumstances (patient-centered care) (45). Given the relative high cost of implementing DOT in community clinics by nurses in developing countries (48,49), trained lay supervisors (50) and patient-nominated family members (51) have been reported to successfully administer DOT in tropical areas. Adequate implementation of DOTS and public control measurements have improved patient adherence to treatment and TB incidence in low-income, high-incidence countries at the national level (15), and at the local level, even in areas of high rate of HIV–TB coinfection (52). In fact, the global success rate for new sputum smear-positive cases on DOTS is 78% against 38% in cases treated under non-DOTS conditions in 1997 (46). Nevertheless, most of the high-burden TB countries located in tropical areas are still below the WHO goals of 70% for DOTS detection rate (percentage of estimated smear-positive cases notified under DOT), and 85% for treatment success (53).

B. Principles of Treatment of Active Pulmonary Tuberculosis

The authors recommend for in-depth reviews of the evidence and basis for TB treatment the following excellent publications: the recent ATS/CDC/ISDA document (44); the chapter on TB chemotherapy in the book entitled *A Clinician's Guide to Tuberculosis* by Dr. Michael D. Iseman (54); the overview of the studies on the treatment of TB undertaken by the British Medical Research Council (BMRC) tuberculosis units, between 1946 and 1986 (55); and the monograph entitled "Interventions for Tuberculosis Control and Elimination" published by Dr. Hans L. Rieder and the IUATLD (56).

The foundations of modern TB treatment is based on decades of extraordinary work carried out by the BMRC and collaborators from around the world (55,57), by the U.S. Public Health Service and the U.S. Veterans Administration (58), and by other groups from developed and developing countries (56). The main BMRC centers outside Britain included sites in tropical and subtropical countries such as Uganda, Kenya, Tanzania, Zambia, Zimbabwe, Madras—India, Hong Kong, Singapore, Trankei—South Africa, Algeria, and others (55). In brief, the main goals for the treatment of TB are the following: to cure the patient of TB; to prevent death from active TB or its late effects; to prevent relapse of TB; to decrease transmission of TB to others; and to prevent the development of acquired drug resistance (46). H, R, Z, ethambutol (E), and streptomycin (S) are considered first-line anti-TB agents; however, thioacetazone (T) is also frequently used in developed countries because of low cost, and but its use is discouraged by the WHO guidelines (46). T has less efficacy than the rifampin-contained regimes, and its use is associated with significant toxicity, especially in HIV-infected populations (54).

In general, an antimicrobial can be categorized as bactericidal or bacteriostatic; however, this concept does not apply well to the different anti-TB agents because their mode of antibacterial action varies with the variable bacterial metabolic state and the different host environment (56). Based on extensive microbiological and clinical trial data, anti-TB agents can be categorized according to the following mode of antibacterial action: (a) early bactericidal activity, defined as drug capacity to kill large amounts of TB bacilli in the first days of treatment; (b) prevention of clinical emergence of drug resistance; and (c) sterilizing activity in disease sites (54,59). The first two types of actions are mostly associated with the success of the regimen at completion of therapy; the sterilizing activity is mostly associated with relapse prevention after completion of treatment (54,59). H has the highest early bactericidal activity, followed by E, R, S, T, and Z in that order (60). H and R have the highest resistance prevention activity followed by S, and E, and in a much lesser degree, Z and T (54,59). Sterilizing activity is the highest with R; sterilization is also high with Z, but intermediate with H and S, and low with E (54,59). Extensive treatment trial data suggest that TB treatment requires the use of no less than three to four anti-TB agents in the initial part of treatment (intensive phase) to achieve a significant bacteriological response (sputum conversion) by the second month of therapy (55–57). The very original use of S as monotherapy in the sanatorium era was associated with the rapid development of S resistance, as early as 3 weeks of treatment (61). The development of acquired drug resistance on monotherapy is felt to be due to the presence of small amount of drug-resistant bacterial mutants within large volumes of bacilli in some of the host environment such as the cavitary lesions (56). The original use of two agent regimens was associated with prolonged treatment courses to achieve successful outcomes (55,62,63), with the potential for development of DR (64), especially in the setting of primary DR to at least one of the agents. The original design of three-drug regimens in the initial phase (i.e., S for the first 6 weeks, plus H and *para*-aminosalicylic in earlier studies) was associated with better treatment outcomes, including subsequent lower rate of relapse, in primary DR and pansensitive TB cases (65). As a result of many years of clinical trials and global epidemiologic data of DR (12), most authorities recommend the use of four-drug regimens with first-line agents, including H and R, and usually P and either E or S in the initial intensive phase (46,54,56), which usually last for 2 months, because of the high incidence of primary isoniazid resistance and other DR, as well as secondary DR in patients previously treated in many developing and tropical countries (12). In terms of the total treatment duration, the original introduction of R in TB treatment allowed the design of effective TB regimens of <12 months (55,66), compared with older treatment regimens (without R) of ≥12 months (55). The introduction of Z, which has mainly anti-TB activity in acidic host environments (i.e., necrotizing lesions), allowed the design of successful TB treatment regimens of even shorter duration (6-month total) (55). The use of Z for 2 months was as effective as the use of Z for 4 or 6 months (55). Treatment regimens of less than 4 months total have failed to achieve good treatment outcomes such as unacceptable high relapse rates (55).

A continuation phase follows the intensive phase, and it attempts to sterilize the residual foci of MTB infection, this phase usually includes H and another anti-TB drug(s) with sterilizing activity, and usually last 4 months to allow enough time to eradicate the low-metabolic-state bact erial remnants (54,56). A prolonged continuation phase (i.e., 6–7 months) is recommended when P is not used in the intensive phase, a rifamycin (i.e., R) is not used in the continuation phase, and/or the patient has a cavitary TB associated with a lack of AFB sputum conversion by the second month of treatment (45). TB treatment regimen without R in the continuation phase has been tested for setting where the use of this drug is not financially feasible and/or lack of DOT implementation could increase chances to develop DR, including rifampin-DR (R-DR). The first three East Africa BMRC studies established the efficacy of the affordable 8-month regimen 2SHRZ/TH, which is frequently used in developing countries that have a low incidence of HIV–TB coinfection. However, WHO discourages the use of T-contained regimens (46) because they have been associated with significant risk of toxicity in HIV-infected individuals, including cases of lethal toxic epidermal necrolysis (67). A more recent study from India also reported a reasonable efficacy of a self-administered 8-month regimen using E and H in the continuation phase (2HREZ/EH) (68). However, a cost-effectiveness analysis from the World Bank and the WHO favored the use of short course (6 months) TB regimens in the long-term because of lower failure and relapse rates (69).

Short-course intermittent dosage regimens were designed and tested in an attempt to decrease the intensity and frequency of DOT, to increase patient adherence to treatment, and to reduce cost (56). Even though, bi-weekly regimens have proven to be as effective as thrice-weekly and daily regimens under protocol conditions (55) and in developed countries (70), the WHO recommends the use of thrice-weekly regimens under DOT conditions because of the potential transient interruption of therapy and risk of treatment failure in case of missing doses in the biweekly regimens (46,56). In fact, in HIV-infected patients, especially the ones with CD4 ≤100 cells/μL, risk of failure or relapse has increased with development of acquired R-DR by using rifamycin-containing TB regimens administrated bi-weekly and once-weekly in their continuation phase (71,72). For this reason, most authorities recommend the use of R (or rifabutin) in the continuation phase by daily or thrice-weekly dosage in advanced HIV-infected individuals (45,46). WHO also recommends the use of R along with DOT because of the possibility of potential development of R-DR in the setting of poor patient adherence to treatment under non-DOT conditions (46). Treatment of R-DR and MDR-TB cases are associated with poorer treatment outcomes using short-course regimens designed for pansensitive TB cases (73). In fact, a case-control study from Peru found 75% of patients failing a short-course TB treatment ($2HREZ/4H_2R_2$) have MDR-TB, and lack of sputum AFB-smear conversion at 2 months can predict treatment failure, and therefore can detect potential MDR-TB cases (74).

C. Treatment of Extrapulmonary Tuberculosis

In general, extrapulmonary forms of TB are treated in the same way with standard short-course regimens as pulmonary TB forms (45,46,54). However, E and S can be interchanged in the initial phase, as in the case of TB meningitis (46), and the length of time of the continuation phase can be extended depending of the patient's presentation and clinical circumstances (54). In TB lymphadenitis, 6-month (Z2H6R6) regimen is as effective as the 9-month regimens (Z2H9R9 and E2H9R9) in patients with pansensitive organisms (75). TB of the spine, another frequent form of extrapulmonary TB, which is associated with significant disability, is also effectively treated with 6-month short-course therapy including H and R throughout the regimen (76,77). Although surgical debridement and radical operation have shown no additional benefit in comparison to anti-TB treatment alone (77), spinal surgery may be indicated in some cases, such as persistent and recurrent neurological symptoms, instability of the spine and cord-compression signs (45). TB of the central nervous system (CNS), especially TB meningitis is treated with anti-TB agents that can cross the blood–brain barrier (BBB) in disease state (56), H and Z cross well BBB; R and S cross less effectively the BBB, but their CSF levels are usually above the MIC for pansensitive MTB (56,78). E penetrates poorly into normal meninges or in the absence of meningeal inflammation (79), and the WHO do not recommend E in the treatment of TB meningitis (46); however, other experts do (45). Pleural TB and most forms of extrapulmonary TB can be treated effectively with standard short-course (6-month) regimens (45). However, the continuation phase of some forms of extrapulmonary TB can be extended for 7 months or more if necessary (54), such as in the case of CNS TB and some forms of bone and joint TB (45). The use of systemic steroids, in addition to effective standard short-course TB therapy, is recommended only for cases of pericardial TB and symptomatic TB meningitis (45). In fact, a randomized double-blind study in symptomatic TB pericarditis patients showed better outcomes by adding oral steroids for 11 weeks to full anti-TB treatment in South Africa (80). Another prospective study showed benefits of adjunct treatment with 6-week oral steroids in patients with TB pericarditis and HIV coinfection in Zimbabwe (81). In a randomized, double-blind, placebo-controlled trial in Vietnam the use of adjunctive treatment with dexamethasone improved survival in patients over 14 years of age with CNS/meningeal TB but probably did not prevent severe disability (163); in addition, several nonrandomized trials have showed benefit of systemic steroids as adjunct treatment for CNS/meningeal TB patients, particularly in the ones with decreased level of consciousness (45,82).

D. Treatment of Sputum AFB Smear-Negative Tuberculosis

A common scenario in developing countries is the presentation of respiratory symptomatic patients with chest X-ray findings suggestive of TB (i.e., apical infiltrates often associated with volume loss), with multiple negative sputum AFB smears, suggesting less extensive (paucibacillary) forms of pulmonary TB (54,55). Two BRMC Hong Kong studies addressed prospectively this type of sputum AFB smear-negative patients with very-short-course treatment regimens (83,84). The first study found that more than 50% of this type of patients will develop TB in 5 years follow-up, and the 2 and 3 months of treatment regimens had unacceptable high relapse rates in treating sputum AFB smear-negative and culture-positive cases (83). A second BRMC prospective study included sputum AFB smear-negative ($\times 5$), culture-negative, with diagnosis of TB by clinical-radiological response, and treated with 3 months daily $H + R + P + S$ (3HRPS), 3 months thrice weekly $H + R + P + S$ ($3I_3R_3P_3S$) and $4H_3R_3P_3S_3$ (84). The study also included another group of patients with AFB smear-negative cases with positive AFB cultures, in which the patients were treated with 4HRPS, $4H_3R_3P_3S$, and $6H_3R_3P_3S$ (84). Low relapse rates were found with all 4- and 6-month treatment regimens, regardless of the initial follow-up AFB culture results (84). However, slightly higher relapse rates were found among patients having H and/or S DR (84). In contrast, there are no data to support the use of 4-month TB treatment for sputum AFB smear-negative in HIV+TB coinfection, and therefore this very short regimen is not recommended. Of note, HIV + TB-coinfected patients can have sputum AFB smears-negative, culture-positive in a higher proportion of patients compared to HIV-seronegative individuals infected with TB (43% vs. 24%), as described in Zambia (85).

E. Treatment of Silicotuberculosis

Pulmonary TB is usually more difficult to treat in the setting of significant underlying silicosis (86). The coexistence of these two conditions (silico-TB) is not an uncommon scenario in many parts of the world where workers are exposed to silica and TB is prevalent; those locations includes

Escalante and Jones

subtropical areas such as in Hong Kong (87), India (88), Taiwan (89), Thailand (90), South Africa (91), and some parts of the Americas (92,93). A randomized trial in Hong Kong ($6H_3R_3P_3S$ vs. $8H_3R_3P_3S$) showed that a 6-month regimen was poorly effective compared to an 8-month regimen (94). $8H_3R_3P_3S$ was still less effective compared to similar therapeutic trials results in non-silico-TB cases (relapse rates around 7%) (54,55). For these reasons, silico-TB is recommended to be treated with extended treatment regimens of more than 50% of the standard duration (54).

F. Fixed-Dose Combination Treatment

The WHO also recommends the use fixed-dose combinations (FDC) anti-TB drug formulations, because of the potential advantage of a more straightforward anti-TB dosage in an attempt to decrease prescription errors, and the possibility to increase patient adherence to treatment due to a lesser burden of number of pills to the patient (46). Potential disadvantages of FDC are over- and under-dosage, and difficulties to rechallenge patients experiencing side effects to one or more of the individual agents (46). FDC may not be easily implemented at the individual level, but it has many advantages as part of larger TB control program strategy (95).

G. WHO Proposed TB Treatment Regimens for Low-Income, High-Incidence Countries (46)

1. Active pulmonary TB (WHO category I): Sputum AFB smear-positive, and sputum AFB smear-negative patients with extensive parenchymal involvement, severe concomitant HIV coinfection, and severe forms of extrapulmonary TB: *2HRZE(or S)/4HR*: Daily or thrice a week H + R + Z + E (or S) for 2 months in the intensive phase; followed by daily or thrice a week H+R for 4 months in the continuation phase (all under DOT conditions) is the preferred regimen. Alternatively, daily H+E for 6 months in the continuation phase under DOT or non-DOT conditions (2HRZE(or S)/6HE). S should be used for E in meningeal TB (continuation phase with H+R can be prolonged to 7 months in meningeal TB cases).

2. Previously treated sputum AFB smear-positive pulmonary TB (WHO category II): includes "retreatment regimen" for relapse, treatment after interruption of therapy, and treatment failure: *2HRZES/1HRZE/5HRE*: Initial phase composed by 2 months of daily or thrice weekly H + R + Z + E + S, followed by 1 month of daily or thrice weekly H + R + Z + E; followed by a continuation phase with daily or thrice weekly H + R + E for 5 months (all under DOT), initial drug susceptibility testing is also recommended whenever is possible for possibility of DR.

3. New sputum AFB smear-negative pulmonary TB and less severe forms of extrapulmonary TB (WHO category III): *2HRZE(or S)/4HR*: The same as for WHO category I, except that E (or S) could be omitted during the initial phase of treatment for patient with noncavitary, sputum AFB smear-negative, HIV-seronegative, pansensitive pulmonary TB, and young children with primary TB.

4. "Chronic" and MDR-TB cases (WHO category IV): Specially designed standardized or individualized treatment regimens under close supervision. Expert consultation is recommended. Contacts of patients with proven MDR-TB should also have early sputum AFB cultures and drug susceptibilities

H. HIV Infection and Treatment of Active Tuberculosis

In general, standard rifampin-based, short-course, daily or thrice weekly anti-TB regimens are recommended for the treatment of TB+HIV-coinfected patients (45,46,56). These recommendations are based on prospective controlled and observational trials showing acceptable rates of relapse using standard short-course regimes in patients with TB+HIV coinfection (45,56,96). However, a review of the most relevant studies suggest that 6-month regimens had different cure rate and relative low treatment effectiveness despite having similar relapse rates, and most of the studies showed a significant all-cause mortality (range 20–41.1%) (96). In fact, the increased mortality in HIV + TB coinfection is largely due to opportunistic infections other than TB in Africa (97,98). One randomized trial from Central Africa showed better treatment outcomes with an extended (12-month) regimen compared with a 6-month one (recurrent rate of 3% vs. 9%, respectively); however, nonadherence issues, differences in CD4+ counts, and potential exogenous reinfection could have influenced the results of this study and others (46,96,99). The use of non-rifampin based anti-TB regimens have been associated with poor treatment outcomes in African patients with TB+HIV coinfection (100). Anti-TB drugs malabsorption and low serum drug concentrations have been described in TB+HIV-coinfected patients (101,102), which can be associated with poor response to therapy (101) and potential development of DR (103). However, anti-TB drugs malabsorption appears not to be a widespread problem among TB + HIV-coinfected patients in Africa (71,104). The management of HIV and TB coinfection is complicated by potential drug interactions between the rifamycins and antiretroviral therapy (ART). In addition, immune reconstitution syndromes, manifested by paradoxical clinical and/or radiological worsening, may also occur during anti-TB and ARV therapy, and these paradoxical reactions can be more often seen in TB+HIV-coinfected patient on ARV compared with HIV-seronegative TB patients and TB+HIV-coinfected ones without ART (104). Expert opinion suggests the use of systemic steroids for 1–2 weeks as treatment of symptomatic paradoxical reactions (45).

A study in the United States suggests that intermittent (once or twice weekly) therapy, including H and a rifamycin, increases the risk for acquired rifamycin resistance among TB patients with advanced HIV coinfection (71). Current guidelines recommend that patients with HIV+TB and CD4+ cell counts $<100/mm^3$ not be treated with highly intermittent (i.e., once or twice weekly) regimens (45). These patients should receive daily therapy during the intensive phase and at least three doses a week during the continuation phase administered by DOT (105). In addition, a prospective randomized study in Haiti, showed a reduced rate of recurrent TB in TB+HIV-coinfected patients taking H for 1 year after a 6-month anti-TB treatment in comparison to TB+HIV coinfection patients taking placebo (8). HIV-seronegative patients also had a low rate of recurrent TB after short-course therapy in a high incidence area such as Haiti. Symptomatic TB+HIV-coinfected patients appeared to have higher chances to develop recurrent TB after completion of short-course therapy (8).

The advent of highly active ART has dramatically improved the clinical outcome of HIV infection, decreasing death and opportunistic infections by 60–90% (106). The initiation of ART prior to the completion of anti-TB therapy improves outcomes in patients coinfected with TB+HIV in Asia and Africa (107,108). The risk for TB infection is further reduced in HIV-infected patients in ART in developed countries (109,110). Revised WHO guidelines recommend that for patients with CD4+ cells <200, ART be started as soon as TB treatment is tolerated (between 2 weeks and 2 months), and efaverenz (EFZ) containing regimens are recommended (111). For patients with CD4+ cells between 200 and $350\,mm^3$, it is recommended that ART be started after the initiation phase of TB therapy (unless severely immuncompromised), with EFZ containing regimens, or nevirapine (NVP) containing regimens in case of rifampicin-free continuation phase TB treatment regimen (111). For patients with CD4 cells $>350\,mm^3$, it is recommended that ART be deferred. In the absence of CD4 cell counts, it is recommended that ART be started on TB + HIV-coinfected patients (111). Timing of ART initiation should be up to clinical judgment based on other signs of immunodeficiency (111). Despite these WHO-proposed ART recommendations, cost-effectiveness analysis suggests a much better value for the invested money with interventions targeting on prevention of HIV infection and treatment of TB cases in Africa (112).

Because of possible drug interactions, dose adjustments may be necessary when ART is administered with rifamycin-based regimens for the treatment of TB (45,105). R is a potent cytochrome P450 inducer that can cause enhanced drug metabolism in patients and may lead to subtherapeutic levels of many protease inhibitors (PIs) and non-nucleoside reverse transcriptase inhibitors (NNRTIs) (105). Updated guidelines for the use of

rifamycins for the treatment of TB among HIV-infected patients taking protease inhibitors or non-nucleoside reverse transcriptase inhibitors were
recently published by the CDC (105). The CDC recommends the use of
R in limited situations in patients on ART regimens, including efavirenz
(increased to 800 mg) and two nucleoside reverse transcriptase inhibitors
(NRTIs) (105). The CDC also recommends the use of rifabutin, a less
potent inducer of cytochrome P450, as a substitute for R for TB patients
on ART (105). For patients on efavirenz, it is recommended that rifabutin
be increased to 450 mg/day or 600 mg 3×/week) (105). Although it is
expensive and not readily available in most tropical countries, rifabutin
potentially allows for more treatment options in patients receiving ART
(113). Rifabutin-based regimens appear to be as effective as rifampin-based
regimens for patients with TB and *Mycobacterium africanum* infection coinfected with HIV in Africans (114).

The success of the DOTS strategy for treating TB could serve as a
model for implementing ART in developing countries (115). Expert panels
have been suggested that TB+HIV-coinfected TB patients could receive
anti-TB drugs and ARV drugs in TB or HIV clinics (111). A joint approach
to treat TB patients with antiretrovirals could potentially be beneficial for
the treatment of both infections. However, this proposed approach
will require safely testing and validation in the field before widespread
recommendations.

I. Treatment of MDR-TB Infection

Treatment for MDR-TB requires the use of second-line agents and is more
costly, and usually associated with more drug toxicity, and more extended
treatment regimens compared to standard short-course regimens for pansensitive TB patients (116). Treatment for MDR-TB, especially in their
chronic forms, is usually associated with suboptimal treatment outcomes
as compared to treatment of pansensitive TB cases even in developed
countries settings (117). Standardized retreatment regimens were designed to
treat patients who failed standard regimens for nonadherence issues, were
treated incompletely in the past, or relapse to first-line treatment regimes,
in settings where the chances for MDR-TB were low and access to reliable
drug-susceptibility testing was limited (46,55). In the past, patients who
relapse usually were still drug-sensitive to first-line agents and standardized
retreatment regimes were successful (55). However, there is increasing prevalence of DR in patients previously treated in some areas of the world (12),
and standardized retreatment regimes may no longer be effective in those
scenarios (118). In fact, except for a few retrospective studies (119,120),
treatment outcomes for MDR-TB with standardized short-course, retreatment, and empirical regimens have been disappointed in developing and
tropical countries (14,73,121–124). Cost-benefit model analysis favored

the use of individualized treatment regimens based on good-quality drug-susceptibility testing (125), which is the standard of care in developed countries (45), instead of empirical treatment regimens commonly used in developing countries (116). Recently, an optimized and individualized treatment approach for MDR-TB cases using DOT (DOT-Plus) was associated with relatively better treatment outcomes in Peru (126) compared to prior studies with similar populations (14,121). Prior to the internationally funded implementation of "DOT-Plus" in Peru, the Peruvian TB control program used individualized and standardized under DOT strategy for MDR-TB cases, but lacked adequate financial resources to implement a comprehensive treatment program for MDR-TB cases, including reliable laboratory support and good availability of second-line anti-TB drugs (personal communication). Among the interventions to implement effective DOT-Plus in Peru, those included improvement of already existing DOT infrastructure and resources, supporting the involved medical and nonmedical personnel, assuring availability of second-line anti-TB drugs early during the therapy, optimizing drug-susceptibility testing and reporting, enhancing mechanisms of community-base support for patients and their families, and warranting appropriate level of funding for the duration of the program (126,127). However, the potential implementation of MDR-TB treatment programs under DOTS-Plus, in already a well-run DOTS program, could theoretically shift significant resources from DOTS programs targeting mostly pansensitive TB cases towards DOTS-Plus for MDR-TB cases, potentially weakening existing pansensitive DOTS program coverage (128).

Ideally, treatment regimens for MDR-TB require an expert consultation usually planned in a referral center (45,56,116). The treatment regimen chosen should be individualized based on reliable drug susceptibility testing, and patient's response and tolerance to therapy should be closely monitored and followed up because of potential significant drug side effects (45,116). This type of comprehensive treatment plan is expensive and very difficult to be carried out in resource-poor settings (116,129); however, new international initiatives are under way to enable countries with resource-poor settings to have availability of second-line drugs, financial and technical assistance to manage MDR-TB cases under TB control programs conditions (DOTS-Plus) (130,131). There is controversy about the optimal number (3,4,5, or 6) of anti-TB agents to be used for the initial phase of the MDR-TB treatment regimens (45,115,132,133). In the absence of randomized data, prior prospective treatment trials designed without effective first-line agents in their regimens could help us to conceptualize a reasonable therapeutic strategy (55). A BMRC East Africa trial tested daily three-drug treatment regimes with and without R (6SHR, 6SHZ, 6SHT, 6SH, 2STH/16TH) in pansensitive TB cases (134); relapse rates were much better with 6SHR (3%), and 6SHZ (8%), but 6SHT and 6HT regimens were associated with 22% and 29% relapse rates, respectively (134). The standard daily 18-month (2STH/16TH) comparison regimen used at the time had a relapse rate of 3% (134). These data suggest that in the absence of R and Z, short-course three-drug regimens including H and S had sub-optimal treatment outcomes, and these relatively weak therapeutic regimens required extended treatment courses to be effective. In addition, in the absence of H because of suspected acquired H resistance, the use of two-drug second-line retreatment regimen (effectively without H and R) were associated with poor treatment outcomes at 12 months (55). All these data suggest that in the absence of H and R, the use of only two-drug second-line treatment regimens is inadequate, more so if no first-line agents are used. However, in the absence of H+R, a retreatment regimen using three drugs, but including two other first-line and second-line agents (E + Z + cycloserine), was associated with favorable treatment outcomes in Hong Kong under protocol conditions (55,160). These data suggest that in the absence of H + R, retreatment regimes for susceptible E and Z TB strains could be successfully treated with three-drug EZ-containing regimens. However, the effectiveness of three-drug retreatment regimens for all first-line resistant TB is unknown, and there are concerns about potential poor long-term outcomes and development of further acquired resistance in the field (amplification effect) (132), especially in cases with significant cavitary and fibrotic disease with large bacterial load. Current expert opinion favored the use of five to six anti-TB drugs for which the MTB isolate is susceptible to, especially in chronic-cavitary forms, and in the presence of resistance to all first-line agents (45,116). Treatment outcomes of chronic forms of MDR-TB (117) are not as good as treatment outcomes of more acute MDR-TB forms, even in the presence of HIV coinfection (135,136), as described in developed countries studies. Besides aminoglycosides, capreopycin, and other second-line agents, most fluoroquinolones (FQ) have shown significant activity against pansensitive TB and MDR-TB strains (137–139). Successful MDR-TB treatment regimens using FQ have been reported but no prospective randomized studies are available (121,141–143). However, recent reports of FQ resistance have been described (144,145). In addition, expert opinion recommends surgical treatment for resectable and localized forms of chronic MDR-TB in adequate surgical candidates, more so if the disease can be at least partially contained by medical treatment (45,116). However, surgical treatment requires a specialized surgical expertise, dedicated postoperative care, and individualized MDR-TB treatment follow-up for this type of difficult cases (116), conditions that are probably not readily available in most resources-poor countries. MDR-TB treatment duration is usually extended; expert opinion recommends continuation of treatment for at least 2 years after achieving sputum AFB culture conversion (45,116). Chronic forms of MDR-TB should be followed up after treatment completion for potential relapse (117).

J. Adjuvant Immunotherapy in Tuberculosis

Researchers have attempted to upregulate the patient's immune response to TB infection to improve treatment outcomes with short-course anti-TB regimens. Trial results have been disappointing for *Mycobacterium vacae* vaccination (146,147), interleukin-12 (148), and anti-TNFα treatments (149) in blinded randomized studies in Africa, despite preliminary favorable data. However, inhaled γ-interferon has been reported to temporarily improve body weight, CT scan findings, and sputum bacteriology testing in MDR-TB cases (150). Inhaled γ-interferon is expensive and no long-term outcome data are available at the time. Treatment of coexisting intestinal parasitic disease could potentially be beneficial not only to improve nutritional status but also to shift theoretically the Th2 immune response associated with parasitic conditions, towards a more effective Th1 response against TB infection (151,161). Malnutrition and vitamin D deficiency are associated with increased susceptibility to TB (152). Adequate nutritional support, including adequate vitamin supplementation (153), is probably a good immunotherapy option in resource-poor countries. Screening for HIV coinfection and ART is also recommended if this therapeutic option is available in resource-poor settings (111).

IV. Future Directions

The main goal of global tuberculosis (TB) control in the next decade is to dramatically reduce TB deaths, TB incidence, and to limit the average duration of illness (26) and ongoing transmission, especially in areas of high prevalence of TB + HIV coinfection (154). The best possible application of short-course therapy has the potential to decrease the TB burden by more than 50% in 10 years (26). However, common therapeutic errors (155) and nonuniversal application of DOTS continue increasing the risk for DR and MDR-TB, further complicating resource-poor countries in their efforts to control TB in their communities (personal communication). In some urban resource-poor countries, new strategies integrating private practitioners in TB control programs are under way (162). International technical and financial supports to further expand the DOTS implementation in high TB prevalence communities are also in progress, potentially limiting further spread of DR (130,131). High incidence TB + HIV countries pose a particular and enormous challenge, which require different strategies to control TB compared to low-HIV prevalence countries (154). Integrations of TB and HIV public health efforts and individual treatment interventions have been suggested, but further validation studies in resource-poor countries are needed (111,154). Although DOTS alone has been felt to be unlikely to control tuberculosis in sub-Saharan Africa, containment of spread of DR is a major accomplishment in those populations (154). Moreover, new and more intensive strategies are needed to interrupt on-going transmission and prevention of reactivation TB + HIV-infected populations (154). The emergence of DR is threatening TB control efforts in various areas of the world, including subtropical areas in Asia, the Americas, and Africa, but also in the former Soviet Union (156). Optimization of current treatment strategies with shortened and more simplified treatment regimens could improve the implementation of DOTS and further containing the emergence of DR (156). Improvement in access to adequate laboratory testing and second-line agents for regional specialized centers could further help to implement treatment program for DR patients in many resource-poor countries (157). Research in new and affordable techniques to optimize the prompt detection of DR cases in the field could further enhance efforts to control this problem (158). More research is also needed in development and validation of new effective anti-TB agents, and in a different class of agents that could effectively enhance protective human immune response and containment against TB infection, and potentially treating DR infections immunologically (156). Along these lines, an effective TB vaccine will greatly enhance prevention efforts in populations at risk for TB infection and disease progression (159). In fact, intensive research and validation studies with new TB vaccines candidates are under way (159). Finally, in the absence of an effective TB vaccine, tuberculosis infection will probably persist in many areas of our planet for much longer.

References

1. Dye C, Scheele S, Dolin P, Pathania V, Raviglione MC, for the WHO Global Surveillance, Monitoring Project. Global burden of tuberculosis; estimated incidence, prevalence and mortality by country. JAMA 1999; 282:677–686.
2. Anonymous. Global Tuberculosis Control. WHO Report 2001. Geneva: World Health Organization, 2001.
3. Anonymous. AIDS Epidemic Update: December 2000. Geneva: UNAIDS, 2000.
4. Anonymous. Report on the Global HIV/AIDS Epidemic, June 2000. Geneva: UNAIDS, 2000.
5. Bleed D, Dye C, Raviglione MC. Dynamics and control of the global tuberculosis epidemic. Curr Opin Pulm Med 2000; 6:174–179.
6. Raviglione MC, Harries AD, Msiska R, Wilkinson D, Nunn P. Tuberculosis and HIV: current status in Africa. AIDS 1997; 11(suppl B):S115–S123.
7. Small PM, Shafer RW, Hopewell PC, Singh SP, Murphy MJ, Desmond E, Sierra MF, Schoolnik GK. Exogenous reinfection with multidrug-resistant *Mycobacterium tuberculosis* in patients with advanced HIV infection. N Engl J Med 1993; 328:1137–1144.
8. Fitzgerald DW, Desvarieux M, Severe P, Joseph P, Johnson WD Jr, Pape JW. Effect of post-treatment isoniazid on prevention of recurrent tuberculosis in HIV-1-infected individuals: a randomized trial. Lancet 2000; 356:1470–1474.

9. Del Amo J, Malin AS, Pozniak A, De Cock KM. Does tuberculosis accelerate the progression of HIV disease? Evidence from basic science and epidemiology. AIDS 1999; 13:1151–1158.

10. Mukadi YD, Maher D, Harries A. Tuberculosis case fatality rates in high HIV prevalence populations in sub-Saharan Africa. AIDS 2001; 15:143–152.

11. Anonymous. Prevention and treatment of tuberculosis among patients infected with human immunodeficiency virus: principles of therapy and revised recommendations. Centers for Disease Control and Prevention. Morb Mortal Wkly Rep 1998; 47:1–58.

12. Pablos-Mendez A, Raviglione MC, Laszlo A, Binkin N, Rieder HL, Bustreo F, Cohn DL, Lambregts-van Weezenbeek CS, Kim SJ, Chaulet P, Nunn P. Global surveillance for antituberculosis-drug resistance, 1994–1997. World Health Organization-International Union against Tuberculosis and Lung Disease Working Group on Anti-Tuberculosis Drug Resistance Surveillance. N Engl J Med 1998; 338:1641–1649.

13. Quy HT, Lan NT, Borgdorff MW, Grosset J, Linh PD, Tung LB, van Soolingen D, Raviglione M, Co NV, Broekmans J. Drug resistance among failure and relapse cases of tuberculosis: is the standard re-treatment regimen adequate?. Int J Tuberc Lung Dis 2003; 7:631–636.

14. Suarez PG, Floyd K, Portocarrero J, Alarcon E, Rapiti E, Ramos G, Bonilla C, Sabogal I, Aranda I, Dye C, Raviglione M, Espinal MA. Feasibility and cost-effectiveness of standardised second-line drug treatment for chronic tuberculosis patients: a national cohort study in Peru. Lancet 2002; 359: 1980–1989.

15. Suarez PG, Watt CJ, Alarcon E, Portocarrero J, Zavala D, Canales R, Luelmo F, Espinal MA, Dye C. The dynamics of tuberculosis in response to 10 years of intensive control effort in Peru. J Infect Dis 2001; 184:473–478.

16. Furin JJ, Mitnick CD, Shin SS, Bayona J, Becerra MC, Singler JM, Alcantara F, Castanieda C, Sanchez E, Acha J, Farmer PE, Kim JY. Occurrence of serious adverse effects in patients receiving community-based therapy for multidrug-resistant tuberculosis. Int J Tuberc Lung Dis 2001; 5:648–655.

17. Yew WW, Chan CK, Chau CH, Tam CM, Leung CC, Wong PC, Lee J. Outcomes of patients with multidrug-resistant pulmonary tuberculosis treated with ofloxacin/levofloxacin-containing regimens. Chest 2000; 117:744–751.

18. Colditz GA, Brewer TF, Berkey CS, Wilson ME, Burdick E, Fineberg HV, Mosteller F. Efficacy of BCG vaccine in the prevention of tuberculosis. Meta-analysis of the published literature. JAMA 1994; 271:698–702.

19. Brewer TF, Colditz GA. Relationship between bacille Calmette-Guerin (BCG) strains and the efficacy of BCG vaccine in the prevention of tuberculosis. Clin Infect Dis 1995; 20:126–135.

20. Wilson ME, Fineberg HV, Colditz GA. Geographic latitude and the efficacy of bacillus Calmette-Guerin vaccine. Clin Infect Dis 1995; 20:982–991.

21. O'Brien KL, Ruff AJ, Louis MA, Desormeaux J, Joseph DJ, McBrien M, Coberly J, Boulos R, Halsey NA. Bacillus Calmette-Guerin complications in children born to HIV-1-infected women with a review of the literature. Pediatrics 1995; 95:414–418.

22. Talbot EA, Perkins MD, Silva SF, Frothingham R. Disseminated bacille Calmette-Guerin disease after vaccination: case report and review. Clin Infect Dis 1997; 24:1139–1146.

23. Cohn DL. Use of the bacille Calmette-Guerin vaccination for the prevention of tuberculosis: renewed interest in an old vaccine. Am J Med Sci 1997; 313:372–376.

24. Thaithumyanon P, Thisyakorn U, Punnahitananda S, Praisuwanna P, Ruxrungtham K. Safety and immunogenicity of bacillus Calmette-Guerin vaccine in children born to HIV-1 infected women. Southeast Asian J Trop Med Public Health 2000; 31:482–486.

25. Sterling TR, Brehm WT, Moore RD, Chaisson RE. Tuberculosis vaccination versus isoniazid preventive therapy: a decision analysis to determine the preferred strategy of tuberculosis prevention in HIV-infected adults in the developing world. Int J Tuberc Lung Dis 1999; 3:248–254.

26. Dye C. Tuberculosis 2000–2010: control, but not elimination. Int J Tuberc Lung Dis 2000; 4(12 suppl 2):S146–S152.

27. Shingadia D, Novelli V. Diagnosis and treatment of tuberculosis in children. Lancet Infect Dis 2003; 3:624–632.

28. Claessens NJ, Gausi FF, Meijnen S, Weismuller MM, Salaniponi FM, Harries AD. Screening childhood contacts of patients with smear-positive pulmonary tuberculosis in Malawi. Int J Tuberc Lung Dis 2002; 6:362–364.

29. Whalen CC, Johnson JL, Okwera A, Hom DL, Huebner R, Mugyenyi P, Mugerwa RD, Ellner JJ. A trial of three regimens to prevent tuberculosis in Ugandan adults infected with the human immunodeficiency virus. Uganda-Case Western Reserve University Research Collaboration. N Engl J Med 1997; 337:801–808.

30. Bucher HC, Griffith LE, Guyatt GH, Sudre P, Naef M, Sendi P, Battegay M. Isoniazid prophylaxis for tuberculosis in HIV infection: a meta-analysis of randomized controlled trials. AIDS 1999; 13:501–507.

31. Bell JC, Rose DN, Sacks HS. Tuberculosis preventive therapy for HIV-infected people in sub-Saharan Africa is cost-effective. AIDS 1999; 13:1549–1556.

32. Johnson JL, Nyole S, Okwera A, Whalen CC, Nsubuga P, Pekovic V, Huebner R, Wallis RS, Mugyenyi PN, Mugerwa RD, Ellner JJ. Instability of tuberculin and candida skin test reactivity in HIV-infected Ugandans. The Uganda-Case Western Reserve University Research Collaboration. Am J Respir Crit Care Med 1998; 158:1790–1796.

33. Gordin F, Chaisson RE, Matts JP, Miller C, de Lourdes Garcia M, Hafner R, Valdespino JL, Coberly J, Schechter M, Klukowicz AJ, Barry MA, O'Brien RJ. Rifampin and pyrazinamide vs isoniazid for prevention of tuberculosis in HIV-infected persons: an international randomized trial. Terry Beirn Community Programs for Clinical Research on AIDS, the Adult AIDS Clinical Trials Group, the Pan American Health Organization, and the Centers for Disease Control and Prevention Study Group. JAMA 2000; 283:1445–1450.

34. Centers for Disease Control and Prevention (CDC), American Thoracic Society. Update: adverse event data and revised American Thoracic Society/CDC recommendations against the use of rifampin and pyrazinamide

for treatment of latent tuberculosis infection—United States, 2003. MMWR Morb Mortal Wkly Rep 2003; 52:735–739.

35. Quigley MA, Mwinga A, Hosp M, Lisse I, Fuchs D, Porter JDH, Godfrey-Faussett P. Long-term effect of preventive therapy for tuberculosis in a cohort of HIV-infected Zambian adults. AIDS 2001; 15:215–222.

36. Lugada ES, Watera C, Nakiyingi J, Elliott A, Brink A, Nanyunja M, French N, Antivelink L, Gilks C, Whitworth J. Operational assessment of isoniazid prophylaxis in a community AIDS service organization in Uganda. Int J Tuberc Lung Dis 2002; 6:326–331.

37. Sacks LV, Pendle S, Orlovic D, Blumberg L, Constantinou C. A comparison of outbreak- and nonoutbreak-related multidrug-resistant tuberculosis among human immunodeficiency virus-infected patients in a South African hospital. Clin Infect Dis 1999; 29:96–101.

38. de Kantor IN, Latini O, Barrera L. Resistance and multiresistance to antitubercular drugs in Argentina and in other Latin American countries [Spanish]. Medicina (B. Aires) 1998; 58:202–208.

39. Gonzalez Montaner LJ, Alberti F, Palmero D. Multidrug-resistant tuberculosis associated with AIDS (kinetics of nosocomial epidemics of multidrug-resistant tuberculosis associated with AIDS. Possible transformation into endemic disease) [French]. Bull Acad Natl Med 1999; 183:1085–1094.

40. Campos PE. Multidrug-resistant *Mycobacterium tuberculosis* in HIV-infected persons, Peru. Emerg Infect Dis 2003; 9:1571–1578.

41. Silva VM, Cunha AJ, Oliveira JR, Figueira MM, Nunes ZB, DeRiemer K, Kritski AL. Medical students at risk of nosocomial transmission of *Mycobacterium tuberculosis*. Int J Tuberc Lung Dis 2000; 4:420–426.

42. Garcia-Garcia ML, Jimenez-Corona A, Jimenez-Corona ME, Ferreyra-Reyes L, Martinez K, Rivera-Chavira B, Martinez-Tapia ME, Valenzuela-Miramontes E, Palacios-Martinez M, Juarez-Sandino L, Valdespino-Gomez JL. Factors associated with tuberculin reactivity in two general hospitals in Mexico. Infect Control Hosp Epidemiol 2001; 22:88–93.

43. Harries AD, Maher D, Nunn P. Practical and affordable measures for the protection of health care workers from tuberculosis in low-income countries. Bull World Health Organ 1997; 75:477–489.

44. Yanai H, Limpakarnjanarat K, Uthaivoravit W, Mastro TD, Mori T, Tappero JW. Risk of *Mycobacterium tuberculosis* infection and disease among health care workers, Chiang Rai, Thailand. Int J Tuberc Lung Dis 2003; 7:36–45.

45. Blumberg HM, Burman WJ, Chaisson RE, Daley CL, Etkind SC, Friedman LN, Fujiwara P, Grzemska M, Hopewell PC, Iseman MD, et al. American Thoracic Society, Centers for Disease Control and Prevention and the Infectious Diseases Society: treatment of tuberculosis. Am J Respir Crit Care Med 2003; 167:603–662.

46. Maher D, Chaulet P, Spinaci S, Harries A. Treatment of Tuberculosis: Guidelines for National Programmes. 2nd ed. WHO/TB/97.220. World Health Organization, Geneva, Switzerland, 1997.

47. Enarson DA, Rieder HL, Arnadottir T, Trébucq A. In: Management of Tuberculosis. A Guide for Low Income Countries. 5th ed. Paris: International Union against Tuberculosis and Lung Disease, 2000:1–89.

48. Wyss K, Kilima P, Lorenz N. Cost of tuberculosis for households and health-care providers in Dar es Salaam, Tanzania. Trop Med Int Health 2001; 6: 60–68.
49. Bevan E. Tuberculosis treatment is expensive for patients in developing countries. BMJ 1997; 315:187–188.
50. Wilkinson D. High-compliance tuberculosis treatment program in a rural community. Lancet 1994; 343:647–648.
51. Manders A, Banerjee A, van den Borne HW, Harries AD, Kok GJ, Salaniponi FM. Can guardians supervise tuberculosis treatment as well as health workers? A study of adherence during the intensive phase. Int J Tuberc Lung Dis 2001; 5:838–842.
52. Kelly PM. Local problems, local solutions: improving tuberculosis control at the district level in Malawi. Bull World Health Org 2001; 79:111–117.
53. Dye C, Watt CJ, Bleed D. Low access to a highly effective therapy: a challenge for international tuberculosis control. Bull World Health Org 2002; 80:437–444.
54. Iseman MD. Tuberculosis chemotherapy, including directly observed therapy. In: A Clinician's Guide to Tuberculosis. Philadelphia, PA, USA: Lippincott Williams &Wilkins, 2000:271–321.
55. Fox W, Ellard GA, Mitchinson DA. Studies on the treatment of TB undertaken by the British Medical Research Council tuberculosis units, 1946–1986, with relevant subsequent publications. Int J Tuberc Lung Dis 1999; 3(suppl 2):S231–S279.
56. Rieder HL. Interventions for Tuberculosis Control and Elimination. Paris: International Union against Tuberculosis and Lung Disease, 2002:1–215.
57. Iseman Md, Sbarbaro JA. Short-course chemotherapy of tuberculosis. Hail Britannia (and friends). Editorial. Am Rev Respir Dis 1991; 143:697–698.
58. O'Brien RJ, Vernon AA. New tuberculosis drug development. How can we do better? (Editorial). Am J Respir Crit Care Med 1998; 157:1705–1707.
59. Mitchison DA. The action of antituberculosis drugs in short-course chemotherapy. Tubercle 1985; 66:219–225.
60. Jindani A, Aber VR, Edwards EA, Mitchison DA. The early bactericidal activity of drugs in patients with pulmonary tuberculosis. Am Rev Respir Dis 1980; 121:939–949.
61. British Medical Research Council. Streptomycin treatment of pulmonary tuberculosis. A Medical Research Council investigation. Br Med J 1948; 2: 769–783.
62. Medical Research Council. Treatment of pulmonary tuberculosis with streptomycin and para-aminosalicylic acid. Br Med J 1950; 2:1073–1085.
63. Fox W, Southerland I. A five-year assessment of patients in a controlled trial of streptomycin, para-aminosalicylic acid, and streptomycin plus para-aminosalicylic acid, in pulmonary tuberculosis. Q J Med 1956; 25:221–243.
64. Medical Research Council. Emergence of bacterial resistance in pulmonary tuberculosis under treatment with isoniazid, streptomycin plus PAS, and streptomycin plus isoniazid. Lancet 1953; 2:217–307.
65. Medical Research Council. Long-term chemotherapy in the treatment of chronic pulmonary tuberculosis with cavitation. Tubercle 1962; 43:201–267.
66. Fox W. The current status of short-course chemotherapy. Tubercle 1979; 60:177–190.

67. Nunn P, Kibuga D, Gathua S, Brindle R, Imalingat A, Wasunna K, Lucas S, Gilks C, Omwega M, Were J, et al. Cutaneous hypersensitivity reactions due to thiacetazone in HIV-1 seropositive patients treated for tuberculosis. Lancet 1991; 337:627–630.
68. Tuberculosis Research Centre Chennai. A controlled clinical trial of oral short-course regimens in the treatment of sputum-positive pulmonary tuberculosis. Int J Tuberc Lung Dis 1997; 1:509–517.
69. Murray CJL, Styblo K, Rouillon A. Tuberculosis in developing countries: burden, interventions and cost. Bull Int Union Tuberc Lung Dis 1990; 65:33–74.
70. Cohn DL, Catlin BJ, Peterson KL, Judson FN, Sbarbaro JA. A 62-dose, 6-month therapy for pulmonary and extrapulmonary tuberculosis. A twice-weekly, directly observed, and cost-effective regimen. Ann Intern Med 1990; 112:407–415.
71. Vernon A, Burman W, Benator D, Khan A, Bozeman L. Acquired rifamycin monoresistance in patients with HIV-related tuberculosis treated with once-weekly rifapentine and isoniazid. Tuberculosis Trials Consortium. Lancet 1999; 353:1843–1847.
72. El-Sadr WM, Perlman DC, Matts JP, Nelson ET, Cohn DL, Salomon N, Olibrice M, Medard F, Chirgwin KD, Mildvan D, Jones BE, Telzak EE, Klein O, Heifets L, Hafner R. Evaluation of an intensive intermittent-induction regimen and duration of short-course treatment for human immunodeficiency virus-related pulmonary tuberculosis. Terry Beirn Community Programs for Clinical Research on AIDS (CPCRA) and the AIDS Clinical Trials Group (ACTG). Clin Infect Dis 1998; 26:1148–1158.
73. Espinal MA, Kim SJ, Suarez PG, Kam KM, Khomenko AG, Migliori GB, Baez J, Kochi A, Dye C, Raviglione MC. Standard short-course chemotherapy for drug-resistant tuberculosis: treatment outcomes in 6 countries. JAMA 2000; 283:2537–2545.
74. Chavez Pachas AM, Blank R, Smith Fawzi MC, Bayona J, Becerra MC, Mitnick CD. Identifying early treatment failure on category I therapy for pulmonary tuberculosis in Lima Ciudad, Peru. Int J Tuberc Lung Dis 2004; 8:52–58.
75. Campbell IA, Ormerod LP, Friend JA, Jenkins PA, Prescott RJ. Six months versus nine months chemotherapy for tuberculosis of lymph nodes: final results. Respir Med 1993; 87:621–623.
76. Medical Research Council. A 15-year assessment of controlled trials of the management of tuberculosis of the spine in Korea and Hong Kong. Thirteenth Report of the Medical Research Council Working Party on Tuberculosis of the Spine. J Bone Joint Surg Br 1998; 80-B:456–462.
77. Medical Research Council. Five-year assessment of controlled trials of short-course chemotherapy of 6, 9, or 18 months duration for spinal tuberculosis in patients ambulatory from the start or undergoing radical surgery. Fourteenth Report of the Medical Research Council Working Party on Tuberculosis of the Spine. Int Orthop 1999; 23:73–81.
78. Ellard GA, Humphries MJ, Allen BW. Cerebrospinal fluid drug concentrations and the treatment of tuberculous meningitis. Am Rev Respir Dis 1993; 148: 650–655.

79. Place VA, Pyle MM, De la Huerga J. Ethambutol in tuberculous meningitis. Am Rev Respir Dis 1969; 99:783–785.

80. Strang JI, Kakaza HH, Gibson DG, Allen BW, Mitchison DA, Evans DJ, Girling DJ, Nunn AJ, Fox W. Controlled clinical trial of complete open surgical drainage and of prednisolone in treatment of tuberculous pericardial effusion in Transkei. Lancet 1988; 2:759–764.

81. Hakim JG, Ternouth I, Mushangi E, Siziya S, Robertson V, Malin A. Double blind randomised placebo controlled trial of adjunctive prednisolone in the treatment of effusive tuberculous pericarditis in HIV seropositive patients. Heart 2000; 84:183–188.

82. Girgis NI, Farid Z, Kilpatrick ME, Sultan Y, Mikhail IA. Dexamethasone adjunctive treatment for tuberculous meningitis. Pediatr Infect Dis J 1991; 10:179–183.

83. Hong Kong Chest Service/Tuberculosis Research Centre, Madras/British Medical Research Council. A control trial of 2-month, 3-month, and 12-month regimens of chemotherapy for sputum-smear negative pulmonary tuberculosis: results at 60 months. Am Rev Respir Dis 1984; 130:23–28.

84. Hong Kong Chest Service/Tuberculosis Research Centre, Madras/British Medical Research Council. A controlled trial of 3-month, 4-month, and 6-month regimens of chemotherapy for sputum-smear negative pulmonary tuberculosis: results at 5 years. Am Rev Respir Dis 1989; 139:871–876.

85. Elliott AM, Namaambo K, Allen BW, Luo N, Hayes RJ, Pobee JO, McAdam KP. Negative sputum smear results in HIV-positive patients with pulmonary tuberculosis in Lusaka, Zambia. Tuber Lung Dis 1993; 74:191–194.

86. Snider DE Jr. The relationship between tuberculosis and silicosis. Am Rev Respir Dis 1978; 118:455–460.

87. Chang KC, Leung CC, Tam CM. Tuberculosis risk factors in a silicotic cohort in Hong Kong. Int J Tuberc Lung Dis 2001; 5:177–184.

88. Jindal SK, Aggarwal AN, Gupta D. Dust-induced interstitial lung disease in the tropics. Curr Opin Pulm Med 2001; 7:272–277.

89. Lin TP, Suo J, Lee CN, Lee JJ, Yang SP. Short-course chemotherapy of pulmonary tuberculosis in pneumoconiotic patients. Am Rev Respir Dis 1987; 136:808–810.

90. Aungkasuvapala N, Juengprasert W, Obhasi N. Silicosis and pulmonary tuberculosis in stone-grinding factories in Saraburi, Thailand. Med Assoc Thai 1995; 78:662–669.

91. Sonnenberg P, Murray J, Glynn JR, Thomas RG, Godfrey-Faussett P, Shearer S. Risk factors for pulmonary disease due to culture-positive *M. tuberculosis* or nontuberculous mycobacteria in South African gold miners. Eur Respir J 2000; 15:291–296.

92. Mendes R. Epidemiologic study of pulmonary silicosis in the southeast region of Brazil, based on a survey of patients hospitalized in tuberculosis hospitals. Rev Saude Publica 1979; 13:7–19.

93. Pinell LF. Incidence of silicosis and silicotuberculosis in Bolivian miners. Epidemiological study. Bull Int Union Tuberc 1976; 51(1 Pt 2):615–620.

94. Hong Kong Chest Service/Tuberculosis Research Centre/British Medical Research Council. A controlled trial of 6 and 8 months of antituberculous

chemotherapy in the treatment of patients with silicotuberculosis in Hong Kong. Am Rev Respir Dis 1991; 143:262–267.

95. Chaulet P. Implementation of fixed-dose combinations in tuberculosis control: outline of responsibilities. Int J Tuberc Lung Dis 1999; 3(11 suppl 3): S353–S357.

96. El-Sadr WM, Perlman DC, Denning E, Matts JP, Cohn DL. A review of efficacy studies of 6-month short-course therapy for tuberculosis among patients infected with human immunodeficiency virus: differences in study outcomes. Clin Infect Dis 2001; 32:623–632.

97. Connolly C, Reid A, Davies G, Sturm W, McAdam KP, Wilkinson D. Relapse and mortality among HIV-infected and uninfected patients with tuberculosis successfully treated with twice weekly directly observed therapy in rural South Africa. AIDS 1999; 13:1543–1517.

98. Murray J, Sonnenberg P, Shearer SC, Godfrey-Faussett P. Human immunodeficiency virus and the outcome of treatment for new and recurrent pulmonary tuberculosis in African patients. Am J Respir Crit Care Med 1999; 159: 733–740.

99. Perriens JH, St Louis ME, Mukadi YB, Brown C, Prignot J, Pouthier F, Portaels F, Willame JC, Mandala JK, Kaboto M, et al. Pulmonary tuberculosis in HIV-infected patients in Zaire. A controlled trial of treatment for either 6 or 12 months. N Engl J Med 1995; 332:779–784.

100. Okwera A, Whalen C, Byekwaso F, Vjecha M, Johnson J, Huebner R, Mugerwa R, Ellner J. Randomised trial of thiacetazone and rifampicin-containing regimens for pulmonary tuberculosis in HIV-infected Ugandans. The Makerere University-Case Western University Research Collaboration. Lancet 1994; 344:1323–1328.

101. Berning SE, Huitt GA, Iseman MD, Peloquin CA. Malabsorption of antituberculosis medications by a patient with AIDS. N Engl J Med 1992; 327: 1817–1878.

102. Peloquin CA, Nitta AT, Burman WJ, Brudney KF, Miranda-Massari JR, McGuinness ME, Berning SE, Gerena GT. Low antituberculosis drug concentrations in patients with AIDS. Ann Pharmacother 1996; 30:919–925.

103. Patel KB, Belmonte R, Crowe HM. Drug malabsorption and resistant tuberculosis in HIV-infected patients. N Engl J Med 1995; 332:336–337.

104. Narita M, Ashkin D, Hollender ES, Pitchenik AE. Paradoxical worsening of tuberculosis following antiretroviral therapy in patients with AIDS. Am J Respir Crit Care Med 1998; 158:157–161.

105. Centers for Disease Control and Prevention. Updated guidelines for the use of rifamycins for the treatment of tuberculosis among HIV-infected patients taking protease inhibitors or nonnucleoside reverse transcriptase inhibitors. Version 1.20.04. www.cdc.gov/nchstp/tb/tb_hiv_drugs/TOC.htm

106. Kirk O, Gatell JM, Mocroft A, Pedersen C, Proenca R, Brettle RP, Barton SE, Sudre P, Phillips AN. Infections with *Mycobacterium tuberculosis* and *Mycobacterium avium* among HIV-infected patients after the introduction of highly active antiretroviral therapy. EuroSIDA Study Group JD. Am J Respir Crit Care Med 2000; 162(3 Pt 1):865–872.

107. Hung CC, Chen MY, Hsiao CF, Hsieh SM, Sheng WH, Chang SC. Improved outcomes of HIV-1-infected adults with tuberculosis in the era of highly active antiretroviral therapy. AIDS 2003; 17:2615–2622.

108. Seyler C, Anglaret X, Dakoury-Dogbo N, Messou E, Toure S, Danel C, Diakite N, Daudie A, Inwoley A, Maurice C, Tonwe-Gold B, Rouet F, N'Dri-Yoman T, Salamon R. ANRS 1203 Study Group. Medium-term survival, morbidity and immunovirological evolution in HIV-infected adults receiving antiretroviral therapy, Abidjan, Cote d'Ivoire. Antivir Ther 2003; 8:385–393.

109. Jones JL, Hanson DL, Dworkin MS, DeCock KM. Adult/Adolescent Spectrum of HIV Disease Group. HIV-associated tuberculosis in the era of highly active antiretroviral therapy. The Adult/Adolescent Spectrum of HIV Disease Group. Int J Tuberc Lung Dis 2000; 4:1026–1031.

110. Girardi E, Antonucci G, Vanacore P, Libanore M, Errante I, Matteelli A, Ippolito G. Gruppo Italiano di Studio Tubercolosi e AIDS (GISTA). Impact of combination antiretroviral therapy on the risk of tuberculosis among persons with HIV infection. AIDS 2000; 14:1985–1991.

111. Scano F. Anitretroviral therapy and tuberculosis control: a powerful combination to reach the "3 by 5" target. IUATLD Conference, Paris, 2003. www.who.int/gtb/TBHIV/symposium_paris_31oct03/.

112. Creese A, Floyd K, Alban A, Guinness L. Cost-effectiveness of HIV/AIDS interventions in Africa: a systematic review of the evidence. Lancet 2002; 359:1635–1643.

113. Narita M, Stambaugh JJ, Hollender ES, Jones D, Pitchenik AE, Ashkin D. Use of rifabutin with protease inhibitors for human immunodeficiency virus-infected patients with tuberculosis. Clin Infect Dis 2000; 30:779–783.

114. Schwander S, Rusch-Gerdes S, Mateega A, Lutalo T, Tugume S, Kityo C, Rubaramira R, Mugyenyi P, Okwera A, Mugerwa R. A pilot study of antituberculosis combinations comparing rifabutin with rifampicin in the treatment of HIV-1 associated tuberculosis. A single-blind randomized evaluation in Ugandan patients with HIV-1 infection and pulmonary tuberculosis. Tuber Lung Dis 1995; 76:210–218.

115. Adams G, Addo M, Aldovini A, et al. Consensus statement on antiretroviral treatment for AIDS in poor countries. Inter AIDS Soc USA 2001; 9:14–26.

116. Iseman MD. Drug-resistant tuberculosis. In: A Clinician's Guide to Tuberculosis. Philadelphia, PA, USA: Lippincott Williams &Wilkins, 2000:271–321.

117. Goble M, Iseman MD, Madsen LA, Waite D, Ackerson L, Horsburgh CR Jr. Treatment of 171 patients with pulmonary tuberculosis resistant to isoniazid and rifampin. N Engl J Med 1993; 328:527–532.

118. Espinal MA. Time to abandon the standard retreatment regimen with first-line drugs for failures of standard treatment. Int J Tuberc Lung Dis 2003; 7:607–608.

119. Heldal E, Arnadottir T, Cruz JR, Tardencilla A, Chacon L. Low failure rate in standardised retreatment of tuberculosis in Nicaragua: patient category, drug resistance and survival of 'chronic' patients. Int J Tuberc Lung Dis 2001; 5:129–136.

120. Salaniponi FM, Nyirenda TE, Kemp JR, Squire SB, Godfrey-Faussett P, Harries AD. Characteristics, management and outcome of patients with

recurrent tuberculosis under routine programme conditions in Malawi. Int J Tuberc Lung Dis 2003; 7:948–952.

121. Escalante P, Cordero L, Yi A, Accinelli R. Enoxacin in the retreatment of pulmonary tuberculosis. Am Rev Respir Dis Crit Care 1997; 155(suppl):A562.

122. Lan NTN, Lademarco MF, Binkin NJ, Tung LB, Quy HT, Cj NV. A case series: initial outcome of persons with multidrug-resistant tuberculosis after treatment with the WHO standard retreatment regimen in Ho Chi Minh City, Vietnam. Int J Tuberc Lung Dis 2001; 5:575–578.

123. Migliori GB, Espinal M, Danilova ID, Punga VV, Grzemska M, Raviglione MC. Frequency of recurrence among MDR-tB cases 'successfully' treated with standardised short-course chemotherapy. Int J Tuberc Lung Dis 2002; 6:858–864.

124. Kritski AL, Rodrigues de Jesus LS, Andrade MK, Werneck-Barroso E, Vieira MA, Haffner A, Riley LW. Retreatment tuberculosis cases. Factors associated with drug resistance and adverse outcomes. Chest 1997; 111: 1162–1167.

125. Escalante P, Accinelli R, Awe R, Beck JR. Retreatment of pulmonary tuberculosis in a developing country: a decision analysis. Am Rev Respir Dis Crit Care 1997; 155(suppl):A562.

126. Mitnick C, Bayona J, Palacios E, Shin S, Furin J, Alcantara F, Sanchez E, Sarria M, Becerra M, Fawzi MC, Kapiga S, Neuberg D, Maguire JH, Kim JY, Farmer P. Community-based therapy for multidrug-resistant tuberculosis in Lima, Peru. N Engl J Med 2003; 348:119–128.

127. Palacios E, Guerra D, Llaro K, Chalco K, Sapag R, Furin J. The role of the nurse in the community-based treatment of multidrug-resistant tuberculosis (MDR-TB). Int J Tuberc Lung Dis 2003; 7:343–346.

128. Sterling TR, Lehmann HP, Frieden TR. Impact of DOTS compared with DOTS-plus on multidrug resistant tuberculosis and tuberculosis deaths: decision analysis. BMJ 2003; 326:574.

129. Mwinga A. Drug-resistant tuberculosis in Africa. Ann N Y Acad Sci 2001; 953:106–112.

130. Pablos-Mendez A, Gowda DK, Frieden TR. Controlling multidrug-resistant tuberculosis and access to expensive drugs: a rational framework. Bull World Health Organ 2002; 80:489–495.

131. Mukherjee JS, Rich ML, Socci AR, Joseph JK, Viru FA, Shin SS, Furin JJ, Becerra MC, Barry DJ, Kim JY, Bayona J, Farmer P, Smith Fawzi MC, Seung KJ. Programmes and principles in treatment of multidrug-resistant tuberculosis. Lancet 2004; 363:474–481.

132. Caminero JA, de March P. Statements of ATS, CDC, and IDSA on treatment of tuberculosis (letter). Am J Respir Crit Care Med 2004; 169:316–317.

133. Iseman MD. Statements of ATS, CDC, and IDSA on treatment of tuberculosis (author reply). Am J Respir Crit Care Med 2004; 169:317.

134. East Africa/British Medical Research Council. Results at 5 years of a controlled comparison of a 6-month and a standard 18-month regimen chemotherapy for pulmonary tuberculosis. Am Rev Respir Dis 1977; 116:3–8.

135. Telzak EE, Sepkowitz K, Alpert P, Mannheimer S, Medard F, el-Sadr W, Blum S, Gagliardi A, Salomon N, Turett G. Multidrug-resistant tuberculosis in patients without HIV infection. N Engl J Med 1995; 333:907–911.

136. Turett GS, Telzak EE, Torian LV, Blum S, Alland D, Weisfuse I, Fazal BA. Improved outcomes for patients with multidrug-resistant tuberculosis. Clin Infect Dis 1995; 21:1238–1244.
137. Alangaden GJ, Lerner SA. The clinical use of fluoroquinolones for the treatment of mycobacterial diseases. Clin Infect Dis 1997; 25:1213–1221.
138. Sirgel FA, Botha FJ, Parkin DP, Van de Wal BW, Schall R, Donald PR, Mitchison DA. The early bactericidal activity of ciprofloxacin in patients with pulmonary tuberculosis. Am J Respir Crit Care Med 1997; 156(3 Pt 1): 901–905.
139. Sirgel FA, Donald PR, Odhiambo J, Githui W, Umapathy KC, Paramasivan CN, Tam CM, Kam KM, Lam CW, Sole KM, Mitchison DA. A multicentre study of the early bactericidal activity of anti-tuberculosis drugs. J Antimicrob Chemother 2000; 45:859–870.
140. Tsukamura M, Nakamura E, Yoshii S, Amano H. Therapeutic effect of a new antibacterial substance ofloxacin (DL8280) on pulmonary tuberculosis. Am Rev Respir Dis 1985; 131:352–356.
141. Chan ED, Laurel V, Strand MJ, Chan JF, Huynh ML, Goble M, Iseman MD. Treatment and outcome analysis of 205 patients with multidrug-resistant tuberculosis. Am J Respir Crit Care Med 2004; 169:1103–1109.
142. Yew WW, Chan CK, Leung CC, Chau CH, Tam CM, Wong PC, Lee J. Comparative roles of levofloxacin and ofloxacin in the treatment of multidrug-resistant tuberculosis: preliminary results of a retrospective study from Hong Kong. Chest 2003; 124:1476–1481.
143. Richeldi L, Covi M, Ferrara G, Franco F, Vailati P, Meschiari E, Fabbri LM, Velluti G. Clinical use of levofloxacin in the long-term treatment of drug resistant tuberculosis. Monaldi Arch Chest Dis 2002; 57:39–43.
144. Perlman DC, El Sadr WM, Heifets LB, Nelson ET, Matts JP, Chirgwin K, Salomon N, Telzak EE, Klein O, Kreiswirth BN, Musser JM, Hafner R. Susceptibility to levofloxacin of *Myocobacterium tuberculosis* isolates from patients with HIV-related tuberculosis and characterization of a strain with levofloxacin monoresistance. Community Programs for Clinical Research on AIDS 019 and the AIDS Clinical Trials Group 222 Protocol Team. AIDS 1997; 11:1473–1478.
145. Tupasi TE, Quelapio MI, Orillaza RB, Alcantara C, Mira NR, Abeleda MR, Belen VT, Arnisto NM, Rivera AB, Grimaldo ER, Derilo JO, Dimarucut W, Arabit M, Urboda D. DOTS-Plus for multidrug-resistant tuberculosis in the Philippines: global assistance urgently needed. Tuberculosis (Edinb) 2003; 83:52–58.
146. Mwinga A, Nunn A, Ngwira B, Chintu C, Warndorff D, Fine P, et al. *Mycobacterium vaccae* (SRL172) immunotherapy as an adjunct to standard antituberculosis treatment in HIV-infected adults with pulmonary tuberculosis: a randomized placebo-controlled trial. Lancet 2002; 360:1050.
147. de B, Garner P. *Mycobacterium vaccae* immunotherapy for treating tuberculosis (Cochrane Review). Cochrane Database Syst Rev 2003; (1):CD001166.
148. Johnson JL, Ssekasanvu E, Okwera A, Mayanja H, Hirsch CS, Nakibali JG, et al. Randomized trial of adjunctive interleukin-2 in adults with pulmonary tuberculosis. Am J Respir Crit Care Med 2003; 168:185–191.

149. Wallis RS, Nsubuga P, Whalen C, Mugerwa RD, Okwera A, Oette D, Jackson JB, Johnson JL, Ellner JJ. Pentoxifylline therapy in human immunodeficiency virus-seropositive persons with tuberculosis: a randomized, controlled trial. J Infect Dis 1996; 174:727–733.

150. Condos R, Rom WN, Schluger NW. Treatment of multidrug-resistant pulmonary tuberculosis with interferon-gamma via aerosol. Lancet 1997; 49:1513–1515.

151. Bentwich Z, Kalinkovich A, Weisman Z, Borkow G, Beyers N, Beyers AD. Can eradication of worms change the face of AIDS and tuberculosis? Immunol Today 1999; 20:485–487.

152. Chan TY. Vitamin D deficiency and susceptibility to tuberculosis [comment]. Calcif Tissue Int 2000; 66:476–478.

153. Bellamy R. Evidence of gene-environment interaction in development of tuberculosis [comment]. Lancet 2000; 355:588–589.

154. De Cock KM, Chaisson RE. Will DOTS do it? A reappraisal of tuberculosis control in countries with high rates of HIV infection. Int J Tuberc Lung Dis 1999; 3:457–465.

155. Mahmoudi A, Iseman MD. Pitfalls in the care of patients with tuberculosis. Common errors and their association with the acquisition of drug resistance. JAMA 1993; 270:65–68.

156. Iseman MD. Tuberculosis therapy: past, present and future. Eur Respir J Suppl 2002; 36:87s–94s.

157. Dye C, Williams BG, Espinal MA, Raviglione MC. Erasing the world's slow stain: strategies to beat multidrug-resistant tuberculosis. Science 2002; 295:2042–2046.

158. Fisher M. Diagnosis of MDR-TB: a developing world problem on a developed world budget. Expert Rev Mol Diagn 2002; 2:151–159.

159. Ginsberg AM. What's new in tuberculosis vaccines? Bull World Health Org 2002; 80:483–488.

160. Hong Kong Tuberculosis Treatment Services/Brompton Hospital/British Medical Research Council. A controlled trial of daily and intermittent rifampin plus ethambutol in the retreatment of patients with pulmonary tuberculosis: results up to 30 months. Tubercle 1975; 56:179–189.

161. Elias D, Wolday D, Akuffo H, Petros B, Bronner U, Britton S. Effects of deworming on human T-cell responses to mycobacterial antigens in helminth-exposed individuals before and after bacilli Calmette-Guérin (BCG) vaccination. Clin Exp Immunol 2001; 123:219–255.

162. Chaudhury RR, Thatte U. Beyond DOTS: avenues ahead in the management of tuberculosis. Natl Med J India 2003; 16:321–327.

163. Thwaites GE, Nguyen DB, Nguyen HD, Hoang TQ, Do TT, Nguyen TC, Nguyen QH, Nguyen TT, Nguyen NH, Nguyen TN, Nguyen NL, Nguyen HD, Vu NT, Cao HH, Tran TH, Pham PM, Nguyen TD, Stepniewska K, White NJ, Tran TH, Farrar JJ. Dexamethasone for the treatment of tuberculous meningitis in adolescents and adults. N Engl J Med 2004; 351:1741–1751.

Index